COLOR ATLAS AND SYNOPSIS:
Gastrointestinal Pathology

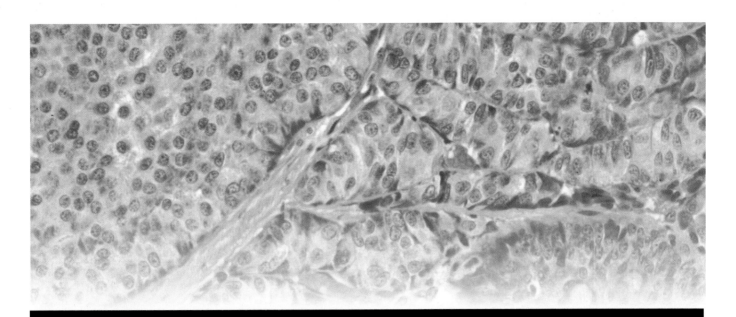

COLOR ATLAS AND SYNOPSIS:
Gastrointestinal Pathology

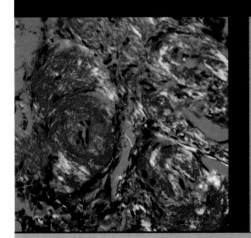

Shu-Yuan Xiao, MD
Professor
Department of Pathology
Division of Biological Sciences
University of Chicago
Chicago, Illinois

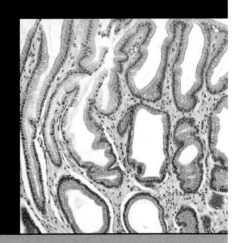

Mc
Graw
Hill
Education

New York   Chicago   San Francisco   Athens   London   Madrid   Mexico City
Milan   New Delhi   Singapore   Sydney   Toronto

Color Atlas and Synopsis: Gastrointestinal Pathology

1 2 3 4 5 6 7 8 9 0   CTP/CTP   20 19 18 17 16 15

ISBN: 978-0-07-182046-2
MHID: 0-07182046-9

Notice

Medicine is an ever-changing science. As new research and clinical experience broaden our knowledge, changes in treatment and drug therapy are required. The authors and the publisher of this work have checked with sources believed to be reliable in their efforts to provide information that is complete and generally in accord with the standards accepted at the time of publication. However, in view of the possibility of human error or changes in medical sciences, neither the authors nor the publisher nor any other party who has been involved in the preparation or publication of this work warrants that the information contained herein is in every respect accurate or complete, and they disclaim all responsibility for any errors or omissions or for the results obtained from use of the information contained in this work. Readers are encouraged to confirm the information contained herein with other sources. For example and in particular, readers are advised to check the product information sheet included in the package of each drug they plan to administer to be certain that the information contained in this work is accurate and that changes have not been made in the recommended dose or in the contraindications for administration. This recommendation is of particular importance in connection with new or infrequently used drugs.

This book was set in Minion Pro by Cenveo® Publisher Services.
The editors were Alyssa Fried and Christie Naglieri.
The production supervisor was Richard Ruzycka.
Project management was provided by Vastavikta Sharma, Cenveo Publisher Services.
The index was prepared by Michael Ferreira.
China Translation & Printing Services, Ltd. was the printer and binder.

This book is printed on acid-free paper.

Library of Congress Cataloging-in-Publication Data

Color atlas and synopsis : gastrointestinal pathology / edited by
Shu-Yuan Xiao. —1 ed.
    p. ; cm.
Gastrointestinal pathology
Includes bibliographical references.
ISBN 978-0-07-182046-2 (hardcover : alk. paper)—ISBN 0-07-182046-9
(hardcover : alk. paper)
I. Xiao, Shu-Yuan, editor.   II. Title: Gastrointestinal pathology.
[DNLM: 1. Gastrointestinal Diseases—pathology—Atlases. WI 17]
RC802.9
616.3'307—dc23
                                2015030066

To my mother and father,
my wife, Fang,
and my children, Stephanie and Emily

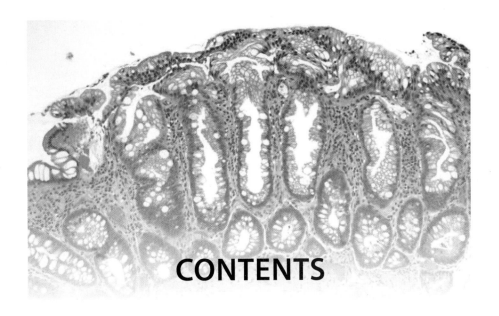

CONTENTS

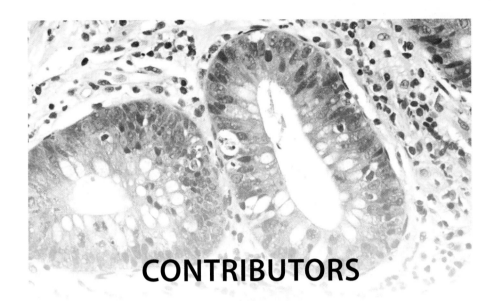

CONTRIBUTORS

Lindsay Alpert, MD
Fellow, Department of Pathology
The University of Chicago Medicine
Chicago, Illinois
*Chapter 2: GI Biopsies in Transplant
Settings*

Nhu Thuy Can, MD
Fellow, Department of Pathology
The University of Chicago Medicine
Chicago, Illinois
*Chapter 28: Infectious and Other
Colitis*

Giovanni De Petris, MD
Associate Professor of Pathology
Mayo Clinic College of Medicine
Mayo Clinic in Arizona
Scottsdale, Arizona
*Chapter 9: Barrett Esophagus and
Adenocarcinoma*

David E. Fleischer
Professor of Medicine
Mayo Clinic College of Medicine
Consultant, Division of
Gastroenterology
Mayo Clinic Arizona, Scottsdale,
Arizona
*Chapter 9: Barrett Esophagus and
Adenocarcinoma*

Deborah A. Giusto, MD
Associate Pathologist
4path Pathology Services
Justice, Illinois
*Chapter 21: Small Bowel Polyps and
Nodules*

David Hernandez Gonzalo, MD
Assistant Professor
Department of Pathology
University of Florida, Gainesville
School of Medicine
Gainesville, Florida
*Chapter 13: Reactive (Chemical)
Gastropathy*

Shriram Jakate, MD
Professor of Pathology
Rush University Medical School
Chicago, Illinois
Chapter 31: Inflammatory Lesions

Nora Joseph, MD
Staff Pathologist
Associate Director, Molecular Genetic
Pathology
Department of Pathology and Labora-
tory Medicine
NorthShore University HealthSystem
Evanston, Illinois
*Chapter 7: Molecular and Other
Ancillary Tests For GI Tumors*

Heewon Kwak, MD
Resident, Department of Pathology
The University of Chicago Medicine
Chicago, Illinois
*Chapter 17: Gastric Neuroendocrine
Tumors and Other Rare Tumors;
Chapter 23: Other Small Bowel
Tumors*

Michael S. Landau
Assistant Professor
Department of Pathology
University of Pittsburgh Medical
Center, Pittsburgh, Pennsylvania
Chapter 24: Appendicitis

Jingmei Lin, MD, PhD
Assistant Professor
Department of Pathology and
Laboratory Medicine
Indiana University School of Medicine
Indianapolis, Indiana
*Chapter 32: HPV-Associated Squamous
Lesions*

Xiuli Liu, MD, PhD
Associate Professor and Staff
Department of Anatomic Pathology
Cleveland Clinic
Cleveland, Ohio
*Chapter 10: Squamous Cell Carcinoma
and Other Miscellaneous Malignancies
of the Esophagus; Chapter 26:
Ulcerative Colitis and Complications
of Ileal Pouch–Anal Anastomosis;
Chapter 27: Surveillance Biopsies
of Inflammatory Bowel Disease for
Dysplasia; Chapter 29: Colon Polyps*

Reetesh K. Pai, MD
Associate Professor
Department of Pathology
University of Pittsburgh Medical
Center
Pittsburgh, Pennsylvania
*Chapter 24: Appendicitis; Chapter 25:
Neoplasms of the Appendix*

Rish K. Pai, MD, PhD
Assistant Professor and Staff
Department of Anatomic Pathology
Robert J. Tomsich Pathology and
Laboratory Medicine Institute
Cleveland, Ohio
*Chapter 13: Reactive (Chemical)
Gastropathy*

Safia Salaria, MD
Assistant Professor of Pathology
Vanderbilt University Medical Center
Nashville, Tennessee
Chapter 14: Hypertrophic Gastropathy

Chanjuan Shi, MD, PhD
Assistant Professor of Pathology
Vanderbilt University Medical Center
Nashville, Tennessee
*Chapter 6: Gastrointestinal
Neuroendocrine Tumors*

Katherine Sun, MD, PhD
Clinical Associate Professor
Department of Pathology
Langone Medical Center
New York University
New York, New York
Chapter 20: Small Bowel Infections

Mary Kay Washington, MD
Professor of Pathology
Vanderbilt University Medical Center
Nashville, Tennessee
*Chapter 6: Gastrointestinal
Neuroendocrine Tumors;
Chapter 14: Hypertrophic
Gastropathy*

Emma Whitcomb, MD
Clinical Assistant Professor
Department of Pathology and
Laboratory Medicine
University of Calgary
Calgary, Canada
*Chapter 22: Small Bowel
Adenocarcinoma*

Lei Zhao, MD, PhD
Assistant Professor
Department of Pathology
University of Alabama at Birmingham
Birmingham, Alabama
*Chapter 5: Gastrointestinal Stromal
Tumors and Other
Mesenchymal Tumors*

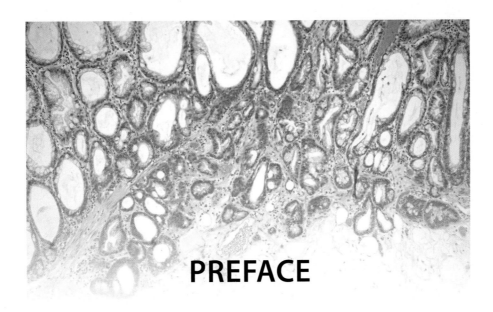

PREFACE

When I was first asked to produce a volume on gastrointestinal (GI) pathology in late 2011, I could not help but wonder if, considering the many excellent books already written on the topic, it was really necessary for me to write yet another one. What could I possibly add? I remember remarking to my editor, Alyssa Fried, "This will be a big challenge. It'll add so much to my busy schedule!" She replied, "Well, why can't this be a good opportunity instead of a challenge?"

After speaking to colleagues and my family, it occurred to me that this indeed would be a great opportunity for me to sort through more than a decade's worth of experience practicing GI pathology and to share this experience with an audience. Even if only 10 people in the world ultimately read this book, that experience would be amplified 10 times. And, if nothing else, then perhaps some of the photomicrographs might be nice to examine or prove useful as teaching illustrations. So, I started writing a book proposal. The result is this volume.

When I was a resident, I thought that if I could just memorize everything I read from textbooks—some of them considered "bibles" in surgical pathology—I would know all the facts about a disease and could make a firm diagnosis in every case. In these books, papers were cited and statistics were listed to support the facts and diagnostic criteria. However, the longer I practice, the less assured I feel about certainties in diagnostic pathology. It has gradually come to me that we do not know much about most diseases and are not always sure about the known "facts." We even cannot be sure about some of the statistics. For example, in the lists of facts written about lymphocytic gastritis, some volumes state that a certain percentage of lymphocytic gastritis is due to *Helicobacter pylori* infection. But how were the cases defined in the studies that generated the figure? Should these cases be considered *H. pylori*–induced lymphocytic gastritis, or should they be considered lymphocytic gastritis with superimposed *H. pylori* infection? The two alternatives lead to fundamentally different statistics and thus clinical outcomes.

The former condition would respond to anti–*H. pylori* treatment, while the latter would not. If a study did not make such a distinction, the data are impossible to apply.

Another issue with statistics relates to how frequently a certain entity occurs in a certain site or age group. Knowing these figures contributes to our knowledge as informed practitioners. However, applying that knowledge may sometimes hamper our diagnoses. For example, we have learned that sessile serrated polyps (SSPs) are more frequent in the right colon than in the left. It is not uncommon in our practice for a small lesion that may have some features of an SSP to be called an SSP if it is from the right colon and a hyperplastic polyp if it is from the rectum. The end result is to make the original statement even stronger when subsequent case analysis is performed, while making SSPs in the rectum even more "rare." Because we are morphologists and there are defined histologic criteria for a particular diagnostic entity, such locational information should not influence our decision making.

Due to these considerations, my intention is to not cite too many statistics in this book, as statistics based on a population really do not directly contribute to a histologic diagnosis in an individual case and instead offer a false sense of assurance based on probability.

As practicing pathologists, we usually encounter a certain pattern of tissue injury that may be due to one of several possible diseases, or we are given a biopsy with a particular clinical purpose that dictates a more or less predefined set of questions to be addressed. A quick reference text centered on these kinds of tasks will offer unique value. For example, faced with a patient with a clinical history of celiac disease who is not responding to standard treatment, what questions does the clinician have in mind when sending a duodenal biopsy specimen? These questions are unlikely to be written on the requisition forms in most instances. What histologic features do we need to comment on in the pathology report? What ancillary studies should be performed on this biopsy to best address the clinician's concerns? What are other differential diagnoses that commonly occur in these patients that need to be considered or excluded? Instead of creating another large volume of text that details every disease of the GI tract, the modest goal of this book is to provide a "field-guide-type" but in-depth discussion of selected diagnostic entities that are commonly encountered or carry crucial clinical significance, while anticipating potential concerns/questions from clinicians. By outlining some of the more frequently encountered clinicopathological entities and problem situations, this book can function as an easily accessible tool for practicing pathologists.

Despite all the new advances in high-throughput molecular testing and ever-increasing data sets for personalized medicine, our daily practices are still dominated by a light microscope. At the cellular or tissue level, as revealed by light microscopy, the patterns of response to injury in a particular tissue are limited. Many diseases share overlapping histologic features; that is, a particular disease will not have its "own" special set of microscopic features. An honest and realistic approach by the pathologist would be to render a histologic diagnosis with a list of diseases that share this histology pattern when additional clinical information is not available, or to render his or her opinion if other relevant clinical information has been provided. For example, both graft-vs-host disease involving the GI tract and injury associated with immunosuppressive drugs, such as mycophenolate, may occur in patients after a transplant. These entities are often microscopically indistinguishable. We must keep this lack of specificity in mind and render a descriptive diagnosis, such as "toxic-ischemic type" (see Chapter 1) or "apoptotic-type" injury, and then include a list of potential etiologies for this histologic pattern. The clinician can then rely on other information or parameters to "tilt" the differential balance toward one diagnosis over the others and make the appropriate corresponding clinical decisions. Handling such cases and producing a concise but useful pathology report requires a combination of art and science. The prerequisite for this approach is, of course, the ability to recognize a general pattern of injury, and knowing the correct list of diseases that share the pattern. One of the features of this book is to provide algorithms for using additional, readily obtainable information to help reach the correct diagnosis.

This book deals with some of the most frequently encountered clinical specimens and questions. The first few chapters deal with special topics not limited to any single site, followed by chapters on specific anatomic sites. The general approach of each chapter is to start with several main histologic patterns in a given anatomic site and then provide a discussion of conditions that likely enter the differential diagnosis for these histologic patterns. A practical algorithm is included when applicable. It is not the aim of this book to list and discuss all the common GI diseases or some of the more straightforward diagnoses. *Helicobacter pylori* gastritis, for instance, is not covered in great detail, as this rarely poses much of a diagnostic challenge.

In this book, ample references to microscopic images are made. In the case of many diagnostic entities, mere verbal descriptions (no matter how elegantly made) are not always enough to convey the full message, so visual examples in the form of photomicrographs provide easy and useful illustrations. This feature is especially important for chapters dealing with histologically challenging (confusing) entities, such as dysplasia in inflammatory bowel disease (IBD). Any one-paragraph outline of microscopic features of IBD-associated dysplasia would be insufficient and unsatisfactory to practicing pathologists because these lesions can take many different forms; the only effective way to recognize them is by seeing examples, including pictures.

Changes in practice are becoming the rule rather than the exception, as rapid progress in research has led to the development of new diagnostic approaches and treatment modalities. These continuing changes call for frequent updates in the practice of diagnostic pathology, with pathology reports tailored to meet new and additional clinical requirements. Faced with this challenge, I also plan to offer a digital version of this volume, which will allow for more frequent updates as necessary and serve as a more accessible option for readers.

Shu-Yuan Xiao, M.D.

ACKNOWLEDGMENTS

I would like to acknowledge the following scholars who shared my passion for this project and contributed excellent chapters to this book independently and collaboratively: Xiuli Liu, Kay Washington, Giovanni De Petris, Reetesh K. Pai, Shriram Jakate, Jingmei Lin, Katherine Sun, Lindsay Alpert, Aimee Kwak, Emma Whitcomb, Nhu Thuy Can, Nora Joseph, Chanjuan Shi, Safia Nawazish Salaria, David E. Fleischer, Rish K. Pai, David Hernandez Gonzalo, Lei Zhao, Deborah Giusto and Michael S. Landau. I also thank John Hart, who trained me as a gastrointestinal and liver pathology fellow and continues to be a wonderful colleague. Over the years, I have worked with many residents and fellows whose inquisitive questions have helped me maintain continuous curiosity regarding pathology. They are the reason I enjoy working in an academic setting.

In addition, I would like to thank the following colleagues for sharing cases or photomicrographs used in this book: Thomas Krausz (Figure 11-13); Hanlin Wang (Figures 16-23 and 17-2); Katherine Sun (Figures 16-29 and 23-6); Nhu Thuy Can (Figure 20-5); Xiuli Liu (Figures 23-16 and 28-8); John Hart (Figure 5-1); and Elisabeth Montgomery (Figure 5-25). I also thank Lindsay Alpert for her help in proofreading several of the chapters.

Finally, my family—Fang, Stephanie, Emily, and Mango the cat—also deserve special thanks for inspiring, encouraging, and supporting this endeavor. I have been busy with this book project for over 2 years, and they have graciously supported me along the way.

Shu-Yuan Xiao, M.D.

■ ABOUT THE AUTHOR

Dr. Shu-Yuan Xiao has been practicing and teaching diagnostic gastrointestinal pathology since 1999. He received a medical degree from Wuhan University School of Medicine in Wuhan, China. He has previously served as J. E. Fogarty Visiting Fellow and Visiting Associate at the National Institutes of Health; National Research Council Senior Research Associate at the US Army Medical Research Institute for Infectious Diseases; Professor of Pathology and Internal Medicine at the University of Texas Medical Branch; and Professor and Co-Chief of gastrointestinal pathology at Cornell Medical College. Currently, he is Professor of Pathology at the University of Chicago. Dr. Xiao has contributed to more than 130 peer-reviewed papers, 14 book chapters and reviews, and another reference book, *Liver Pathology* (2014).

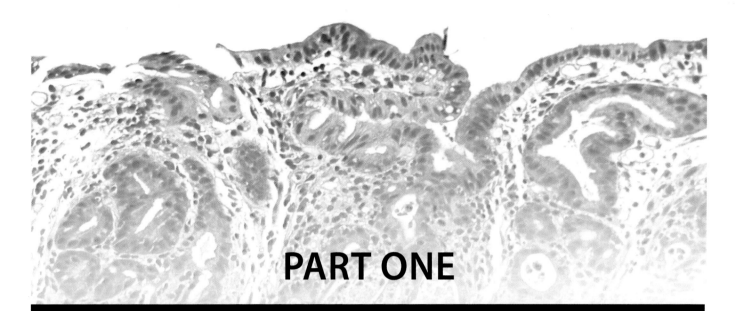

PART ONE

GENERAL TOPICS

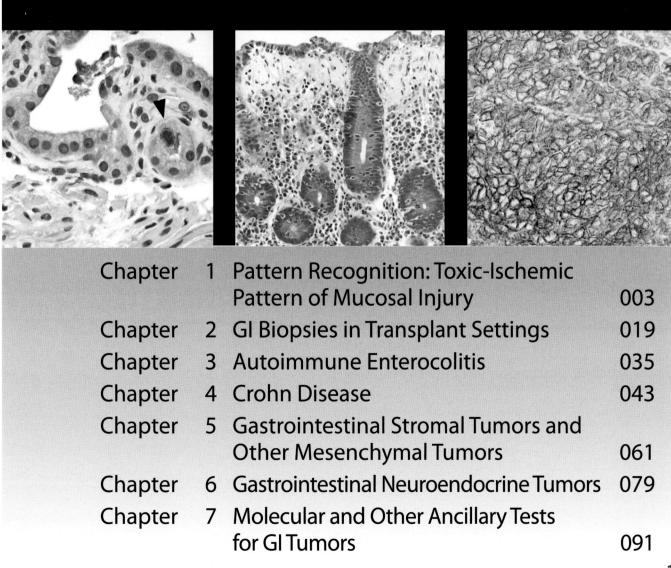

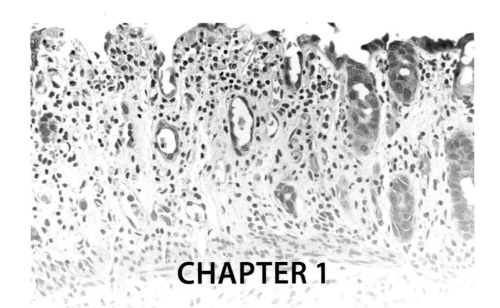

CHAPTER 1

Pattern Recognition: Toxic-Ischemic Pattern of Mucosal Injury

INTRODUCTION

Pattern recognition plays an important role in our daily diagnostic practice. Pathologists employ it either intentionally or subconsciously. Although it may sound mechanistic, pattern recognition does not imply a lack of sophistication; it differs from "picture matching." In diagnostic pathology, pattern recognition is the process of quickly or intuitively picking out the most relevant set of information from a large array of data contained in a single section stained with hematoxylin-eosin (H&E). It takes years of training and practice (and perhaps a little bit of conditioning).

In this chapter, the concept of histologic pattern recognition in diagnostic pathology is introduced. In particular, a practically useful pattern, the toxic-ischemic pattern (TIP) of mucosal injury (Figure 1-1), is described in detail. Quickly and correctly recognizing this pattern can help the pathologist narrow down the list of differential diagnoses and improve the efficiency of diagnostic tasks.

As opposed to pattern recognition, another strategy is to start with observing and analyzing individual structural or cellular changes. Focusing solely on individual cytologic parameters is important, but these features often lack specificity and may be meaningless when taken out of context. For example, what is the significance of finding one or two mitotic figures? They represent ongoing cellular turnover or proliferation, which can be seen in a physiological, inflammatory, or

neoplastic process. It is the surrounding microenvironment (an associated array of other changes) that allows one to determine which process is at the root of these findings. What is the significance of finding neutrophils in the mucosa? Can it only represent a primary inflammatory process? As illustrated in Figure 1-2, the location of the neutrophilic infiltrate varies depending on the background pathogenesis. Evidently, one has to consider this finding in its specific context. On the other hand, to look at everything in a section and take into consideration every single piece of information, one would have to spend hours evaluating a single slide. In the end, it would be impossible to reach a conclusion if one did not look at the big picture; that is, the pattern.

WHAT IS PATTERN RECOGNITION?

It is difficult to provide a single definition for pattern recognition because it may mean different things in different fields of study. A description from Wikipedia about pattern recognition algorithms used in computer science states that they "generally aim to provide a *reasonable* answer for all possible inputs and to perform 'most likely' matching of the inputs, taking into account their statistical variation," and they are "opposed to *pattern matching* algorithms, which look for exact matches in the input with pre-existing patterns." To reach this goal, the computer has to be programmed and "trained." Similarly, the human brain has to go through a

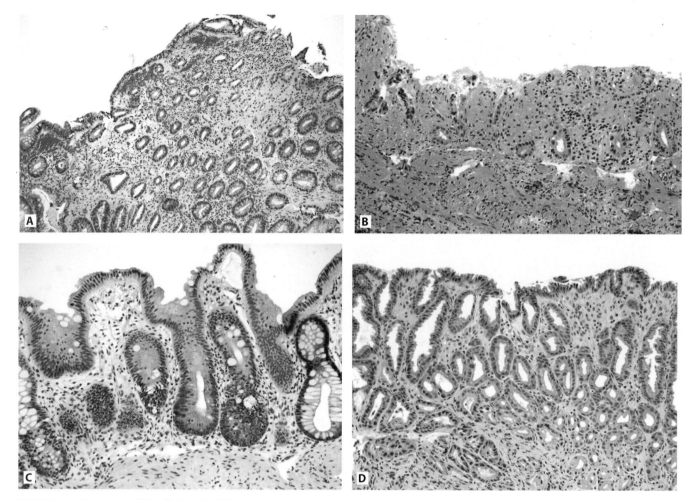

FIGURE 1-1. Examples of TIP of injury. **A.** Colonic mucosa with atrophy and mucin depletion in the surface epithelium and superficial crypts, with focal sloughing (right upper corner). The lamina propria is replaced by dense fibrinous and fibrous stroma. Note the relative sparsity of inflammatory infiltration. This mild change may represent nonsteroidal anti-inflammatory drug (NSAID) or other drug-induced injury or early ischemia (as in mucosal prolapse). **B.** Ischemic colitis. There is near-complete crypt destruction except for the most basal portion, with lamina propria fibrosis. **C.** Crypt damage by increased apoptosis in graft-versus-host disease. There is a lack of inflammatory infiltration. **D.** NSAID-induced gastropathy with erosion, atrophy, or "shrinkage" of the foveolar epithelium and a more "solid" lamina propria with relative lack of inflammatory infiltration.

training process; however, the human brain is much more powerful than a computer.

Pattern recognition has been used frequently in device-aided diagnostics and is the basis for the design of such systems.[1–6] However, the discussion in this chapter focuses on histologic pattern recognition. In diagnostic pathology, the process of pattern recognition may be the first step in the workup of most cases. For example, when viewing an H&E-stained slide microscopically, one can form a general impression of whether the pathologic process is neoplastic (Figure 1-3), inflammatory (Figure 1-4), or reactive (Figure 1-5) in the first few seconds. There are exceptions, which are the more difficult cases with overlapping features (Figure 1-6). This ability to recognize pathologic processes is predominantly based on the overall low-power

microscopic findings. To an untrained eye, the picture on a histologic slide is just a random mixture of colors and shapes and thus is patternless. The hidden beauty can only be recognized and appreciated by a trained anatomic pathologist. The pathologist not only is able to pick out the relevant information (ignoring the rest as "noise") but also needs to form a differential diagnosis consisting of a limited number of disorders based on statistics or likelihood, rather than considering unlimited possibilities. Occasionally, the untrained eye can recognize certain things in H&E-stained tissue sections that have nothing to do with the diagnosis (Figure 1-7).

A pattern is something that can be recognized at a glance, requiring no scrutiny. It by definition is not highly specific either pathologically or etiologically. Many diseases

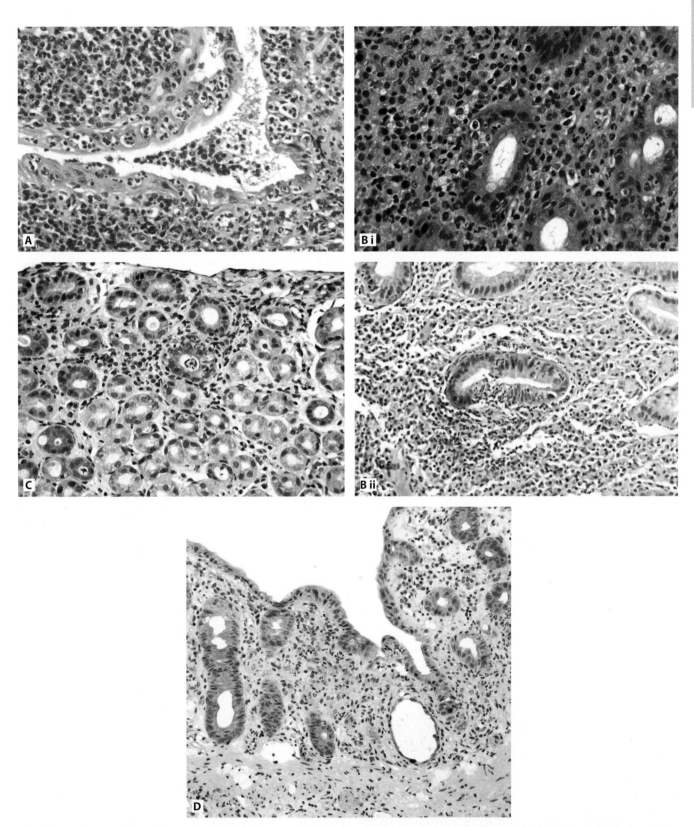

FIGURE 1-2. Neutrophilic infiltration in different diseases. **A.** Marked intraepithelial neutrophilic infiltrate in ulcerative colitis. **B.** Intraepithelial infiltrate in *Helicobacter pylori* gastritis. **C.** Focal neutrophilic infiltration in alcoholic gastropathy. **D.** Neutrophilic infiltration in the lamina propria in ischemic colitis.

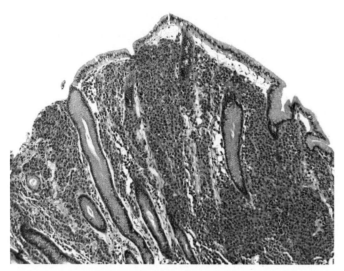

FIGURE 1-3. Neoplastic pattern in melanoma involving the stomach. Sheets of monotonous cells expand the lamina propria.

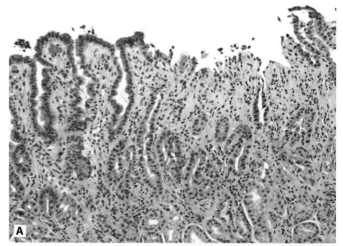

share a common pattern, and one disease may manifest in several different patterns. Therefore, a pattern only provides a general guide regarding what other elements should be evaluated. For example, *lymphocytic gastritis* is a pattern diagnosis. It is characterized by significant lamina propria infiltration of mixed inflammatory cells and infiltration of the epithelium by lymphocytes. This pattern may be seen in some cases of *Helicobacter pylori* infection, in autoimmune gastritis (Chapter 12), in patients with celiac disease (Chapter 18), in autoimmune enterocolitis (Chapter 3), and in several other conditions. Similarly, it has been increasingly recognized that collagenous colitis is also a pattern diagnosis because it is the histologic manifestation of autoimmune enterocolitis (Chapter 3), collagenous sprue, drug-induced enterocolitis (Chapter 28), or an idiopathic disorder.

FIGURE 1-4. Inflammatory pattern in colonic mucosa involved by salmonella infection. The lamina propria infiltration consists of mixed inflammatory cells. Crypt abscesses are also present.

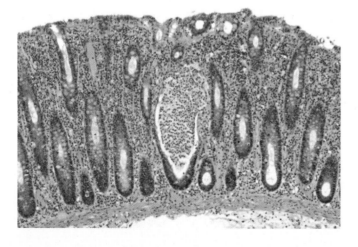

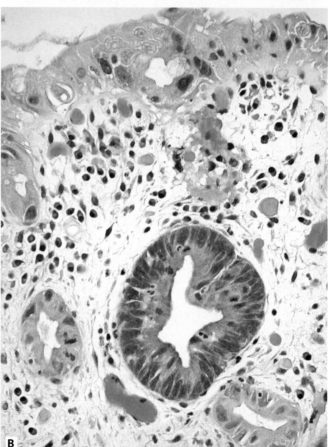

FIGURE 1-5. Reactive pattern. **A.** Chemical gastropathy with mostly epithelial changes and fibrosis of the lamina propria. There is a relative lack of cellular infiltration. **B.** Reactive atypia of the colonic surface and crypt epithelia due to radiation injury.

WHAT IS THE TOXIC-ISCHEMIC PATTERN?

Toxic-ischemic pattern can be recognized by a characteristic combination of epithelial injury and lamina propria changes (Figure 1-1). As the name implies, it is characteristically seen in either ischemic or toxin/drug-induced injuries.[7]

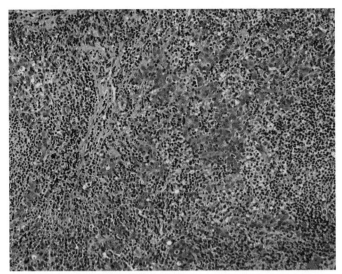

FIGURE 1-6. Mixed neoplastic and inflammatory pattern in medullary carcinoma of the stomach. Prominent lymphocytic infiltration is seen in the background of poorly differentiated syncytial tumor cells.

Some bacterial infections can cause mucosal injury through release of toxins as well. Viruses may directly cause cytopathic changes or cause host cytokine release, leading to a similar toxic epithelial or endothelial injury.[8–10]

Microscopically, a spectrum of epithelial injuries may be seen in TIP, ranging from mucin depletion to atrophy (shrinkage) to loss of surface or glandular epithelial cells (Figure 1-8). The severity of these changes increases from the base of the crypts or glands to the surface, because the surface is subject to a higher concentration of toxic exposure, and it is further away from the diminishing blood supply due to the hairpin-like configuration of the vasculature, or both (Figure 1-9). In some cases, this manifests as superficial necrosis, with preservation of the lower portion or base of the crypts. Some crypts may have a withered appearance, meaning they appear dilated with flattening of the epithelium and luminal accumulation of debris (Figure 1-10). Crypt apoptosis is often seen. Due to this feature, the phrase

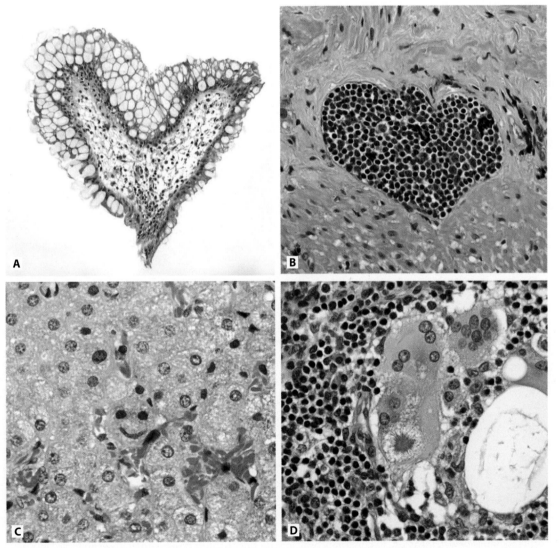

FIGURE 1-7. Things that laypeople would recognize: **A.** "Heart" (colonic mucosa). **B.** "Heart" (lymphoid aggregate). **C.** "A smiling hepatocyte." **D.** Both a layperson and a pathologist may recognize this as an asteroid body.

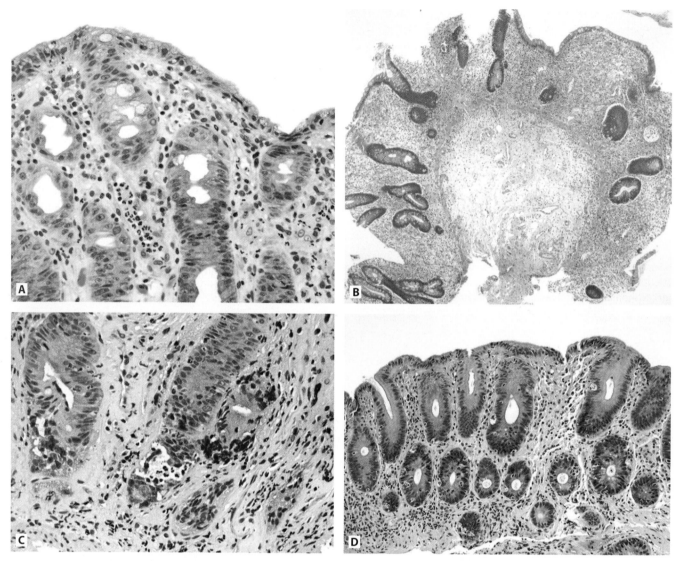

FIGURE 1-8. Epithelial changes in TIP. **A.** Mucin depletion and glandular atrophy (ischemic colitis). **B.** Loss of surface epithelial cells and glands. **C and D.** Apoptosis of crypt or gland epithelial cells, fibrosis in lamina propria.

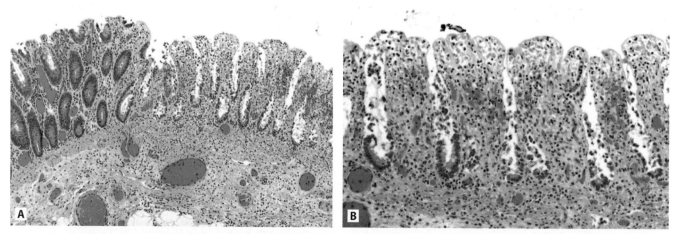

FIGURE 1-9. Acute ischemic bowel disease. **A.** Ischemic mucosal necrosis due to thrombosis, with uniform epithelial loss of the surface and the upper portion of crypts. Note the sharp demarcation from the adjacent unaffected area. **B.** Higher-power view showing preservation of the crypt base and lack of significant inflammatory infiltration.

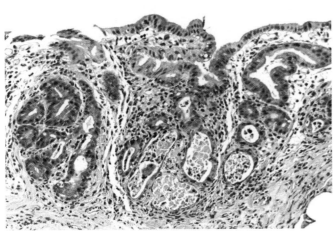

FIGURE 1-10. Gastric mucosa with withered glands containing debris, due to severe apoptosis, in graft-versus-host disease.

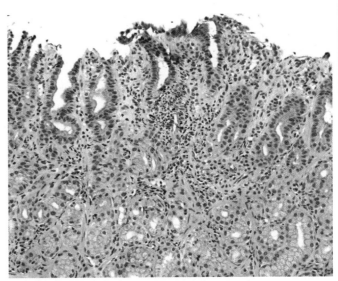

FIGURE 1-12. Neutrophilic infiltration as response to surface erosion in gastropathy induced by a NSAID. Other than the focal active infiltration, there is only minimal background inflammation.

apoptotic pattern of injury has also been used.[11] Depending on the duration of injury at the time of examination, the lamina propria can range from being "empty" to occasionally containing varying degrees of mixed inflammatory infiltration, including neutrophils (Figure 1-11). However, this inflammatory cellular infiltration is usually not prominent. When the lamina propria is expanded or "stuffed" with mononuclear cellular infiltration, an inflammatory process should be considered instead. It should be emphasized that infiltration by neutrophils in the lamina propria may be a secondary response to mucosal injury rather than a primary inflammatory disease (gastritis, enteritis, or colitis) when there is compromise of the surface protective barrier (Figure 1-12). Therefore, seeing neutrophils in the mucosa is not a reason to exclude the TIP. In the TIP of injury of longer duration (such as in ischemia), the lamina propria exhibits

FIGURE 1-11. Ischemic enteritis. The lamina propria contains neutrophils as part of the response to mucosal necrosis.

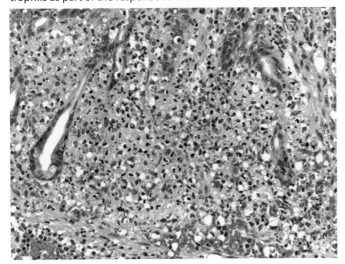

fibrinoid material or collagen deposition (early fibrosis) (Figures 1-1B, 1-13).

There are several reasons the descriptor *toxic-ischemic* is used for a pattern that can be associated with many different diseases. First, the pattern observed in bona fide ischemic colitis shares many of the microscopic features seen in mucosal injuries associated with Shiga toxin–producing bacteria, such as *Escherichia coli* O157:H7[12,13] and drugs.[14,15] For example, in typical ischemic colitis, the mucosa exhibits destruction of the superficial layer with relative preservation of the crypt base, withering of crypts, and dense fibrinoid change or fibrosis (depending on the duration of injury) of the lamina propria (Figures 1-1B, 1-9). These are similar to the changes seen in some cases of *Clostridium difficile* colitis or enterohemorrhagic *E. coli* O157 colitis. Pathogenically, part of the mechanism by which ischemia causes cell death is related to a local toxic effect from various cytokines or increased reactive oxygen species[16] released by inflammatory cells that are recruited to the site of ischemia.[11] Second, this type of change is not unique to the colon. Similar features can be seen in other segments of the gastrointestinal (GI) tract, such as the stomach (Figures 1-1D, 1-10); therefore, it represents a histopathologic pattern common to the GI tract in general. Third, not infrequently what we diagnose as ischemic colitis in biopsies does not correlate with a clinically confirmed case of ischemia, which can lead to confusion.[17,18] These lesions are best grouped under the name *toxic-ischemic pattern of injury*. From a practical standpoint, recognizing this pattern of mucosal injury greatly facilitates the development of a differential list when examining slides and helps one select the proper diagnostic algorithms, thereby leading to the proper histopathologic diagnosis.

It must be clarified that a pure TIP is only rarely seen. Depending on the underlying etiology, location of the lesion,

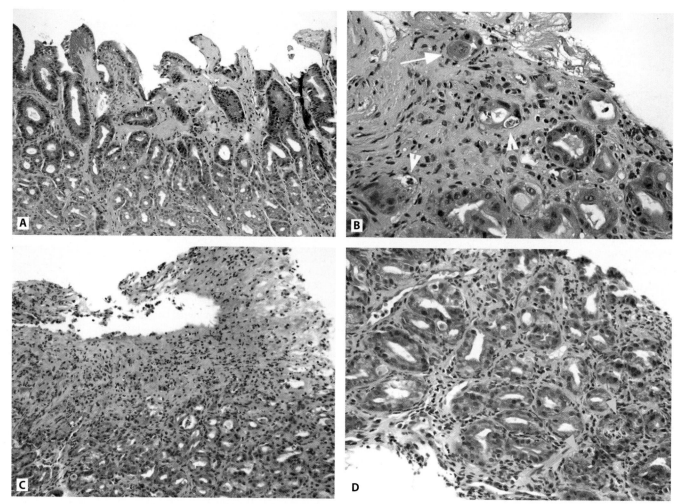

FIGURE 1-13. Gastric mucosal injury with TIP. **A.** Lamina propria fibrosis in reactive gastropathy. **B.** Severe gastropathy with an ulcer associated with a NSAID. Note the regenerative change of the residual glands, with apoptosis (arrowheads) and an abnormal mitotic figure (arrow). **C.** Ischemic ulceration of the gastric mucosa. **D.** High-power view showing degenerative changes of glands with cellular debris in some glandular lumens (arrowheads). Note the relative sparsity of inflammatory infiltration in the lamina propria.

and duration of the injury, each case may exhibit different additional changes, which help to further stratify the differential diagnoses without masking the common denominator of TIP. For example, in colon biopsies, at one end of the spectrum is ischemic necrosis due to vascular compromise (Figures 1-1B, 1-9), and at the other, *C. difficile* colitis, which sometimes has a more prominent inflammatory component (Chapter 28). In true ischemia, the oxygen supply to the affected mucosal tissue is compromised by vasculitis or thromboemboli, leading to partial or full-thickness mucosal necrosis or total infarction (Figure 1-9). On the other hand, with toxic damage from bacteria or other sources, there may be vasoconstriction, vascular degeneration, spasm, leakage, or other dysfunction,[19–21] leading to limited or transient ischemia, in addition to direct cytotoxic effects.[13] Therefore, injuries related to a primary vascular disorder (true ischemia) and "toxins" interact and merge, resulting in this hybrid terminology. Rarely, in a severely obstructed

colon, the pathology takes the form of an ischemic pattern due to diffuse and gradually diminished blood flow to the mucosa from increased luminal pressure. Therefore, even though the microscopic image of TIP may be uniform, the underlying diseases may be diverse.

As mentioned, although TIP lesions do not start as an inflammatory process initially, neutrophilic infiltration does occur in some cases as a secondary response to chemotactic factors released due to local cellular damage (Figures 1-2C, 1-2D, and 1-11). In contrast to primary inflammatory conditions, in which neutrophils infiltrate the epithelium, in toxic-ischemic injury the neutrophils are more predominantly located in the lamina propria (Figure 1-11).

The following are brief descriptions of several diseases that microscopically manifest as a TIP of injury. Many of these conditions are also discussed further in their relevant context in other chapters.

ISCHEMIC MUCOSAL INJURY

Ischemic mucosal injury is well represented by ischemic colitis[22] or enteritis. Ischemic gastritis is also encountered rarely[23,24] (Figures 1-13C, 1-13D). Diminished or total lack of blood supply to a segment of the bowel due to either vasculitis or thromboemboli leads to mucosal or transmural necrosis (an infarct). The process affects the superficial portion of the mucosa most severely and has less effect on the base of the crypts or glands. For this reason, except for cases of total transmural infarction, the basal zone of the mucosa is retained but has a peculiar "diminished" appearance: The glands appear small, and the epithelium is atrophic (Figure 1-9). Some of the glands exhibit a withered appearance (Figure 1-2D). The lamina propria is solid appearing and fibrotic. There is usually a lack of significant mononuclear cellular infiltration. However, focal or prominent neutrophilic infiltration can be seen (Figures 1-2D, 1-9) as the superficial necrosis leads to both physical and functional breakdown of the natural mucosal defenses, resulting in release of chemotactic factors. After a longer duration of partial ischemia, there is crypt or gland "dropout," leaving "empty" spaces in the lamina propria (stroma only) (Figure 1-1B). Residual glands or crypts exhibit regenerative changes or architectural distortion, including shortening or atrophy, basal budding, and branching (Figure 1-14).

FIGURE 1-14. Chronic ischemic colitis. **A.** Dense fibrosis in the lamina propria. **B.** Regenerative changes of residual crypts with architectural distortion.

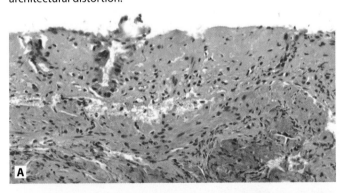

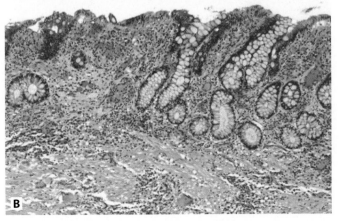

When the diagnosis of ischemic colitis is under consideration, the location of the biopsy can be helpful. There are two watershed regions in the colon, the sigmoid and the splenic flexure, that are more susceptible to ischemia. Due to duplication of the vasculature, ischemia of the rectum is rare. However, a TIP of injury is not unusual in mucosal biopsies from this region due to the common occurrence of mucosal prolapse, which likely causes strangulation of the submucosal blood vessels (Figure 1-15), as opposed to a true ischemic colitis.

Diagnosis of ischemic injury in mucosal biopsies depends on recognition of the characteristic microscopic pattern (i.e., TIP) and proper clinical correlation because thromboemboli or other vascular blockages are rarely present in the specimen. In some diseases, such as multiple superficial mucosal ulcerations in microangiopathic hemolytic anemia, microthrombi can be readily demonstrated in the submucosal vessels in the biopsies (Figure 1-16).

RADIATION-INDUCED MUCOSAL INJURY

Radiation causes GI mucosal injury through two main mechanisms: (1) direct injury to susceptible cells, mostly the gut epithelial cells, and (2) injury to arterial blood vessels, leading to subacute or chronic ischemia to the mucosa. The histologic changes vary depending on the dose and duration of exposure. For example, mild radiation injury of the rectosigmoid colon mucosa may result in slight crypt architectural distortion and capillary vessel dilation (Figure 1-17), sometimes with microthrombi. Severe injury causes superficial ulceration (Figure 1-18). Subacute or chronic changes manifest as loss of crypts or glands, crypt hypertrophy (Figure 1-19), or marked crypt architectural distortion (Figure 1-20). Radiation-induced cytologic changes are evident in vascular endothelial cells and fibroblasts and are characterized by enlarged nuclei with hyperchromasia. One of the more prominent findings is the subendothelial myxoid degeneration and thickening of arterioles in the submucosa, which is usually seen in the direct field of exposure to radiation.

Differentiation from Ischemic Mucosal Injury
Focally, radiation-induced mucosal injury may be indistinguishable from chronic ischemic change. Clinical history certainly is of great help in distinguishing the two conditions. In addition, certain microscopic findings, particularly cytologic and nuclear atypia of stromal cells and subendothelial or medial myxoid or foamy changes, are clues to this etiology.

Differentiation from Inflammatory Bowel Disease
Some features described for radiation-induced injury (crypt loss, architectural distortion) are part of the histologic spectrum of Crohn disease or ulcerative colitis. In contrast to the last conditions, radiation injury usually lacks significant inflammatory cellular infiltrate or active inflammation involving the crypts or glands. In other words,

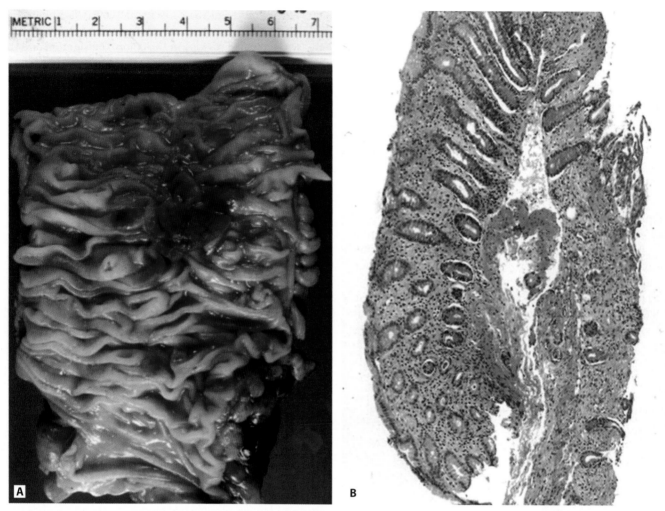

FIGURE 1-15. Rectal mucosal prolapse with ischemic changes. **A.** One side of the prolapsed fold exhibits erythematous changes and erosion. **B.** Microscopically, one side of the lesion (right) demonstrates typical ischemic superficial necrosis with lamina propria fibrosis; the opposite side of the lesion exhibits slight crypt hyperplasia.

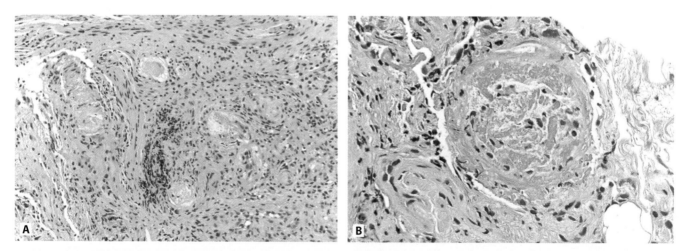

FIGURE 1-16. Microangiopathic hemolytic anemia. Multiple small, shallow ulcers were seen endoscopically in the duodenum and jejunum. **A.** Biopsies of the ulcers revealed microthrombi in the small submucosal blood vessels, sometimes accompanied by endothelial injury and hyperplasia. **B.** High-power view of a prominent thrombus.

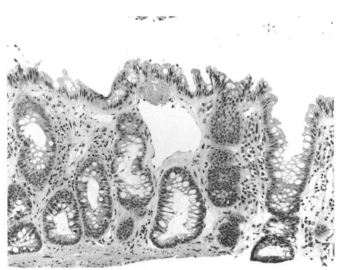

FIGURE 1-17. Radiation-related mucosal injury showing mild crypt distortion and dilated capillary vessels with microthrombi.

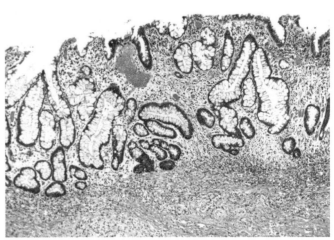

FIGURE 1-20. Radiation-related mucosal injury indicating degenerative changes in the surface epithelium and marked crypt distortion with lamina propria fibrosis and capillary vessel dilation.

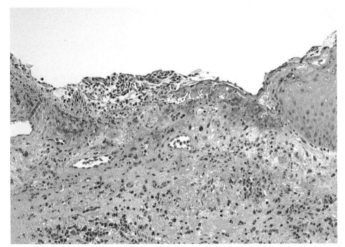

FIGURE 1-18. Radiation injury to the anorectal junctional mucosa, with ulceration and reactive atypia of stromal cells.

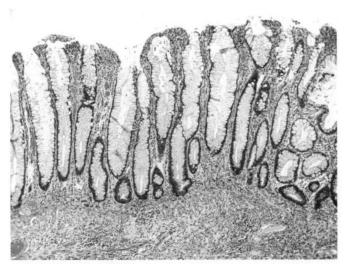

FIGURE 1-19. Radiation-related mucosal injury with colonic crypt hypertrophy.

although inflammatory bowel diseases are characterized by an inflammatory histologic pattern, radiation injury is that of a toxic (radiation) and ischemic (secondary to vascular injury) pattern (TIP).

◼ MUCOSAL PROLAPSE

Mucosal prolapse is most commonly seen in the rectosigmoid region, as mentioned previously,[25–28] but any region of the colon or GI tract can be involved. Some examples of hyperplastic polyps in the gastric mucosa are also mucosal prolapse.[29,30] Prolapse occurring in the rectosigmoid region, when large, may be accompanied by surface erosion or ulceration; hence some cases were given a clinical diagnosis of *solitary rectal ulcer syndrome*.[25,26] With increased use of endoscopy, more cases of small or minute mucosal prolapse are encountered, which show less-severe histologic changes.

The typical mucosal prolapse results in a polyp, or a prominent redundant mucosal fold (Figure 1-15). Due to traumatic impact by the luminal contents of the bowel as well as chronic vascular strangulation by mechanical pulling on the submucosa of the redundant fold,[26] the surface of the lesion incurs ischemic changes (Figure 1-15) similar to that of chronic ischemic colitis. The example in Figure 1-21 of a portion of prolapsed mucosa demonstrates superficial sloughing of the mucosa, atrophy and withering of the base of crypts, and lamina propria fibrosis. Occasionally, the reactive glandular hyperplasia or regeneration can be marked, with active fibrotic changes in the prolapsed lamina propria, giving rise to an irregular nodular endoscopic presentation and microscopic resemblance to invasive adenocarcinoma (Figure 1-22).

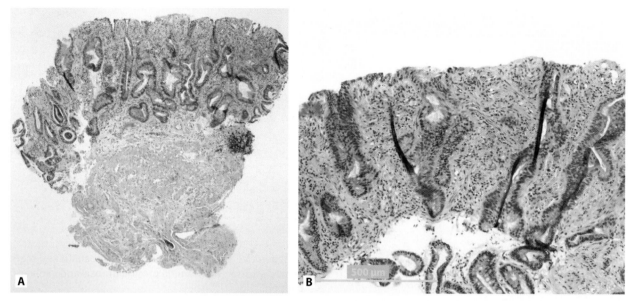

FIGURE 1-21. Rectal mucosal prolapse. **A.** There is superficial mucosal damage. In response to the ischemic injury, the crypts exhibit regenerative changes with architectural distortion. **B.** High-power view showing epithelial degeneration with mucin depletion and lamina propria fibrosis.

It should be pointed out that many cases of diminutive mucosal prolapse do not show ischemic change but exhibit slight crypt elongation or irregularity (Figure 1-23) that is often indistinguishable from normal mucosa. Biopsies of this lesion are often given a diagnosis of an inflammatory-type polyp, although for the most part there is no real increase in the lamina propria inflammatory infiltrate. These should more appropriately be called *early mucosal prolapse* or *minute prolapse polyp*.

The distinction of mucosal prolapse from true ischemic colitis depends on the clinical and endoscopic context.

■ BACTERIAL TOXIN-INDUCED MUCOSAL INJURY

Two bacteria account for most cases of enterocolitis that exhibit a TIP of mucosal injury: *C. difficile*[31-33] and *E. coli* O157:H7 (Chapter 28).[12,13] Both bacteria can cause superficial

FIGURE 1-22. Rectal mucosal prolapse. **A.** Chronic injury and regenerative response due to prolapse led to marked hyperplasia and lamina propria fibrosis. The epithelium otherwise exhibits mucin depletion. **B.** Some areas show markedly distorted crypts surrounded by active fibroblastic proliferation that mimics the desmoplasia of invasive carcinoma.

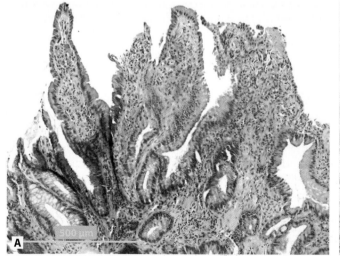
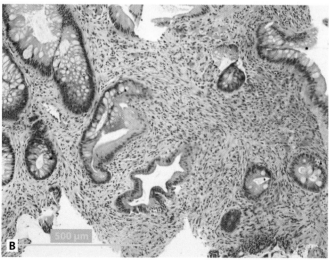

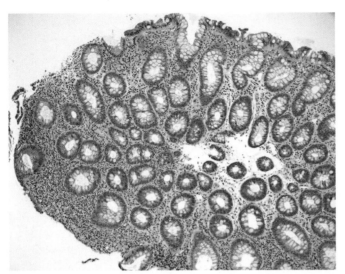

FIGURE 1-23. Inflammatory type polyp in the colon. This polypoid lesion exhibits nonspecific lamina propria inflammatory infiltration with slight crypt change.

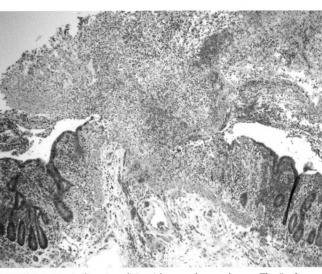

FIGURE 1-25. Ischemic colitis with pseudomembrane. The "volcano eruption"–like appearance of the necroinflammatory exudate mimics that of *Clostridium difficile* colitis.

or full-thickness mucosal necrosis, and *C. difficile* may be accompanied by a characteristic fibrinopurulent adherent exudate at the necrotic foci, giving rise to pseudomembranes (Chapter 28).[12,13] When mucosal necrosis is not full thickness, the residual mucosa exhibits the TIP (Figure 1-24). Similarly, some cases of enterohemorrhagic *E. coli* O157 infection can manifest as an ischemic mucosal injury pattern and may be mistaken for ischemic colitis (Chapter 28).

Conversely, ischemic colitis may occasionally exhibit the histologic changes of pseudomembranes (Figure 1-25).

VIRAL-INDUCED MUCOSAL INJURY

Several viruses that infect the GI tract, such as cytomegalovirus (CMV) and adenovirus, can lead to either a predominantly inflammatory pattern or TIP. For example, CMV can cause reactive gastropathy in some immunocompromised patients without significant inflammatory infiltration (Figure 1-26) or it can cause CMV colitis with a mucosal infiltrate mimicking inflammatory bowel disease (Chapter 28).

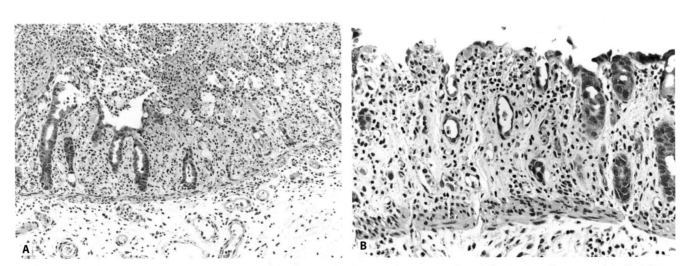

FIGURE 1-24. *Clostridium difficile* colitis with TIP changes. **A.** Superficial mucosal necrosis with an inflammatory fibrous exudate. **B.** Adjacent areas showing TIP changes with loss of surface epithelium and loss of crypts but no significant inflammatory infiltration in the lamina propria, a picture that is indistinguishable from acute ischemic colitis.

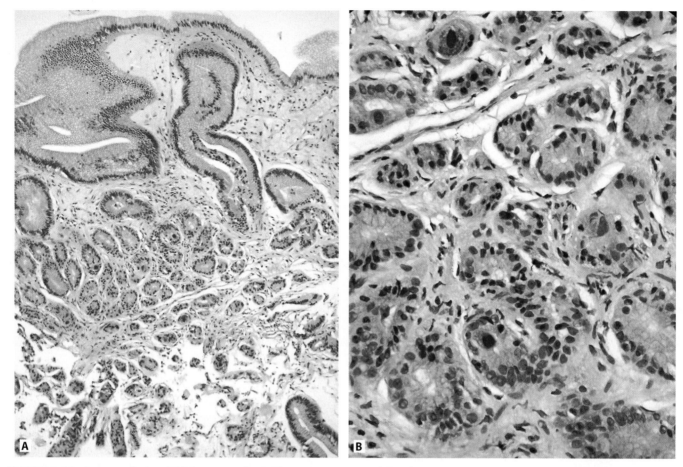

FIGURE 1-26. Cytomegalovirus (CMV) gastropathy. **A.** The gastric mucosa exhibits foveolar hyperplasia without inflammatory infiltration. **B.** Multiple large CMV inclusion bodies are evident in the glandular epithelium.

In gastric biopsies, CMV infection often causes a microscopic pattern of reactive/chemical gastropathy. This gastropathy is characterized by injury to the superficial epithelial compartment, including erosion or ulceration, hyperplasia of the foveolar layer with reactive changes, and a lack of dense mononuclear cell infiltration of the lamina propria. A careful search may allow for identification of typical CMV inclusions. Differential diagnoses include bile reflux, uremic gastropathy, other chemicals or drugs (nonsteroidal anti-inflammatory drugs, doxycycline, mycophenolate), and graft-versus-host disease.

Regardless of the pattern, the histologic hallmark is the CMV-induced cytopathic effect in the form of cytomegaly, large cytoplasmic basophilic granules, and typical nuclear inclusions (Figure 1-26). Adenovirus infection can also cause a TIP mucosal injury, which is characterized by mucosal injury that includes a malnourished epithelium exhibiting superficial necrosis, crypt apoptosis, an empty lamina propria, fibrinoid change of the lamina propria, and withered crypts (Chapter 2). Adenovirus infection may also manifest in an inflammatory histologic pattern.

CYTOTOXIC DRUG-RELATED MUCOSAL INJURY

As is discussed in several other chapters, certain immunosuppressive drugs (eg, mycophenolate mofetil, CellCept®) and targeted-therapy drugs[34,35] may cause GI mucosal injury in the form of TIP, as characterized by prominent apoptosis and occasionally crypt withering, without significant background inflammatory infiltration. Long-term injury may lead to significant loss of crypts (Figure 1-27).

DIFFERENTIAL CONSIDERATIONS FOR DIFFERENT SITES WITH TIP

In summary, the TIP of injury is a type of microscopic mucosal change that suggests a short list of potential diagnoses. When recognized and applied appropriately, TIP is a useful guide for the formation of a differential diagnosis and further workup. Table 1-1 lists conditions that should be considered or investigated when a TIP of injury is encountered; these are grouped by the portion of the GI tract involved.

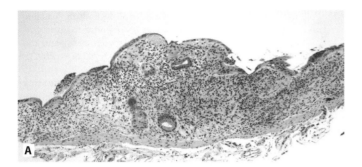

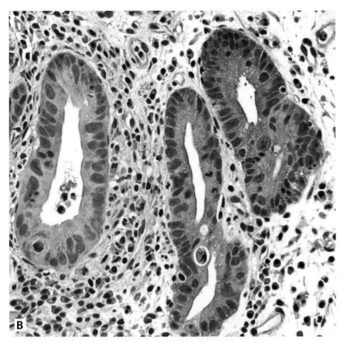

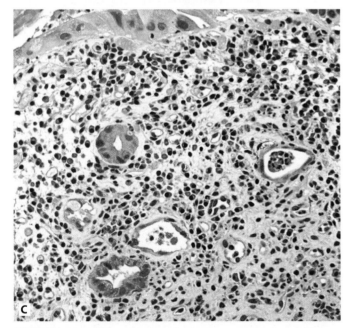

FIGURE 1-27. CellCept®-induced colonic mucosal injury. **A.** There is prominent crypt loss. **B.** Crypt apoptosis is indicative of ongoing toxic injury. **C.** Crypt withering is also evident.

TABLE 1-1. Differential diagnoses for toxic-ischemic pattern of injury.

Esophagus
  Pill esophagitis
  Mechanical injury (stent-induced injury)
  Radiation

Stomach
  Nonsteroidal anti-inflammatory drugs
  Other drugs (doxycycline, immunosuppressive therapy, chemotherapy)
  Alcohol gastropathy
  Cytomegalovirus gastropathy
  Amyloidosis
  Graft-versus-host disease
  Uremic gastropathy
  Ischemia

Small bowel
  Ischemic bowel disease
  Drug-induced enteropathy
  Graft-versus-host disease
  Viral infection
  Rejection (small-bowel transplant)

Colon
  Ischemic colitis
  Mucosal prolapse
  Clostridium difficile colitis
  Shiga toxin-producing bacteria colitis
  Graft-versus-host disease
  Radiation colitis

■ REFERENCES

1. Stauch G, Muenzenmayer C. Computational pathology and telepathology: SY05-1 pattern recognition in telepathology. *Pathology*. 2014;46(Suppl 2):S6. PMID: 25188189.

2. Webster JD, Michalowski AM, Dwyer JE, et al. Investigation into diagnostic agreement using automated computer-assisted histopathology pattern recognition image analysis. *J Pathol Inform*. 2012;3:18. PMID: 22616030. PMCID: 3352619.

3. Hipp J, Smith SC, Cheng J, et al. Optimization of complex cancer morphology detection using the SIVQ pattern recognition algorithm. *Anal Cell Pathol*. 2012;35(1):41–50. PMID: 21988838.

4. Adsay V, Logani S, Sarkar F, Crissman J, Vaitkevicius V. Foamy gland pattern of pancreatic ductal adenocarcinoma: a deceptively benign-appearing variant. *Am J Surg Pathol*. 2000;24(4):493–504. PMID: 10757396.

5. Braak H, Braak E. Morphological criteria for the recognition of Alzheimer's disease and the distribution pattern of cortical changes related to this disorder. *Neurobiol Aging*. 1994;15(3):355–356; discussion 79–80. PMID: 7936061.

6. Montironi R, Scarpelli M, Pisani E, Ansuini G, Mariuzzi GM. Histomorphometry and pattern recognition analysis of urothelial papillary lesions. *Tumori.* 1984;70(5):463–466. PMID: 6506232.

7. Xiao SY, Zhao L, Hart J, Semrad CE. Gastric mucosal necrosis with vascular degeneration induced by doxycycline. *Am J Surg Pathol.* 2013;37(2):259–263. PMID: 23060354.

8. Waldman WJ, Knight DA. Cytokine-mediated induction of endothelial adhesion molecule and histocompatibility leukocyte antigen expression by cytomegalovirus-activated T cells. *Am J Pathol.* 1996;148(1):105–119. PMID: 8546198. PMCID: 1861599.

9. Hamilton ST, Scott G, Naing Z, et al. Human cytomegalovirus-induces cytokine changes in the placenta with implications for adverse pregnancy outcomes. *PloS One.* 2012;7(12):e52899. PMID: 23300810. PMCID: 3534118.

10. Bolovan-Fritts CA, Trout RN, Spector SA. Human cytomegalovirus-specific CD4+-T-cell cytokine response induces fractalkine in endothelial cells. *J Virol.* 2004;78(23):13173–13181. PMID: 15542669. PMCID: 525022.

11. Trump BF, Berezesky IK, Chang SH, Phelps PC. The pathways of cell death: oncosis, apoptosis, and necrosis. *Toxicol Pathol.* 1997;25(1):82–88. PMID: 9061857.

12. Kelly J, Oryshak A, Wenetsek M, Grabiec J, Handy S. The colonic pathology of *Escherichia coli* O157:H7 infection. *Am J Surg Pathol.* 1990;14(1):87–92. PMID: 2403759.

13. Griffin PM, Olmstead LC, Petras RE. *Escherichia coli* O157:H7-associated colitis. A clinical and histological study of 11 cases. *Gastroenterology.* 1990;99(1):142–149. PMID: 2188868.

14. Berenguer J, Cabades F, Gras MD, Pertejo V, Rayon M, Sala T. Ischemic colitis attributable to a cleansing enema. *Hepatogastroenterology.* 1981;28(3):173–175. PMID: 7250900.

15. Deana DG, Dean PJ. Reversible ischemic colitis in young women. Association with oral contraceptive use. *Am J Surg Pathol.* 1995;19(4):454–462. PMID: 7694947.

16. Takeda M, Shirato I, Kobayashi M, Endou H. Hydrogen peroxide induces necrosis, apoptosis, oncosis and apoptotic oncosis of mouse terminal proximal straight tubule cells. *Nephron.* 1999;81(2):234–238. PMID: 9933761.

17. Carlson RM, Madoff RD. Is "ischemic" colitis ischemic? *Dis Colon Rectum.* 2011;54(3):370–373. PMID: 21304312.

18. Mosli M, Parfitt J, Gregor J. Retrospective analysis of disease association and outcome in histologically confirmed ischemic colitis. *J Dig Dis.* 2013;14(5):238–243. PMID: 23419044.

19. Grandel U, Bennemann U, Buerke M, et al. Staphylococcus aureus alpha-toxin and Escherichia coli hemolysin impair cardiac regional perfusion and contractile function by activating myocardial eicosanoid metabolism in isolated rat hearts. *Crit Care Med.* 2009;37(6):2025–2032. PMID: 19384217.

20. Stenger KO, Windler F, Karch H, von Wulffen H, Heesemann J. Hemolytic-uremic syndrome associated with an infection by verotoxin producing *Escherichia coli* 0111 in a woman on oral contraceptives. *Clin Nephrol.* 1988;29(3):153–158. PMID: 3282732.

21. Walmrath D, Ghofrani HA, Rosseau S, et al. Endotoxin "priming" potentiates lung vascular abnormalities in response to *Escherichia coli* hemolysin: an example of synergism between endo- and exotoxin. *J Exp Med.* 1994;180(4):1437–1443. PMID: 7931076. PMCID: PMC2191678.

22. Brandt LJ, Feuerstadt P, Blaszka MC. Anatomic patterns, patient characteristics, and clinical outcomes in ischemic colitis: a study of 313 cases supported by histology. *Am J Gastroenterol.* 2010;105(10):2245–2252; quiz 53. PMID: 20531399.

23. Richieri JP, Pol B, Payan MJ. Acute necrotizing ischemic gastritis: clinical, endoscopic and histopathologic aspects. *Gastrointest Endosc.* 1998;48(2):210–212. PMID: 9717792.

24. Force T, MacDonald D, Eade OE, Doane C, Krawitt EL. Ischemic gastritis and duodenitis. *Dig Dis Sci.* 1980;25(4):307–310. PMID: 7389531.

25. Levine DS. "Solitary" rectal ulcer syndrome. Are "solitary" rectal ulcer syndrome and "localized" colitis cystica profunda analogous syndromes caused by rectal prolapse? *Gastroenterology.* 1987;92(1):243–253. PMID: 3536653.

26. Lonsdale RN. Microvascular abnormalities in the mucosal prolapse syndrome. *Gut.* 1993;34(1):106–109. PMID: 8432438. PMCID: 1374110.

27. Warren BF, Davies JD. Prolapse-induced inflammatory polyps of the colorectum and anal transition zone. *Histopathology.* 1994;24(2):201–202. PMID: 8181820.

28. Kang YS, Kamm MA, Engel AF, Talbot IC. Pathology of the rectal wall in solitary rectal ulcer syndrome and complete rectal prolapse. *Gut.* 1996;38(4):587–590. PMID: 8707093. PMCID: 1383120.

29. Gencosmanoglu R, Sen-Oran E, Kurtkaya-Yapicier O, Tozun N. Antral hyperplastic polyp causing intermittent gastric outlet obstruction: case report. *BMC Gastroenterol.* 2003;3:16. PMID: 12831404. PMCID: 166166.

30. Vesoulis Z, Naik N, Maseelall P. Histopathologic changes are not specific for diagnosis of gastric antral vascular ectasia (GAVE) syndrome: a review of the pathogenesis and a comparative image analysis morphometric study of GAVE syndrome and gastric hyperplastic polyps. *Am J Clin Pathol.* 1998;109(5):558–564. PMID: 9576573.

31. King A, Rampling A, Wight DG, Warren RE. Neutropenic enterocolitis due to *Clostridium septicum* infection. *J Clin Pathol.* 1984;37(3):335–343. PMID: 6699196. PMCID: 498711.

32. Lima AA, Innes DJ, Jr, Chadee K, Lyerly DM, Wilkins TD, Guerrant RL. *Clostridium difficile* toxin A. Interactions with mucus and early sequential histopathologic effects in rabbit small intestine. *Lab Invest.* 1989;61(4):419–425. PMID: 2507823.

33. Chumbler NM, Farrow MA, Lapierre LA, et al. *Clostridium difficile* toxin B causes epithelial cell necrosis through an autoprocessing-independent mechanism. *PLoS Pathog.* 2012;8(12):e1003072. PMID: 23236283. PMCID: 3516567.

34. Pessi MA, Zilembo N, Haspinger ER, et al. Targeted therapy-induced diarrhea: a review of the literature. *Crit Rev Oncol Hematol.* 2014;90(2):165–179. PMID: 24373918.

35. Cappell MS. Colonic toxicity of administered drugs and chemicals. *Am J Gastroenterol.* 2004;99(6):1175–1190. PMID: 15180742.

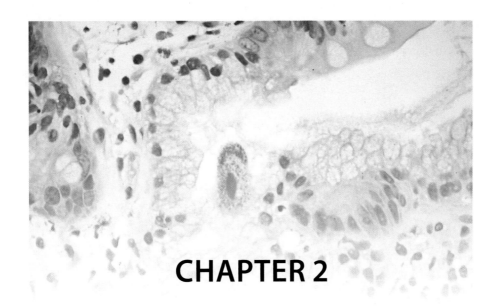

CHAPTER 2

GI Biopsies in Transplant Settings

Lindsay Alpert and Shu-Yuan Xiao

■ OVERVIEW

As solid-organ and stem cell transplantation have increasingly been utilized in the management of a variety of benign and malignant conditions, the frequency with which pathologists encounter gastrointestinal (GI) biopsies from this patient population has risen. These biopsies are usually obtained when a transplant patient presents with GI symptoms, but in some cases, they may be collected as part of a surveillance protocol, as is routine following small-bowel transplantation. Transplant patients are susceptible to a number of GI disorders, some of which are not specific to this population and instead may be seen in association with a variety of medical conditions; opportunistic infections and drug-induced injury are included in this category. However, there are several disorders that are unique to the transplant population and deserve special consideration, including graft-versus-host disease (GVHD), post-transplantation lymphoproliferative disorder (PTLD), and allograft rejection. Therefore, the pathologist must be aware of a wide range of disorders when examining biopsies from transplant patients. This chapter reviews the major entities encountered in GI biopsies from transplant patients and provides a framework for considering diagnoses in the differential based on the histologic features present.

■ GRAFT-VERSUS-HOST DISEASE

Graft-versus-host disease is a common complication of hematopoietic stem cell transplantation and represents a significant source of morbidity and mortality in the transplant population. The underlying pathogenesis of GVHD involves graft recognition of host cells as foreign due to genetic differences between the donor and the recipient, without a corresponding rejection of graft cells by the immunosuppressed host. The subsequent graft lymphocyte attack on host cells targets the transplant recipient's skin, GI tract, and liver. Occasionally, recipients of solid-organ transplants may also develop GVHD as a result of donor lymphocytes passively transferred within transplanted organs.[1] Patients with acute GI GVHD present with nausea, vomiting, anorexia, diarrhea, and abdominal pain, typically within the first 100 days post-transplantaion. In severe cases, paralytic ileus and intestinal hemorrhage may occur.[2] Endoscopic findings range from normal mucosa to edematous, erythematous, friable, and severely ulcerated mucosa, although these findings do not always correspond with the degree of changes seen histologically.

Microscopic Features of Acute GVHD

Apoptosis of epithelial cells is the histologic hallmark of acute GVHD and affects the regenerative compartment of the crypts and glands of the GI tract.[1] Apoptotic cells are vacuolated and filled with karyorrhectic debris (Figure 2-1), bearing a resemblance to pieces of popcorn, which is why they are often referred to as "popcorn lesions." These apoptotic epithelial cells can be seen in a number of conditions affecting the GI tract, as discussed further in this chapter, and are therefore nonspecific, but the presence of these cells is required to make the diagnosis of GVHD.

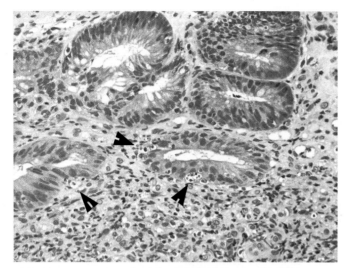

FIGURE 2-1. Apoptotic bodies. High-power view of colonic mucosa with vacuolated crypt epithelial cells containing karyorrhectic debris (arrowheads). These apoptotic cells are often described as "popcorn lesions."

TABLE 2-1.	Histologic grading of acute GVHD.
Grade	Histologic features
I	Single epithelial cell apoptosis
II	Destruction of single crypts/glands with apoptotic crypt abscesses
III	Focal mucosal necrosis with ulceration and loss of contiguous crypts/glands
IV	Diffuse mucosal necrosis with denudation

Most cases of GI GVHD involve the large intestine, with apoptosis of single epithelial cells at the base of crypts the earliest histologic finding. Subsequently, there is progression to crypt destruction with crypt withering and dilation, often containing intraluminal apoptotic debris (Figure 2-2).[1,3] Eventually, mucosal ulceration and diffuse mucosal necrosis may occur. While histologic grading of acute GVHD is not universally performed, the most commonly used grading system stratifies these features as shown in Table 2-1. Unfortunately, the correlation between histologic grade and endoscopic and clinical features of acute GVHD is generally poor, although the degree of crypt loss has been associated with more severe clinical disease and steroid refractoriness.[3]

Although GVHD is thought to be mediated by graft lymphocytes attacking the host's epithelium, on histologic examination of GI biopsies, intraepithelial lymphocytes are not as prominent as might be expected. This lack of visual evidence of lymphocyte-induced damage suggests that rather than lymphocytes directly causing apoptosis in the host epithelium, the graft's lymphocytes trigger a cascade of events that ultimately result in epithelial apoptosis. In addition to this lack of intraepithelial inflammation, acute GI GVHD has classically been described as displaying a paucity of inflammatory cells in the lamina propria. Depending on the timing of the biopsies, this lack of inflammation may in part be due to chemotherapeutic ablation of the host immune system prior to transplantation. However, many cases of acute GVHD do exhibit significant inflammation, which could be partially explained by recent advances in cytoreductive regimens. The background infiltrate in these cases generally consists of mononuclear cells, eosinophils, and occasional neutrophils (Figure 2-3). Such cases may show significant histologic overlap with infectious colitis, a condition that must be excluded, as is discussed further in this chapter. Finally, mucosal endocrine cells may appear prominent in some cases of GVHD.

FIGURE 2-2. Acute graft-versus-host disease (GVHD) involving colonic mucosa. **A.** Colonic mucosa with dilated, focally withered crypts containing intraluminal apoptotic debris. **B.** High-power view of colonic mucosa displaying a withered, dilated crypt with apoptotic debris in its lumen.

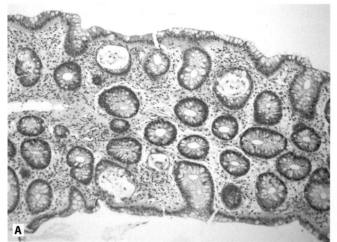

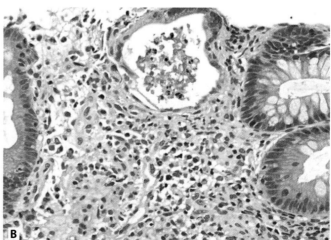

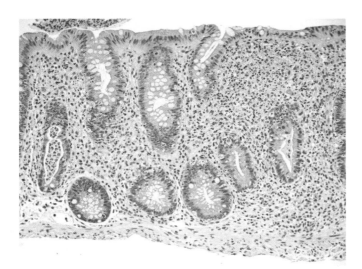

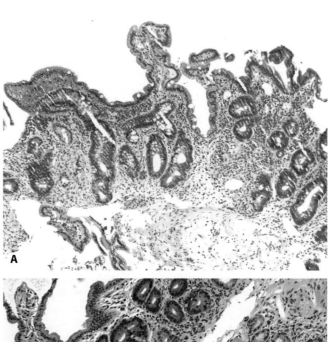

FIGURE 2-3. Acute GVHD involving colonic mucosa. The mucosa demonstrates both brisk apoptosis of crypt epithelial cells and significant active inflammation, with neutrophils infiltrating the lamina propria and epithelium. Infectious etiologies were excluded using immunohistochemical stains.

The small-bowel mucosa displays similar features when involved by acute GVHD, with changes ranging from individual apoptotic bodies to crypt dropout with progressive ulceration (Figure 2-4). The apoptotic epithelial cells are most prominent in the neck region and at the base of crypts (Figure 2-4A), and the associated villous blunting is often subtle. The duodenum may display significant activity, including numerous intraepithelial neutrophils, when involved by GVHD, and in such cases infectious etiologies must again be excluded. In severe cases, pericapillary hemorrhage as a result of endothelial injury may also be seen, although this finding is generally not diagnostically useful as indistinguishable changes can occur due to biopsy trauma.[1]

In the stomach, apoptotic epithelial cells and destruction of glands with intraluminal eosinophilic material (Figure 2-5) are the major findings of acute GVHD.[2] Apoptosis affects the cells in the neck region of the glands of the gastric body but is seen deeper in the glands of the gastric antrum. As in the duodenum, a neutrophilic infiltrate may be present, raising concern for infectious sources of gastritis, which must be excluded. Changes due to proton pump inhibitor (PPI) therapy should also be considered in gastric biopsies when evaluating for GVHD, as these medications can cause gland dilation in the gastric body mucosa as well as apoptosis of epithelial cells in the gastric antrum. However, because apoptosis due to PPIs has been shown to be restricted to the gastric antrum, the presence of apoptotic epithelium in the gastric body supports the diagnosis of GVHD over PPI effect.[2]

While esophageal involvement by acute GVHD is uncommon, the histologic features are similar to those seen in the skin, with mucosal desquamation and apoptosis of basal cells (Figure 2-6). Often, only nonspecific findings, such as inflammation or granulation tissue, are present, in which case infectious conditions must be ruled out.

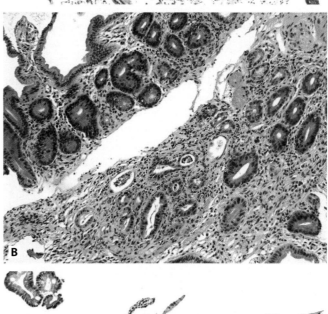

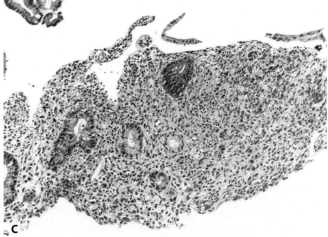

FIGURE 2-4. Acute GVHD involving duodenal mucosa. **A.** Small-bowel mucosa with numerous apoptotic bodies most prominent in the neck region and at the base of crypts. **B.** A slightly more advanced case of acute GVHD with a focus of withering crypts containing intraluminal apoptotic debris. **C.** In this severe case of acute GVHD, there is extensive crypt dropout and erosion of the overlying surface epithelium. The remaining crypts contain scattered apoptotic bodies.

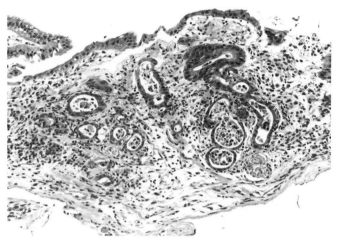

FIGURE 2-5. Acute GVHD involving gastric mucosa, which has dilated, withered glands contain intraluminal eosinophilic material and apoptotic debris.

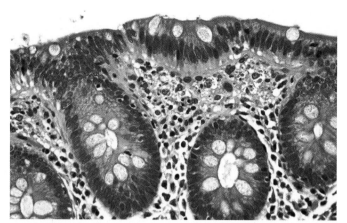

FIGURE 2-7. Colonic mucosa with apoptotic cells in the superficial lamina propria caused by bowel preparation prior to colonoscopy.

Histologic Diagnosis of Acute GVHD

The minimum criteria for the histologic diagnosis of acute GVHD are not well established. The diagnosis is largely dependent on the clinical setting and symptoms, with certain histologic findings supportive of the clinical diagnosis. The minimum histologic findings needed for the diagnosis of acute GVHD at various institutions range from a single apoptotic epithelial cell per biopsy piece to several crypts or glands involved by apoptosis. In the proper clinical setting, it is reasonable to suggest the possibility of acute GVHD when 1–2 crypts or glands display apoptotic epithelial cells, and the diagnosis is even more likely if 3 or more crypts or glands are involved. Apoptosis involving the surface subepithelial zone in itself is insufficient for the diagnosis of acute GVHD,

FIGURE 2-6. Acute GVHD involving the esophagus. Squamous epithelium with apoptotic epithelial cells most prominent in the basal layers. Dyskeratotic cells are occasionally seen (arrowhead). Spongiosis and intraepithelial lymphocytes are prominent.

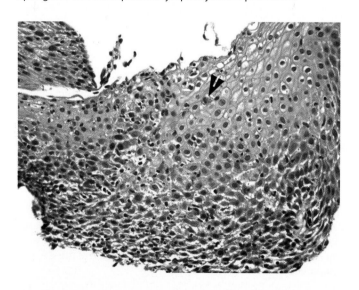

as this process can be the result of bowel preparation regimens alone (Figure 2-7). Because of the patchy nature of this condition, several sections of each biopsy should be examined when assessing for evidence of acute GVHD, although recommendations on the precise number of sections that should be examined vary. Confounding factors such as infections and drug reactions should always be considered and excluded whenever possible; however, these conditions may coexist with GVHD, so their presence does not rule out the possibility of concurrent GVHD.[4,5]

Chronic GVHD

Chronic GVHD was initially defined as GVHD occurring over 100 days following transplantation, but after a National Institutes of Health (NIH) consensus conference in 2005, the classification of chronic GVHD transitioned to classification based largely on clinical findings. The only diagnostic feature of chronic GVHD in the GI tract as defined by the 2005 criteria is the presence of esophageal webs.[6,7] Gastric involvement by severe GVHD may lead to atrophic gastritis with intestinal metaplasia (see Chapter 12). The histologic features seen in colonic biopsies from patients with chronic GVHD include mucosal architectural distortion, lymphoplasmocytic infiltration, Paneth cell metaplasia, and lamina propria and submucosal fibrosis, which are nonspecific findings that can be seen in numerous conditions, including inflammatory bowel disease. In transplant patients, these features can represent the sequelae of acute GVHD and may be characterized by marked crypt loss, leaving large areas with an "empty" lamina propria, often accompanied by ongoing damage in the form of epithelial cell apoptosis.[4] Identification of these histological changes in the proper clinical setting can support the clinical diagnosis of chronic GI GVHD.

Diagnostic Challenges and Differential Diagnosis

The diagnosis of GVHD is complicated by several factors, including a number of conditions with overlapping features that occur in the transplant patient population. Reduced-intensity conditioning regimens and improvements in GVHD prophylaxis have led to a decreased incidence of acute GVHD along with detection of disease at earlier stages, resulting in an increase in cases with subtle manifestations that make definitive histologic diagnosis of acute GVHD difficult.[1,5] In addition, the nonuniform nature of GVHD makes the detection of this condition challenging when the disease is mild and a small number of areas are sampled.[4]

As mentioned previously, a wide range of factors can produce epithelial cell apoptosis in the GI tract, including pre-transplant conditioning regimens, infections, and commonly used post-transplant medications, such as mycophenolate mofetil (MMF). Chemotherapeutic agents used prior to transplantation are known to cause diffuse apoptosis of the gut epithelium, which has been documented as late as 30 days post-transplant. For this reason, assessment of acute GVHD in the first month following transplantation is especially problematic.[1,5]

Infectious agents such as cytomegalovirus (CMV), adenovirus, and cryptosporidium are also well-known causes of apoptosis in the GI tract, and infectious conditions, particularly CMV, are often on the clinical differential for GI disturbances in immunosuppressed transplant recipients. If infection is clinically suspected or severe mucosal injury is found but no viral inclusions are identified histologically, immunohistochemical stains should be used to exclude infectious etiologies.[1] Acute GVHD and GI infections can also occur simultaneously in this immunosuppressed patient population. In cases of infectious gastroenteritis, the possibility of concurrent GVHD should be suspected when epithelial cell apoptosis is extensive (Figure 2-8).[5]

Significant histologic overlap also exists between GVHD and toxicity from various medications, especially immunosuppressive therapies such as the antimetabolite drug MMF (CellCept®). MMF is used to prevent and treat acute allograft rejection and GVHD. Unfortunately, GI toxicity, usually in the form of diarrhea, is a common side effect of this drug.[8] Colonic biopsies from affected patients often show epithelial cell apoptosis in crypts, sometimes in association with a mixed inflammatory infiltrate and focal ulceration (see the section on CMV). The clinical and histologic similarity between GVHD and MMF-induced colitis is problematic, as transplant patients are frequently at risk for both conditions, and the two diagnoses differ significantly in their therapeutic implications. Although the entire GI system may be affected by MMF toxicity, the histologic effects seen in the upper portion of the GI tract are mostly those of mucosal irritation, such as ulcerative esophagitis, reactive gastropathy, and duodenal ulcers. Therefore, the finding of extensive apoptosis at more proximal sites is likely the result of GVHD rather than MMF toxicity.[9] Recent data also suggest that cases with prominent eosinophilic infiltrates but no endocrine cell aggregates or apoptotic microabscesses are more likely due to MMF toxicity than GVHD.[8]

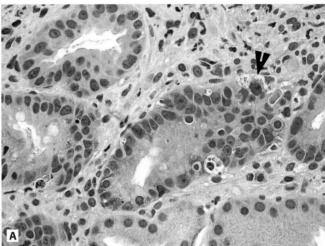

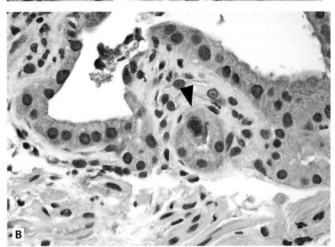

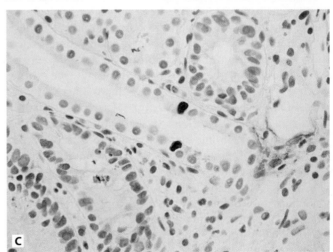

FIGURE 2-8. Acute GVHD and adenoviral infection simultaneously involving the small bowel. **A.** Small-bowel mucosa with numerous apoptotic crypt epithelial cells consistent with involvement by acute GVHD. A crypt epithelial cell with an enlarged, smudgy, and dark nucleus and a perinuclear halo is also present (arrowhead), indicating a concurrent adenovirus infection. **B.** A separate field from the same biopsy shows another epithelial cell with a smudgy, basophilic intranuclear inclusion (arrowhead). **C.** Immunohistochemical staining for adenovirus confirmed the presence of adenoviral inclusions in the epithelial cells.

DRUG-INDUCED INJURY

Gastrointestinal toxicity is a side effect of a variety of medications, as discussed in Chapter 1, and transplant patients often require treatment with multiple drugs, some of which are particularly known for their propensity to cause GI damage. Chief among these medications is the immunosuppressant MMF (see preceding section), although other immunosuppressive drugs commonly used in transplant patients, such as tacrolimus (FK506), are also known to cause injury to the GI tract. Unfortunately, much of the histologic evidence of this damage is nonspecific and significantly overlaps with other conditions encountered in the transplant setting, making a definitive pathologic diagnosis of drug-induced injury difficult.

Mycophenolate Mofetil

Mycophenolate mofetil is an immunosuppressant drug that commonly plays a role in the prophylactic and therapeutic regimens for both stem cell and solid-organ transplant patients.[8] MMF is approved by the Food and Drug Administration (FDA) for the prevention of organ rejection in combination with cyclosporine and corticosteroids in kidney, heart, and liver transplant recipients. In addition, the drug is used to treat rejection in patients who have had a heart or liver transplant and can also be administered to prevent and treat GVHD following stem cell and solid-organ transplantation.

Mycophenolate mofetil is a prodrug that undergoes hepatic conversion to mycophenolic acid. The active form of the drug inhibits inosine monophosphate dehydrogenase, an enzyme in the de novo pathway of purine synthesis. As the de novo pathway is the main source of purine synthesis for lymphocytes, T- and B-lymphocyte proliferation is selectively decreased by MMF.[10] Unfortunately, enterocytes also use the de novo pathway for much of their purine synthesis, and it is therefore not surprising that the main adverse effect of MMF therapy is GI toxicity.[10] GI symptoms occur in approximately half of patients treated with MMF and typically manifest as chronic diarrhea, sometimes accompanied by nausea, vomiting, and abdominal pain. Conditions in the clinical differential often include GVHD (as discussed previously), infectious colitis, and inflammatory bowel disease. On endoscopy, findings are generally nonspecific and range from normal mucosa to edematous, friable, and ulcerated mucosa.[11]

Histologically, GI biopsies from patients with MMF toxicity also display a variety of changes. In the colon, common features of acute and subacute MMF-induced mucosal injury include mildly dilated, "withered" crypts with an atrophic epithelial lining and intraluminal debris (Figure 2-9), as well as crypt epithelial apoptosis (Figure 2-10). Some cases also exhibit a prominent neutrophilic or eosinophilic infiltrate (Figure 2-11). When ongoing damage with partial healing occurs, lamina propria edema, crypt architectural distortion, and regenerative atypia of the epithelium may be seen

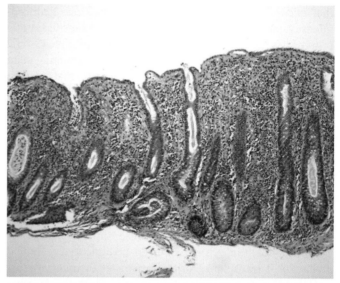

FIGURE 2-9. Mucosal injury induced by MMF. Colonic mucosa with atrophic surface epithelium, mildly dilated crypts, and active colitis with crypt abscesses.

(Figure 2-12).[9,10,12] These histologic findings in MMF-induced mucosal damage are often patchy, but they tend to be more pronounced in the right colon than in the left colon.[10,12]

The damage due to MMF toxicity is nonspecific and can be difficult to differentiate from other entities in the transplant setting. As discussed, apoptotic crypt epithelium combined with a hypocellular lamina propria can closely resemble GVHD, which is often also considered in these patients and has opposing therapeutic implications. The presence of an eosinophilic infiltrate without associated endocrine cell aggregates or apoptotic microabscesses has recently been shown to support a diagnosis of MMF toxicity over GVHD.[8] However, exceptions to this rule exist, so definitive histologic distinction between these entities is not always possible.[8]

FIGURE 2-10. Mucosal injury induced by MMF. Colonic mucosa with crypt epithelial cell apoptosis (arrowhead) and focal withering of crypts.

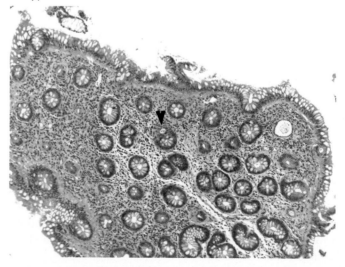

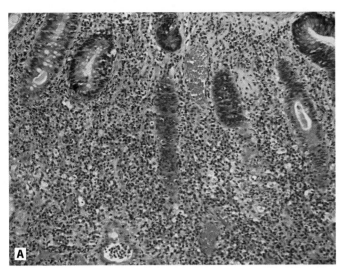

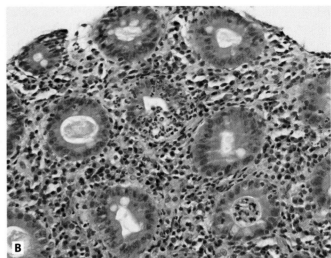

FIGURE 2-11. Mucosal injury in the colon induced by MMF. **A.** Active colitis with dense neutrophilic and eosinophilic infiltration of the lamina propria and extensive cryptitis with focal crypt abscess formation. **B.** High-power view of colonic mucosa from the same patient displaying cryptitis and a crypt abscess.

Alternatively, if a neutrophilic lamina propria infiltrate is seen along with cryptitis and crypt abscesses, sources of infectious colitis must be considered. In such cases, organisms such as CMV and adenovirus should be excluded immunohistochemically if no viral inclusions are identified on sections stained with hematoxylin and eosin (H&E).

Although less common, MMF can also cause pathologic changes in the upper GI tract, which are largely the result of mucosal irritation. Ulcerative esophagitis may be present, and biopsies of the stomach often reveal reactive gastropathy with foveolar hyperplasia and edema and fibromuscular replacement of the lamina propria (Figure 2-13A). Some cases exhibit an active gastritis with a neutrophilic infiltrate (Figure 2-13B),

FIGURE 2-12. Mucosal injury in the colon induced by mycophenolate mofetil (MMF). The colonic mucosa in this case shows architectural distortions with loss of crypts as well as lamina propria edema. The epithelium displays reactive atypia with hyperchromatic, irregularly shaped, enlarged nuclei. This pattern of histologic features suggests long-standing MMF toxicity with partial healing.

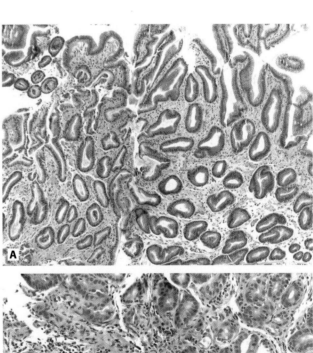

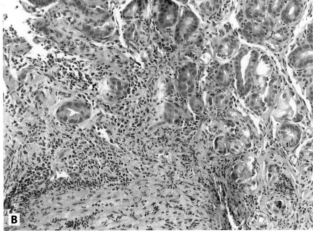

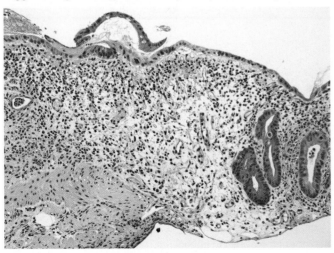

FIGURE 2-13. Mucosal injury in the stomach induced by MMF. **A.** This biopsy shows reactive gastropathy in the antrum with a fibrotic-appearing lamina propria. **B.** A different field from the same biopsy reveals a focus of active antral gastritis with neutrophils infiltrating the lamina propria and epithelium.

and active duodenitis with ulcer formation may also be seen. Apoptotic epithelial cells are frequently detected, although this finding is nonspecific.[13] As mentioned previously, extensive apoptosis in the upper GI tract is more likely the result of GVHD than MMF toxicity, although consideration of both entities is of utmost importance when examining upper GI biopsies from transplant patients.[9]

Tacrolimus

Tacrolimus (FK506) is an immunosuppressant drug of the calcineurin inhibitor class, which, like cyclosporine, functions by preventing T-cell activation induced by interleukin (IL) 2. Tacrolimus is commonly used in the management of graft rejection in transplant patients.[14] This drug is FDA approved for rejection prophylaxis in kidney, heart, and liver transplant recipients, and it is also used to prevent rejection following lung and small-bowel transplantation. In addition, tacrolimus can be administered as prophylaxis against or treatment of GVHD in stem cell transplant recipients.

Patients receiving this drug have been found to occasionally develop eosinophilic GI disease, which is thought to result from the drug's ability to increase intestinal permeability, leading to enhanced exposure to food allergens. Also, tacrolimus is known to elevate immunoglobulin (Ig) E levels, possibly by altering cytokine production. Patients with tacrolimus-induced eosinophilic GI disease typically present with vomiting, diarrhea, hematochezia, and poor oral intake.[15] GI biopsies display varying degrees of eosinophilic infiltration involving the mucosa of the esophagus, stomach, small intestine, or colon.[14] The inflammatory infiltrate may range from scattered eosinophils to eosinophilic abscess formation (Figure 2-14). While eosinophilic GI disease has multiple potential etiologies, it is important to consider tacrolimus as the causative agent in transplant patients who develop GI symptoms with a mucosal eosinophilic infiltrate on biopsy.

◼ OPPORTUNISTIC INFECTIONS

In addition to the GI injury caused by drugs used in transplant recipients, these medications significantly suppress the immune system, resulting in increased susceptibility to a variety of GI infections. Among these, viral infections, particularly CMV infection, are most commonly encountered, although almost any viral, bacterial, fungal, or parasitic infection can occur in this immunocompromised patient population. This section focuses on the common viral, fungal, and bacterial GI pathogens seen in transplant recipients; it also highlights some rare organisms that have recently emerged in these patients.

Cytomegalovirus

Cytomegalovirus is one of the most important pathogens in the post-transplant setting. CMV-negative recipients of organs from CMV-positive donors are at greatest risk of infection, although viral reactivation in CMV-positive recipients is

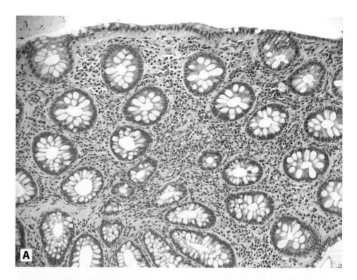
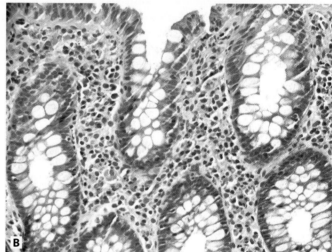
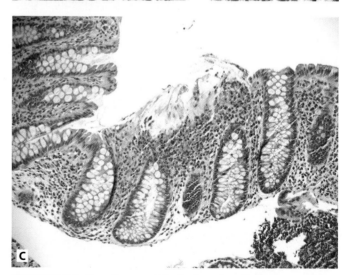

FIGURE 2-14. Tacrolimus toxicity in the colon. **A.** Numerous eosinophils are seen infiltrating the lamina propria of the colon, with focal involvement of the crypt epithelium. **B.** High-power view showing the eosinophilic lamina propria infiltrate as well as occasional eosinophils in the crypt and surface epithelium. **C.** An eosinophilic abscess is seen in the superficial colonic mucosa with necrosis of the overlying epithelium.

not uncommon. While prophylactic regimens have lowered the rate of CMV infection in transplant patients overall, late-onset infections after cessation of antiviral therapy is encountered with increasing frequency.[16]

Patients with tissue-invasive CMV infection of the GI tract typically present with abdominal pain and diarrhea; severe cases may result in perforation and hemorrhage. Patients with upper GI involvement may report dysphagia and odynophagia. The colon is the most common site of GI involvement, although the esophagus, stomach, and small bowel may also be affected.[17] On endoscopic examination, the classic findings are well-circumscribed, "punched-out" ulcers, although this finding is nonspecific and the clinical presentation and endoscopic appearance can overlap significantly with GVHD.[18]

A wide range of histological findings may be present in cases of CMV infection of the GI tract in transplant patients. Mucosal ulceration is often seen and may be associated with necrosis and granulation tissue. The accompanying mixed inflammatory infiltrate, usually containing many neutrophils, is highly variable in intensity and depends on the degree of immunosuppression present in the patient. Crypt atrophy and apoptosis of epithelial cells are also common findings (Figure 2-15A) and may add to the diagnostic confusion between CMV infection and GVHD.

Cytomegalovirus has a predilection for infecting endothelial and stromal cells, although it is not uncommonly seen in glandular epithelial cells as well (Figure 2-15B). Because infected cells can be sparse, examination of additional H&E sections is recommended in the appropriate clinical setting and when histological findings are suggestive of CMV infection. Immunohistochemical staining for CMV should also be used to identify viral inclusions in such cases and to confirm the diagnosis.

Adenovirus

Like CMV, adenovirus is a common source of infectious gastroenteritis and colitis in transplant patients and should be considered in the differential when such patients present with GI complaints. Adenoviral infection of the GI tract is most frequently seen following hematopoietic stem cell transplantation and has a strong predilection for the pediatric population.[19] However, solid-organ transplant recipients, especially liver and small-bowel transplant patients, are also at risk for adenoviral infections involving the GI tract, with a higher rate of infection again seen in pediatric patients.[20–22] Patients with acute GVHD also appear to be at increased risk of adenovirus infection, likely as a result of the increased immunosuppressant therapy administered in such patients.[19,23,24] Patients with adenoviral infections of the GI tract typically present early in the post-transplant period with persistent diarrhea, often accompanied by fever.[19] Endoscopic findings are nonspecific and include abnormalities such as mucosal erythema, edema, and granularity.[23] The colon is most commonly affected, but other sites in the GI tract that may be involved include the stomach, small bowel, gallbladder, and appendix.

Histologic changes of adenoviral infection in the GI tract include surface sloughing, apoptosis, and viral inclusions. Varying degrees of inflammation may be seen, and mild villous blunting is often present in cases with small-bowel involvement. Adenovirus inclusions are intranuclear and are usually found in surface epithelial cells, especially goblet cells. The inclusions typically appear smudgy and basophilic (Figure 2-16); in some cases, crescent-shaped inclusions can be seen. Cells infected by adenovirus are normal in size, although their nucleus is usually enlarged. Infected cells may be sparse and difficult to detect on H&E sections, so immunohistochemical staining for adenovirus is recommended to rule out infection in transplant patients with acute GVHD or

FIGURE 2-15. Cytomegalovirus colitis. **A.** This patient had extensive crypt epithelial cell apoptosis, and alone this finding is indistinguishable from the changes seen in GVHD. **B.** However, other fields from the patient's colon biopsies revealed findings diagnostic of CMV infection, including this enlarged epithelial cell with a central intranuclear inclusion and granular, basophilic cytoplasmic inclusions.

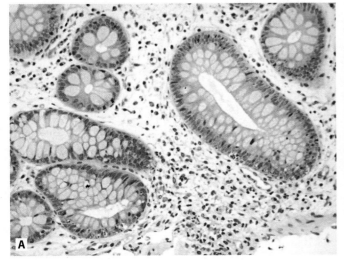
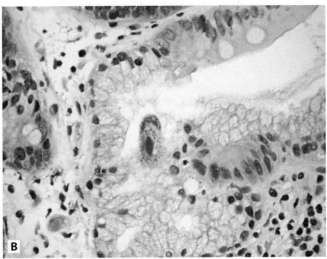

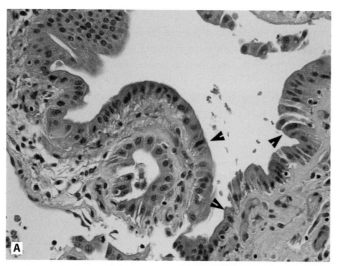
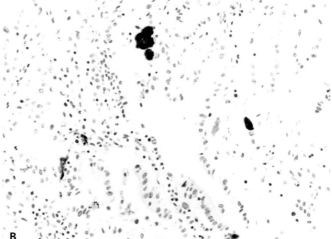

FIGURE 2-16. Adenoviral infection of the gallbladder. **A.** The epithelial lining of the gallbladder contains scattered cells with slightly enlarged nuclei and a smudgy, basophilic appearance (arrowheads). **B.** An immunohistochemical stain for adenovirus confirmed the presence of adenoviral inclusions in these cells.

a history of persistent diarrhea, as well as for confirmation if viral inclusions are identified. In cases with concurrent acute GVHD, infected cells are most commonly detected in areas not involved by the histologic changes of GVHD.[23]

Fungi

In addition to the viral infections discussed, the immunocompromised status of transplant recipients also increases their risk for certain fungal infections. In the early post-transplant period, *Candida* esophagitis is commonly encountered.[25] As in other immunocompromised states, transplant patients with esophagitis due to *Candida* infection typically present with odynophagia. Endoscopic examination reveals white plaques that are easily removed to reveal ulcerated mucosal. Histologically, yeast and pseudohyphae are seen in the superficial layers of the squamous epithelium and are usually associated with active inflammation, often with necrosis (see Chapter 8). Periodic acid–Schiff (PAS) and Gomori methamine silver (GMS) stains will highlight the fungal organisms.

Recently, infections with fungal organisms of the class *Zygomycetes* have emerged as a threat in transplant recipients. Lung and liver transplant patients are most likely to be affected; additional risk factors include concurrent diabetes mellitus, renal failure, or high-dose corticosteroid therapy. Disseminated forms of the disease may involve the GI tract, with cases of gastric, colonic, esophageal, and hepatic zygomycosis reported.[25] Patients with GI zygomycosis present with abdominal pain, nausea, vomiting, GI bleeding, or fever.[26,27] Patients with infections due to organisms of the *Mucor* genus may present with an ischemic colitis picture, as these organisms have a particular predilection for blood vessels.[28] Therefore, zygomycosis should be considered in all transplant patients presenting with signs of bowel ischemia. On endoscopic examination, shallow ulcers are usually present, often with necrotic borders, and mucosal edema and friability can also be seen.[26,27] Microscopic examination of biopsied tissue reveals broad, nonseptate hyphae that appear "ribbon-like" and branch at varying angles. Detection of the organisms is enhanced by PAS and GMS stains.

Clostridium difficile

Infections with the spore-forming bacterium *Clostridium difficile* have been on the rise over the last decade, and transplant patients, especially recipients of hematopoietic stem cell transplants, have a particularly high risk of infection.[29] Reported rates of *C. difficile* infections in transplant patients range from 5% to 23% and are highest within the first year post-transplant , likely due to increased immunosuppressant and antimicrobial therapy and prolonged exposure to health care facilities.[28] In addition, there appears to be an association between *C. difficile* infection and acute GVHD, although the reason for this association is not fully understood.[30]

Symptoms of *C. difficile* infection include watery diarrhea, abdominal pain, and fever; transplant recipients may also exhibit a more fulminant course and present with toxic megacolon, ileus, or septic shock.[28] Importantly, the classic yellow-white, adherent colonic pseudomembranes seen endoscopically in patients with *C. difficile* infection are sometimes absent in transplant recipients.[29] Histologically, these pseudomembranes manifest as a volcano-shaped eruption of mucin containing parallel lines of neutrophils overlying dilated, degenerating colonic crypts (see Chapter 28). In transplant patients presenting with persistent diarrhea and evidence of nonspecific colitis without pseudomembranes on endoscopic or histologic examination, the diagnosis of *C. difficile* colitis can be made based on laboratory assays that detect *C. difficile* toxins or the toxigenic *C. difficile* organism itself in stool samples.

POST-TRANSPLANT LYMPHOPROLIFERATIVE DISORDERS

Post-transplant lymphoproliferative disorders represent a diverse group of lymphoid proliferations that occur following solid-organ or hematopoietic stem cell transplantation. Most forms of PTLD consist of polyclonal B-cell or monoclonal B- or T-cell proliferations induced by Epstein-Barr virus (EBV) that occur in the setting of decreased T-cell immune surveillance. PTLD is more common after solid-organ transplantation than after stem cell transplantation, with incidence rates of approximately 10% and 1%, respectively.[31,32] Within solid-organ transplants, the incidence is highest following small-bowel transplantation, with reported rates of 10%–30%.[33-35] The incidence following transplantation of other solid organs ranges from 2%–10% following lung transplantation, to 1%–6% following heart transplant, to 1%–5% following liver or kidney transplants.[31-33,35] The variation in incidence of PTLD following transplantation of different solid organs can largely be attributed to the intensity of immunosuppression required to avoid organ rejection and the quantity of lymphoid tissue transplanted with the organ.[33] Additional risk factors for PTLD include young age, EBV negativity at transplant, and antithymocyte globulin therapy.[32-35]

Post-transplant lymphoproliferative disorder is most often encountered within the first 2 years following transplantation but can occur at any time. Late-onset PTLD is associated with a higher rate of EBV negativity and a tendency for aggressive disease.[33,35] Both lymph nodes and extranodal sites may be involved by PTLD. GI involvement is frequently seen, especially in late-onset cases, with rates of GI involvement ranging from 25% to 53%. Within the GI tract, the small bowel is the most common site of involvement by PTLD, followed by the right colon.[33,36]

Patients with PTLD of the GI tract may present with abdominal pain, GI bleeding, vomiting, diarrhea, or weight loss. Endoscopically, PTLD lesions are usually raised and rubbery, with associated mucosal erythema and ulceration. Luminal narrowing and stricture formation may be seen.[31,37]

The World Health Organization (WHO) classification divides PTLD lesions into four categories: early lesions, polymorphic PTLD, monomorphic PTLD, and classical Hodgkin lymphoma–like PTLD. Early lesions contain a mixture of cell types predominantly consisting of small lymphocytes with associated plasma cells and immunoblasts. These lesions typically assume an infectious mononucleosis-like or plasmacytic hyperplasia pattern. The underlying tissue's architecture is preserved, and the lesions are usually polyclonal, although occasionally small clonal or oligoclonal populations of B cells are detected. Polymorphic PTLD lesions also contain a mixture of cells, but the underlying tissue's architecture is effaced by a mixture of lymphocytes of varying size, atypical immunoblasts, plasma cells, and Reed-Sternberg–like cells. These lesions are monoclonal, mostly EBV positive, and common in children.[32] Monomorphic PTLD lesions fulfill the criteria

of a non-Hodgkin lymphoma (other than an indolent B-cell neoplasm) or a plasma cell neoplasm. GI tract involvement by PTLD is most commonly of the monomorphic type, with the majority being diffuse large B-cell lymphomas (DLBCLs).[33,36] Such DLBCL lesions contain sheets of large B cells that are positive for CD19, CD20, and CD79a, as well as EBV in many cases (Figure 2-17). Monomorphic PTLD can also take the form of a T- or natural killer (NK)–cell lymphoma, in which case the rate of EBV positivity is much lower. The final category of PTLD, classical Hodgkin lymphoma–like PTLD, is rare and should contain Reed-Sternberg cells with the typical CD30-positive, CD15-positive, CD45-negative, CD20-negative immunophenotype.

Given the variability in time of onset and clinical presentation of PTLD, as well as its proclivity for the GI tract,

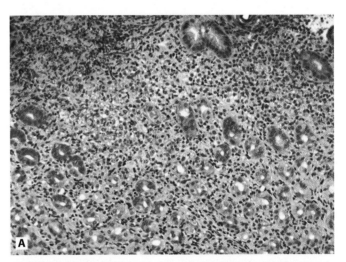

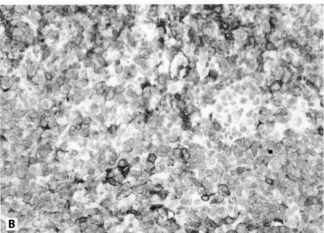

FIGURE 2-17. Monomorphic PTLD, diffuse large B-cell lymphoma. **A.** The gastric mucosa is infiltrated and effaced by a monomorphous population of medium-to-large, atypical lymphoid cells. **B.** The cells express the B-cell antigen CD19. **C.** They are also strongly CD79a positive, further supporting their B-cell origin. **D.** In situ hybridization for Epstein-Barr virus-encoded small RNAs (EBER) shows strong hybridization signals in the tumor cells, which confirms that this PTLD is EBV related.

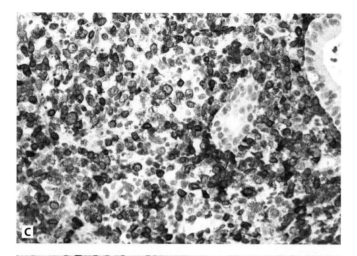

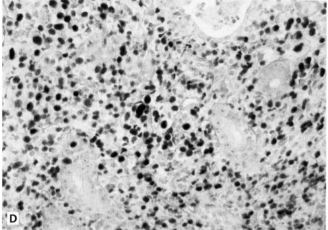

FIGURE 2-17. *(Continued)*

this condition should be considered in all transplant patients presenting with GI symptoms. Awareness of the range of histologic appearances of PTLD is crucial to ensure early recognition of this entity. In cases of suspected PTLD, immunohistochemical stains for B-cell and T-cell markers and in situ hybridization for EBV should be obtained to further characterize the lesion. Testing for clonal B-cell and T-cell rearrangements may also be useful in establishing the diagnosis, although clonality is not a requirement for the diagnosis of PTLD.

■ REJECTION IN SMALL-BOWEL TRANSPLANTATION

Over the past several decades, small-bowel transplantation has become an increasingly utilized therapeutic option in the management of short-gut syndrome in children. While the success of such procedures has risen in recent years, allograft rejection continues to pose a challenge and remains a leading cause of small-bowel transplant failure.[38] Small-bowel transplants are particularly susceptible to rejection because of the high concentration of immunogenic lymphoid tissue within this organ.[39] Various forms of rejection, including

hyperacute rejection, acute humoral and cellular rejection, and chronic rejection, may be seen, and these complications range in onset from the immediate post-transplant period to years after the procedure.

Assessment of biopsies from multiple areas of the transplanted bowel is recommended when evaluating small-intestine allografts for rejection, as the process can be quite focal. In addition, comparison of transplanted tissue to tissue from native organs can assist in the differentiation of rejection from more widespread processes like GVHD, PTLD, and infections.[40,41] In the early post-transplant period, protocol biopsies are often obtained, but after the first several months, endoscopy with biopsy is generally performed only in symptomatic patients.[39]

Hyperacute and Accelerated Acute Rejection

Hyperacute and accelerated acute rejection occur within days following transplantation due to pre-formed recipient antibodies directed against the donor organ. These antibodies lead to vascular injury, which results in formation of thrombi and ultimately ischemia. Histologically, the involved bowel shows congested vessels with marginating neutrophils and an associated mixed inflammatory infiltrate and necrosis. However, this form of rejection is rarely seen in small-bowel transplants due to the extensive recipient-donor cross-matching performed prior to transplantation.[38]

Acute Cellular Rejection

Acute cellular rejection is the most common form of rejection seen following small-bowel transplantation. Often, no inciting factor can be identified, although the development of acute cellular rejection can sometimes be linked to a recent infection or lack of compliance with immunosuppressive regimens.[40] Patients typically present during the first two months following transplantation with nonspecific symptoms, including fever, vomiting, increased fecal output, and abdominal pain and distension, often accompanied by signs of malabsorption.[39,40] However, in some cases evidence of acute cellular rejection is detected on protocol biopsies in asymptomatic patients (subclinical acute rejection).[38,42] Endoscopic findings include mucosal edema, hyperemia, granularity, erosions, and ulcerations.[39] The ileum is often the site of most severe involvement.[38]

Histologically, acute cellular rejection consists of a combination of apoptotic epithelial cells, inflammatory infiltration, and/or architectural distortion. Based on the extent and combination of these features, acute cellular rejection is graded as indeterminate, mild, moderate, or severe.[38,41] A key element of this grading system is the apoptotic body count, which is the total number of apoptotic epithelial cells, or epithelial cells containing fragmented nuclear debris, found in 10 consecutive crypts. This count should be performed within the area identified as most severely involved.[39]

The indeterminate grade is used for cases that show features of acute cellular rejection but do not meet the criteria for mild rejection. Apoptosis of crypt epithelial cells is present, but the apoptotic body count is less than 6, the recommended cutoff for a definitive diagnosis.[41] In mild acute rejection, the crypt epithelium displays reactive changes, including depletion of mucin, cytoplasmic basophilia, and nuclear enlargement, as well as increased apoptotic bodies, with 6 or more apoptotic epithelial cells present in 10 consecutive crypts. There is a predominantly mononuclear inflammatory infiltrate in the lamina propria, but the surface epithelium remains intact (Figure 2-18). Vascular congestion and stromal edema may be present. When crypt apoptosis becomes more confluent and focal loss of crypts is encountered, the grade of acute cellular rejection is raised to moderate. The lamina propria infiltrate is usually more prominent in such cases, and marked villous blunting, vascular congestion, and stromal edema are often

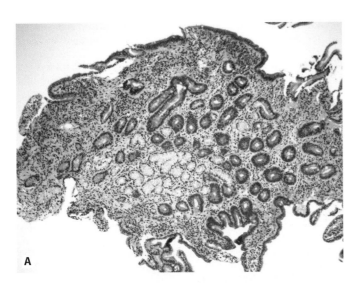

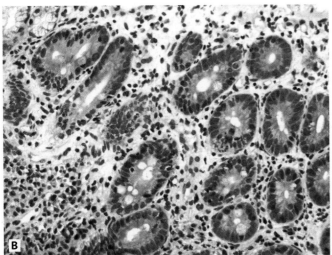

FIGURE 2-18. Mild acute cellular rejection. **A.** In this low-power view of the small-bowel mucosa, a mononuclear inflammatory infiltrate is seen in the lamina propria, and there is focal architectural distortion with villous blunting (top half of the field). **B.** A higher-power view from the same biopsy reveals several apoptotic crypt epithelial cells, a required feature for the diagnosis of acute cellular rejection.

seen. In addition, focal erosion of the surface epithelium may be present. Finally, a diagnosis of severe acute cellular rejection is appropriate when there is extensive damage of crypts with diffuse erosion or ulceration of the surface epithelium. Paradoxically, apoptotic epithelial cells may be less prominent in severe acute cellular rejection due to the widespread loss of crypts. The inflammatory infiltrate is dense and often contains a neutrophilic component due to the lack of overlying epithelium.[39,41]

While acute rejection should always be considered in small-bowel transplant recipients presenting with GI complaints, the clinical and histological features of this condition again lack specificity; therefore, a number of other entities should be included in the differential. Viral enteritis, especially enteritis caused by adenovirus infection, can mimic acute cellular rejection due to the presence of epithelial cell apoptosis and lamina propria inflammation. Therefore, a careful search for adenoviral inclusions and consideration of immunohistochemical staining for adenovirus and other infectious agents is warranted in these patients.[39] In addition, because the hallmark of GVHD is epithelial apoptosis and GVHD has been described in small-bowel transplant recipients, this entity must be considered in cases displaying significant apoptosis. Similarly, certain immunosuppressant medications are known to cause apoptosis of epithelial cells, and evaluation for potential drug-induced mucosal injury is therefore also necessary in these patients.[40] Comparing biopsies from the small-bowel allograft to those taken from the patient's native bowel may be helpful in this regard. Cases of acute cellular rejection will typically reveal apoptosis and inflammation largely confined to the transplanted intestine, while infections and drug-induced injury will usually result in histologic changes in both the transplanted and native tissues, and the changes of GVHD will primarily involve the patient's native organs.[39]

Antibody-Mediated Rejection

Antibody-mediated rejection in small-bowel transplants can occur as an isolated phenomenon or in association with acute cellular rejection. Patients with antibody-mediated rejection either develop alloantibodies against donor antigens following transplantation or experience a rise in donor-specific antibodies that were present at low levels prior to transplantation. This form of rejection is most often encountered early after transplantation, frequently within the first 2 weeks post-transplant.[38] Clinical features of antibody-mediated rejection include abdominal pain and distension, diarrhea, and weight loss, which overlap with the presentation of a multitude of conditions seen in transplant patients.[43]

Small-bowel transplants involved by antibody-mediated rejection display varying degrees of vascular congestion and inflammation, often accompanied by extravasation of red blood cells into the lamina propria. Both small and large arteries can be involved by vasculitis, although large-vessel vasculitis cannot usually be identified in biopsy specimens. It is important to keep in mind that cellular rejection can also produce vasculitis; therefore, evidence of a concomitant rise in donor-specific antibodies is needed to diagnose antibody-mediated rejection. Immunohistochemical stains, particularly C4d staining, and immunofluorescence for immunoglobulin and complement deposition can also be used to support the diagnosis of antibody-mediated rejection.[38] However, studies of C4d staining in mucosal biopsies from small-bowel transplants have found that such staining is not specific; therefore, reliance on this feature for the diagnosis of antibody-mediated rejection is not recommended.[43]

Chronic Rejection

As the survival of small-bowel grafts improves, chronic rejection is becoming an increasingly frequent problem and is currently one of the main causes of late intestinal transplant loss. Unfortunately, chronic rejection is often difficult to diagnose clinically due to its insidious onset and nonspecific symptoms, which include persistent diarrhea and, later, protein-losing enteropathy. Endoscopic findings include a firm-appearing bowel with irregularly flattened villi and focal ulceration, although these features may not be identifiable until late in the course of the disease.[38,39]

Microscopically, the diagnostic finding of chronic rejection is vasculopathy consisting of concentric intimal hyperplasia, medial hypertrophy, and adventitial fibrosis of small-to-large arteries. These changes can be found in the mesenteric, serosal, and submucosal vasculature. Because these regions are not typically sampled by endoscopic biopsies, biopsies from small-bowel transplants suspected to have chronic rejection may only reveal secondary changes of ischemia, such as lamina propria fibrosis, villous blunting, and crypt dropout, sometimes accompanied by mucosal ulceration. If such features are noted, the possibility of chronic rejection should be raised. The presence of these histologic changes in biopsies from the transplanted bowel and not in those from adjacent native tissues is supportive of the diagnosis of chronic rejection.[38] However, mucosal biopsies are often insufficient to confirm the diagnosis of chronic rejection, and in many clinically suspected cases, the diagnosis can only be made on full-thickness biopsies or at explantation of failed grafts.[39]

■ SUMMARY

Solid-organ and hematopoietic stem cell transplant recipients frequently experience GI symptoms that require endoscopic evaluation with biopsies. GI biopsies from these patients may display a wide range of histologic features, including architectural distortion, epithelial cell apoptosis, crypt loss, and lamina propria infiltrates. Because most of these morphologic features are not specific on their own, the pathologist must consider them in combination with the results of special and immunohistochemical stains and information from the patient's clinical history, such as type of transplant and level of immunosuppression. Pathologists should be aware of the key histologic features of diseases commonly encountered in transplant patients: GVHD, drug-induced injury, opportunistic infections, PTLD, and rejection. They must also keep in mind that these patients can develop non–transplant-related GI disorders, such as inflammatory bowel disease and ischemic colitis. In addition, close communication with the clinical team is crucial in these complex cases. By carefully considering the pathologic and clinical factors described in this chapter, the pathologist can ensure that the correct diagnosis is made, allowing the patient to receive the proper medical care.

■ REFERENCES

1. Washington K, Jagasia M. Pathology of graft-versus-host disease in the gastrointestinal tract. *Hum Pathol*. 2009;40(7):909–917.
2. Welch DC, Wirth PS, Goldenring JR, Ness E, Jagasia M, Washington K. Gastric graft-versus-host disease revisited: does proton pump inhibitor therapy affect endoscopic gastric biopsy interpretation? *Am J Surg Pathol*. 2006;30(4):444–449.
3. Melson J, Jakate S, Fung H, Arai S, Keshavarzian A. Crypt loss is a marker of clinical severity of acute gastrointestinal graft-versus-host disease. *Am J Hematol*. 2007;82(10):881–886.
4. Shulman HM, Kleiner D, Lee SJ, et al. Histopathologic diagnosis of chronic graft-versus-host disease: National Institutes of Health Consensus Development Project on Criteria for Clinical Trials in Chronic Graft-versus-Host Disease: II. Pathology Working Group Report. *Biol Blood Marrow Transplant*. 2006;12(1):31–47.
5. Nguyen CV, Kastenberg DM, Choudhary C, Katz LC, DiMarino A, Palazzo JP. Is single-cell apoptosis sufficient for the diagnosis of graft-versus-host disease in the colon? *Dig Dis Sci*. 2007;53(3):747–756.
6. Lee SJ, Flowers M. Recognizing and managing chronic graft-versus-host disease. *Hematology Am Soc Hematol Educ Program*. 2008;134–141.
7. Vigorito AC, Campregher PV, Storer BE, et al. Evaluation of NIH consensus criteria for classification of late acute and chronic GVHD. *Blood*. 2009;114(3):702–708.
8. Star KV, Ho VT, Wang HH, Odze RD. Histologic features in colon biopsies can discriminate mycophenolate from GVHD-induced colitis. *Am J Surg Pathol*. 2013;37(9):1319–1328.
9. Parfitt JR, Jayakumar S, Driman DK. Mycophenolate mofetil-related gastrointestinal mucosal injury: variable injury patterns, including graft-versus-host disease-like changes. *Am J Surg Pathol*. 2008;32(9):1367–1372.
10. Lee S, de Boer WB, Subramaniam K, Kumarasinghe MP. Pointers and pitfalls of mycophenolate-associated colitis. *J Clin Pathol*. 2012;66(1):8–11.
11. Selbst MK, Ahrens WA, Robert ME, Friedman A, Proctor DD, Jain D. Spectrum of histologic changes in colonic biopsies in patients treated with mycophenolate mofetil. *Mod Pathol*. 2009;22(6):737–743.
12. Al-Absi AI, Cooke CR, Wall BM, Sylvestre P, Ismail MK, Mya M. Patterns of injury in mycophenolate mofetil–related colitis. *Transplant Proc*. 2010;42(9):3591–3593.
13. Nguyen T, Park JY, Scudiere JR, Montgomery E. Mycophenolic acid (CellCept and Myofortic) induced injury of the upper GI tract. *Am J Surg Pathol*. 2009;33(9):1355–1363.
14. Saeed SA, Integlia MJ, Pleskow RG, et al. Tacrolimus-associated eosinophilic gastroenterocolitis in pediatric liver transplant recipients: role of potential food allergies in pathogenesis. *Pediatr Transplant*. 2006;10(6):730–735.
15. Lee JH, Park HY, Choe YH, Lee S-K, Lee Il S. The development of eosinophilic colitis after liver transplantation in children. *Pediatr Transplant*. 2007;11(5):518–523.

16. Eid AJ, Razonable RR. New developments in the management of cytomegalovirus infection after solid organ transplantation. *Drugs.* 2010;70(8):965–981.

17. Talmon GA. Histologic features of cytomegalovirus enteritis in small bowel allografts. *Transplant Proc.* 2010;42(7):2671–2675.

18. Mills AM, Guo FP, Copland AP, Pai RK, Pinsky BA. A comparison of CMV detection in gastrointestinal mucosal biopsies using immunohistochemistry and PCR performed on formalin-fixed, paraffin-embedded tissue. *Am J Surg Pathol.* 2013;37(7):995–1000.

19. de Mezerville MHN, Tellier R, Richardson S, Hébert D, Doyle J, Allen U. Adenoviral infections in pediatric transplant recipients. *Pediatr Infect Dis J.* 2006;25(9):815–818.

20. Ison MG, Green M, the AST Infectious Diseases Community of Practice. Adenovirus in solid organ transplant recipients. *Am J Transplant.* 2009;9:S161–S165.

21. Hoffman JA. Adenovirus infections in solid organ transplant recipients. *Curr Opin Organ Transplant.* 2009;14(6):625–633.

22. Lee LY, Ison MG. Diarrhea caused by viruses in transplant recipients. *Transplant Infect Dis.* 2014;16(3):347–358.

23. Shayan K, Saunders F, Roberts E, Cutz E. Adenovirus enterocolitis in pediatric patients following bone marrow transplantation: report of 2 cases and review of the literature. *Arch Pathol Lab Med.* 2003;127(12):1615–1618.

24. Ison MG. Adenovirus infections in transplant recipients. *Clin Infect Dis.* 2006;43(3):331–339.

25. Ponticelli C, Passerini P. Gastrointestinal complications in renal transplant recipients. *Transplant Int.* 2005;27:305–316.

26. Almyroudis NG, Sutton DA, Linden P, Rinaldi MG, Fung J, Kusne S. Zygomycosis in solid organ transplant recipients in a tertiary transplant center and review of the literature. *Am J Transplant.* 2006;6(10):2365–2374.

27. Do GW, Jung SW, Jun J-B, Seo JH, Nah YW. Colonic mucormycosis presented with ischemic colitis in a liver transplant recipient. *World J Gastroenterol.* 2013;19(22):3508–3511.

28. Honda H, Dubberke ER. *Clostridium difficile* infection in solid organ transplant recipients. *Curr Opin Infect Dis.* 2014;27(4):336–341.

29. Alonso CD, Marr KA. *Clostridium difficile* infection among hematopoietic stem cell transplant recipients: beyond colitis. *Curr Opin Infect Dis.* 2013;26(4):326–331.

30. Alonso CD, Kamboj M. *Clostridium difficile* infection (CDI) in solid organ and hematopoietic stem cell transplant recipients. *Curr Infect Dis Rep.* 2014;16(8):414.

31. Grivas PD. Post-transplantation lymphoproliferative disorder (PTLD) twenty years after heart transplantation: a case report and review of the literature. *Med Oncol.* 2010;28(3):829–834.

32. Al-Mansour Z, Nelson BP, Evens AM. Post-transplant lymphoproliferative disease (PTLD): risk factors, diagnosis, and current treatment strategies. *Curr Hematol Malig Rep.* 2013;8:173–183.

33. Cruz RJ Jr, Ramachandra S, Sasatomi E, et al. Surgical management of gastrointestinal posttransplant lymphoproliferative disorders in liver transplant recipients. *Transplant J.* 2012;94(4):417–423.

34. Nassif S, Kaufman S, Vahdat S, Yazigi N. Clinicopathologic features of post-transplant lymphoproliferative disorders arising after pediatric small bowel transplant. *Pediatr Transplant.* 2013;17:765–773.

35. Lo RC-L, Chan S-C, Chan K-L, Chiang AK-S, Lo C-M, Ng IO-L. Post-transplant lymphoproliferative disorders in liver transplant recipients: a clinicopathological study. *J Clin Pathol.* 2013;66(5):392–398.

36. Wudhikarn K, Holman CJ, Linan M, et al. Post-transplant lymphoproliferative disorders in lung transplant recipients: 20-yr experience at the University of Minnesota. *Clinical Transplant.* 2010;25(5):705–713.

37. O'Connor JA, Cogley C, Burton M, Lancaster-Weiss K, Cordle RA. Posttransplantation lymphoproliferative disorder: endoscopic findings. *J Pediatr Gastroenterol Nutr.* 2000;31(4):458.

38. Ruiz P. Updates on acute and chronic rejection in small bowel and multivisceral allografts. *Current Opin Organ Transplant.* 2014;19:293–302.

39. Remotti H, Subramanian S. Small-bowel allograft biopsies in the management of small-intestinal and multivisceral transplant recipients: histopathologic review and clinical correlations. *Arch Pathol Lab Med.* 2012;136(7):761–771.

40. Ruiz P. How can pathologists help to diagnose late complications in small bowel and multivisceral transplantation? *Current Opin Organ Transplant.* 2012;17(3):273–279.

41. Ruiz P, Bagni A, Brown R, et al. Histological criteria for the identification of acute cellular rejection in human small bowel allografts: results of the pathology workshop at the VIII International Small Bowel Transplant Symposium. *Transplant Proc.* 2004;36(2):335–337.

42. Ruiz P, Takahashi H, Delacruz V, et al. International grading scheme for acute cellular rejection in small-bowel transplantation: single-center experience. *Transplant Proc.* 2010;42(1):47–53.

43. Gerlach UA, Lachmann N, Sawitzki B, et al. Clinical relevance of the de novo production of anti-HLA antibodies following intestinal and multivisceral transplantation. *Transplant Int.* 2013;27(3):280–289.

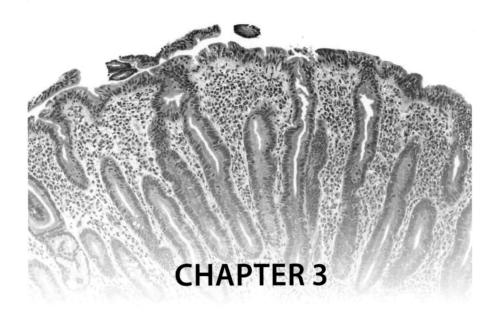

CHAPTER 3

Autoimmune Enterocolitis

INTRODUCTION

Several gastrointestinal inflammatory diseases, including ulcerative colitis, Crohn disease, celiac disease, and microscopic colitis, share pathogenic mechanisms involving abnormalities in host immunity. These disorders have well-defined clinical and histological features and are discussed in separate chapters. Autoimmune enterocolitis (AIEC) is a group of protracted diarrheic disorders that are associated with other autoimmune conditions as well as one or more types of autoantibodies in the blood. The disease is characterized clinically by severe refractory diarrhea and malabsorption and histologically by small-bowel villous atrophy and other abnormalities. These signs and symptoms are unresponsive to strict dietary control and often require immunosuppressive therapy.

The more commonly used term *autoimmune enteropathy* (AIE) was first introduced to describe a condition seen in a subset of pediatric patients with severe refractory diarrhea and pathologic changes mainly involving the small bowel.[1,2] However, it soon became evident that in most cases, the small-bowel disease is accompanied by colonic or gastric involvement.[3–8] Therefore, the term *autoimmune enterocolitis* seems to better reflect the clinicopathologic spectrum of the disease[8] and is being increasingly used in clinical practice. Another term that is rarely used is *generalized autoimmune gut disorder* (GAGD).[6,9]

Autoimmune enterocolitis should be considered to represent a group of heterogeneous diseases that share immunologic and histologic abnormalities. Its association with

autoantibodies varies among patients. Association with other autoimmune disorders can be identified in most patients; these conditions include bullous pemphigoid, autoimmune hepatitis, rheumatoid arthritis, systemic vasculitis, and many others.[4,10–13] Venous thrombosis is also seen in some patients.[14,15] Familial involvement is present in some cases.[11,12,16]

Several forms of AIEC exist: (1) the pediatric disease of immune dysregulation, polyendocrinopathy, AIE, X-linked syndrome (IPEX); (2) an isolated autoimmune gastrointestinal form of AIE in children; and (3) adult AIEC.

PEDIATRIC-ONSET AUTOIMMUNE ENTEROPATHY

Historically, AIE referred to a severe protracted diarrhea that failed to respond to total parenteral nutrition (TPN) or other dietary restrictions and was associated with other autoimmune disorders. Avery et al[17] described a subgroup of infants 3 months of age or younger who had diarrhea without apparent cause that was refractory to treatment and had a high mortality rate. The term *intractable (protracted) diarrhea of early infancy* was applied to this condition. Biopsy studies in these patients have demonstrated total villous atrophy with crypt hyperplasia or hypoplasia in the small bowel.[16–20] Some children were initially considered to have celiac disease, as they had positive celiac serology and severe villous blunting, but these children had no response to a gluten-free diet (GFD) or steroids. In some of these cases, circulating antibodies to gut enterocytes had been demonstrated,[1,5,20] so the disorder was considered to be autoimmune in nature.[1] In addition, a tendency for familial clustering was evident.[1,16]

Powell et al described a series of 17 boys with AIE, which suggested X-linked transmission.[21] Subsequently, other studies identified further association between the early onset of severe diarrhea and diabetes mellitus or other endocrinopathies. Cases meeting these descriptions are thus considered a special form of AIE known as IPEX syndrome.[22–24]

Recent genetic studies identified that mutations in the *FOXP3* gene are mainly responsible for the pathogenesis of IPEX. Normally expressed in CD4[+]/CD25[+] regulatory T cells, defects in this gene lead to hyperactivation of T cells and autoimmunity.[24,25] However, it should be noted that *FOXP3* is not the only gene that is responsible for the pathogenesis of this disorder.

Pediatric patients with AIE who lack the underlying X-linked syndrome may be of either gender. Two of 5 cases in the original series by Davidson et al[16] were female. Some cases have a familial association. Another syndromic form of pediatric AIEC is *autoimmune polyendocrinopathy–candidiasis–ectodermal dystrophy* (APECED), which is related to mutations in the *AIRE* gene. More recently, Singhi et al[26] described findings from 14 pediatric patients, including 6 males and 8 females, with age of onset ranging from birth to 16 years old. About 70% of patients had an immunodeficiency disorder or another autoimmune-related disease (one of which was IPEX), and 80% had antienterocyte antibodies. Histologically, 80% of cases had small bowel-predominant changes, including villous blunting, crypt hyperplasia, increased crypt apoptosis, and increased lamina propria inflammatory infiltration (Figure 3-1). Only 21% of cases exhibited marked intraepithelial lymphocytosis. Of note, half of the patients had cryptitis or crypt abscesses, indicating a superimposed active inflammation. In addition, goblet cell or Paneth cell depletion was present in half of the cases, and crypt apoptosis was found in colonic biopsies of all patients. Most of the patients responded to immunosuppressive therapy (such as FK506). A mortality rate of 21% was found for the group.[26]

Thus, it is evident that AIE in children is a clinically, pathologically, and pathogenically heterogeneous group of diseases. Diagnosis and treatment of AIE as well as workup for underlying genetic and immunologic abnormalities should therefore be tailored to each patient's unique situation.

ADULT AUTOIMMUNE ENTEROCOLITIS

Initially, AIE was considered a disease of children. Adult patients with chronic diarrhea that could not be diagnosed as another well-defined disease or was refractory to treatment for such diseases were gradually recognized as having a form of autoimmune gastrointestinal disorder. One of the first series of adult cases was reported by Corazza et al[5] In this series, 4 women were found to have subtotal villous atrophy and an increase in intraepithelial lymphocytes (IELs) but were unresponsive to a GFD. All patients tested positive for

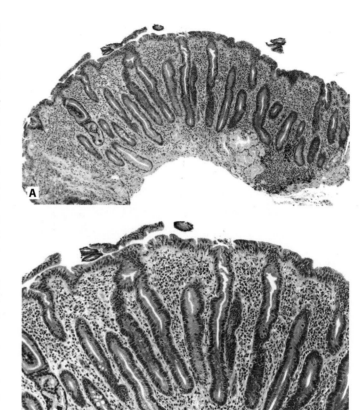

FIGURE 3-1. Autoimmune enteropathy in duodenum, celiac-like pattern. **A.** Complete villous blunting and crypt hyperplasia, accompanied by inflammatory infiltration in the lamina propria and mild increase in intraepithelial lymphocytes. **B.** High-power view further demonstrating nearly complete goblet cell depletion and loss of Paneth cells.

antienterocyte antibodies. These observations were further supported by other studies, leading to the recognition that there is an adult form of AIEC.[6,13,27,28]

In the series of 14 patients described by Akram et al,[28] there is an essentially equal male-to-female distribution, with a median age of 55 years. Among these cases, 93% had a positive presence of antienterocyte or anti–goblet cell antibodies.

In adult AIEC, gastric involvement in the form of atrophic gastritis,[6] and colonic involvement[29] are present in many patients. Some cases are associated with a thymoma.[30] In patients with clinical evidence of malabsorption and villous atrophy and intraepithelial lymphocytosis of the small-bowel mucosa (Figure 3-2) that are refractory to treatment, serologic testing for antienterocyte antibodies and anti–goblet cell antibodies should be performed. It is not uncommon in adult patients with AIEC that colonic biopsies exhibit features of collagenous colitis. However, these features are often accompanied by goblet cell depletion and significant crypt apoptosis (Figure 3-3). Other changes, such as marked crypt withering, may also be present (Figure 3-4).

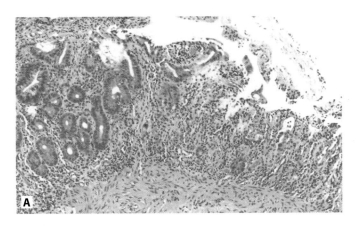

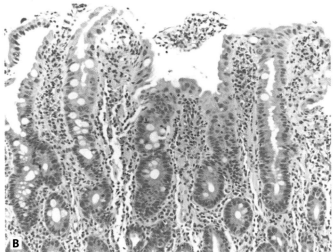

FIGURE 3-2. Autoimmune enteropathy in duodenum, with erosion. **A.** There is focal surface erosion with loss of villi and crypts. Residual Paneth cells are seen on the left side. **B.** Partial villous blunting and crypt hyperplasia with only patchy, mildly increased intraepithelial lymphocytes.

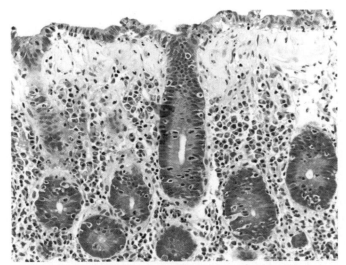

FIGURE 3-3. Autoimmune colitis, collagenous colitis pattern. Colonic biopsies all exhibit marked thickening of the subepithelial collagen layer and goblet cell depletion. However, there is also significant crypt apoptosis.

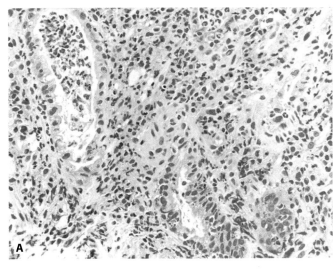

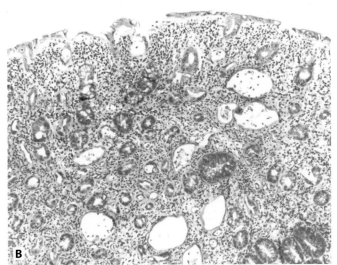

FIGURE 3-4. Autoimmune colitis with severe crypt apoptosis (**A**) and "withered" crypts (**B**).

SEROLOGY

Various autoantibodies had been found in patients with AIE; however, the most commonly seen are antienterocyte antibodies.[11,28,31] Some patients may have anti–goblet cell antibodies as well.[4,28,32,33] These autoantibodies are neither specific nor highly sensitive. That is, some patients with AIEC have negative test results for antienterocyte antibodies; low levels of antienterocyte antibodies have also been found in patients with celiac disease or Crohn disease. Occasionally, patients have antinuclear antibodies (ANAs) or other types of autoantibodies. The presence of an autoantibody mentioned in a patient with other clinical and pathological manifestations of AIEC strongly supports the diagnosis.

HISTOLOGIC CHANGES

Early descriptions of the histology of AIEC included villous blunting and variable intraepithelial lymphocytosis involving the duodenal mucosa (Figures 3-1 and 3-2). Additional histological features, such as increased apoptosis of crypt cells and reduction of Paneth cells and endocrine cells, were also noted (Figures 3-1B and 3-2).[4,29] Subsequently, it was found that in some patients there is also a reduction or depletion of goblet cells in the colorectal mucosa.[4,13,29]

The histologic findings vary significantly among individual patients. In most patients, one of three patterns may predominate in the small bowel, namely, graft-versus-host disease–like, celiac-like, and goblet cell depletion type. However, this classification is an oversimplification. Biopsies usually show a variety of other findings in addition to one of these main histologic patterns, such as lamina propria inflammatory infiltrate, cryptitis, or crypt abscesses. A significant proportion of patients is likely to have a mixed pattern that would be hard to "classify" (Figures 3-5 and 3-6).[8] A patient may exhibit a graft-versus-host disease–like injury in the small bowel and lymphocytic gastritis in the stomach (Figure 3-5). Some of the abnormalities, including severe crypt loss, may resolve after immunosuppressant treatment (Figure 3-6).

The manifestations of colonic involvement also vary among different patients. In some patients, it may be a nonspecific pattern of colitis, with marked inflammatory infiltration in the lamina propria, a patchy increase in IELs and neutrophils, and mild goblet cell loss (Figure 3-7). In other patients, the colonic involvement may be in the pattern of lymphocytic or collagenous colitis, usually accompanied by marked crypt apoptosis (Figure 3-3). Severe apoptosis eventually leads to crypt withering (Figure 3-4) and crypt loss. In addition, active neutrophilic infiltration is not uncommon (Figures 3-8 and 3-9).

FIGURE 3-5. Autoimmune enteropathy. A 30-year-old man with nausea and weight loss was found to have protein-losing enteropathy and a positive serology for antinuclear antibody. There were multiple duodenal ulcers seen on endoscopy. **A.** Duodenum with near-total crypt loss and villous blunting, resembling crypt loss due to severe graft-versus-host disease. **B.** Duodenum, residual crypts with increase in IELs and total loss of Paneth cells. **C.** Terminal ileum with loss of crypts and goblet cell depletion. **D.** Gastric mucosa with increased lamina propria plasma cell infiltration and increased IELs.

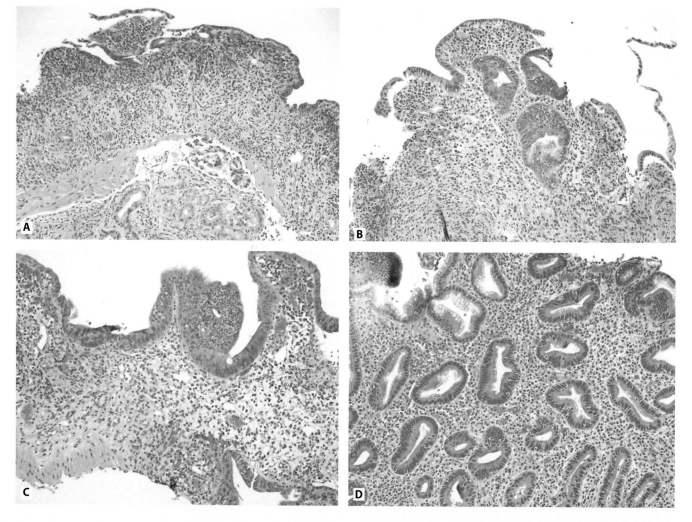

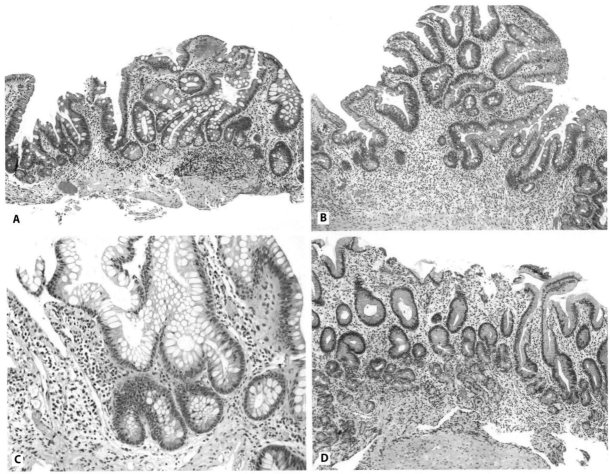

FIGURE 3-6. Same patient as in Figure 3-5 after a course of tacrolimus treatment. **A.** Duodenum demonstrating partially regenerated villi and crypts with recovered goblet cells and Paneth cells. **B.** There is reduction of the lamina propria inflammatory infiltration. Regenerative change toward the base of crypts is evident. **C.** Terminal ileum with similar regeneration of crypts and villi. **D.** Gastric antrum with residual intraepithelial lymphocytes.

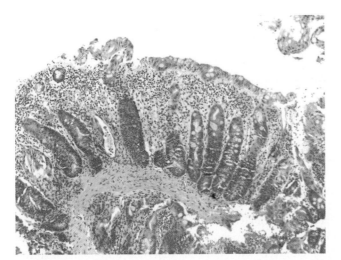

FIGURE 3-7. Autoimmune colitis, nonspecific active pattern. There is a prominent mixed inflammatory infiltrate in the lamina propria and patchy neutrophilic infiltration of the crypt epithelium. There is mild goblet cell depletion and rare degenerating, atrophic crypts.

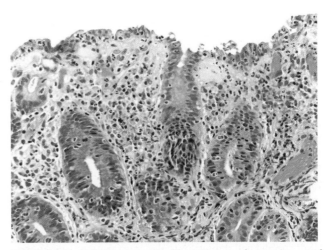

FIGURE 3-8. Collagenous colitis-like pattern with superimposed neutrophilic infiltration. Neutrophils are most evident infiltrating the surface epithelium.

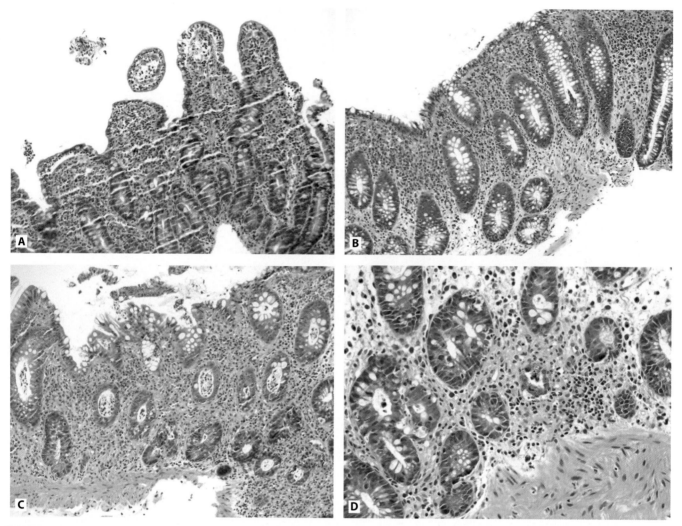

FIGURE 3-9. Autoimmune enterocolitis. In this patient, the duodenal biopsy reveals partial villous atrophy and mild crypt hyperplasia, with an increase in intraepithelial lymphocytes mimicking celiac disease (**A**). The colonic mucosa demonstrates a pattern of lymphocytic colitis, but there is superimposed active cryptitis (**B**). Other areas of the colon exhibit crypt withering (**C**), which on high power manifests as brisk apoptotic bodies in the crypt epithelium (**D**).

When the gastric mucosa is involved, the findings may range from nonspecific inactive gastritis to lymphocytic gastritis (Figures 3-5D and 3-6D) to collagenous gastritis to atrophic gastritis.

It should be noted that small-intestinal and colonic involvements in the same patient do not necessarily take on the same pattern. In addition, there is no correlation between the histologic pattern and the patient's age or background genetic defect. For example, all three patterns can be seen in pediatric[34] or adult patients.[8] However, some studies seem to suggest that in pediatric patients, the celiac-like pattern predominates[26] and lymphocytic colitis is only seen rarely. Colonic goblet cell depletion is also less frequent in pediatric patients (2 of 14 cases in one series).[26]

DIAGNOSIS

As an uncommon disease, AIEC is not usually the first diagnostic consideration in a patient who presents with the symptoms as described above. Many diseases that are more common manifest similarly. Therefore, in these patients, the diagnosis of AIEC is suspected only after exclusion of other diseases, particularly in adults.

In children who develop severe intractable diarrhea that is unresponsive to TPN in the first 6 months of life, AIE should always be included in the differential diagnosis. For older children with chronic diarrhea and malabsorption that are not improved with dietary control or even steroids, the diagnosis of AIE needs to be considered, even if the patient has positive celiac serology (Chapter 18). In pediatric patients, the positivity rate for antienterocyte antibody is fairly high, and detection of this antibody should help make the diagnosis in the proper clinical and pathologic setting. As described, biopsies of the small bowel often reveal various degrees of villous blunting, crypt hyperplasia or hypoplasia, and crypt apoptosis in a background of variable amounts of lamina propria inflammatory infiltration (Figures 3-1 and 3-2). An increase in IELs may be present as well. Goblet cell and endocrine cell loss also have diagnostic value if identified (Figures 3-1 and 3-2).

In adult patients with the symptoms mentioned, a variety of diseases are usually considered initially, including celiac disease, refractory sprue, lymphocytic colitis, and collagenous colitis (Figure 3-8). However, histologic analysis from small-bowel and colonic biopsies may reveal features that are more commonly seen in AIEC than in these other diseases, such as diffuse goblet cell depletion and crypt apoptosis (Figures 3-3 and 3-4).

The diagnosis of AIEC is made only with the integration of clinical, laboratory, endoscopic, and pathologic findings. In general, factors supporting the diagnosis of AIEC include protracted diarrhea associated with small-bowel villous atrophy, lack of response to strict dietary control, evidence of autoimmunity in the form of serum autoantibodies, and other autoimmune disorders. In many patients, pediatric or adult, response to immunosuppressive treatment also contributes to the confirmation of the diagnosis.

Detection of either antienterocyte or anti–goblet cell antibodies is of great help in the proper clinicopathologic setting. However, development of these antibodies is most likely a secondary response and not part of the pathogenesis of the disease; these antibodies are neither specific nor highly sensitive for the disease. Therefore, the presence of either antibody is not required for the diagnosis of AIEC.

■ DIFFERENTIAL DIAGNOSIS

Refractory Sprue

As discussed, many patients with AIEC may be initially diagnosed and treated as having celiac sprue, but they show no improvement with strict adherence to a GFD and are thus labeled as having refractory sprue (Chapter 18). These patients should undergo serological testing for enterocyte and goblet cell antibodies. Histologically, significant crypt apoptosis favors the diagnosis of AIEC.

Collagenous Colitis

Classic cases of collagenous colitis are characterized by chronic watery diarrhea, normal endoscopic findings, and a diffuse increase in IELs accompanied by a prominent subepithelial collagen layer. Any deviation from this typical "picture" is cause for caution in making the diagnosis. While most collagenous colitis is idiopathic, the current understanding is that the histologic pattern of collagenous

colitis may be associated with several diseases, including but not limited to drug-induced injury, collagenous sprue, and AIEC. Therefore, in patients who are not responding to standard treatment for collagenous colitis, the possibility of AIEC should be entertained, with attention given to microscopic features such as diffuse goblet cell depletion and crypt apoptosis and serologic testing for autoantibodies, as mentioned previously.

■ DRUG-INDUCED COLITIS

In adult patients, particularly the elderly, drug-induced enterocolitis should be considered first and investigated with a detailed drug history, including the use of nonsteroidal anti-inflammatory drugs (NSAIDs), olmesartan, and related drugs (Chapter 28).[35] Symptomatic and often histologic improvement usually occurs soon after the cessation of the suspected drug.

Common Variable Immune Deficiency

Rarely, AIEC occurs in patients with common variable immune deficiency (CVID).[26] There can be significant clinical and histologic overlap between CVID and AIEC, including chronic diarrhea, malabsorption, concurrent chronic atrophic gastritis, and microscopic colitis. About 75% of patients with CVID can have increased IELs, and 50% show villous atrophy of the small-bowel mucosa. However, CVID is characterized by depletion of plasma cells and lymphoid hyperplasia. In contrast, the presence of prominent crypt apoptosis raises the possibility of AIEC, particularly if the patients do not respond to immunoglobulin replacement therapy or steroid therapy.[26,36]

■ TREATMENT

Patients diagnosed with AIEC are treated with immunosuppressive drugs.[37,38] Patients may respond variably to tacrolimus,[39,40] infliximab,[41,42] or other agents. However, maintenance of response has been suboptimal, and these treatments have many side effects. Therefore, accurate diagnosis is essential to avoid under- or overtreatment of these patients.

■ REFERENCES

1. Walker-Smith JA, Unsworth DJ, Hutchins P, Phillips AD, Holborow EJ. Autoantibodies against gut epithelium in child with small-intestinal enteropathy. *Lancet*. 1982;1(8271):566–567. PMID: 6120421.
2. Unsworth DJ, Walker-Smith JA. Autoimmunity in diarrhoeal disease. *J Pediatr Gastroenterol Nutr*. 1985;4(3):375–380. PMID: 4020570.
3. Hill SM, Milla PJ, Bottazzo GF, Mirakian R. Autoimmune enteropathy and colitis: is there a generalised autoimmune gut disorder? *Gut*. 1991;32(1):36–42. PMID: 1991636. PMCID: PMC1379210.
4. Moore L, Xu X, Davidson G, Moore D, Carli M, Ferrante A. Autoimmune enteropathy with anti-goblet cell antibodies. *Hum Pathol*. 1995;26(10):1162–1168. PMID: 7557954.

5. Corazza GR, Biagi F, Volta U, Andreani ML, De Franceschi L, Gasbarrini G. Autoimmune enteropathy and villous atrophy in adults. *Lancet*. 1997;350(9071):106–109. PMID: 9228963.

6. Mitomi H, Tanabe S, Igarashi M, et al. Autoimmune enteropathy with severe atrophic gastritis and colitis in an adult: proposal of a generalized autoimmune disorder of the alimentary tract. *Scand J Gastroenterol*. 1998;33(7):716–720. PMID: 9712235.

7. Carroccio A, Volta U, Di Prima L, et al. Autoimmune enteropathy and colitis in an adult patient. *Dig Dis Sci*. 2003;48(8):1600–1606. PMID: 12924654.

8. Masia R, Peyton S, Lauwers GY, Brown I. Gastrointestinal biopsy findings of autoimmune enteropathy: a review of 25 cases. *Am J Surg Pathol*. 2014;38(10):1319–1329. PMID: 25188868. PMCID: NIHMS613877. PMC4162848.

9. Leon F, Olivencia P, Rodriguez-Pena R, et al. Clinical and immunological features of adult-onset generalized autoimmune gut disorder. *Am J Gastroenterol*. 2004;99(8):1563–1571. PMID: 15307878.

10. Jenkins HR, Jewkes F, Vujanic GM. Systemic vasculitis complicating infantile autoimmune enteropathy. *Arch Dis Child*. 1994;71(6):534–535. PMID: 7726616. PMCID: PMC1030094.

11. Lachaux A, Bouvier R, Cozzani E, et al. Familial autoimmune enteropathy with circulating anti-bullous pemphigoid antibodies and chronic autoimmune hepatitis. *J Pediatr*. 1994;125(6 Pt 1):858–862. PMID: 7996356.

12. Lachaux A, Loras-Duclaux I, Bouvier R. Autoimmune enteropathy in infants. Pathological study of the disease in two familial cases. *Virchows Arch*. 1998;433(5):481–485. PMID: 9849864.

13. Casis B, Fernandez-Vazquez I, Barnardos E, et al. Autoimmune enteropathy in an adult with autoimmune multisystemic involvement. *Scand J Gastroenterol*. 2002;37(9):1012–1016. PMID: 12374224.

14. Pirisi-Hauck NC, Foss HD, Baier J, Kurunczi S. Simultaneous occurrence of autoimmune enteropathy and recurrent deep venous thrombosis. *J Pediatr Gastroenterol Nutr*. 2000;30(3):324–329. PMID: 10749421.

15. Ranta A, Mokanahalli R. Cerebral venous thrombosis in autoimmune enteropathy. *N Z Med J*. 2010;123(1309):108–110. PMID: 20186248.

16. Davidson GP, Cutz E, Hamilton JR, Gall DG. Familial enteropathy: a syndrome of protracted diarrhea from birth, failure to thrive, and hypoplastic villus atrophy. *Gastroenterology*. 1978;75(5):783–790. PMID: 100367.

17. Avery GB, Villavicencio O, Lilly JR, Randolph JG. Intractable diarrhea in early infancy. *Pediatrics*. 1968;41(4):712–722. PMID: 5643979.

18. Rossi TM, Lebenthal E, Nord KS, Fazili RR. Extent and duration of small intestinal mucosal injury in intractable diarrhea of infancy. *Pediatrics*. 1980;66(5):730–735. PMID: 6776476.

19. Stern M, Gruttner R, Krumbach J. Protracted diarrhoea: secondary monosaccharide malabsorption and zinc deficiency with cutaneous manifestations during total parenteral nutrition. *Eur J Pediatr*. 1980;135(2):175–180. PMID: 6778699.

20. Fisher SE, Boyle JT, Holtzapple P. Chronic protracted diarrhea and jejunal atrophy in an infant. Cimetidine-associated stimulation of jejunal mucosal growth. *Dig Dis Sci*. 1981;26(2):181–186. PMID: 7460719.

21. Powell BR, Buist NR, Stenzel P. An X-linked syndrome of diarrhea, polyendocrinopathy, and fatal infection in infancy. *J Pediatr*. 1982;100(5):731–737. PMID: 7040622.

22. Ruemmele FM, Brousse N, Goulet O. Autoimmune enteropathy: molecular concepts. *Curr Opin Gastroenterol*. 2004;20(6):587–591. PMID: 15703687.

23. Ruemmele FM, Moes N, de Serre NP, Rieux-Laucat F, Goulet O. Clinical and molecular aspects of autoimmune enteropathy and immune dysregulation, polyendocrinopathy autoimmune enteropathy X-linked syndrome. *Curr Opin Gastroenterol*. 2008;24(6):742–748. PMID: 19122524.

24. Gambineri E, Perroni L, Passerini L, et al. Clinical and molecular profile of a new series of patients with immune dysregulation, polyendocrinopathy, enteropathy, X-linked syndrome: inconsistent correlation between forkhead box protein 3 expression and disease severity. *J Allergy Clin Immunol*. 2008;122(6):1105–1112.e1. PMID: 18951619.

25. Moes N, Rieux-Laucat F, Begue B, et al. Reduced expression of FOXP3 and regulatory T-cell function in severe forms of early-onset autoimmune enteropathy. *Gastroenterology*. 2010;139(3):770–778. PMID: 20537998.

26. Singhi AD, Goyal A, Davison JM, Regueiro MD, Roche RL, Ranganathan S. Pediatric autoimmune enteropathy: an entity frequently associated with immunodeficiency disorders. *Mod Pathol*. 2014;27(4):543–553. PMID: 24051695.

27. Ryan BM, Kelleher D. Refractory celiac disease. *Gastroenterology*. 2000;119(1):243–251. PMID: 10889175.

28. Akram S, Murray JA, Pardi DS, et al. Adult autoimmune enteropathy: Mayo Clinic Rochester experience. *Clin Gastroenterol Hepatol*. 2007;5(11):1282–1290;quiz 45. PMID: 17683994. PMCID: NIHMS34012 PMC2128725.

29. Al Khalidi H, Kandel G, Streutker CJ. Enteropathy with loss of enteroendocrine and paneth cells in a patient with immune dysregulation: a case of adult autoimmune enteropathy. *Hum Pathol*. 2006;37(3):373–376. PMID: 16613334.

30. Mais DD, Mulhall BP, Adolphson KR, Yamamoto K. Thymoma-associated autoimmune enteropathy. A report of two cases. *Am J Clin Pathol*. 1999;112(6):810–815. PMID: 10587704.

31. Colletti RB, Guillot AP, Rosen S, et al. Autoimmune enteropathy and nephropathy with circulating anti-epithelial cell antibodies. *J Pediatr*. 1991;118(6):858–864. PMID: 2040920.

32. Rogahn D, Smith CP, Thomas A. Autoimmune enteropathy with goblet-cell antibodies. *J R Soc Med*. 1999;92(6):311–312. PMID: 10472291. PMCID: PMC1297216.

33. Hori K, Fukuda Y, Tomita T, et al. Intestinal goblet cell autoantibody associated enteropathy. *J Clin Pathol*. 2003;56(8):629–630. PMID: 12890820. PMCID: PMC1770039.

34. Patey-Mariaud de Serre N, Canioni D, Ganousse S, et al. Digestive histopathological presentation of IPEX syndrome. *Mod Pathol*. 2009;22(1):95–102. PMID: 18820676.

35. Marthey L, Cadiot G, Seksik P, et al. Olmesartan-associated enteropathy: results of a national survey. *Aliment Pharmacol Ther*. 2014;40(9):1103–1109. PMID: 25199794.

36. Malamut G, Verkarre V, Suarez F, et al. The enteropathy associated with common variable immunodeficiency: the delineated frontiers with celiac disease. *Am J Gastroenterol*. 2010;105(10):2262–2275. PMID: 20551941.

37. Seidman EG, Lacaille F, Russo P, Galeano N, Murphy G, Roy CC. Successful treatment of autoimmune enteropathy with cyclosporine. *J Pediatr*. 1990;117(6):929–932. PMID: 2246696.

38. Sanderson IR, Phillips AD, Spencer J, Walker-Smith JA. Response to autoimmune enteropathy to cyclosporin A therapy. *Gut*. 1991;32(11):1421–1425. PMID: 1752480. PMCID: PMC1379182.

39. Steffen R, Wyllie R, Kay M, Kyllonen K, Gramlich T, Petras R. Autoimmune enteropathy in a pediatric patient: partial response to tacrolimus therapy. *Clin Pediatr*. 1997;36(5):295–299. PMID: 9152557.

40. Daum S, Sahin E, Jansen A, et al. Adult autoimmune enteropathy treated successfully with tacrolimus. *Digestion*. 2003;68(2–3):86–90. PMID: 14581765.

41. von Hahn T, Stopik D, Koch M, Wiedenmann B, Dignass A. Management of severe refractory adult autoimmune enteropathy with infliximab and tacrolimus. *Digestion*. 2005;71(3):141–144. PMID: 15785040.

42. Elwing JE, Clouse RE. Adult-onset autoimmune enteropathy in the setting of thymoma successfully treated with infliximab. *Dig Dis Sci*. 2005;50(5):928–932. PMID: 15906770.

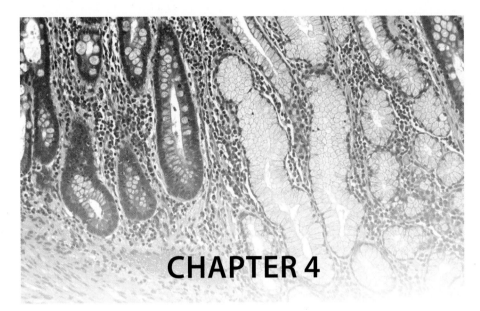

CHAPTER 4

Crohn Disease

■ INTRODUCTION

The underlying pathology of Crohn disease is that of chronic relapsing inflammation, often accompanied by granulomas, ulcers, fistulas, and fibrosis. The anatomic distribution of inflammation is regional and segmental in a discontinuous pattern. Any segments of the gastrointestinal (GI) tract can be involved, including the upper GI tract,[1-3] but disease of the terminal ileum is most common. The last often occurs with concurrent cecal involvement. A significant subset of patients has disease limited to the colon. Upper GI tract involvement more commonly causes focal gastritis[1,2] followed by duodenal injury,[1,2] and is relatively more common in pediatric patients.[4] In addition to the GI tract, patients with Crohn disease may have extra-GI involvement, such as of the skin or the oral or genital mucosa. Other autoimmune disorders occur as complications in some patients.

Pathologically, the Crohn lesions range from subtle mucosal inflammatory infiltration to erosion, ulcer, fissure, transmural inflammation, abscess, and fistula. Repeated ulceration causes fibrosis of the submucosa or muscularis propria, leading to scarring and thickening of the bowel wall and stricture formation. Stenosis and obstruction may also be related to local fistula formation and adhesions between loops of bowel.

Due to its "global" involvement of the GI tract, this chapter on Crohn disease is placed in the General Topics section. The common microscopic abnormalities and features unique to individual segments (esophagus, stomach, duodenum, jejunum and ileum, and colon) are discussed. Long-term complications, including dysplasia and adenocarcinoma, are also briefly discussed.

■ MACROSCOPIC FEATURES

When involving the upper GI tract, Crohn disease usually manifests as mucosal erosions or ulcerations. In the small bowel, the disease can cause mucosal ulceration, stricture (Figure 4-1), intramural abscess, fistula, and perforation[5,6] due to transmural inflammation and fibrosis. Free perforation can also occur in colonic Crohn disease,[5] as well as stenosis.[7,8] Adenocarcinomas can occur as a later complication of Crohn enteritis or colitis.[9-15] Rectal and perineal involvement can be seen in up to one-third of patients, with changes ranging from skin tags, fissures, fistulas, perineal abscesses, and anal canal strictures.[6,16,17]

■ MICROSCOPIC FEATURES

Pathology of the GI tract in Crohn disease can be observed in either mucosal biopsies or resected specimens (small bowel and colon). Because Crohn disease is usually a transmural inflammatory process, the pathologic changes involve all layers of the bowel wall. Biopsies allow only lesions of the mucosa and submucosa to be observed; all the abnormalities can be seen in resected specimens.

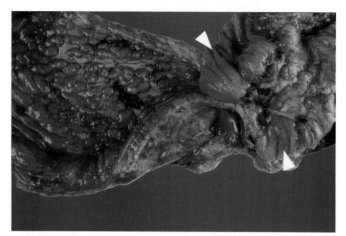

FIGURE 4-1. Active Crohn enteritis. Resection of a strictured small-bowel segment, with mucosal cobblestoning (left side), marked wall thickening in the narrowed area, and linear ulcer to the right. Note relatively normal-appearing mucosa (arrowheads).

In the early phases, the involved mucosa exhibits focal active inflammation: infiltration of the lamina propria by a mixture of lymphocytes and plasma cells and infiltration of surface or crypt epithelium by neutrophils (cryptitis) (Figure 4-2A) or crypt abscesses (Figure 4-2B). In most patients, the changes of active disease are accompanied by changes of chronicity or chronic mucosal injury due to repeated episodes of mucosal damage and ineffective crypt repair. In acute self-limited colitis or enteritis, injury or destruction to crypts usually does not leave behind chronic changes due to proper regeneration within the native stromal framework from stem cells present in the base of crypts. This gives rise to essentially normal but "replenished" mucosa. However, if the regenerative process is interrupted before completion by repeated episodes of injury the newly formed crypts or villi take irregular forms (*aborted or ineffective regeneration*), with dilation or branching of the crypts (Figure 4-2C) and shortening or complete loss of villi. Some crypts may never be replaced due to complete destruction,

FIGURE 4-2. Microscopic lesions seen in Crohn disease. **A.** Cryptitis: neutrophils infiltrating epithelium of the crypts; the lamina propria also contains mixed inflammatory infiltration consisting of plasma cells, lymphocytes, and some eosinophils. **B.** Crypt abscess: a partially ruptured crypt (center) contains a cluster of neutrophils mixed with necrotic debris. **C.** Crypt branching. **D.** Loss of crypts in the left side of the field. Also note Paneth cell metaplasia (cells with bright pink granular cytoplasm) at the base in some of the crypts in this left colon biopsy.

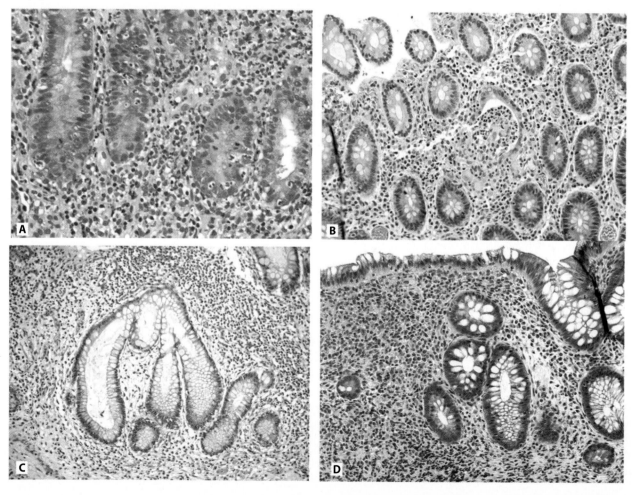

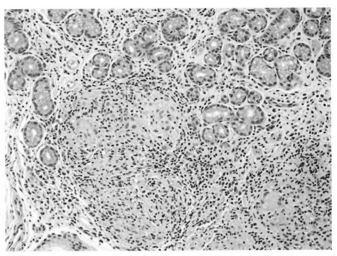

FIGURE 4-3. Well-formed epithelioid and giant cell granulomas.

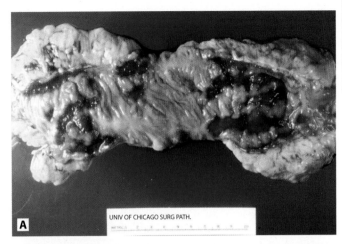

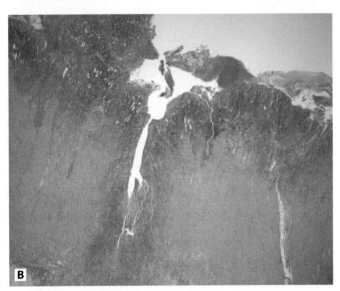

FIGURE 4-5. **A.** Crohn colitis with linear ulcers. Multiple longitudinal ulcers are apparent on the mucosa of this opened segmental resection. Note the intervening mucosa is essentially normal. **B.** Microscopic view of a deep ulcer extending almost through the muscularis propria, surrounded by marked inflammation.

including the progenitor cells, leaving behind empty spaces within the lamina propria (crypt loss) (Figure 4-2D). Therefore, chronicity of small-bowel lesions consists of focal flattening or loss of villi, and that of both small-bowel and colon lesions includes crypt branching, dilation (*crypt architectural distortion*), and loss. It should be noted that such changes of chronicity may be subtle and patchy, sometimes making it difficult to appreciate microscopically. Occasionally, epithelioid or giant cell granulomas can accompany these changes (Figure 4-3).

In severely active lesions, the mucosal injury progresses to superficial erosion or ulcer, particularly over large lymphoid follicles, leading to aphthous ulcers (Figure 4-4). With progression, these small, shallow ulcers can expand and coalesce, forming irregular or linear ulcers (Figure 4-5A). One of the characteristics of Crohn disease is that ulceration can be narrow but extend deep to the submucosa or superficial muscularis propria, giving rise to fissuring ulcers (Figure 4-5B). Inflammation and ulceration in Crohn disease often lead to

submucosal fibrosis, which can be responsible for focal thickening accompanied by hypertrophy of nerves in the submucosal or myenteric plexus.

As mentioned, the inflammation in Crohn disease is often transmural, particularly when involving the small bowel. This manifests as prominent lymphoid follicles or granulomas with lymphocytic infiltration in submucosa and muscularis propria (*lymphoid beading*) (Figure 4-6). Some of the lesions develop into abscesses or sinus tracts and progress to fistula tracts, extending to involve adjacent bowel segments or other structures that have adhesions. In addition, serosal involvement eventually leads to fibrosis and adhesions, often with adipose tissue wrapping on the involved segment, giving rise to "creeping fat" lesions (see the section on the colon), on the antimesenteric side of the serosa.

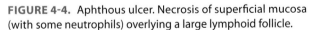

FIGURE 4-4. Aphthous ulcer. Necrosis of superficial mucosa (with some neutrophils) overlying a large lymphoid follicle.

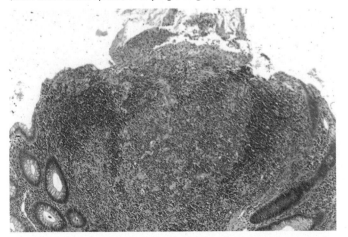

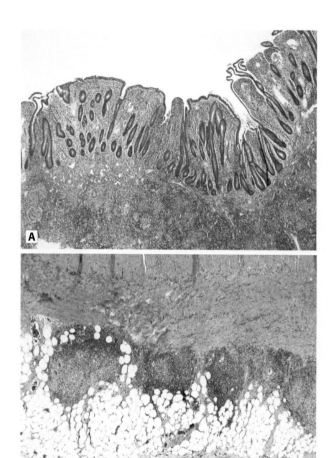

FIGURE 4-6. Transmural inflammation. **A.** Coalesced lymphoid follicles mixed with granulomas in the submucosa (muscularis propria also involved but not shown) of this resected segment of small bowel. The inflamed mucosa exhibits total villous blunting with crypt hypertrophy. **B.** Subserosal lymphoid beading.

Another important microscopic feature of Crohn disease is the development of pyloric gland metaplasia (PGM) (Figure 4-7). This occurs when the crypts are replaced as part of the repair process by complex, neutral-mucin glands similar to that in gastric cardia, antrum, or pylorus. In some cases, PGM is prominent and extensive, likely resulting from overgrowth or hyperplasia. PGM is usually seen in the setting of chronic mucosal injury and is most frequently described in Crohn enteritis. Some authors have suggested that in an appropriate clinical setting, the finding of PGM in the terminal ileum is pathognomic for Crohn enteritis. However, similar changes can be seen in injury induced by nonsteroidal anti-inflammatory drugs (NSAIDs) or other mucosal injuries (discussed in "Differential Diagnosis"). Although PGM is more frequently associated with small-bowel lesions, it can occasionally occur in colonic Crohn as well.

Vascular abnormalities can be seen in Crohn disease,[18] but prominent vasculitis or microthrombi of arterioles are

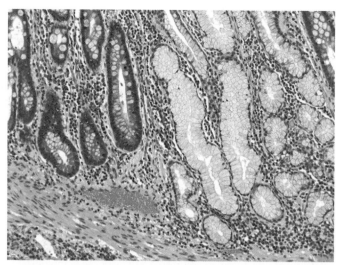

FIGURE 4-7. Pyloric gland metaplasia. Typical small-bowel glands (crypts) are seen on the left side of the field. To the right are many tubular mucous glands with pale cytoplasm and flat, basally located nuclei.

usually associated with mucosal ulcers and thus may represent a secondary change.[18]

Within the general pathologic background described, Crohn disease expresses certain histologic features unique to the region of the GI tract involved. These are discussed in the following individual sections.

Esophagus

Esophageal Crohn disease is rare.[19,20] When involved, the esophageal mucosa may have ulcers, erythema or erosions, or strictures. Fistulas can also occur.[21] Histologically, most lesions exhibit focal, chronic, active inflammation of the squamous epithelium, characterized by lymphocytic or neutrophilic infiltration and sometimes eosinophils, intercellular edema (spongiosis), erosion, and ulceration[19,20,22] (Figure 4-8). Granulomas may be seen when lamina propria is included in the biopsy.[20] Lymphocytic infiltration is also prominent in the lamina propria, which sometimes forms a band-like concentration at the epithelium-stromal junction (Figure 4-8). As these changes are rather nonspecific, other more common diseases need to be excluded, such as infectious, drug-induced, and reflux esophagitis causes.

Stomach

Chronic active gastritis occurring in patients with Crohn disease can be due to superimposed *Helicobacter pylori* infection or as part of Crohn disease.[23,24] The latter usually exhibits multifocal microscopic chronic inflammation,[23,25,26] with the background mucosa largely unremarkable, a pattern termed *focally enhanced gastritis* (FEG)[27] (Figure 4-9A). The inflammation is mainly a mixture of lymphocytes, plasma

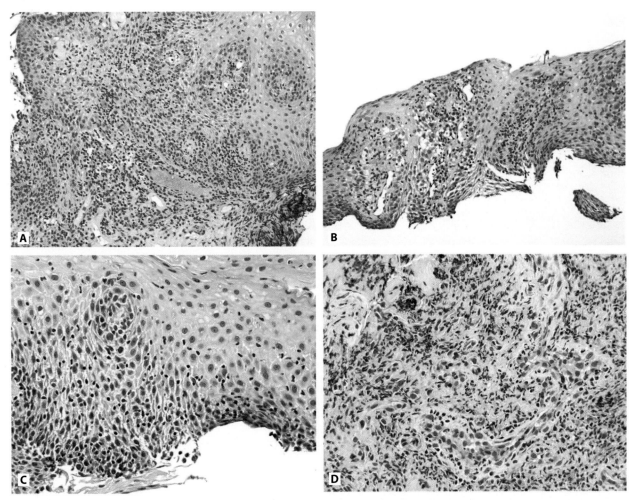

FIGURE 4-8. Crohn disease involving esophagus. **A.** Marked focal lymphocytic infiltration. **B.** Marked spongiosis of the squamous epithelium. **C.** Mild infiltration of the squamous epithelium by lymphocytes and some neutrophils, with intercellular edema at the basal zone. **D.** Ulcer base characterized by granulation tissue with mixed inflammatory infiltration.

cells, and histiocytes surrounding a single gland or a cluster of glands (Figure 4-9B), but more advanced lesions may show destruction of the glands by neutrophils (Figure 4-9C). Epithelioid and giant cell granulomas can be seen as well (Figure 4-9D). Prolonged involvement may lead to focal loss of glands, accompanied by endocrine cell hyperplasia. Even though the neutrophilic infiltration is similar to microscopic activity of chronic *H. pylori* gastritis, no organisms or positive immunohistochemical stains for *H. pylori* can be identified in these lesions.

Duodenum

In most cases, the mucosal changes in the duodenum are nonspecific, ranging from focal injury mimicking peptic injury to increased intraepithelial lymphocytosis accompanied by focal villous atrophy.[1,2,26,28–30] Therefore, when only these changes are identified in a mucosal biopsy, they are not helpful for histologic diagnosis of Crohn disease. However, in some patients, there may be focal gland-destroying chronic active duodenitis (Figure 4-10), sometimes with granulomas. As described, small-bowel Crohn disease may be accompanied by PGM. However, because pyloric glands are morphologically almost indistinguishable from the Brunner's glands that are normally present in the duodenal mucosa, this feature is hard to appreciate and cannot be reliably used for diagnosis.

Jejunum and Ileum

Although Crohn disease most frequently involves the distal 15 to 20 cm of the ileum, any segment of small bowel can be affected. Small-bowel Crohn disease is most commonly associated with adhesion, wall thickening, and stricture, which can be multiple in some cases,[6] often resulting in bowel obstruction. Small-bowel Crohn disease can also lead to spontaneous perforation and peritonitis.[5,31] Although most patients have focal disease, diffuse Crohn jejunoileitis can also occur, more frequently in younger patients.[32]

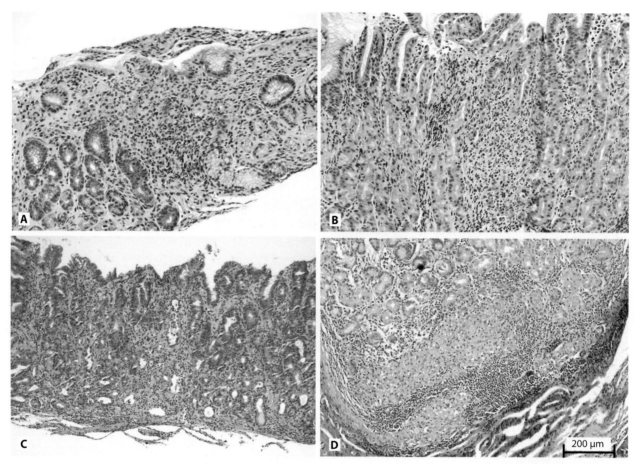

FIGURE 4-9. Crohn gastritis. **A.** Focally enhanced gastritis: inflammatory cells forming a cluster surrounding 1 or 2 glands. The adjacent background is otherwise unremarkable. **B.** Inflammation with neutrophils destroying glands focally. **C.** Evident loss of gastric glands due to active inflammation. **D.** Large, well-formed epithelioid granulomas at the base of the mucosa.

Histologically, early mucosal lesions consist of focal loss or atrophy of villi, focal infiltration of surface and crypt epithelium by neutrophils, and erosion or ulceration (Figure 4-11), which is endoscopically described as an aphthous ulcer. In patients with longer duration of the disease, mucosal architectural changes are more evident, with active inflammation (Figure 4-12A) or granulomas and PGM (Figure 4-12B). Occasionally in a biopsy, the only abnormality may be a well-formed submucosal granuloma with an otherwise-normal mucosal background (Figure 4-12C).

Resected small-bowel specimens usually contain pathologic changes that are more advanced, including single or multifocal ulcers, accompanied by focal or extensive PGM. In addition, the mucosa may show prominent inflammatory polyps or pseudopolyps with deep fissuring ulcers. Focal fibrosis and thickening of the bowel wall are accompanied by hyperplasia of nerve bundles or neural plexus. In the ulcer base or adjacent areas, nonspecific vascular injury may be seen. Rarely, the thickened and strictured segment may harbor an adenocarcinoma[9,12,13,33,34] (discussed in the section on dysplasia and adenocarcinoma).

Colon

Colonic involvement by Crohn disease can be a part of enterocolitis or as isolated Crohn colitis. The cecum is most commonly involved. Colon-only involvement occurs in about 25% of patients. It is usually in the form of multifocal, irregularly distributed mucosal lesions, including crypt architectural distortion, crypt loss (Figure 4-13A), isolated granuloma (Figure 4-13B), inflammatory polyps (Figure 4-13C), with a variable degree of activity (Figure 4-13D). Occasionally, diffuse colitis occurs,[35,36] which grossly and microscopically can be similar to ulcerative colitis (UC) (Figure 4-14A). In the last situation, it is common to find deep ulcers or transmural inflammation on careful examination of the resected specimen. Hypertrophy of the mural neural plexus (Figure 4-14B) and serosal adhesion by adipose tissue ("fat wrapping") (Figure 4-14C) can be identified as well. These features are suggestive of Crohn disease and can be helpful in distinguishing Crohn colitis from UC.

In many patients, particularly those who have received treatment, the colonic lesions are mild, with a patchy, multifocal distribution, and exhibit the usual mucosal changes

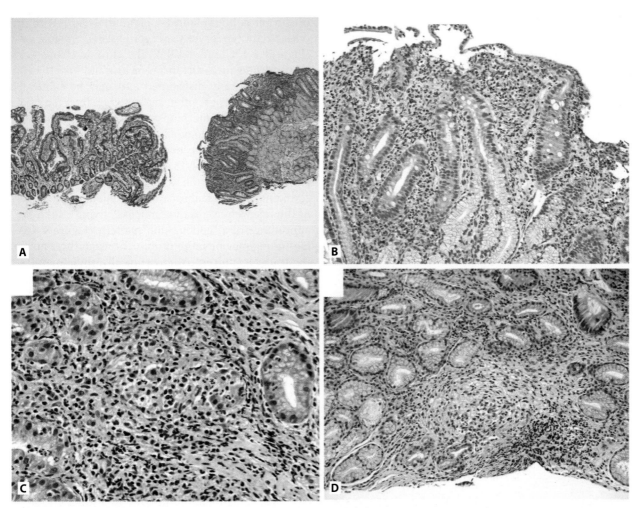

FIGURE 4-10. Crohn duodenitis. **A.** A biopsy contains fragments of completely normal duodenal mucosa (left) and mucosa with marked crypt hyperplasia with complete blunting of villi (even for mucosa overlying Brunner's glands). **B.** Higher magnification showing active inflammation. **C.** Focal active inflammation causing destruction of glands. Note a mixed infiltration consisting of lymphocytes, plasma cells, and many neutrophils, with residual epithelial cells of the gland. **D.** An epithelioid granuloma in the base of the mucosa.

FIGURE 4-11. Early Crohn enteritis involving terminal ileum: biopsy of an aphthous erosion. **A.** Focal inflammatory infiltration associated with villous and crypt architectural change. **B.** Higher power view showing mixed inflammatory cells, including many plasma cells and eosinophils (vs. a lymphoid aggregate) and scattered intraepithelial neutrophils.

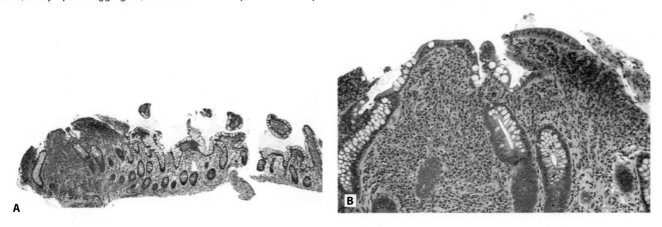

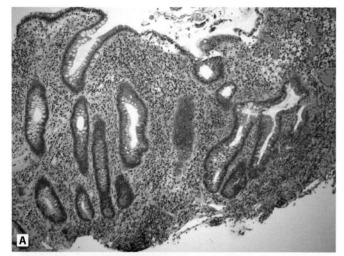

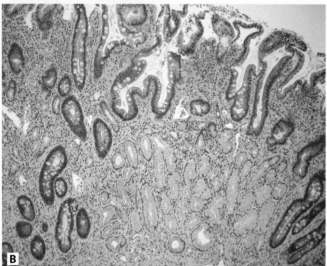

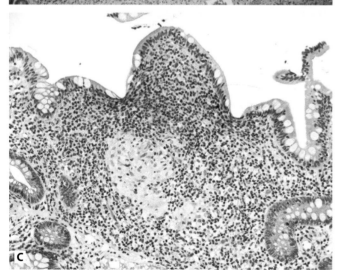

FIGURE 4-12. Crohn enteritis. **A.** Mildly active Crohn enteritis involving terminal ileum. **B.** Quiescent Crohn enteritis with pyloric gland metaplasia. **C.** A well-formed epithelioid and giant cell granuloma in the small-bowel mucosa. Although the villi directly overlying the granuloma are slightly shortened, the overall mucosal structure is maintained. There is no active disease.

of chronic colitis (Figures 4-13A and 4-13B), with or without activity (eg, cryptitis, crypt abscess, erosion, or ulcer) (Figures 4-13C and 4-13D). The chronic changes, such as crypt architectural distortion or loss and Paneth cell metaplasia, are focally distributed and may be subtle. Foci of abnormal crypts are often separated by intervening normal mucosa in the same biopsy fragment. Compared to UC, the mucosal pathologic changes are usually milder. However, in severe cases, deep, "knife-like" ulcers can occur (Figures 4-14A and 4-15). When the involvement is extensive and inflammation severely active, parallel linear and serpiginous ulcers alternate with edema and hyperplasia of the intervening residual mucosa, giving rise to the gross appearance of a "cobblestone" pattern (Figure 4-16). Cobblestoning may be more prominent when there are coexisting transverse ulcers. Microscopically, these manifest as an actively inflamed ulcer base and marked crypt architectural distortion in the adjacent mucosa.

Intramural abscess or fistula is less common in the colon as opposed to the small bowel. However, rectal or perianal diseases may lead to frequent fistula formation (Figure 4-17A). It should be noted that the epithelial lining can extend deep into a fistula tract, often showing marked reactive changes (Figure 4-17B). This has implications as discussed regarding the distinction from adenocarcinoma in the material that follows.

Anal and Perianal Areas

Anal or perianal disease is common in patients with Crohn disease, who sometimes can develop vaginal mucosal disease, with inflammation, fissures, or fistula. The squamous mucosa shows focal or diffuse chronic active inflammation with granulomas. For further discussion of anal and perianal diseases, please refer to Chapter 31.

Involvement of Other Sites

Nearly half of patients with Crohn disease can have involvement of, or present with, lesions of the oral cavity, such as vesicular lesions or aphthous ulcers. Microscopically, these lesions consist of chronic inflammation, often mixed with noncaseating granulomas, as in the GI tracts. Focal inflammation, erosion, or ulcer may involve the genital mucosa. A rectovaginal fistula may form in female patients.

■ SPECIAL CONSIDERATIONS OF CROHN HISTOPATHOLOGY

Displaced Glands or Epithelium

As a result of repeated deep ulceration or fistula formation (Figures 4-17A and 4-17B), followed by re-epithelialization or mucosal regeneration, fibrosis, and microdiverticulum, residual mucous glands may be formed and entrapped ("left behind") in the deep layers of the bowel wall (Figure 4-18), including the submucosa, muscularis propria, or subserosa. When prominent and with mucin accumulation, these may

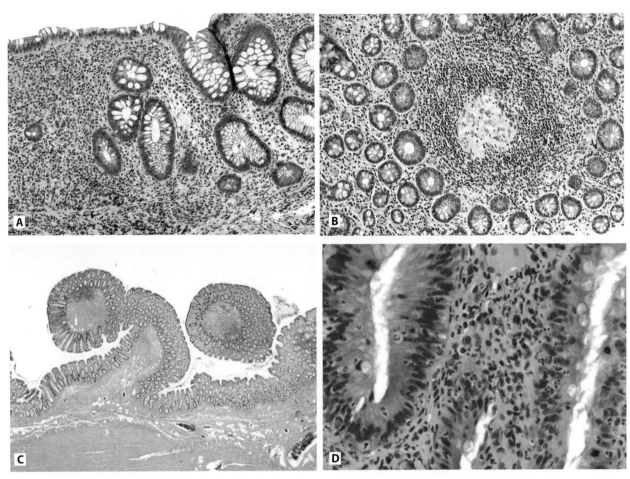

FIGURE 4-13. Crohn colitis. **A.** Crypt architectural distortion, Paneth cell metaplasia, and focal loss of crypts. **B.** A rim of lymphoid tissue surrounding an epithelioid granuloma. **C.** Inflammatory polyps. **D.** Inflammatory infiltration with cryptitis.

become cystically dilated and give rise to enteritis cystica profunda or focal colitis cystica profunda. An important microscopic feature is the presence of the normal lamina propria surrounding these entrapped glands. Sometimes, the displaced glands may be associated with marked fibrosis, causing focal bowel wall thickening or a mass lesion. Differentiation between this process and invasive adenocarcinoma is usually straightforward because benign displaced glands exhibit bland, nondysplastic epithelium associated with lamina propria and lack desmoplasia, a histologic hallmark of invasive carcinoma. However, in rare cases, the distinction may be extremely challenging or even impossible because sometimes cancer can be well differentiated and show no evident epithelial atypia. In addition, increased intraluminal pressure due to accumulation of mucin may destroy the lining epithelium, resulting in mucin leaking into the stroma and inciting a fibroblastic reaction that may be indistinguishable from desmoplasia.

Dysplasia and Adenocarcinoma in Crohn Disease

Long-standing mucosal inflammation in Crohn disease carries increased risk for dysplasia and eventually the development of adenocarcinoma.[11,34,37–44] Understandably, patients develop adenocarcinoma at a younger age than the general population.[11] The overall incidence of the neoplastic transformation in Crohn disease is much lower than in UC due to the segmental and regional distribution of the former, with less-extensive involvement of the mucosal surface. However, there appears to be no difference in risk of malignant transformation in a given involved segment. Increased risk is associated with younger age at diagnosis of Crohn disease, longer disease duration, and longer interval between the exams.[42] Therefore, similar to patients with UC, patients with Crohn disease should be subject to endoscopic surveillance for early detection of dysplasia or cancer.[45,46] Dysplasia occurring in Crohn disease may resemble that in UC,[37,44] such as crypt overgrowth, nuclear hyperchromasia, and pseudostratification of elongated nuclei (Figure 4-19A). Sometimes the nuclear atypia is expressed as marked hyperchromasia, enlargement, and haphazard arrangement, mainly in the lower portion of crypts (Figure 4-19B). High-grade dysplasia may exhibit complex glandular architecture, including a cribriform pattern and aberrant histophenotype (Figure 4-19C).

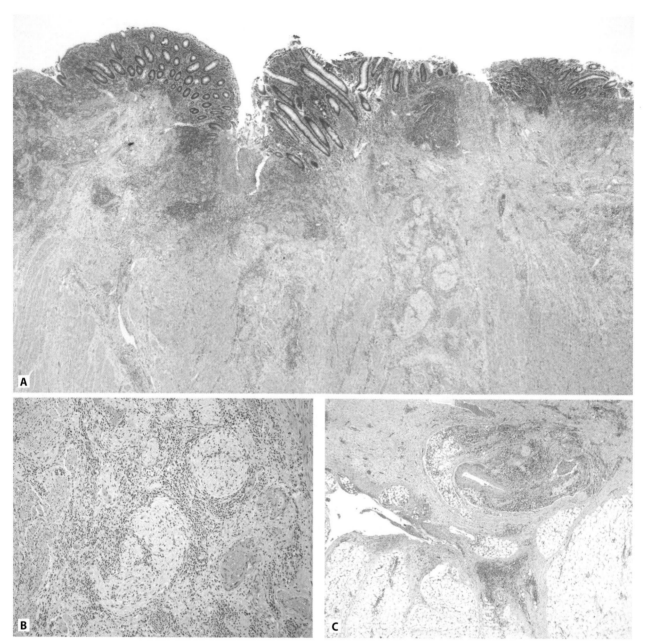

FIGURE 4-14. A case of diffuse Crohn colitis. **A.** Extensive mucosal architectural distortion with superficial and deep ulcers and fibrosis of the submucosa. **B.** Higher magnification of nerve hypertrophy. **C.** Adhesion of fat to the serosa at site of inflammation (fat wrapping).

Although less well characterized, dysplasia occurring in the small bowel may exhibit additional unique features. It can manifest as a polypoid lesion with villous dysplasia[40] or with surface serrated changes. Interestingly, in patients with Crohn colorectal carcinomas, dysplastic foci can be identified distant from the cancer (recognized independently from carcinoma), while in small-bowel carcinomas, dysplasia can only be identified adjacent to the cancer,[39] reflecting the difficulty in recognizing dysplasia in the small bowel. In some cases of frank small-bowel adenocarcinomas, the surface epithelium totally lacks classic adenomatous change.

In addition, small-bowel adenocarcinomas occurring in Crohn disease have certain unique characteristics compared to those occurring without a Crohn disease background, including younger age at diagnosis and higher frequency of ileal location.[9,12,13,33,34,38,39,47–49] Many of these tumors are identified incidentally in resected specimens[34,39] and often occur in a stricture[13,31,34] or previous strictureplasty site.[12] Although some tumors exhibit histologic features of the "usual" intestinal adenocarcinomas, many exhibit features resembling gastric tubular-type adenocarcinoma (Figure 4-20),[9,49] including expression of *MUC5AC*

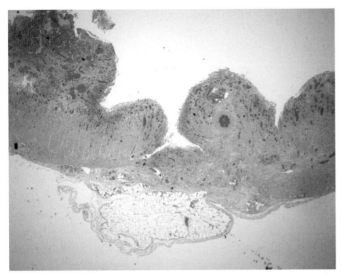

FIGURE 4-15. A deep fissuring ulcer, nearly resulting in perforation.

and *MUC6* immunohistochemically.[49] Tumors of this morphology are frequently associated with extensive PGM, suggesting a pyloric metaplasia-tumorigenesis pathway, as described in Chapter 22.

■ HISTOLOGIC ASSESSMENT

Histologic Diagnosis

Diagnosis of Crohn disease for the most part is based on microscopic examination of *mucosal* biopsies from patients with the appropriate clinical symptoms and radiologic and endoscopic findings suspicious for the disease. Therefore, some of the pathologic features described, particularly those involving deeper layers of the intestinal wall, such as transmural inflammation, intramural abscess, deep granulomas, and lymphoid "beading," are not practical for this purpose.

The initial biopsies are usually obtained to confirm a clinical working diagnosis, although rarely systematic upper and lower GI endoscopic biopsies may show microscopic

FIGURE 4-16. Cobblestone change of extensively ulcerated colon mucosa.

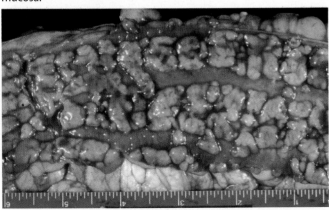

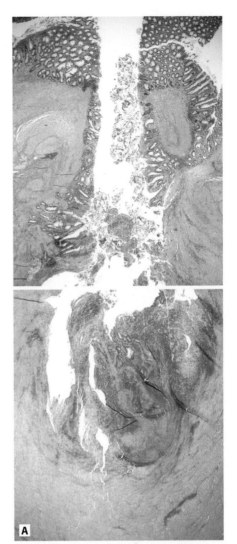

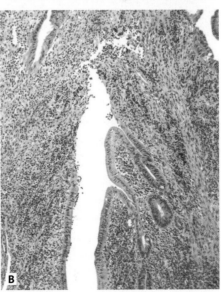

FIGURE 4-17. Rectal involvement by Crohn disease. **A.** A rectal fistula, with partial mucosal lining and re-epithelialization toward the deeper portion. The morphology indicates a start from a diverticulum. **B.** Higher-power view showing reepithelialization of the fistula tract, with marked epithelial atypia.

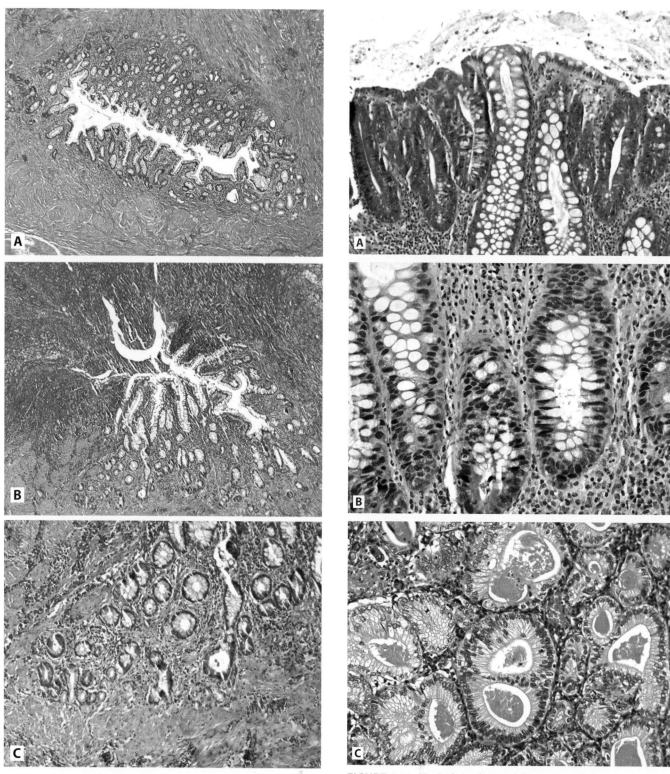

FIGURE 4-18. Re-epithelialization of terminal ileum fistula tract. **A.** This section was obtained away from the bowel lumen of a fistula tract deep in the wall, re-epithelialized by mucosa similar to small-bowel mucosa but with no normal villi. **B.** Secondary inflammation causing focal ulceration of the re-epithelialization mucosa of the fistula. **C.** The chronic inflammation also contains focal pyloric gland metaplasia.

FIGURE 4-19. **A.** Crohn colitis with low-grade dysplasia. The two crypts at the center of the field are normal. The crypts on both sides show nuclear hyperchromasia, elongation, and overlap, with loss of mucin content in the cytoplasm. **B.** Low-grade dysplasia mainly involving the basal zone of crypts. **C.** Crohn enteritis with high-grade dysplasia. The glands exhibit gastric pyloric morphology but with nuclear atypia and marked proliferation and focal cribriform changes.

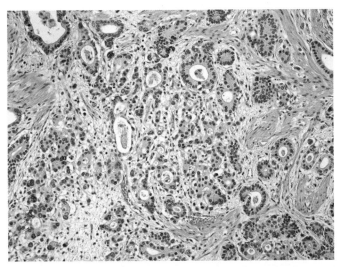

FIGURE 4-20. Adenocarcinoma arising from Crohn enteritis. Large and small malignant glands are invading the muscularis propria. There are also individual clusters of cells not forming glands.

changes characteristic of Crohn disease in a patient otherwise not clinically suspected for the disease. This includes multifocal, noncontinuous mucosal architectural distortion, often with granulomas. It cannot be overemphasized that no matter how strong the histologic evidence is, a diagnosis of Crohn disease should not be made without proper clinical correlation. This is because the pathologic features described are nonspecific and can be seen in a variety of other diseases. For clinicians, it is important to submit the clinical history and detailed endoscopic description along with the biopsy specimens so that meaningful histologic interpretation can be rendered.

In classic Crohn disease cases, multiple biopsies from the colon may show various microscopic findings, ranging from entirely normal mucosa to marked crypt architectural distortion with active inflammation. For the most part, biopsies from endoscopically abnormal areas exhibit typical changes of chronic active colitis, but endoscopic and microscopic discrepancy is not uncommon. Convincing changes of chronic colitis include crypt architectural distortion (shortening, branching, budding, irregular dilatation) or crypt loss. Often, the intervening regions with completely normal crypts can be seen, representing microscopic "skip" lesions. Depending on the inflammatory activity, there may be scattered cryptitis, crypt abscess, erosion, or overt ulceration. In the distal colon (from the splenic flexure), the presence of Paneth cells is abnormal (Paneth cell metaplasia). When the biopsies lack overt crypt architectural distortions, identification of Paneth cell metaplasia can aid the diagnosis of chronic colitis. In addition, granulomas not directly associated with a ruptured crypt are helpful in the diagnosis. Due to the scattered and uneven distribution, granulomas are identified more often in resected specimens than in biopsies. They are more frequently in the colon than in the small bowel. To increase

diagnostic confidence, particularly for the initial diagnosis, biopsies from the terminal ileum are critical when the distinction from UC is not clear.

To establish a diagnosis, it is important to include esophagogastroduodenoscopy (EGD) with biopsies as part of the initial workup, in addition to colonoscopy, even in patients without upper GI symptoms. This increases the diagnostic yield due to the unpredictable and patchy distribution of Crohn disease, particularly in pediatric patients.[50] Not uncommonly, cases are encountered in which the only abnormalities initially identified are from the upper GI biopsies, plus focal active ileitis. The latter alone may not be sufficient to suggest the diagnosis of Crohn disease (see below).

Differential Diagnosis

Ulcerative Colitis

Untreated, classic UC is characterized by diffuse, continuous mucosal inflammation, which is usually superficial and does not involve the submucosa (see also Chapter 26). Microscopically, crypt architectural distortion is prominent and diffuse, without intervening normal crypts. When granulomas are present, they are usually intramucosal and directly associated with a ruptured crypt (*mucin granulomas*) (Figure 4-21). When multiple biopsies are submitted for microscopic examination and the location of each biopsy is known, the pathologist usually can determine if the disease is continuous and diffuse, which greatly help the distinction between Crohn colitis and UC. This is particularly true when a biopsy from the terminal ileum is also included. Except for cases of fulminant colitis, the inflammation in UC is confined to the mucosal layer. Therefore, when marked chronic and active inflammation extends to the submucosa, particularly when submucosal epithelioid

FIGURE 4-21. Intramucosal mucin granuloma in ulcerative colitis. The small granuloma is adjacent to a crypt and contains multinucleate cells mixed with mucin content.

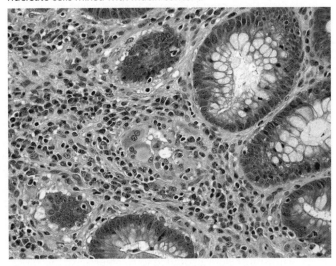

granulomas are seen, the diagnosis of Crohn colitis should be considered over UC.

When inflammation is identified in biopsies from the terminal ileum, one should be cautious in interpreting its significance. If colonic involvement is limited to the distal colon, bona fide active chronic ileitis is more consistent with the diagnosis of Crohn disease. However, if there is pancolitis, with disease activity extending to the cecum, inflammation of distal ileitis more likely represents "backwash ileitis," particularly when there is little evidence of chronicity or granulomas (see also Chapters 19 and 26). Backwash ileitis mostly involves the distal 5 cm of the terminal ileum, although in rare severe forms it can extend beyond 10 cm, and erosion and ulceration may occur.[51] When evident chronic changes are identified, such as deep ulcer, PGM, or epithelioid granulomas, one should seriously entertain the diagnosis of Crohn disease, even in face of pancolitis. As mentioned, some cases of Crohn disease can present in a diffuse pattern, mimicking UC.

By definition, UC is a disease of the colon without small-bowel involvement, except for occasional terminal ileum involvement as backwash ileitis as discussed previously. Nevertheless, rarely a patient with a well-established diagnosis of UC who underwent total colectomy may develop severe upper GI disease (see also Chapter 19), raising questions regarding the diagnosis. This usually occurs shortly after total colectomy (within a month or so),[52-57] in the form of diffuse enteritis,[58] gastritis, and duodenitis[52,54,56](Figure 4-22). Some authors apply the term *ulcerative gastroduodenitis* to this condition. No other clinical or pathologic evidence of Crohn disease can be identified in these patients. It is therefore important to recognize this condition and not erroneously change the diagnosis to Crohn disease.

One of the challenges in distinguishing Crohn disease from UC relates to treated UC. In these cases, colonic biopsies may show focal lack of crypt architectural distortion, similar to the microscopic skip lesions of Crohn colitis. However, a well-established history of UC should help solve the diagnostic dilemma, particularly if a set of previous biopsies showing typical changes of UC is available for review. Sometimes, even though these biopsies may not show crypt branching or loss, careful comparison with truly normal mucosa may reveal the diffuse shortening of the crypts, a result of diffuse mucosal atrophy.

NSAIDs-Induced Injuries

Sometimes a biopsy from the terminal ileum in a symptomatic patient shows the changes of active ileitis, characterized by focal villous architectural change and intraepithelial neutrophilic infiltration. In this scenario, possibilities other than Crohn disease should be considered, such as NSAID-induced injury.

NSAIDs and related drugs are widely used and are responsible for GI tract injury in a significant number of patients. For example, it was found that risk of GI-related death in patients with rheumatoid arthritis taking NSAIDs was 0.2% per year.[59] In a study of patients with duodenal ulcers, while most were attributed to *H. pylori* gastritis, those negative for *H. pylori* were mostly due to NSAID injury,

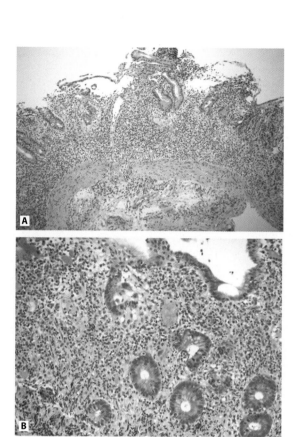

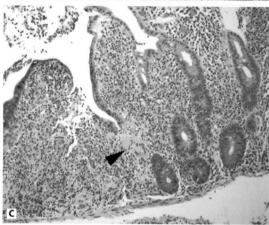

FIGURE 4-22. Post-colectomy diffuse duodenitis in a patient who had confirmed ulcerative colitis and underwent total colectomy. **A.** Diffuse inflation of duodenal mucosa with ulcers. **B.** Marked inflammatory infiltration, with cryptitis, and villous atrophy. **C.** Occasionally, giant cell granulomas can be seen, but they are immediately associated with a mucosal erosion.

followed by oral antibiotics,[60] and rarely, Crohn disease.[61] NSAID use may cause mucosal injuries, including erosions and ulcerations, similar to those of Crohn disease, both in histologic appearance and in distribution (eg, duodenum, ileum, or colon).[62] For most cases, close clinical-pathologic correlation will be helpful in sorting out the etiology. However, NSAID use is significantly underreported by patients,[63] making the differential diagnosis difficult. In adult patients, a finding of focal or patchy mucosal injury in the terminal ileum or colon may suggest the diagnosis of Crohn disease, but a final diagnosis requires other features of the disease, and often a short-term follow-up (cessation of any drug that may cause GI toxicity) is necessary.

There are certain microscopic changes that may help distinguish a Crohn lesion from NSAID injury. For example, the presence of prominent PGM or well-formed epithelioid granulomas favors the diagnosis of Crohn disease (although focal PGM can be seen in some NSAID lesions). Similarly, scattered foci of Paneth cell metaplasia in the distal colon or granulomas are less common in NSAID-induced injury.

Isolated Ileitis

Not uncommonly, in patients who undergo colonoscopy for lower GI symptoms without a clear clinical diagnosis, the only pathology identified is from the terminal ileum, usually in the form of focally active chronic ileitis. There are usually no abnormal findings in the colon. Some of these cases can eventually be attributed to either NSAID-induced ileal injury or Crohn ileitis after thorough clinical workup. Some patients may have a background of another disease, such as Henoch-Schoenlein syndrome[64] or cytomegalovirus infection.[65] In some patients, however, despite careful scrutiny, no clinical history can be elicited to explain these findings. In this scenario, the proper diagnosis should be "isolated ileitis." Currently, the clinical significance of this diagnosis is undetermined. A small number of these patients may be found to have Crohn disease after follow-up.[66]

Another scenario involves patients who have no clinical symptoms but undergo screening colonoscopy and are incidentally found to have erosions or ulcers of the terminal ileum that have microscopically active and sometimes chronic ileitis. If NSAID use is excluded, these cases are properly diagnosed, tentatively, as *isolated asymptomatic ileitis* (IAI). Follow-up studies in such patients usually yielded no clinical consequence[66,67] unless the patients were symptomatic or had findings of concurrent chronic gastritis. But, in such a scenario, they do not qualify for the diagnosis of IAI in the first place because they are neither asymptomatic nor "isolated." To reiterate, if erosions or ulcers are identified in the terminal ileum during a screening colonoscopy for polyps in an otherwise-healthy adult, no concern is necessary clinically.

Infectious Enteritis and Colitis

Granulomatous ileitis is common in patients with tuberculosis (TB), histoplasmosis, and illness from other infectious organisms. Histologically, this may be difficult to distinguish from Crohn ileitis. However, a striking feature of TB is that there are usually prominent epithelioid and giant cell granulomas with central necrosis (caseating necrosis), which is rarely seen in granulomas of Crohn disease. Most important, in an endemic region and in patients at high risk for the infection, clinical history, exposure history, skin tests, radiographic findings, and microbiological tests will ultimately help sort out the possible etiologies and reaching the correct diagnosis. Using polymerase chain reaction testing to detect TB DNA from formalin-fixed, paraffin-embedded tissue specimens also has diagnostic value. Careful examination for fungal organisms, including special stains when a granulomatous lesion is encountered, shall easily help sort out the differential diagnosis, such as that of histoplasmosis.

Other infectious agents may also contribute to chronic, multifocal enteritis or colitis, such as *Schistosomiasis*, *Entamoeba histolytica*, and others. Again, correlation with clinical history and other laboratory studies should help with correct diagnosis.

Surveillance Biopsies for Dysplasia

Colonoscopic surveillance for dysplasia or cancer in CD patients is similar to that for patients with UC.[37,42,45,46,68-72] However, the value and practicality of endoscopic surveillance of the small bowel remains in question.

For surveillance biopsies obtained from the colon, dysplasia can be assessed using the morphologic features described previously,[37,40,44] and the diagnosis should be placed into the categories of negative for dysplasia, indefinite for dysplasia (IND), low-grade dysplasia, or high-grade dysplasia[73] (Figure 4-19). There is usually fair agreement among pathologists in recognizing high-grade dysplasia and specimens negative for dysplasia. Difficulty arises when lesions show features that are suspicious but not overtly diagnostic for dysplasia. For example, when active inflammation is present, there can be cytologic atypia that is reactive in nature but resembles dysplasia. Caution should be taken before a diagnosis of dysplasia is rendered. Sometimes it is not possible to either rule in or rule out dysplasia, and the most appropriate histologic diagnosis should be IND, with a suggestion to repeat the biopsy after treatment of active disease (within 6 months).

Occasionally, instead of typical changes of adenomatous dysplasia, the colonic mucosa may exhibit "unusual" cytologic or architectural changes, including dystrophic goblet cells and surface serrated changes. The former refers to goblet cells that are rounded with mucin droplet displacement to the subnuclear aspect (in contrast to the luminal aspect as in normal goblet cells). The latter refers to changes similar to sessile serrated polyps, with the superficial portion of some crypts showing a sawtoothed configuration. Seeing either of these patterns should prompt obtaining additional tissue sections because sometimes conventional dysplasia may be identified in the basal zone of these crypts. When definite dysplasia cannot be identified in deeper sections, my policy is to alert the clinician for a shorter interval of follow-up to avoid missing a nearby dysplasia or metachronous carcinoma, as the true nature of these lesions is currently unknown. Some authors will label these lesions as IND as well.[74]

In diagnostically challenging cases, some pathologists seek ancillary immunohistochemical stains to help with the assessment for dysplasia. It has been observed that in neoplastic transformation, the epithelial cells may show aberrant cytokeratin (CK) expression or an increase nuclear staining for p53 protein[75,76] (Figure 4-23). Normal colonic epithelium expresses CK20 but not CK7. This pattern is reversed in

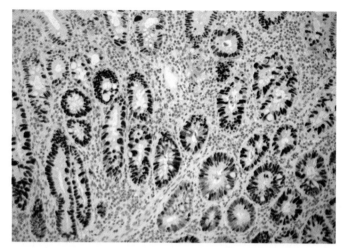

FIGURE 4-23. A focus of low-grade dysplasia with markedly increased nuclear stain for p53 (immunohistochemistry).

some dysplastic foci[69,77-79] (see also Chapter 27). In addition, the cellular proliferative index is often increased in dysplastic epithelium. This can be assessed using immunohistochemical staining for Ki-67. In nondysplastic, regenerative changes, increased Ki-67 nuclear staining is usually confined to the base of the crypts. When this expands to the middle or upper portion of the crypts, it is more likely to be associated with dysplasia. Therefore, when a final decision cannot be made regarding whether the suspicious focus is dysplastic or not, using a combination of these immunohistochemical stains may be helpful. However, it should be noted that the performance of these markers has not been subject to rigorous testing in terms of specificity and sensitivity. Blindly applying these markers without close correlation with hematoxylin and eosin (H&E) histology will likely be misleading. It should be emphasized that histologic evaluation based on a H&E stained section, when a consensus is reached among several expert GI pathologists, is the gold standard; the immunomarkers should only be used to either strengthen or weaken a wavering working diagnosis. In the context of this discussion, immunostains should not be used often, as only a small portion of cases may require this. For example, in a severely inflamed biopsy with features worrisome for dysplasia, a strong and diffuse p53 nuclear staining pattern would alert the pathologist to a diagnosis of dysplasia or at least prompt a consultation. Alternatively, in quiescent colitis without significant reactive changes, diffuse and strong CK7 immunoreactivity should also alert the pathologist to a diagnosis of dysplasia or at least prompt a consultation.

Some authors claim that patients with Crohn disease confined to the small intestine are not considered to have an increased risk for colon cancer, and therefore endoscopic surveillance should be similar to that for the general population. This view has been challenged as there is clearly a higher incidence of small-bowel adenocarcinomas directly arising from the small bowel involved by the disease, usually associated with thickened bowel wall or a stricture, as discussed previously, and colonic Crohn disease may be histologically subtle but still carry increased risk for colon cancer. However, the lack of microscopically identifiable classic dysplastic changes in many cases, and the difficulty in accessing the small bowel in routine procedures, diminishes the value of surveillance of the small intestine.[44] In this regard, recent advances in endoscopic technology, including video capsule endoscopy and double-balloon enteroscopy (DBE), may circumvent some of these challenges in the near future.[80-84]

Intraoperative Assessment for Adenocarcinoma in Strictureplasty or in Resections for Obstruction

Many small-bowel adenocarcinomas in patients with Crohn disease are identified incidentally during histologic examination of a stricture after resection, as described in the previous section. Therefore, frozen section is recommended for any suspected lesions during or after surgery to rule out carcinoma,[34] particularly during a strictureplasty procedure because no tissue would be obtained otherwise and potential carcinoma may be missed and left in the patient. In such a scenario, a biopsy is usually obtained from the stricture, processed for cryostat cutting (frozen section), and examined intraoperatively for dysplasia or carcinoma.[34]

Pathologic Evaluation of Resected Specimens

Most of the resected segments of small bowel will exhibit features of severe Crohn disease, with strictures, obstructions, thickened walls, fissuring ulcers, or sinus tract or fistula formation. It is desirable that the resection margins are without microscopic involvement by the disease. However, intraoperative evaluation of resection margin status is not necessary and not recommended because it is not related to frequency of disease recurrence.[85] The frequency depends more on the distribution of disease and preoperative response to medical treatment. Nevertheless, after examination of the fixed specimens, if a margin is involved by markedly active Crohn disease, it should be recorded and the surgeon notified. Any area with marked thickening or other questionable areas should be thoroughly processed for microscopic examination to rule out adenocarcinoma.

◼ REFERENCES

1. Oberhuber G, Hirsch M, Stolte M. High incidence of upper gastrointestinal tract involvement in Crohn's disease. *Virchows Arch.* 1998;432(1):49-52. PMID: 9463587.
2. Wright CL, Riddell RH. Histology of the stomach and duodenum in Crohn's disease. *Am J Surg Pathol.* 1998;22(4):383-390. PMID: 9537465.
3. Annunziata ML, Caviglia R, Papparella LG, Cicala M. Upper gastrointestinal involvement of Crohn's disease: a prospective study on the role of upper endoscopy in the diagnostic work-up. *Dig Dis Sci.* 2012;57(6):1618-1623. PMID: 22350786.
4. Lenaerts C, Roy CC, Vaillancourt M, Weber AM, Morin CL, Seidman E. High incidence of upper gastrointestinal tract involvement in children with Crohn disease. *Pediatrics.* 1989;83(5):777-781. PMID: 2717294.
5. Greenstein AJ, Mann D, Sachar DB, Aufses AH Jr. Free perforation in Crohn's disease: I. A survey of 99 cases. *Am J Gastroenterol.* 1985;80(9):682-689. PMID: 3898819.

6. Shoesmith JH, Tate GT, Wright CJ. Multiple strictures of the jejunum. *Gut.* 1964;5:132–135. PMID: 14159400.

7. Galandiuk S, Kimberling J, Al-Mishlab TG, Stromberg AJ. Perianal Crohn disease: predictors of need for permanent diversion. *Ann Surg.* 2005;241(5):796–801; discussion 801–802. PMID: 15849515. PMCID: 1357134.

8. Bousvaros A, Antonioli DA, Colletti RB, et al. Differentiating ulcerative colitis from Crohn disease in children and young adults: report of a working group of the North American Society for Pediatric Gastroenterology, Hepatology, and Nutrition and the Crohn's and Colitis Foundation of America. *J Pediatr Gastroenterol Nutr.* 2007;44(5): 653–674. PMID: 17460505.

9. Bearzi I, Ranaldi R. Small bowel adenocarcinoma and Crohn's disease: report of a case with differing histogenetic patterns. *Histopathology.* 1985;9(3):345–357. PMID: 3997089.

10. Petras RE, Mir-Madjlessi SH, Farmer RG. Crohn's disease and intestinal carcinoma. A report of 11 cases with emphasis on associated epithelial dysplasia. *Gastroenterology.* 1987;93(6):1307–1314. PMID: 2824276. Epub 1987/12/01. Eng.

11. Michelassi F, Testa G, Pomidor WJ, Lashner BA, Block GE. Adenocarcinoma complicating Crohn's disease. *Dis Colon Rectum.* 1993;36(7):654–661. PMID: 8348849.

12. Marchetti F, Fazio VW, Ozuner G. Adenocarcinoma arising from a strictureplasty site in Crohn's disease. Report of a case. *Dis Colon Rectum.* 1996;39(11):1315–1321. PMID: 8918446.

13. Dossett LA, White LM, Welch DC, et al. Small bowel adenocarcinoma complicating Crohn's disease: case series and review of the literature. *Am Surgeon.* 2007;73(11):1181–1187. PMID: 18092659.

14. Elriz K, Carrat F, Carbonnel F, Marthey L, Bouvier AM, Beaugerie L. Incidence, presentation, and prognosis of small bowel adenocarcinoma in patients with small bowel Crohn's disease: a prospective observational study. *Inflamm Bowel Dis.* 2013;19(9):1823–1826. PMID: 23702807. Epub 2013/05/25. Eng.

15. Whitcomb E, Liu X, Xiao SY. Crohn enteritis-associated small bowel adenocarcinomas exhibit gastric differentiation. *Hum Pathol.* 2014;45(2):359–367. PMID: 24331840.

16. Lewis RT, Bleier JI. Surgical treatment of anorectal Crohn disease. *Clin Colon Rectal Surg.* 2013;26(2):90–99. PMID: 24436656. PMCID: 3709961.

17. Saadah OI, Oliver MR, Bines JE, Stokes KB, Cameron DJ. Anorectal strictures and genital Crohn disease: an unusual clinical association. *J Pediatr Gastroenterol Nutr.* 2003;36(3):403–406. PMID: 12604983.

18. Shelley-Fraser G, Borley NR, Warren BF, Shepherd NA. The connective tissue changes of Crohn's disease. *Histopathology.* 2012;60(7): 1034–1044. PMID: 22008086.

19. Weinstein T, Valderrama E, Pettei M, Levine J. Esophageal Crohn's disease: medical management and correlation between clinical, endoscopic, and histologic features. *Inflamm Bowel Dis.* 1997;3(2):79–83. PMID: 23282748.

20. Geboes K, Janssens J, Rutgeerts P, Vantrappen G. Crohn's disease of the esophagus. *J Clin Gastroenterol.* 1986;8(1):31–37. PMID: 3701011.

21. Cosme A, Bujanda L, Arriola JA, Ojeda E. Esophageal Crohn's disease with esophagopleural fistula. *Endoscopy.* 1998;30(9):S109. PMID: 9932775.

22. Tobin JM, Sinha B, Ramani P, Saleh AR, Murphy MS. Upper gastrointestinal mucosal disease in pediatric Crohn disease and ulcerative colitis: a blinded, controlled study. *J Pediatr Gastroenterol Nutr.* 2001;32(4):443–448. PMID: 11396811.

23. Halme L, Karkkainen P, Rautelin H, Kosunen TU, Sipponen P. High frequency of *Helicobacter* negative gastritis in patients with Crohn's disease. *Gut.* 1996;38(3):379–383. PMID: 8675090. PMCID: 1383066.

24. Ormand JE, Talley NJ, Shorter RG, et al. Prevalence of *Helicobacter pylori* in specific forms of gastritis. Further evidence supporting a pathogenic role for *H. pylori* in chronic nonspecific gastritis. *Dig Dis Sci.* 1991;36(2):142–145. PMID: 1988256.

25. Danelius M, Ost A, Lapidus AB. Inflammatory bowel disease-related lesions in the duodenal and gastric mucosa. *Scand J Gastroenterol.* 2009;44(4):441–445. PMID: 19110988.

26. Sonnenberg A, Melton SD, Genta RM. Frequent occurrence of gastritis and duodenitis in patients with inflammatory bowel disease. *Inflamm Bowel Dis.* 2011;17(1):39–44. PMID: 20848539.

27. Oberhuber G, Puspok A, Oesterreicher C, et al. Focally enhanced gastritis: a frequent type of gastritis in patients with Crohn's disease. *Gastroenterology.* 1997;112(3):698–706. PMID: 9041230.

28. Weinstein WM. The diagnosis and classification of gastritis and duodenitis. *J Clin Gastroenterol.* 1981;3(Suppl 2):7–16. PMID: 7320471.

29. Schmidt-Sommerfeld E, Kirschner BS, Stephens JK. Endoscopic and histologic findings in the upper gastrointestinal tract of children with Crohn's disease. *J Pediatr Gastroenterol Nutr.* 1990;11(4):448–454. PMID: 2262833.

30. Shen B, Wu H, Remzi F, Lopez R, Shen L, Fazio V. Diagnostic value of esophagogastroduodenoscopy in patients with ileal pouch-anal anastomosis. *Inflamm Bowel Dis.* 2009;15(3):395–401. PMID: 18972552.

31. Freeman HJ. Spontaneous free perforation of the small intestine in Crohn's disease. *Can J Gastroenterol.* 2002;16(1):23–27. PMID: 11826334.

32. Tan WC, Allan RN. Diffuse jejunoileitis of Crohn's disease. *Gut.* 1993;34(10):1374–1378. PMID: 8244104.

33. Senay E, Sachar DB, Keohane M, Greenstein AJ. Small bowel carcinoma in Crohn's disease. Distinguishing features and risk factors. *Cancer.* 1989;63(2):360–363. PMID: 2910443.

34. Barwood N, Platell C. Case report: adenocarcinoma arising in a Crohn's stricture of the jejunum. *J Gastroenterol Hepatol.* 1999;14(11):1132–1134. PMID: 10574144.

35. Matsui T, Yao T, Sakurai T, et al. Clinical features and pattern of indeterminate colitis: Crohn's disease with ulcerative colitis-like clinical presentation. *J Gastroenterol.* 2003;38(7):647–655. PMID: 12898357.

36. Fichera A, McCormack R, Rubin MA, Hurst RD, Michelassi F. Long-term outcome of surgically treated Crohn's colitis: a prospective study. *Dis Colon Rectum.* 2005;48(5):963–969. PMID: 15785882.

37. Korelitz BI, Lauwers GY, Sommers SC. Rectal mucosal dysplasia in Crohn's disease. *Gut.* 1990;31(12):1382–1386. PMID: 2265778.

38. Watermeyer G, Locketz M, Govender D, Mall A. Crohn's disease-associated small bowel adenocarcinoma with pre-existing low-grade dysplasia: a case report. *Am J Gastroenterol.* 2007;102(7):1545–1546. PMID: 17593171.

39. Sigel JE, Petras RE, Lashner BA, Fazio VW, Goldblum JR. Intestinal adenocarcinoma in Crohn's disease: a report of 30 cases with a focus on coexisting dysplasia. *Am J Surg Pathol.* 1999;23(6):651–655. PMID: 10366146.

40. Cuvelier C, Bekaert E, De Potter C, Pauwels C, De Vos M, Roels H. Crohn's disease with adenocarcinoma and dysplasia. Macroscopical, histological, and immunohistochemical aspects of two cases. *Am J Surg Pathol.* 1989;13(3):187–196. PMID: 2465699.

41. Lutgens MW, Vleggaar FP, Schipper ME, et al. High frequency of early colorectal cancer in inflammatory bowel disease. *Gut.* 2008;57(9):1246–1251. PMID: 18337322.

42. Basseri RJ, Basseri B, Vassilaki ME, et al. Colorectal cancer screening and surveillance in Crohn's colitis. *J Crohn's Colitis.* 2012;6(8):824–829. PMID: 22398087.

43. Kiran RP, Khoury W, Church JM, Lavery IC, Fazio VW, Remzi FH. Colorectal cancer complicating inflammatory bowel disease: similarities and differences between Crohn's and ulcerative colitis based on three decades of experience. *Ann Surg.* 2012;252(2):330–335. PMID: 20622662.

44. Simpson S, Traube J, Riddell RH. The histologic appearance of dysplasia (precarcinomatous change) in Crohn's disease of the small and large intestine. *Gastroenterology.* 1981;81(3):492–501. PMID: 7250636.

45. Friedman S, Rubin PH, Bodian C, Harpaz N, Present DH. Screening and surveillance colonoscopy in chronic Crohn's colitis: results of a surveillance program spanning 25 years. *Clin Gastroenterol Hepatol.* 2008;6(9):993–998; quiz 53–54. PMID: 18585966.

46. Baumgart DC. Endoscopic surveillance in Crohn's disease and ulcerative colitis: who needs what and when? *Dig Dis.* 2011;29(Suppl 1):32–35. PMID: 22104750.

47. Fleming KA, Pollock AC. A case of "Crohn's carcinoma." *Gut*. 1975; 16(7):533–537. PMID: 1158190.

48. Palascak-Juif V, Bouvier AM, Cosnes J, et al. Small bowel adenocarcinoma in patients with Crohn's disease compared with small bowel adenocarcinoma de novo. *Inflamm Bowel Dis*. 2005;11(9):828–832. PMID: 16116317.

49. Whitcomb E, Liu X, Xiao S-Y. Crohn's-associated small bowel adenocarcinomas exhibit gastric differentiation. *Mod Pathol*. 2013; 26(Suppl 2):187A.

50. Hummel TZ, ten Kate FJ, Reitsma JB, Benninga MA, Kindermann A. Additional value of upper GI tract endoscopy in the diagnostic assessment of childhood IBD. *J Pediatr Gastroenterol Nutr*. 2012;54(6): 753–757. PMID: 22584746.

51. Haskell H, Andrews CW Jr, Reddy SI, et al. Pathologic features and clinical significance of "backwash" ileitis in ulcerative colitis. *Am J Surg Pathol*. 2005;29(11):1472–1481. PMID: 16224214.

52. Valdez R, Appelman HD, Bronner MP, Greenson JK. Diffuse duodenitis associated with ulcerative colitis. *Am J Surg Pathol*. 2000; 24(10):1407–1413. PMID: 11023103.

53. Korelitz BI, Rajapakse R. Ulcerative duodenitis with ulcerative colitis: is it Crohn's disease or really ulcerative colitis? *J Clin Gastroenterol*. 2001;32(2):97. PMID: 11205662.

54. Terashima S, Hoshino Y, Kanzaki N, Kogure M, Gotoh M. Ulcerative duodenitis accompanying ulcerative colitis. *J Clin Gastroenterol*. 2001;32(2):172–175. PMID: 11205658.

55. Ikeuchi H, Hori K, Nishigami T, et al. Diffuse gastroduodenitis and pouchitis associated with ulcerative colitis. *World J Gastroenterol*. 2006;12(36):5913–5915. PMID: 17007066.

56. Hisabe T, Matsui T, Miyaoka M, et al. Diagnosis and clinical course of ulcerative gastroduodenal lesion associated with ulcerative colitis: possible relationship with pouchitis. *Dig Endosc*. 2010;22(4):268–274. PMID: 21175478.

57. Lin J, McKenna BJ, Appelman HD. Morphologic findings in upper gastrointestinal biopsies of patients with ulcerative colitis: a controlled study. *Am J Surg Pathol*. 2010;34(11):1672–1677. PMID: 20962621.

58. Corporaal S, Karrenbeld A, van der Linde K, Voskuil JH, Kleibeuker JH, Dijkstra G. Diffuse enteritis after colectomy for ulcerative colitis: two case reports and review of the literature. *Eur J Gastroenterol Hepatol*. 2009;21(6):710–715. PMID: 19282770.

59. Fries JF, Williams CA, Bloch DA, Michel BA. Nonsteroidal anti-inflammatory drug-associated gastropathy: incidence and risk factor models. *Am J Med*. 1991;91(3):213–222. PMID: 1892140.

60. Xiao SY, Zhao L, Hart J, Semrad CE. Gastric mucosal necrosis with vascular degeneration induced by doxycycline. *Am J Surg Pathol*. 2013; 37(2):259–263. PMID: 23060354.

61. Borody TJ, George LL, Brandl S, et al. *Helicobacter pylori*-negative duodenal ulcer. *Am J Gastroenterol*. 1991;86(9):1154–1157. PMID: 1882793.

62. Goldstein NS, Cinenza AN. The histopathology of nonsteroidal anti-inflammatory drug-associated colitis. *Am J Clin Pathol*. 1998;110(5): 622–628. PMID: 9802347.

63. Sidhu R, Brunt LK, Morley SR, Sanders DS, McAlindon ME. Undisclosed use of nonsteroidal anti-inflammatory drugs may underlie small-bowel injury observed by capsule endoscopy. *Clin Gastroenterol Hepatol*. 2010;8(11):992–995. PMID: 20692369.

64. Di Perna CD, Vanni S, Allegri L, Manganelli P, Buzio C. Severe glomerulonephritis and isolated ileitis in adult Henoch-Schoenlein purpura. *Clin Nephrol*. 2001;56(6):487–489. PMID: 11770802.

65. Kotler DP, Baer JW, Scholes JV. Isolated ileitis due to cytomegalovirus in a patient with AIDS. *Gastrointest Endosc*. 1991;37(5):571–574. PMID: 1657681.

66. Courville EL, Siegel CA, Vay T, Wilcox AR, Suriawinata AA, Srivastava A. Isolated asymptomatic ileitis does not progress to overt Crohn disease on long-term follow-up despite features of chronicity in ileal biopsies. *Am J Surg Pathol*. 2009;33(9):1341–1347. PMID: 19606015.

67. Petrolla AA, Katz JA, Xin W. The clinical significance of focal enhanced gastritis in adults with isolated ileitis of the terminal ileum. *J Gastroenterol*. 2008;43(7):524–530. PMID: 18648739.

68. Jess T, Loftus EV Jr, Velayos FS, et al. Incidence and prognosis of colorectal dysplasia in inflammatory bowel disease: a population-based study from Olmsted County, Minnesota. *Inflamm Bowel Dis*. 2006;12(8):669–676. PMID: 16917220.

69. Levi GS, Harpaz N. Intestinal low-grade tubuloglandular adenocarcinoma in inflammatory bowel disease. *Am J Surg Pathol*. 2006;30(8):1022–1029. PMID: 16861975.

70. Katsanos KH, Vermeire S, Christodoulou DK, et al. Dysplasia and cancer in inflammatory bowel disease 10 years after diagnosis: results of a population-based European collaborative follow-up study. *Digestion*. 2007;75(2–3):113–121. PMID: 17598963.

71. Ullman T, Odze R, Farraye FA. Diagnosis and management of dysplasia in patients with ulcerative colitis and Crohn's disease of the colon. *Inflamm Bowel Dis*. 2009;15(4):630–638. PMID: 18942763.

72. van Schaik FD, Offerhaus GJ, Schipper ME, Siersema PD, Vleggaar FP, Oldenburg B. Endoscopic and pathological aspects of colitis-associated dysplasia. *Nat Rev Gastroenterol Hepatol*. 2009;6(11):671–678. PMID: 19770847.

73. Riddell RH, Goldman H, Ransohoff DF, Appelman HD, Fenoglio CM, Haggitt RC, et al. Dysplasia in inflammatory bowel disease: standardized classification with provisional clinical applications. *Hum Pathol*. 1983;14(11):931–968. PMID: 6629368.

74. Fenoglio-Preiser CM, Noffsinger AE, Stemmermann GN, Lantz PE, Isaacson PG. *Gastrointestinal Pathology. An Atlas and Text*. 3rd ed. New York, NY: Lippincott Williams & Wilkins; 2008.

75. Walsh SV, Loda M, Torres CM, Antonioli D, Odze RD. P53 and beta catenin expression in chronic ulcerative colitis—associated polypoid dysplasia and sporadic adenomas: an immunohistochemical study. *Am J Surg Pathol*. 1999;23(8):963–969. PMID: 10435567.

76. Marx A, Wandrey T, Simon P, et al. Combined alpha-methylacyl coenzyme A racemase/p53 analysis to identify dysplasia in inflammatory bowel disease. *Hum Pathol*. 2009;40(2):166–173. PMID: 18835622.

77. Tatsumi N, Kushima R, Vieth M, et al. Cytokeratin 7/20 and mucin core protein expression in ulcerative colitis-associated colorectal neoplasms. *Virchows Arch*. 2006;448(6):756–762. PMID: 16609910.

78. Stenling R, Lindberg J, Rutegard J, Palmqvist R. Altered expression of CK7 and CK20 in preneoplastic and neoplastic lesions in ulcerative colitis. *APMIS*. 2007;115(11):1219–1226. PMID: 18092953.

79. Jiang W, Shadrach B, Carver P, Goldblum JR, Shen B, Liu X. Histomorphologic and molecular features of pouch and peripouch adenocarcinoma: a comparison with ulcerative colitis-associated adenocarcinoma. *Am J Surg Pathol*. 2012;36(9):1385–1394. PMID: 22895272.

80. Su MY, Liu NJ, Hsu CM, Chiu CT, Chen PC, Lin CJ. Double balloon enteroscopy—the last blind-point of the gastrointestinal tract. *Dig Dis Sci*. 2005;50(6):1041–1045. PMID: 15986851.

81. Ang D, Luman W, Ooi CJ. Early experience with double balloon enteroscopy: a leap forward for the gastroenterologist. *Singapore Med J*. 2007;48(1):50–60. PMID: 17245517.

82. Kopacova M, Bures J, Vykouril L, et al. Intraoperative enteroscopy: ten years' experience at a single tertiary center. *Surg Endosc*. 2007; 21(7):1111–1116. PMID: 17103268.

83. Chermesh I, Eliakim R. Capsule endoscopy in Crohn's disease—indications and reservations 2008. *J Crohn's Colitis*. 2008;2(2):107–113. PMID: 21172200.

84. Fritscher-Ravens A, Scherbakov P, Bufler P, et al. The feasibility of wireless capsule endoscopy in detecting small intestinal pathology in children under the age of 8 years: a multicentre European study. *Gut*. 2009;58(11):1467–1472. PMID: 19625281.

85. Yamamoto T. Factors affecting recurrence after surgery for Crohn's disease. *World J Gastroenterol*. 2005;11(26):3971–3979. PMID: 15996018.

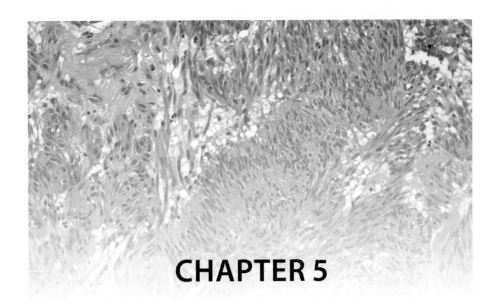

CHAPTER 5

Gastrointestinal Stromal Tumors and Other Mesenchymal Tumors

Lei Zhao and Shu-Yuan Xiao

INTRODUCTION

A gastrointestinal stromal tumor (GIST) is the most commonly encountered mesenchymal tumor of the gastrointestinal (GI) tract. It occurs in all segments of the GI tract and may also occur in the omentum, mesentery, or retroperitoneum as extragastrointestinal GISTs (EGISTs), although some of these are metastases or direct invasion from a GI primary tumor.[1,2] The main diagnostic concern is its distinction from other mesenchymal tumors, including those of smooth muscle, nerve, and fibrovascular origin. There is significant morphological overlap among these tumors; thus, immunostains are usually required for diagnosis. The secondary concern is delineating the underlying mutational status of a tumor, which is related to its response to treatment and biological behavior. The third concern is to recognize features of familial and syndromic GISTs to initiate appropriate genetic counseling and testing.

INTRODUCTION AND CLINICAL FEATURES

A GIST is encountered equally in both genders. Most tumors occur in adults but rare cases occur in children. Historically, the cellular lineage or differentiation was obscure due to aberrant or overlapping morphological and immunohistochemical (IHC) features between neural and muscular phenotypes.

However, it became evident by electron microscopy that most of them lack features of these cell types.[3] Therefore, the generic term *gastrointestinal stromal tumor* was coined,[4] with a suggested link to the interstitial cells of Cajal (ICC) based on cytologic similarities. In 1998, mutations in the receptor tyrosine kinase *KIT* gene were discovered as the underlying genetic abnormality.[5,6] This led to application of a specific IHC marker for tissue diagnosis of GISTs, namely, c-kit, or CD117 (product of the *KIT* gene), and the development of targeted therapy using the kinase inhibitor imatinib (Gleevec®) as standard care for patients with an unresectable, recurrent, or metastatic GIST.

A GIST is encountered in the stomach, small bowel, colon, and esophagus in decreasing frequency. In general, patients present with early satiety, GI bleeding, or fatigue, but signs and symptoms in patients are usually related to the specific location of the tumor. Small-bowel GISTs usually present with GI bleeding. Rarely, spontaneous rupture of a "giant" GIST may cause acute abdomen with hemoperitoneum. Currently, many GISTs, particularly the small-bowel GISTs (about 18% of cases), are discovered incidentally when a patient undergoes image studies or endoscopic examination for other indications.[7]

Most GISTs are sporadic, but some (<5%) may occur in a familial setting or as part of a syndrome, with autosomal dominant inheritance. Patients with neurofibromatosis type I have increased risk of developing GISTs, mostly of the small intestine.[8–10] Epithelioid gastric GISTs occur as part of the Carney triad (CT), which in addition includes paraganglioma and pulmonary chondromas,[11] or Carney-Stratakis syndrome.[12,13] Some kindreds of primary familial GIST syndrome have been reported.[14] In contrast to sporadic tumors, GISTs in Carney-Stratakis syndrome mostly occur in female and younger patients, almost exclusively in the stomach, and may be associated with lymph node metastasis.[13,15,16]

Not uncommonly, occult, microscopic GISTs can be identified, often incidentally, particularly in the elderly.[17–19] These "seedling" GISTs are more commonly found in the stomach and gastroesophageal junction and harbor similar *KIT* mutations as more advanced tumors.

PATHOGENESIS AND GENETIC MUTATIONS

A GIST arises from the ICC or their progenitors, mostly through a gain-of-function mutation in the receptor tyrosine kinase *KIT* gene (in 80% to 95% of cases). A small subset of tumors exhibit mutation in a related gene, platelet-derived growth factor receptor α (PDGFRA).[20] These are nongermline mutations except for the rare familial or syndromic cases. These "driving" mutations lead to constitutively activated downstream signal transduction pathways, with associated activation of signaling intermediates protein kinase B (AKT), mitogen-activated protein kinase (MAPK), and the STAT (signal transducers and activators of transcription) proteins STAT1 and STAT3.[20,21]

Overall, about 10% to 15% of GISTs occurring in adult patients are wild type (wt) for both *KIT* and PDGFRA, as are most pediatric cases. By studying GISTs occurring in Carney-Stratakis syndrome, germline loss-of-function mutations of genes encoding the succinate dehydrogenase (SDH) subunits B, C, or D had been identified,[13,22] as inspired by findings in familial paraganglioma. Further studies identified that a significant proportion of *KIT*-wt and PDGFRA-wt GISTs not associated with paragangliomas also harbor these mutations (in about 12% of cases studied).[23] In addition, loss-of-function germline mutations of the SDHA gene were identified in 2 pediatric GISTs by using a "massively parallel sequencing approach,"[24] a finding confirmed by additional studies.[25,26] Another interesting observation is overexpression of insulin-like growth factor 1 receptor (IGF1R) in some tumors, which are all SDH deficiency associated.[27,28]

Familial hereditary GISTs are characterized by germline mutations of *KIT* or PDGFRA. For example, a p.L576P mutation in *KIT* exon 11 was identified in a familial juvenile-onset GIST kindred, which is characterized by multiple GISTs, skin hyperpigmentation, and esophageal stenosis.[14]

PATHOLOGIC FEATURES AND HISTOLOGIC DIAGNOSIS

A GIST usually manifests as a well-circumscribed mural mass (Figure 5-1) or a mucosal nodule protruding to the lumen (Figure 5-2), which may be accompanied by mucosal

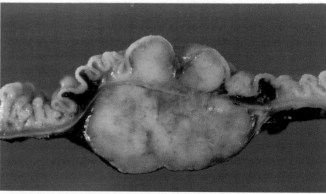

FIGURE 5-1. A small-bowel gastrointestinal stromal tumor as a well-demarcated intramural mass extending into the submucosa in a dumbbell configuration, with a "fleshy" tan, homogeneous cut surface. (Used with permission of Dr. John Hart.)

necrosis and ulceration. The cut surface of a GIST exhibits the generic flesh-colored appearance of a mesenchymal tumor, with a solid texture or focal cystic change when there is necrosis or degeneration (Figure 5-3).

Microscopically, GISTs are composed of spindle cells (Figure 5-4), epithelioid cells, or a mixture of the two types. The cells usually exhibit a "bland" cytology, with abundant fine-granular eosinophilic cytoplasm, elongated nuclei with inconspicuous nucleolus, and fine chromatin (Figure 5-5). Gastric GISTs have a higher tendency for epithelioid morphology (Figure 5-6). Compared to tumors of other sites, there is a higher frequency of PDGFRA mutation or SDH mutation among *KIT*-wt gastric GISTs. More so in small-bowel tumors, a characteristic "skeinoid" fiber can be identified, in the form of dense, elongated hyaline

FIGURE 5-2. A gastric GIST as a mass protruding into the lumen and covered by mucosa, with a central ulcer.

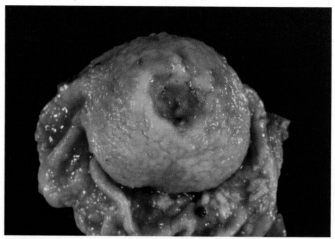

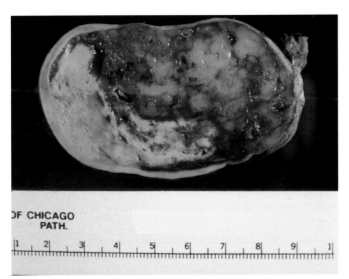

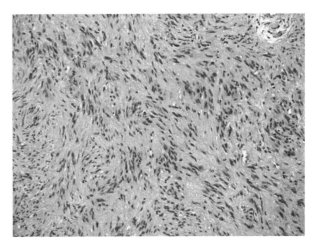

FIGURE 5-5. Small-bowel GIST of spindle cell type. The tumor is bland cytologically, with cells containing fine, granular eosinophilic cytoplasm and small nuclei without atypia.

FIGURE 5-3. A malignant gastrointestinal stromal tumor of the stomach from a 57-year-old man. The mass is well circumscribed, with a tan, hemorrhagic, mottled cut surface consistent with intratumoral necrosis.

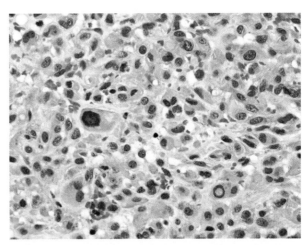

structures (Figure 5-7). GISTs arising from the small bowel are mostly of the spindle cell type, with about 10% of mixed and 5% of epithelioid type.[7] The last tend to be associated malignant features.[7]

The ideal treatment for a localized GIST is complete resection with a clear margin. In patients with proper clinical history and characteristic radiologic findings of a submucosal or mural mass lesion suggestive of GISTs, resections may be performed without a preoperative histologic diagnosis. The final diagnosis is reached by examining the resected specimens, which have the added benefit of ample fresh tissue for mutational analysis. However, in patients with focally

FIGURE 5-6. A gastric GIST with predominantly epithelioid component. Many of the tumor cells contain abundant eosinophilic cytoplasm with an eccentrically located nucleus. There are also occasional binucleated cells and rare cells with an enlarged nucleus.

FIGURE 5-4. Gastric GIST consisting of spindle cells, with focal nuclear palisading and prominent cytoplasmic vacuolization.

FIGURE 5-7. Small-bowel GIST with thick, hyalinized structures, designated "skeinoid" fibers.

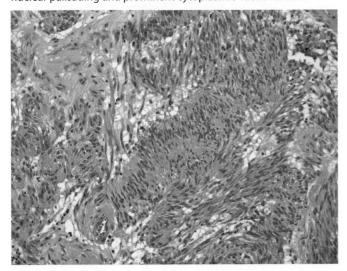

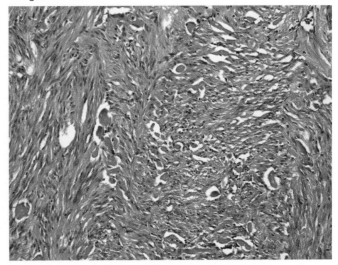

advanced tumors or metastases, effort should be made to reach a definitive diagnosis because of highly effective targeted therapy. One approach is the core needle biopsy guided by endoscopic ultrasound (EUS) (Figure 5-8). EUS-guided fine-needle aspiration (FNA) is also frequently performed and will likely yield sufficient material for IHC stains to reach a definitive diagnosis. However, a drawback of this practice is insufficient tissue for mutational analysis.

Microscopic examination of a biopsied or resected specimen usually demonstrates a characteristic histologic appearance as described. However, the definitive diagnosis cannot be made without IHC study. Certain unique features, if present, may suggest other types of mesenchymal tumors that occur at these sites, leading to a list of possible differential diagnoses (discussed in the section on differential diagnosis). A proper panel of immunostains should be performed (see next section).

FIGURE 5-8. Endoscopic ultrasound-guided needle biopsy of an esophageal mass, demonstrating long, slender spindle tumor cells (**A**) that are diffusely positive for CD117 (**B**) and negative for smooth muscle markers.

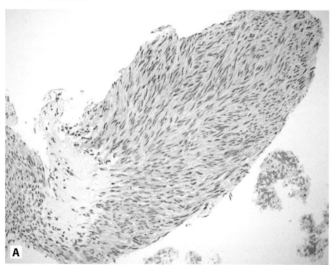

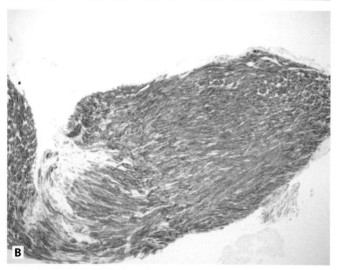

■ IMMUNOHISTOCHEMICAL MARKERS

Several markers had been extensively studied and been described as specific for GIST, but only CD117 has been routinely used in most laboratories. It is positive in most GISTs, including *KIT*-mutated and *KIT*-wt, with both membranous and cytoplasmic staining patterns (Figure 5-9). A dot pattern had been suggested to be prominent in *KIT*-mutated tumors and had been compared to the immunostaining pattern for PDGFRA to predict the underlying mutational status. However, this observation lacks sufficient specificity. As mutational analyses have become routine tests for GISTs, such an attempt to predict mutational status by IHC pattern has become unnecessary and obsolete.

Lack of CD117 immunoreactivity is seen in 5% to 15% of GISTs and 24% of *KIT*-wt tumors (Table 5-1). Using gene expression profiling, West et al in 2004 identified overexpression of a protein, referred to as *discovered on GIST-1* (DOG-1),[29,30] which can be detected immunohistochemically using a rabbit antiserum against the corresponding synthetic peptide. The staining pattern of DOG-1 is usually cytoplasmic or membranous (Figure 5-10). It has been recognized that DOG-1 is a calcium-regulated chloride channel protein,[31,32] encoded by a gene on chromosome 11q13 (other names for the gene are TMEM16A and ORAOV2). In one series,[30] the sensitivity of the antibody clone DOG-1.1 is slightly higher than CD117, although another study showed similar sensitivity for DOG-1 and CD117 (94.4% and 94.7%, respectively). More importantly, DOG-1 is expressed in about 36% of tumors negative for CD117, in all tested cases of GISTs associated with neurofibromatosis 1 (NF1), and in most pediatric GISTs.[33] It should be noted that, overall, still some 2.6% of GISTs are negative for both DOG-1 and CD117.[34]

With a significant proportion of GISTs showing overlap positivity for CD117 and DOG-1, why is it necessary to

FIGURE 5-9. Immunostaining for CD117 of a gastric GIST showing diffuse strong cytoplasmic positivity.

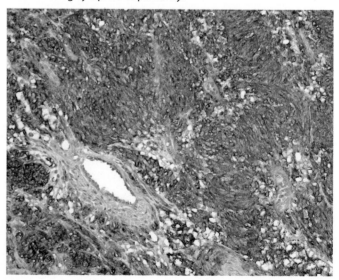

TABLE 5-1. Some features associated with CD117 and DOG-1 immunoreactivity.[a]

GISTs with *KIT* or PDGFRA mutation (overall)	85–90%
GISTs in adult without *KIT* or PDGFRA mutation	10–15%
GISTs in children without *KIT* or PDGFRA mutation	85%
IHC positivity for CD117 (overall)	95%
IHC positivity for DOG-1 (overall)	95%
KIT-mutated GIST	100%
Pediatric GIST	82%
NF1-associated GIST	100%
KIT-wt GIST	36%
PDGFRA-mutated GIST	
IHC positive for CD117	27%
IHC positive for DOG-1	79%

Abbreviations: GIST, gastrointestinal stromal tumor; IHC, immunohistochemical; *NF1*, neurofibromin 1; PDGFRA, platelet-derived growth factor receptor α; wt, wild type.

[a]Data based on multiple studies.[30,33]

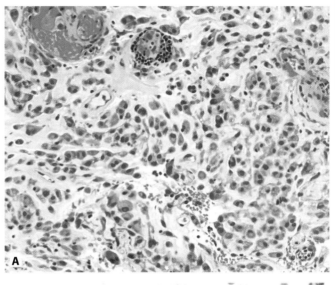

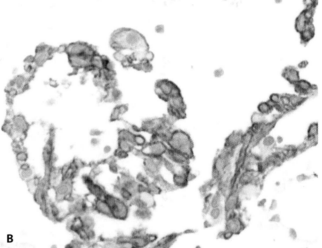

use both markers? The added values of DOG-1 are multiple. First, more than one-third of CD117-negative GISTs can be picked up by positive DOG-1 stain (Figure 5-11). One study showed that 9 of 10 CD117-negative abdominal epithelioid GISTs were positive for DOG-1.[35] Second, some GISTs lose CD117 expression after treatment, making DOG-1 the only positive marker in these cases. Third, several cell types (eg, mast cells, melanocytes, and germ cells) that are not part of a GIST may be positive for CD117 and render a confusing IHC result. These cells are, however, negative for DOG-1. Therefore, adding DOG-1 helps reduce these potentially misleading results and improves the diagnostic specificity. Focal

FIGURE 5-11. A GIST that is negative for CD117 but positive for DOG-1 (discovered on GIST-1). This 8.2-cm gastric mass was from the pre-DOG-1 period. Microscopically, the tumor is mostly epithelioid (**A**). Lack of CD117 staining made the diagnosis difficult. Electron microscopic studies were performed. Mutational analysis showed PDGFRA exon 18 mutation. Subsequently, immunostaining for DOG-1 was performed and showed diffuse positivity (**B**).

FIGURE 5-10. Immunostaining for DOG-1 of an epithelioid gastrointestinal stromal tumor showing strong cytoplasmic positivity with membrane accentuation.

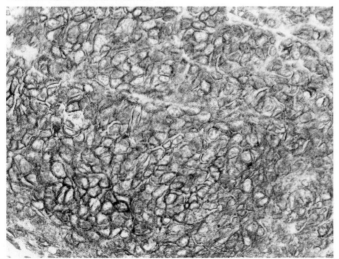

nonspecific staining for CD117 may occur in needle biopsies of other types of tumors; adding DOG-1 in the panel can reduce the risk of an erroneous diagnosis (Figure 5-12). Other tumors, such as uterine-type leiomyomas, synovial sarcomas, and esophageal squamous cell carcinomas, may be focally DOG-1 positive.[34]

Although nonspecific, a significant proportion of GISTs are also positive for CD34; a minority show focal staining for S100, α-smooth muscle actin (SMA), or even desmin. The last may partially be attributed to intermixed or entrapped "native" muscle bundles not uncommonly seen in this tumor. Rare gastric GISTs express synaptophysin as well, particularly in the epithelioid component.

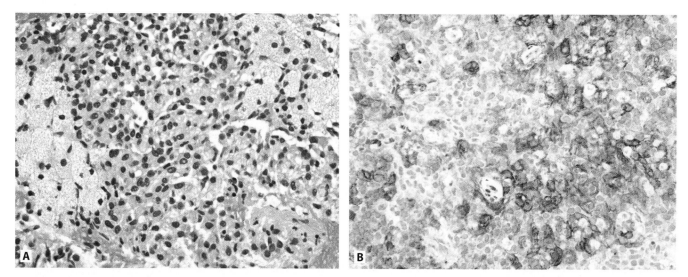

FIGURE 5-12. Needle core biopsy of a large mesenteric mass, a large Schwannoma (**A**), that focally stained positive for CD117 (**B**) but negative for DOG-1 (discovered on GIST-1). Repeat staining on the resected specimen was negative for CD117.

More recently, it had become evident that GISTs in Carney-Stratakis syndrome (Figure 5-13) may exhibit loss of or reduced staining for SDHB (Figure 5-14). Negative or weak staining for SDHB seems to reliably predict mutations of SDHB, SDHC, or SDHD,[36] which can be used to screen patients for further mutational analysis for these genes.[23,37] When negative staining occurs in sporadic GISTs in adults, the tumors usually have morphologic and clinical features

FIGURE 5-13. Gastric GIST from a 17-year-old boy who had a mediastinal paraganglioma and other features of Carney-Stratakis syndrome. The tumor was multifocal in the stomach wall (**A**) with liver metastasis. Tumor cells exhibit plump spindle to epithelioid morphology (**B**), which were immunohistochemically positive for CD117 (**C**), CD34, and DOG-1 (not shown) and completely negative for succinate dehydrogenase (SDH) A (**D**) and SDH B (**E**).

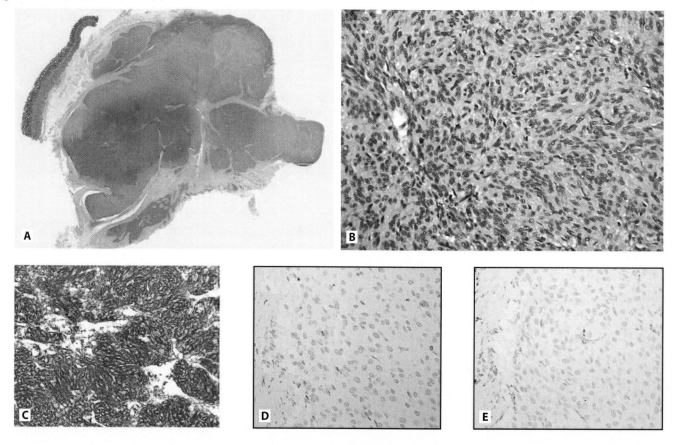

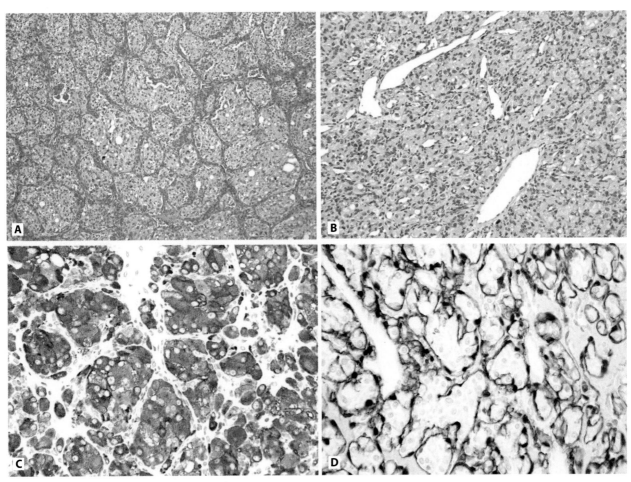

FIGURE 5-14. A mediastinal paraganglioma occurring in the same patient as Figure 5-13. The tumor cells are polygonal to oval and are arranged in nests of cell balls or islands (Zellballen pattern), surrounded by fibrous stroma (**A**, **B**), which contain small, spindle-shaped sustentacular cells. The tumor cells are highlighted by immunostaining for synaptophysin (**C**); immunostaining for S100 highlights the sustentacular cells (**D**).

similar to the pediatric and CSS-type GISTs (Table 5-2). Based on their findings, Gill et al suggested the term *type 2 GIST* (SDHB negative), which accounts for about 3% of all adult GISTs.[37] A significant portion (12%) of *KIT*-wt GISTs in patients without a personal or family history of paraganglioma have germline mutations in SDHB or SDHC. Therefore, it has been recommended that mutational tests be performed.[23] Gastric GISTs with loss of SDHB mostly include cases of younger patient age, female predominance (2:1), with frequent peritoneal and liver metastases, lymphovascular invasion, or lymph node metastases.[38,39] Between 28%[40] and 30%[26] of SDHB-negative gastric GISTs are SDHA deficient. All the SDHA-negative tumors carry an SDHA mutation and no other SDH subunit mutations, indicating that SDHB immunostaining may help identify cases with SDHA mutations as well.[40]

Another interesting observation that may have relevance in differential diagnoses is the overexpression of IGF1R in SDHB-negative GISTs. Immunohistochemically, expression of IGF1R is detected in a vast majority of SDH-deficient GISTs but not SDHB-positive gastric GISTs. A study of more

than 370 intestinal GISTs showed them to be negative for IGF1R, as opposed to other intestinal sarcomas (clear cell sarcoma, leiomyosarcoma, and undifferentiated sarcoma).[41]

■ DIFFERENTIAL DIAGNOSIS

Other non-GIST mesenchymal tumors may be distinguishable from GISTs based on histomorphology. In addition, with the immunomarkers of relative GIST specificity mentioned (in an appropriate context) and other markers, there is usually no difficulty in reaching a correct diagnosis. In our practice, an IHC panel, including CD117, DOG-1, desmin, SMA, and S100, is used in the initial workup.

Leiomyoma

Although most commonly seen in the esophagus, leiomyoma is also commonly seen in the anorectum and, to a lesser degree, the colon. It usually manifests at a younger age (median 30–35 years of age). We usually employ an IHC panel consisting of SMA, desmin, CD117, DOG-1, S100,

TABLE 5-2. Highlights of gastrointestinal stromal tumors (GISTs) occurring in different clinical backgrounds.

Scenario (clinical background)	Genetic abnormality	Clinical features	Site	Pathologic uniqueness	IHC
Sporadic	Somatic mutation in KIT or PDGFRA	No particular trend	Usual	Usual	CD117, DOG-1
Neurofibromatosis type 1 (NF1)	wt KIT or PDGFRA	Affects all age groups, but median age a decade younger than the sporadic	Small bowel	Multiple to numerous; spindle cell, low mitosis	CD117 90%
Carney-Stratakis syndrome (CSS)	Germline mutation in SDH subunit B, C, or D	Affects young women; usually does not respond to imatinib but may respond to sunitib	Stomach, mostly antrum	Multifocal, epithelioid; frequent metastasis, particularly lymph node; ICC hyperplasia	CD117, PDGFRA; loss of SDH subunit proteins
Primary familial GIST syndrome	Autosomal dominant, germline mutation in KIT or PDGFRA	Juvenile onset, other abnormalities		Multifocal	CD117, DOG-1
Pediatric[a] or young adult GIST	KIT or PDGFRA mutation in less than 15%; some with mutation in SDH B, C, or rarely A	Usually does not respond to imatinib but to second-generation kinase inhibitors such as sunitib	Gastric, small intestine	Epithelioid	Loss of SDH subunit proteins; insulin-like growth factor receptor 1
Other wt GIST with no history of paraganglioma	12% germline mutation in SDHB or SDHC, rarely SDH A; 7% adult wt GIST had BRAF mutation	Similar to the above	Gastric predilection; small bowel predilection for BRAF mutated	Epithelioid for gastric; spindle for small bowel tumor	CD117, DOG-1, loss of SDH

Abbreviations: DOG-1, discovered on GIST-1; ICC, interstitial cells of Cajal; IHC, immunohistochemical; PDGFRA, platelet-derived growth factor receptor α; SDH, succinate dehydrogenase; wt, wild type

[a]Studies targeting pediatric GIST likely included a significant proportion of syndromic cases, thus with features overlapping with other groups on this list.

and CD34. Occasionally, a small spindle cell tumor may exhibit focal positive stains for both GIST and leiomyoma markers (Figure 5-15). Careful examination reveals that this represents an evolving GIST with entrapped intratumoral smooth muscle bundles (Figure 5-15). With a quick assumption and immunostaining for a smooth muscle marker for confirmation, this tumor may be mistakenly diagnosed as leiomyoma. In contrast, it should be noted that scattered CD117-positive ICCs may be seen in an otherwise-typical leiomyoma (Figure 5-16).

Gangliocytic Paraganglioma

Gangliocytic paragangliomas (GPGs) are uncommon tumors almost always found in the second portion of the duodenum, and they are mostly benign. Rare cases with lymph node metastasis have been described, but some of the reported cases may in fact have been endocrine tumors. Occasionally, it is associated with von Recklinghausen syndrome (neurofibromatosis type 1). Microscopically, the tumor is characterized by endocrine cells arranged in nests and trabeculae in an organoid pattern, with isolated ganglion cells and Schwann or sustentacular cells (Figure 5-17). Immunohistochemically, the endocrine cells exhibit strong reactivity for synaptophysin, and the spindle Schwann cells do the same for S100. The tumor can be readily differentiated from a GIST

with the help of IHC staining; it is positive for synaptophysin (Figure 5-17) and negative for CD117 and DOG-1.

Schwannoma

Many spindle cell GISTs may exhibit focal microscopic features of Schwannoma, a benign peripheral nerve sheath tumor. True Schwannomas can occur in the GI tract (Figure 5-18). These tumors are usually encapsulated and solitary and demonstrate typical features of the usual cellular Antoni A (nuclear palisading, or Verocay bodies–organoid) (Figure 5-18A) and hypocellular Antoni B areas. Rarely, they have epithelioid areas. The typical IHC profile includes diffuse nuclear positivity for S100 and sometimes glial fibrillary acid protein (GFAP) (Figure 5-19). Most GI Schwannomas also exhibit a characteristic histologic feature of peripheral lymphoid "cuffing" (Figure 5-18B), which is specific for the diagnosis when present. In addition, GI schwannomas may be nonencapsulated, and with only vague palisading, and lack hyalinized blood vessels.

As mentioned, because a GIST can present as an abdominal mass involving the omentum, mesentery, or retroperitoneal compartment, several other entities will enter the differential list, including an inflammatory myofibroblastic tumor (IMT), mesenteric fibromatosis, liposarcoma, and metastatic carcinoma.

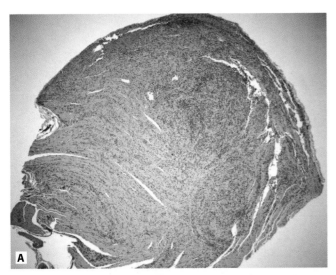

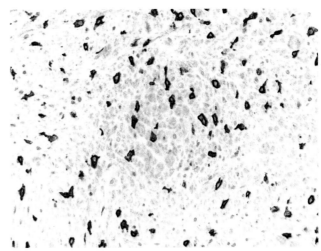

FIGURE 5-16. A gastric leiomyoma with abundant scattered CD117⁺ interstitial cells. Many of these cells are negative for DOG-1 (discovered on GIST-1; not shown), indicating that they are mast cells instead of interstitial cells of Cajal.

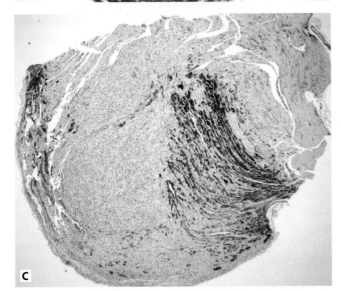

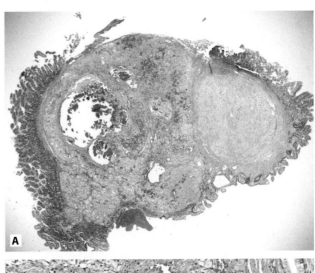

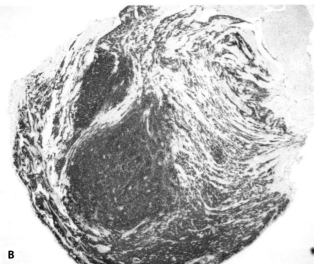

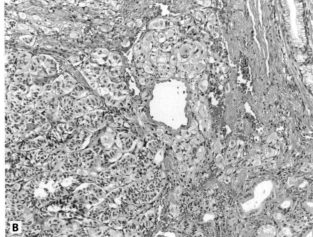

FIGURE 5-15. A small stomach GIST with entrapped native smooth muscle bundles (**A**). While the tumor is mainly positive for CD117 (**B**), focal bundles and strands of muscle cells are high-lighted by α-smooth muscle actin (SMA) (**C**), which may otherwise be interpreted as a GIST positive for both CD117 and SMA.

FIGURE 5-17. Gangliocytic paraganglioma. **A.** This duodenal tumor consists mainly of epithelioid endocrine cells forming a rib-bon, pseudoglands, and nests and another component of spindle cells and ganglion cells. **B.** High-power view of the gangliocytic component next to the endocrine tumor component.

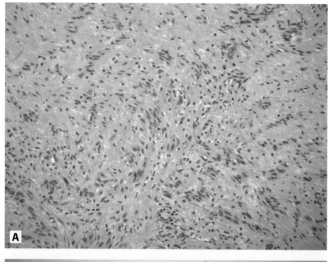

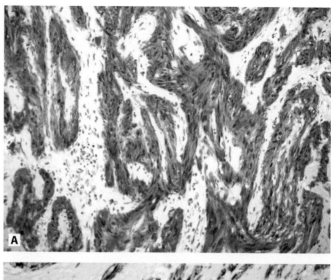

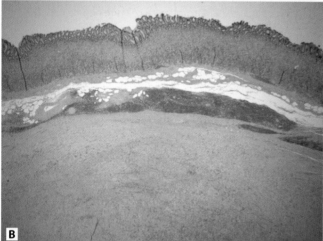

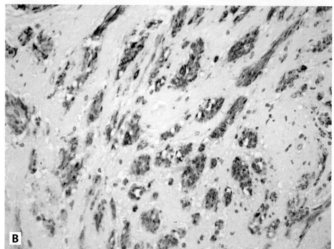

FIGURE 5-18. Cellular Schwannoma of the stomach. The tumor consists of elongated spindle cells with vague palisading (**A**), and capsule formation and peripheral lymphoid aggregates (**B**).

FIGURE 5-19. Cellular Schwannoma, same case as in Figure 5-18. The tumor exhibits positive reactivity immunohistochemically for both S100 (nuclear and cytoplasmic) (**A**) and glial fibrillary acid protein (**B**).

Inflammatory Myofibroblastic Tumor

An IMT consists of myofibroblasts, inflammatory cells, and collagen bundles (Figure 5-20). Immunohistochemically, the cells are negative for CD117, but staining for anaplastic lymphoma kinase (ALK) is positive in about 50% of cases (particularly in the pediatric population).

Ganglioneuroma

A ganglioneuroma is characterized by clusters of ganglion cells in fascicles of Schwann cells, and it most commonly occurs in the posterior mediastinum and retroperitoneum and rarely in adrenal glands. It often presents as a large, encapsulated, firm mass. Diagnostically, this is usually not confused with a GIST due to the clinical symptoms associated with it, including hypertension and diarrhea. However, this tumor may occur as mucosal polyps in the colon or small intestine. The microscopic workup may include GIST as a differential diagnosis.

It resembles neurofibroma except for the clusters of ganglion cells (Figure 5-21). Immunohistochemically, the tumor cells are positive for S100 and synaptophysin.

Intra-Abdominal Fibromatosis

Intra-abdominal fibromatosis occurs either sporadically or as part of familial adenomatous polyposis (FAP) or Gardner's syndrome. Histologically, it is characterized by spindle cells arranged in long, sweeping fascicles mixed with dense collagenous matrix and thin-walled blood vessels (Figure 5-22A). One of the IHC features is the nuclear accumulation of β-catenin in about 75% of cases (Figure 5-22B).

Calcifying Fibrous Tumor

A calcifying fibrous tumor (CFT) is a benign mesenchymal tumor composed of hyalinized fibrous tissue with scarce spindle cells and focal calcifications. It is most commonly

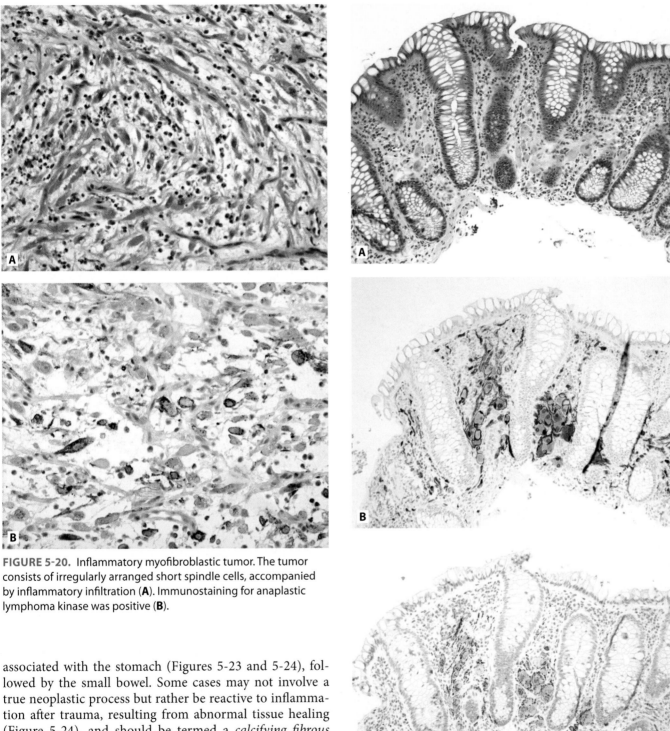

FIGURE 5-20. Inflammatory myofibroblastic tumor. The tumor consists of irregularly arranged short spindle cells, accompanied by inflammatory infiltration (**A**). Immunostaining for anaplastic lymphoma kinase was positive (**B**).

associated with the stomach (Figures 5-23 and 5-24), followed by the small bowel. Some cases may not involve a true neoplastic process but rather be reactive to inflammation after trauma, resulting from abnormal tissue healing (Figure 5-24), and should be termed a *calcifying fibrous pseudotumor*.[42] The diagnosis of sclerosing GIST should be ruled out with immunostains before the diagnosis is made. IHC markers are all negative except for focal CD34 staining. No mutations can be identified.[43]

Gastroblastoma

A gastroblastoma is a recently described epitheliomesenchymal biphasic stomach tumor.[44–46] It seems to occur in young adults. Although histologically essentially indistinguishable

FIGURE 5-21. Ganglion neuroma. This colon polyp intramucosally contained a cluster of ganglion cells intermixed with neurofibers (**A**). The neurofibers are highlighted by positive immunostains for S100 (**B**), synaptophysin (**C**), as well as neurofilaments (not shown).

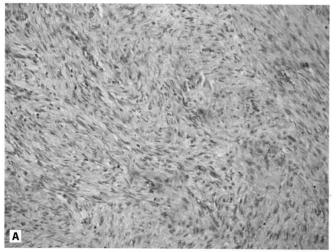

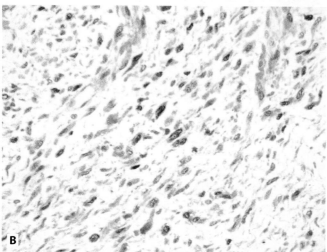

FIGURE 5-22. Intra-abdominal fibromatosis (desmoid tumor). **A.** The tumor consists of uniform bland spindle cells with small nuclei characteristic of fibroblasts. **B.** Immunostaining for β-catenin demonstrates nuclear positivity in a desmoid tumor.

FIGURE 5-23. Perigastric calcifying fibrous pseudotumor. This large perigastric mass was from a 64-year-old man with a preoperative diagnosis of a gastrointestinal stromal tumor. It demonstrates a well-circumscribed mass in the perigastric adipose tissue. There is extensive central tumor degeneration and hemorrhage in the periphery.

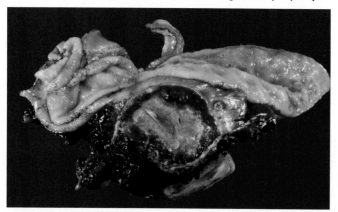

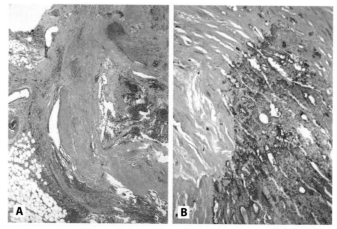

FIGURE 5-24. Microscopically, the tumor in Figure 5.23 consists of residual large vascular channels (**A**) in addition to the central degeneration, with a fibrous reaction forming a "capsule" with calcification (**B**). The lesion was negative for both CD117 and DOG-1 (discovered on GIST-1).

from GISTs, it is characterized by oval or spindled cells and clusters/cords of epithelial cells (Figure 5-25). Immunohistochemically, the epithelial component expresses cytokeratin AE1/3 and partly CK7 but is negative for CK20 and EMA. The spindle cell component is positive for vimentin (Figure 5-26) and CD10 but is negative for CD117, CD34, SMA, desmin, and S100. Although this has been reported as a low-grade malignant epitheliomesenchymal tumor, the true biological nature is unknown as this identification was only based on 3 cases. More recently, a similar tumor was reported to occur in the duodenum.[46]

Clear Cell Sarcoma-like Tumor of the Gastrointestinal Tract or Malignant Gastrointestinal Neuroectodermal Tumor

A clear cell sarcoma-like tumor of the gastrointestinal tract (CCSLTGT), or malignant gastrointestinal neuroectodermal tumor (GNET). This tumor consists of spindle or epithelioid cells, with features closely resembling those of clear cell sarcoma of tendons and aponeuroses (CCSTA) of soft part (Figure 5-27), but lacks melanocytic markers HMB45 and Melan-A.[47] These tumors harbor cytogenetic changes similar to CCSTA, involving Ewing sarcoma breakpoint region 1 gene (*EWSR1*) and a fusion partner *CREB1* or *ATF1*.[48,49] Immunohistochemically, they express S100 protein, SOX10, and vimentin and lack HMB45, Melan-A, smooth muscle markers, and GIST markers (Figure 5-27). A majority of cases are positive for neural markers synaptophysin or CD56 (Figure 5-27).[50] Electron microscopically, there is lack of melanosomes[49,50] but evidence of neural differentiation in studied cases, including interdigitating processes, dense core granules, and clear vesicles reminiscent of synaptic bulbs.[47,50] Therefore, the term *GNET* was recently proposed.[50]

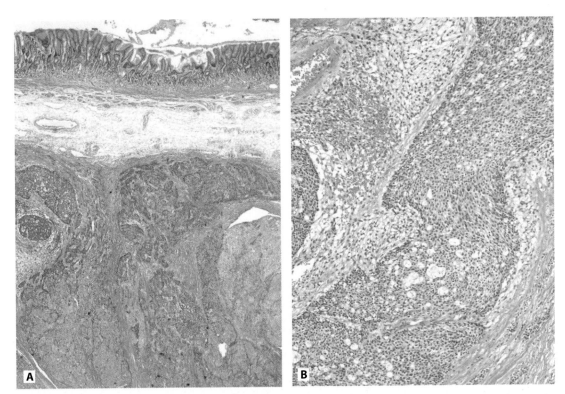

FIGURE 5-25. Gastroblastoma. **A.** This intramural well-circumscribed mass extends to the submucosa; it consists of nests, sheets, and cords of epithelial cells, with dense and loose mesenchyma. **B.** Higher magnification demonstrates a heterologous stromal component, including a myxoid reticular pattern; there is vesicular degeneration in the epithelial component, and there are rounded hyalinized globules. (Used with permission of Dr. Elizabeth Montgomery.)

Perivascular Epithelioid Cell Neoplasm

A perivascular epithelioid cell neoplasm (PEComa) consists of nests of epithelioid cells that express both melanocytic and smooth muscle markers, including Melan-A, HMB45, SMA, and desmin, among others. Angiomyolipoma of the kidney and liver and lymphangioleiomyomatosis and clear cell "sugar" tumor of the lung also belong to this group. Although

FIGURE 5-26. Gastroblastoma immunohistochemistry. **A.** The epithelial component is strongly and diffusely positive for pancytokeratin. **B.** The mesenchymal component is positive for vimentin. (Used with permission of Dr. Elizabeth Montgomery.)

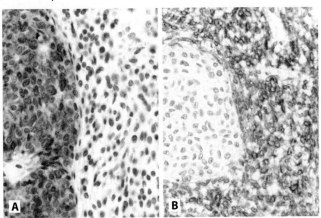

most PEComas are benign, some are locally aggressive; some may metastasize to the liver, lung, and lymph nodes, among other places. These tumors can involve mucosa and submucosa or muscularis propria, with extension to the mesentery, similar to GIST. Morphologically, some GISTs may mimic PEComa; the latter rarely can be positive for CD117. However, expression of Melan-A or HMB45 distinguishes PEComa from a GIST. Sporadic and tuberous sclerosis complex–associated PEComa may respond to mTOR (mammalian target of rapamycin) inhibitors, making it critical to reach an accurate diagnosis.

Immunohistochemical stains play a critical role in the diagnosis of GISTs and similar tumors. Nevertheless, it cannot be overemphasized that no matter how specific some immunomarkers may seem, their specificity is only relevant in a well-defined clinicopathologic context. A proper working differential diagnosis needs to be formed before the IHC stains are interpreted. Errors arise when individual stains are taken out of context. For example, in small biopsies, several metastatic tumors to the GI tract can express CD117 and may be mistaken for GIST, such as melanoma (particularly the spindle cell type),[51,52] germ cell tumors, angiosarcoma, and some colonic neuroendocrine carcinomas.[53] In one series, 12 of 16 anorectal melanomas were positive for CD117.[52] With recognition of the unique morphology on good hematoxylin and eosin (H&E) sections and application of a proper panel

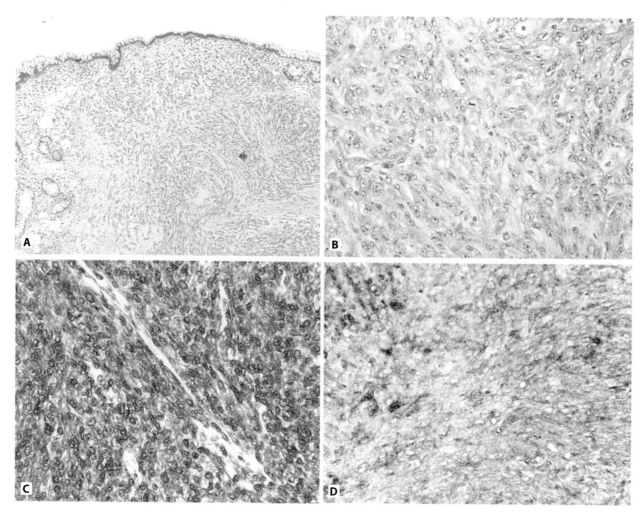

FIGURE 5-27. Malignant gastrointestinal neuroectodermal tumor. **A.** This tumor involves the small-bowel wall, extending to the mucosa. **B.** The tumor consists of epithelioid and spindle cell components, with round-to-oval vesicular nuclei, pale eosinophilic and clear cytoplasm, and occasional mitosis. **C.** Immunostaining for S100 is strongly positive. **D.** Immunostaining for synaptophysin is weakly positive. The tumor is negative for gastrointestinal stromal tumor markers, Melan-A, HMB45, and smooth muscle markers (not shown).

of IHC markers, including cytokeratin, melanocytic markers, and so on, these usually do not cause a diagnostic problem. Another pitfall is a mixed normal component in tumors. Some GI leiomyomas contain scattered to numerous dendritic ICC that stain for both CD117 and DOG-1 (Figure 5-16). Also, some small GISTs may contain focal areas of desmin-positive bands of smooth muscle cells, as entrapped normal muscularis propria in an evolving GIST (Figure 5-15), and should not be mistaken for a leiomyoma. Another well-known technical pitfall is that, for CD117 staining, when antigen retrieval is used, a desmoid tumor can show positive staining.

After imatinib mesylate treatment, some GISTs can acquire desmin expression and lose CD117, posing a diagnostic dilemma. In addition, even though in general desmin is more specific than SMA and caldesmon for indicating a smooth muscle tumor, it may be positive in some epithelioid GISTs (some 30% of *KIT*-negative GISTs were focally positive for desmin in one series). With both CD117 and DOG-1 in

the panel, this is less of a concern. Other changes associated with treatment include rhabdomyoblastic differentiation.[54]

Occasionally, when a superficial mucosa biopsy is performed for a larger tumor, the small portion of the evidently epithelioid tumor may be mixed with mucosal glands, mimicking a poorly differentiated adenocarcinoma. If no relevant clinical and endoscopic information were provided, as often is the case in our daily practice, particularly in an off-site commercial laboratory, a misdiagnosis may occur. Again, applying a panel of IHC stains would readily resolve the problem.

There have been ongoing arguments for limiting the number of immunostains to reduce cost, with the belief that experienced pathologists can rely more on characteristic features in H&E sections, with only one or two positive "confirming" immunomarkers for the diagnosis. This is neither scientifically sound nor cost-effective. Naturally, the more "senior" one becomes, the more confidence one puts in one's ability to make a diagnosis based on H&E sections. However, most mistakes are rather due to overconfidence than lack of experience. For GI mesenchymal tumors, the morphologic and IHC overlaps are so great that the final diagnosis should never be based on a heroic gut feeling of the good pathologist, however famous he or she may be, and should be based on a comprehensive set of immunomarkers that cover all the possible bases.

MUTATIONAL ANALYSIS

Two-thirds of GISTs harbor mutations in exon 11 of the *KIT* gene, which encodes the juxtamembrane domain. The mutations disrupt the secondary structure that normally functions to prevent the kinase activation loop from swinging into the active conformation. Less commonly affected are exon 9 and exon 13. Performing mutational analysis not only confirms the diagnosis, which may be necessary in tumors negative for both CD117 and DOG-1 on IHC, but also, more importantly, influences treatment decisions.[55] GISTs that do not carry *KIT* or PDGFRA mutations are more resistant to imatinib mesylate treatment.[15,16] The exon 11 mutated tumors respond well to imatinib, whereas exon 9 mutated tumors may benefit from a higher dose of the drug (800 mg/d as opposed to the standard 400 mg/d) in terms of progression-free survival.[56] On the other hand, although *KIT* mutation in exon 11 generally confers susceptibility to imatinib, deletional mutations of exon 11, particularly of codon 557 or 558, have been associated with poorer long-term survival.[57,58] A study of 57 GISTs that progressed under imatinib treatment showed that 88% developed secondary drug-resistance mutations in *KIT*,[59] and 34% had 2 or more secondary *KIT* mutations in individual metastases, suggesting that selection/acquisition of secondary mutations within the kinase domain is a common cause of resistance. Another potential benefit of *KIT* mutational analysis is that for *KIT*-wt GISTs, sunitinib malate has been reported to be more potent than imatinib.

All pediatric GISTs should also be subjected first to *KIT* or PDGFRA mutational analysis because tumors with these mutations respond to conventional GIST treatment. For mutated tumors, the guidelines of the National Comprehensive Cancer Network for adult GISTs should be followed. With recent findings of SDH mutations in a subset of GISTs and because tumors with SDH mutations have unique biological features and in general respond poorly to Gleevec treatment, detection of these mutations is recommended for all *KIT*-wt and PDGFRA-wt tumors. Current data indicate that lack of immunostaining for SDHB is predictive for these mutations; therefore, IHC for SDHB may be used as a screening step before mutational analysis is performed.

RISK ASSESSMENT

Traditionally, various morphologic variables have been analyzed as predictors for clinical outcome of GISTs. Some factors associated with high risk for progressive behaviors included invasive growth (infiltrating another organ or

structure), tumor necrosis, proliferative index (percentage MIB-1-positive nuclei; < 4% vs. ≥ 4%, for example), distant metastasis, and positive margins.[58,60] However, differences in case definition and criteria used often led to conflicting conclusions. Only tumor size, mitotic activity, and, to a lesser extent, tumor location have emerged as more reliable behavioral "markers." In general, stomach tumors fare better than small-bowel tumors. Subsequently, an Armed Forces Institute of Pathology (AFIP) study published in 2006 involving a large series of patients from preimatinib age led to the development of a system that provides a prediction score,[60] which was adapted by the College of American Pathologists (CAP).

It should be noted that GISTs occurring in CT or Carney-Stratakis syndrome are less predictable using the consensus risk assessment system.[16] These include the so-called type 2 GISTs as proposed by Gill et al (those occurring in pediatric patients and those in the CT).[37] As discussed, these type 2 tumors are negative for mitochondrial protein SDHB. These tumors often arise in the stomach, are multifocal, and demonstrate a coarsely lobulated growth pattern.[37] Type 2 GISTs have a tendency for lymph node metastasis and are more resistant to imatinib therapy. Therefore, a diagnostic comment referring to these features should be provided in the pathology report to emphasize this potential outcome uniqueness.

REFERENCES

1. Miettinen M, Sobin LH, Lasota J. Gastrointestinal stromal tumors presenting as omental masses—a clinicopathologic analysis of 95 cases. *Am J Surg Pathol.* 2009;33(9):1267–1275. PMID: 19440146.
2. Goh BK, Chow PK, Kesavan SM, Yap WM, Chung YF, Wong WK. A single-institution experience with eight CD117-positive primary extragastrointestinal stromal tumors: critical appraisal and a comparison with their gastrointestinal counterparts. *J Gastrointest Surg.* 2009;13(6):1094–1098. PMID: 19238492.
3. Mazur MT, Clark HB. Gastric stromal tumors. Reappraisal of histogenesis. *Am J Surg Pathol.* 1983;7(6):507–519. PMID: 6625048.
4. Saul SH, Rast ML, Brooks JJ. The immunohistochemistry of gastrointestinal stromal tumors. Evidence supporting an origin from smooth muscle. *Am J Surg Pathol.* 1987;11(6):464–473. PMID: 3035954.
5. Hirota S, Isozaki K, Moriyama Y, et al. Gain-of-function mutations of c-kit in human gastrointestinal stromal tumors. *Science.* 1998;279(5350):577–580. PMID: 9438854.
6. Nakahara M, Isozaki K, Hirota S, et al. A novel gain-of-function mutation of c-kit gene in gastrointestinal stromal tumors. *Gastroenterology.* 1998;115(5):1090–1095. PMID: 9797363.
7. Miettinen M, Makhlouf H, Sobin LH, Lasota J. Gastrointestinal stromal tumors of the jejunum and ileum: a clinicopathologic, immunohistochemical, and molecular genetic study of 906 cases before imatinib with long-term follow-up. *Am J Surg Pathol.* 2006;30(4):477–489. PMID: 16625094.
8. Andersson J, Sihto H, Meis-Kindblom JM, Joensuu H, Nupponen N, Kindblom LG. *NF1*-associated gastrointestinal stromal tumors have unique clinical, phenotypic, and genotypic characteristics. *Am J Surg Pathol.* 2005;29(9):1170–1176. PMID: 16096406.
9. Takazawa Y, Sakurai S, Sakuma Y, et al. Gastrointestinal stromal tumors of neurofibromatosis type I (von Recklinghausen's disease). *Am J Surg Pathol.* 2005;29(6):755–763. PMID: 15897742.
10. Miettinen M, Fetsch JF, Sobin LH, Lasota J. Gastrointestinal stromal tumors in patients with neurofibromatosis 1: a clinicopathologic and molecular genetic study of 45 cases. *Am J Surg Pathol.* 2006;30(1):90–96. PMID: 16330947.

11. Carney JA, Sheps SG, Go VL, Gordon H. The triad of gastric leiomyosarcoma, functioning extra-adrenal paraganglioma and pulmonary chondroma. *N Engl J Med.* 1977;296(26):1517–1518. PMID: 865533.

12. Carney JA, Stratakis CA. Familial paraganglioma and gastric stromal sarcoma: a new syndrome distinct from the Carney triad. *Am J Med Genet.* 2002;108(2):132–139. PMID: 11857563.

13. Pasini B, McWhinney SR, Bei T, et al. Clinical and molecular genetics of patients with the Carney-Stratakis syndrome and germline mutations of the genes coding for the succinate dehydrogenase subunits SDHB, SDHC, and SDHD. *Eur J Hum Genet.* 2008;16(1):79–88. PMID: 17667967.

14. Neuhann TM, Mansmann V, Merkelbach-Bruse S, et al. A novel germline KIT mutation (p.L576P) in a family presenting with juvenile onset of multiple gastrointestinal stromal tumors, skin hyperpigmentations, and esophageal stenosis. *Am J Surg Pathol.* 2013;37(6):898–905. PMID: 23598963.

15. Agaimy A, Wunsch PH. Lymph node metastasis in gastrointestinal stromal tumours (GIST) occurs preferentially in young patients < or = 40 years: an overview based on our case material and the literature. *Langenbecks Arch Surg.* 2009;394(2):375–381. PMID: 19104826.

16. Zhang L, Smyrk TC, Young WF Jr, Stratakis CA, Carney JA. Gastric stromal tumors in Carney triad are different clinically, pathologically, and behaviorally from sporadic gastric gastrointestinal stromal tumors: findings in 104 cases. *Am J Surg Pathol.* 2010;34(1):53–64. PMID: 19935059.

17. Abraham SC, Krasinskas AM, Hofstetter WL, Swisher SG, Wu TT. "Seedling" mesenchymal tumors (gastrointestinal stromal tumors and leiomyomas) are common incidental tumors of the esophagogastric junction. *Am J Surg Pathol.* 2007;31(11):1629–1635. PMID: 18059218.

18. Agaimy A, Wunsch PH, Hofstaedter F, et al. Minute gastric sclerosing stromal tumors (GIST tumorlets) are common in adults and frequently show c-KIT mutations. *Am J Surg Pathol.* 2007;31(1):113–120. PMID: 17197927.

19. Muenst S, Thies S, Went P, Tornillo L, Bihl MP, Dirnhofer S. Frequency, phenotype, and genotype of minute gastrointestinal stromal tumors in the stomach: an autopsy study. *Hum Pathol.* 2007;42(12):1849–1854. PMID: 21658742.

20. Heinrich MC, Corless CL, Duensing A, et al. PDGFRA activating mutations in gastrointestinal stromal tumors. *Science.* 2003;299(5607):708–710. PMID: 12522257.

21. Duensing A, Medeiros F, McConarty B, et al. Mechanisms of oncogenic KIT signal transduction in primary gastrointestinal stromal tumors (GISTs). *Oncogene.* 2004;23(22):3999–4006. PMID: 15007386.

22. Perry CG, Young WF Jr, McWhinney SR, et al. Functioning paraganglioma and gastrointestinal stromal tumor of the jejunum in three women: syndrome or coincidence. *Am J Surg Pathol.* 2006;30(1):42–49. PMID: 16330941.

23. Janeway KA, Kim SY, Lodish M, et al. Defects in succinate dehydrogenase in gastrointestinal stromal tumors lacking KIT and PDGFRA mutations. *Proc Natl Acad Sci U S A.* 2011;108(1):314–318. PMID: 21173220.

24. Pantaleo MA, Astolfi A, Indio V, et al. SDHA loss-of-function mutations in KIT-PDGFRA wild-type gastrointestinal stromal tumors identified by massively parallel sequencing. *J Natl Cancer Inst.* 2011;103(12):983–987. PMID: 21505157.

25. Italiano A, Chen CL, Sung YS, et al. SDHA loss of function mutations in a subset of young adult wild-type gastrointestinal stromal tumors. *BMC Cancer.* 2012;12:408. PMID: 22974104.

26. Dwight T, Benn DE, Clarkson A, et al. Loss of SDHA expression identifies SDHA mutations in succinate dehydrogenase-deficient gastrointestinal stromal tumors. *Am J Surg Pathol.* 2013;37(2):226–233. PMID: 23060355.

27. Chou A, Chen J, Clarkson A, et al. Succinate dehydrogenase-deficient GISTs are characterized by IGF1R overexpression. *Mod Pathol.* 2012;25(9):1307–1313. PMID: 22555179.

28. Belinsky MG, Rink L, Flieder DB, et al. Overexpression of insulin-like growth factor 1 receptor and frequent mutational inactivation of SDHA in wild-type SDHB-negative gastrointestinal stromal tumors. *Genes Chromosomes Cancer.* 2013;52(2):214–224. PMID: 23109135.

29. West RB, Corless CL, Chen X, et al. The novel marker, DOG-1, is expressed ubiquitously in gastrointestinal stromal tumors irrespective of KIT or PDGFRA mutation status. *Am J Pathol.* 2004;165(1):107–113. PMID: 15215166.

30. Espinosa I, Lee CH, Kim MK, et al. A novel monoclonal antibody against DOG1 is a sensitive and specific marker for gastrointestinal stromal tumors. *Am J Surg Pathol.* 2008;32(2):210–218. PMID: 18223323.

31. Caputo A, Caci E, Ferrera L, et al. TMEM16A, a membrane protein associated with calcium-dependent chloride channel activity. *Science.* 2008;322(5901):590–594. PMID: 18772398.

32. Yang YD, Cho H, Koo JY, et al. TMEM16A confers receptor-activated calcium-dependent chloride conductance. *Nature.* 2008;455(7217):1210–1215. PMID: 18724360.

33. Liegl B, Hornick JL, Corless CL, Fletcher CD. Monoclonal antibody DOG1.1 shows higher sensitivity than KIT in the diagnosis of gastrointestinal stromal tumors, including unusual subtypes. *Am J Surg Pathol.* 2009;33(3):437–446. PMID: 19011564.

34. Miettinen M, Wang ZF, Lasota J. DOG1 antibody in the differential diagnosis of gastrointestinal stromal tumors: a study of 1840 cases. *Am J Surg Pathol.* 2009;33(9):1401–1408. PMID: 19606013.

35. Yamamoto H, Kojima A, Nagata S, Tomita Y, Takahashi S, Oda Y. KIT-negative gastrointestinal stromal tumor of the abdominal soft tissue: a clinicopathologic and genetic study of 10 cases. *Am J Surg Pathol.* 2011;35(9):1287–1295. PMID: 21836495.

36. Gill AJ, Benn DE, Chou A, et al. Immunohistochemistry for SDHB triages genetic testing of SDHB, SDHC, and SDHD in paraganglioma-pheochromocytoma syndromes. *Hum Pathol.* 2010;41(6):805–814. PMID: 20236688.

37. Gill AJ, Chou A, Vilain R, et al. Immunohistochemistry for SDHB divides gastrointestinal stromal tumors (GISTs) into 2 distinct types. *Am J Surg Pathol.* 2010;34(5):636–644. PMID: 20305538.

38. Miettinen M, Wang ZF, Sarlomo-Rikala M, Osuch C, Rutkowski P, Lasota J. Succinate dehydrogenase-deficient GISTs: a clinicopathologic, immunohistochemical, and molecular genetic study of 66 gastric GISTs with predilection to young age. *Am J Surg Pathol.* 2011;35(11):1712–1721. PMID: 21997692.

39. Doyle LA, Nelson D, Heinrich MC, Corless CL, Hornick JL. Loss of succinate dehydrogenase subunit B (SDHB) expression is limited to a distinctive subset of gastric wild-type gastrointestinal stromal tumours: a comprehensive genotype-phenotype correlation study. *Histopathology.* 2012;61(5):801–809. PMID: 22804613.

40. Miettinen M, Killian JK, Wang ZF, et al. Immunohistochemical loss of succinate dehydrogenase subunit A (SDHA) in gastrointestinal stromal tumors (GISTs) signals SDHA germline mutation. *Am J Surg Pathol.* 2013;37(2):234–240. PMID: 23282968.

41. Lasota J, Wang Z, Kim SY, Helman L, Miettinen M. Expression of the receptor for type I insulin-like growth factor (IGF1R) in gastrointestinal stromal tumors: an immunohistochemical study of 1078 cases with diagnostic and therapeutic implications. *Am J Surg Pathol.* 2013;37(1):114–119. PMID: 22892600.

42. Fetsch JF, Montgomery EA, Meis JM. Calcifying fibrous pseudotumor. *Am J Surg Pathol.* 1993;17(5):502–508. PMID: 8470765.

43. Agaimy A, Bihl MP, Tornillo L, Wunsch PH, Hartmann A, Michal M. Calcifying fibrous tumor of the stomach: clinicopathologic and molecular study of seven cases with literature review and reappraisal of histogenesis. *Am J Surg Pathol.* 2010;34(2):271–278. PMID: 20090503.

44. Miettinen M, Dow N, Lasota J, Sobin LH. A distinctive novel epitheliomesenchymal biphasic tumor of the stomach in young adults ("gastroblastoma"): a series of 3 cases. *Am J Surg Pathol.* 2009;33(9):1370–1377. PMID: 19718790.

45. Shin DH, Lee JH, Kang HJ, et al. Novel epitheliomesenchymal biphasic stomach tumour (gastroblastoma) in a 9-year-old: morphological, ultrastructural and immunohistochemical findings. *J Clin Pathol.* 2010;63(3):270–274. PMID: 20203230. PMCID: 2922722.

46. Poizat F, de Chaisemartin C, Bories E, et al. A distinctive epithe-liomesenchymal biphasic tumor in the duodenum: the first case of duodenoblastoma? *Virchows Arch.* 2012;461(4):379–383. PMID: 22961103.

47. Zambrano E, Reyes-Mugica M, Franchi A, Rosai J. An osteoclast-rich tumor of the gastrointestinal tract with features resembling clear cell sarcoma of soft parts: reports of 6 cases of a GIST simulator. *Int J Surg Pathol.* 2003;11(2):75–81. PMID: 12754623.

48. Covinsky M, Gong S, Rajaram V, Perry A, Pfeifer J. EWS-ATF1 fusion transcripts in gastrointestinal tumors previously diagnosed as malig-nant melanoma. *Hum Pathol.* 2005;36(1):74–81. PMID: 15712185.

49. Antonescu CR, Nafa K, Segal NH, Dal Cin P, Ladanyi M. EWS-CREB1: a recurrent variant fusion in clear cell sarcoma—association with gastrointestinal location and absence of melanocytic differentia-tion. *Clin Cancer Res.* 2006;12(18):5356–5362. PMID: 17000668.

50. Stockman DL, Miettinen M, Suster S, et al. Malignant gastrointestinal neuroectodermal tumor: clinicopathologic, immunohistochemical, ultrastructural, and molecular analysis of 16 cases with a reappraisal of clear cell sarcoma-like tumors of the gastrointestinal tract. *Am J Surg Pathol.* 2012;36(6):857–868. PMID: 22592145.

51. Curtin JA, Busam K, Pinkel D, Bastian BC. Somatic activation of KIT in distinct subtypes of melanoma. *J Clin Oncol.* 2006;24(26):4340–4346. PMID: 16908931.

52. Chute DJ, Cousar JB, Mills SE. Anorectal malignant melanoma: morphologic and immunohistochemical features. *Am J Clin Pathol.* 2006;126(1):93–100. PMID: 16753594.

53. Akintola-Ogunremi O, Pfeifer JD, Tan BR, et al. Analysis of protein expression and gene mutation of c-kit in colorectal neuroendocrine car-cinomas. *Am J Surg Pathol.* 2003;27(12):1551–1558. PMID: 14657715.

54. Liegl B, Hornick JL, Antonescu CR, Corless CL, Fletcher CD. Rhab-domyosarcomatous differentiation in gastrointestinal stromal tumors after tyrosine kinase inhibitor therapy: a novel form of tumor progres-sion. *Am J Surg Pathol.* 2009;33(2):218–226. PMID: 18830121.

55. Heinrich MC, Corless CL, Demetri GD, et al. Kinase mutations and imatinib response in patients with metastatic gastrointestinal stromal tumor. *J Clin Oncol.* 2003;21(23):4342–4349. PMID: 14645423.

56. Debiec-Rychter M, Sciot R, Le Cesne A, et al. KIT mutations and dose selection for imatinib in patients with advanced gastrointestinal stro-mal tumours. *Eur J Cancer.* 2006;42(8):1093–1103. PMID: 16624552.

57. Wardelmann E, Buttner R, Merkelbach-Bruse S, Schildhaus H-U. Mutation analysis of gastrointestinal stromal tumors: increasing sig-nificance for risk assessment and effective targeted therapy. *Virchows Arch.* 2007;451(4):743–749. PMID: 17701051.

58. Iesalnieks I, Rummele P, Dietmaier W, et al. Factors associated with disease progression in patients with gastrointestinal stromal tumors in the pre-imatinib era. *Am J Clin Pathol.* 2005;124(5):740–748. PMID: 16203282.

59. Liegl B, Kepten I, Le C, et al. Heterogeneity of kinase inhibitor resistance mechanisms in GIST. *J Pathol.* 2008;216(1):64–74. PMID: 18623623.

60. Miettinen M, Lasota J. Gastrointestinal stromal tumors: pathology and prognosis at different sites. *Semin Diagn Pathol.* 2006;23(2):70. PMID: S0740-2570(06)00143-2.

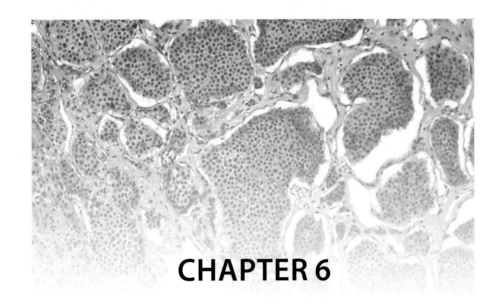

CHAPTER 6

Gastrointestinal Neuroendocrine Tumors

Chanjuan Shi and Kay Washington

OVERVIEW

The term *gastrointestinal neuroendocrine tumor* (GI-NET) refers to a low-grade malignancy arising from the diffuse neuroendocrine system scattered throughout the mucosa of the gut. Such tumors have historically been called "carcinoid tumors," a terminology that has been recognized as archaic and ambiguous and is now by and large replaced by "neuroendocrine tumor" for all gastrointestinal (GI) tract primaries. The term *neuroendocrine* is preferred over the term *endocrine* because of shared antigens between neural elements and these cells of the diffuse endocrine system in the GI tract, such as neuron-specific enolase, chromogranins, protein gene product 9.5, and synaptophysin.[1] The neuroendocrine cells that give rise to GI-NETs are epithelial cells derived from the same stem cells as other epithelial cell lineages in the GI tract, such as enterocytes, Paneth cells, and goblet cells; at least 15 morphologically and functionally distinct GI neuroendocrine cell types producing different hormones have been identified.[2,3] In general, the differentiation pattern of GI-NETs reflects the profile of neuroendocrine cells normally located in that part of the GI tract (Table 6-1).

The designation *GI-NET* is a broad category rather than a specific disease entity. Based on the embryonic origins, this group of tumors has historically been divided into foregut (esophagus, stomach, and duodenum), midgut (jejunum, ileum, appendix, proximal colon), and hindgut (distal colon and rectum) NETs.[4] Even within the same anatomic origin, especially the foregut tumors, they are too heterogeneous to

be considered as a single entity. They have different underlying molecular mechanisms and thereby different biologic behavior and different treatment options (Table 6-2).[5-10] The reported overall 5-year survival for GI-NETs is approximately 90%; however, most patients with this tumor are diagnosed at an advanced/metastatic stage.[11] Surgery is the only curative option for GI-NETs. Inoperable, progressive or symptomatic tumors can be managed by medical interventions. New therapeutic approaches, such as peptide receptor radiotherapy and systemic targeted therapies, are being developed.

EPIDEMIOLOGY

Analysis of over 29,000 gastroenteropancreatic (GEP) NETs reported to the SEER (Surveillance, Epidemiology, and End Results Program) database from 1973 to 2007 has shown that the incidence of these tumors is increasing in the US population, especially for rectal and small-intestinal neuroendocrine tumors (NETs) (Figure 6-1).[5] The increase can be at least partially contributed by improved classification and recognition of the disease as well as increased use of advanced imaging and endoscopic techniques. Based on SEER data, GI-NETs represent 0.5% of all newly diagnosed cancers, 5.4% of all GI malignancies, and 60%–70% of all NETs.[5,11] The median age at diagnosis is 63 years, and the overall incidence of GI-NETs in the period 2003–2007 was 3.22 cases per 100,000 individuals per year.[5] They occurred slightly more commonly in

TABLE 6-1. Gastrointestinal endocrine cells and neuroendocrine tumors in the gastrointestinal tract.

Location	Endocrine cells (product)	Neuroendocrine tumors	Associated condition
Gastric body/fundus	ECL cells (histamine)	Type 1	Chronic atrophic gastritis with ECL cell hyperplasia
	EC cells (serotonin)	ECL cell NET	
	D cells (somatostatin)	Type 2	Duodenal or pancreatic gastrinoma and ZES
	Ghrelin-producing cells	ECL cell NET	(mainly in MEN-1 syndrome) with ECL cell hyperplasia
		Type 3	Atypical carcinoid syndrome; no ECL cell hyperplasia
		ECL cell NET	
		Type 3	Typical carcinoid syndrome
		EC cell NET (rare)	
Gastric antrum	G cells (gastrin)	Type 3 gastrinoma (rare)	ZES
	EC cells (serotonin)	Type 3	Typical carcinoid syndrome
	ECL cells (histamine)	EC cell (rare)	
		Type 3	Atypical carcinoid syndrome
		ECL cell	
Duodenum	D cells	D cell NET	NF1 syndrome
	G cells	(somatostatin-producing NET)	VHL disease
	ECL cells		MEN-1 syndrome
	L cells (GLI/PYY)	Functional G-cell NET	MEN-1 syndrome (25%–33% of the cases); ZES
	CCK, secretin, GIP, and motilin-producing cells	(gastrinoma)	
		Nonfunctional G-cell NET	No ZES
Jejunum	G cells	Gastrinoma	MEN-1 syndrome and sporadic
	EC cells	EC-cell NET	Carcinoid syndrome
	L cells	Nonfunctional NET	
	CCK, secretin, GIP, and motilin-producing cells		
Ileum	EC cells	Serotonin-producing NET	Carcinoid syndrome
	L cells	L-cell NET (very rare)	
	Neurotensin-producing cells		
Appendix	EC cells	EC-cell NET (most common)	Carcinoid syndrome
	L cells	L-cell NET	
		Tubular carcinoid	
Colon	EC cells	EC-cell NET	Carcinoid syndrome
	L cells	L-cell NET (rare)	
Rectum	L cells, EC cells	L-cell NET	

Abbreviations: CCK, cholecystokinin; EC, enterochromaffin; ECL, enterochromaffin-like; GIP, gastric inhibitory polypeptide; GLI, glucagon-like immunoreactivity; MEN 1, multiple endocrine neoplasia 1; NET, neuroendocrine tumor. PYY, peptide YY; ZES, Zollinger-Ellison syndrome.

males than in females (2.78/100,000 vs. 2.35/100,000).[6] In addition, the incidence in blacks (4.44/100,0000) was higher than that in whites (2.32/100,000).[6]

Small-intestinal and rectal NETs are the most common among all GEP-NETs in the United States.[5] The annual age-adjusted rate of small-intestinal NETs is 1.08 cases/100,000/year in the US SEER data, accounting for 18.6% of all NETs between 1973 and 2007 in the pan-SEER registry.[5,9] Similar rates have been reported for rectal NETs. Colonic, gastric, and appendiceal sites represent 7.0%, 6.0%, and 3.1% of total NETs, respectively. Figure 6-2 represents the distribution of GI-NETs based on the SEER data from 2003 to 2007 reported by Lawrence et al.[5] However, in addition to differences in prevalence, the distribution of GI-NETs can be different among different races. For instance, a retrospective study from Taiwan has shown that more than 60% of all NETs are located in the rectum and only 5% in the small intestine.[12] In the United States, rectal NETs are more prevalent among black and Asian populations.[8]

TABLE 6-2. Age-adjusted incidence (per 100,000), age, tumor stage, and prognosis of gastrointestinal neuroendocrine tumors in the US population.

Location	Incidence[a]	Median age at diagnosis (years)	Distal metastasis at diagnosis	Median survival (months)	Five year survival
Stomach	0.33	65	Type 1: 2%–5%	124	Type 1: 96.1%
			Type 2: 10%–30%		Type 2: 60%–75%
			Type 3: 50%–100%		Type 3: <50%
Duodenum	0.25	67	9%	99	81%
Jejunum/ileum	0.82	66	30%	88	68%
Appendix	0.20	47	12%	NR	81%
Colon	0.42	65 (cecum 68)	32% (cecum 44%)	121 (cecum 83)	55%
Sigmoid/rectum	1.05	56	5%	240	89%

[a]Incidence based on the SEER (Surveillance, Epidemiology, and End Results Program) Registry (2000–2007); NR, no reports.

CLINICAL FEATURES

The clinical behavior of GI-NETs varies with their location in the GI tract. Small, nonfunctional tumors are usually clinically silent and may be discovered incidentally. When symptoms are attributable to nonfunctional GI-NETs, they are due to local tumor effects such as GI bleeding, mass obstruction, adhesions, or abdominal fibrosis giving rise to abdominal pain or small-bowel obstruction. Primary gastrinomas may cause uncomplicated/complicated gastric or duodenal ulcers. However, other functional NETs of the GI tract produce endocrine symptoms only when patients have extensive metastatic disease, which releases substantial amounts of biologic active molecules. The carcinoid syndrome (cutaneous flushing of the upper chest, neck, and face; gut hypermotility with diarrhea) occurs in less than 15% of patients with serotonin-producing enterochromaffin (EC) cells NETs.[13] In addition, the atypical carcinoid syndrome (red cutaneous flushing in absence of diarrhea) occurs in patients with a metastatic type 3, histamine-releasing (enterochromaffin-like [ECL] cell) gastric NET. Atypical or typical carcinoid syndrome can be misinterpreted as irritable bowel syndrome, asthma, perimenopausal neurosis, or part of an anxiety or food allergy response.[14,15] For those reasons, failure or delay in diagnosis occurs frequently in patients with GI-NETs.

Diagnostic strategies for patients suspected of having GI-NETs include biochemical testing for urinary 5-hydroxyindoleacetic acid (5-HIAA) and serum testing for elevated chromogranin A levels, followed by localization of

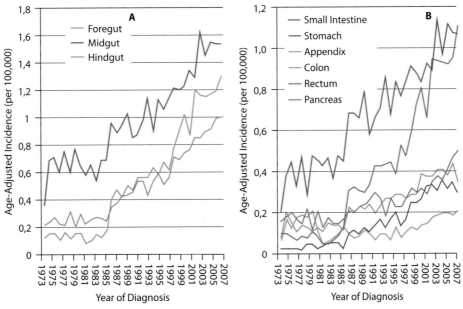

FIGURE 6-1. Increased incidence of gastroenteropancreatic NETs during the period 1973 to 2007. **A.** Increased incidence of foregut, midgut, and hindgut. **B.** Increased incidence in the stomach, small intestinal, appendiceal, colonic, rectal, and pancreatic NETs. (Reproduced with permission from Lawrence B, Gustafsson BI, Chan A, et al. The epidemiology of gastroenteropancreatic neuroendocrine tumors. *Endocrinol Metab Clin North Am.* 2011;40(1):1–18.[5])

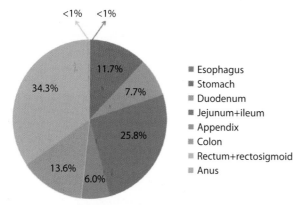

<1%   <1%

- 11.7%
- 7.7%
- 25.8%
- 6.0%
- 13.6%
- 34.3%

- Esophagus
- Stomach
- Duodenum
- Jejunum+ileum
- Appendix
- Colon
- Rectum+rectosigmoid
- Anus

FIGURE 6-2. Distribution of neuroendocrine tumors in the different locations of the gastrointestinal tract.

the tumor by endoscopy, octreoscan scintigraphy, computed tomography (CT), magnetic resonance imaging (MRI), or newer ^{68}Ga-radiolabeled somatostatin analogs (SSAs) combined with positron emission tomographic (PET) imaging. Chromogranin A is the most commonly used neuroendocrine serum marker in diagnosis and monitoring of both nonfunctional and functional NETs.[16] Chromogranin A is elevated in 60%–80% of GEP-NETs; the levels tend to be correlated to tumor burden, tumor location, and degree of differentiation. However, chromogranin A is not specific; for instance, patients on a proton pump inhibitor always have a high level of serum chromogranin A. Elevated chromogranin is also seen in patients with hepatic and renal dysfunction. 5-HIAA is the primary metabolite of serotonin. Urinary 5-HIAA is the primary test for the measurement of serotonin overproduction by serotonin-producing NETs, with a sensitivity of 64% and a specificity of 98% for the tumors.[16] False elevations can be seen in patients consuming tryptophan-/serotonin-rich foods.

The GI-NETs, most commonly ileal tumors, are associated with second primary tumors, usually discovered synchronously, in about 17% of patients. The most common site for second primary tumors is the GI tract, followed by the genitourinary tract and lung. These synchronous tumors are generally of higher grade than the GI-NET, which may be discovered during a staging workup of the associated second primary malignancy.[11,17]

NOMENCLATURE

Since Oberndorfer first described a carcinoid (carcinoma-like) tumor in 1907, the term *carcinoid* has been widely used by many clinicians and pathologists and was even accepted in the first World Health Organization (WHO) classification in 1980. However, the same term has been deprecated because of its failure to encompass the full biological spectrum and site-specific heterogeneity of these tumors, as well as the narrow interpretation of this term to mean a serotonin-producing tumor associated with a carcinoid syndrome.[18] The WHO, while retaining the "carcinoid" terminology in the 2000 publication on classification of tumors of the digestive system,[19] also outlined a three-tier system[20] classifying these neoplasms as well-differentiated NETs of benign or uncertain malignant potential, well-differentiated neuroendocrine carcinoma (NEC), and poorly differentiated NEC. This system had gained more acceptance among European pathologists and was considered more biologically oriented than the umbrella term *carcinoid*, although this terminology can be cumbersome to apply to individual cases. In addition, the system used the unequivocal evidence of malignant behavior, such as local invasion or metastasis, to distinguish between "carcinoma" or "tumor," which may be problematic when an initially localized neuroendocrine "tumor" would be classified as "neuroendocrine carcinoma" if distant metastasis occurred.

Recently, several organizations, including the WHO, the European Neuroendocrine Tumor Society (ENETS), the American Joint Committee on Cancer (AJCC), and the North American Neuroendocrine Tumor Society (NANETS), developed standard nomenclature for NETs to eliminate the confusion and better predict the disease outcome (Table 6-3). All GEP-NETs are classified into two categories: well-differentiated NETs or poorly differentiated NECs based on cell proliferation.[21,22] Although there are some limitations, this classification shows significant prognostic improvement and is now widely used in clinical and research settings.

PATHOLOGY

The pathology report for a resected NET should include (1) location and tumor type; (2) a definition of the differentiation grade using WHO 2010 classification of NETs of

TABLE 6-3. World Health Organization (WHO) 1980, 2000, and 2010 classification of neuroendocrine neoplasms of the gastrointestinal tract.

WHO 1980	*WHO 2000*	*WHO 2010*	
Carcinoid	WD endocrine tumors of benign or uncertain malignant potential	WD NET	Grade 1: Mitosis < 2/10 HPFs and/or Ki67 ≤ 2%
	WD endocrine carcinoma		Grade 2: Mitosis 2-20/10 HPFs and/or Ki67 3%–20%
	PD NEC	PD NEC: Mitosis > 20/10 HPFs and/or Ki67 > 20%	Small-cell carcinoma
			Large-cell NEC

Abbreviations: HPFs, high-power fields; NEC, neuroendocrine carcinoma; NET, neuroendocrine tumor; PD, poorly differentiated; WD, well differentiated.

the digestive system; (3) the presence of additional histologic features (focality, tumor necrosis, vascular or perineural invasion); (4) TNM staging system stage; (5) resection margin status; and (6) results of tests for hormonal production only for confirmation of hormonal syndrome.[23,26]

WHO 2010 Grading System

The ENETS proposed a uniform classification for all GEP-NETs in 2006 and 2007: All NETs are classified as well-differentiated NETs or poorly differentiated NECs based on mitotic rate and Ki67 index.[27,28] The ENETS grading system was entirely adopted by the new WHO classification. In the WHO 2010 classification, GI-NETs are graded as (1) grade 1 well-differentiated NETs (Ki ≤ 2% and mitoses < 2/10 high-power fields (HPFs); Figure 6-3); (2) grade 2 well-differentiated NETs (Ki 3%–20% or mitoses 2–20/10 HPFs; Figure 6-4); and (3) grade 3, high-grade NECs (Ki67 > 20% or mitoses > 20/10 HPFs) (Table 6-3). High-grade NECs are

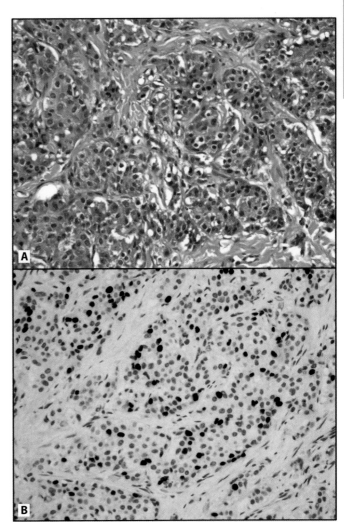

FIGURE 6-4. Well-differentiated neuroendocrine tumor, World Health Organization grade 2. **A.** Hematoxylin and eosin stain (original magnification ×200). **B.** Ki67 immunohistochemical stain showing a Ki67 between 10% and 20% (original magnification ×100).

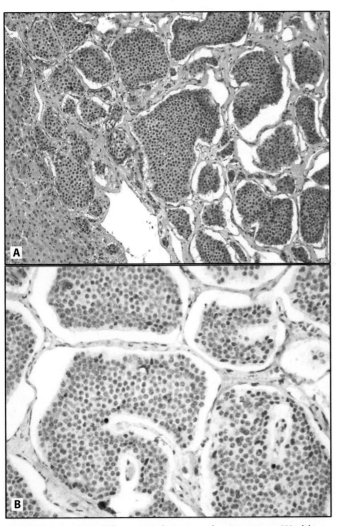

FIGURE 6-3. Well-differentiated neuroendocrine tumor, World Health Organization grade 1. **A.** Hematoxylin and eosin stain (original magnification ×100). **B.** Ki67 immunohistochemical stain showing a Ki67 index less than 2% (original magnification ×200).

further grouped into small-cell carcinoma (Figure 6-5) and large-cell NECs (Figure 6-6).[29]

It is recommended that mitoses be counted in 50 HPFs and Ki67 index be determined by counting 500–2000 tumor cells to ensure accuracy. Due to frequent intratumor heterogeneity of NETs, the Ki67 index should be evaluated in the highest labeling area ("hot spot") by scanning at low power, which might represent the most aggressive component of the tumors.[24] Discrepancy between mitotic rate and Ki67 index is not uncommon. In such cases, the higher grade should be assigned.[24] In addition, several studies have observed that the Ki67 grade is always greater than the mitotic grade if the two proliferation indices point to different grades. Therefore, it has been suggested that Ki67 index alone is sufficient to grade NETs.

A small group of NETs shows the typical morphology of well-differentiated NETs but with a high Ki67 (usually between 20% and 50%) and a low mitotic rate (usually much

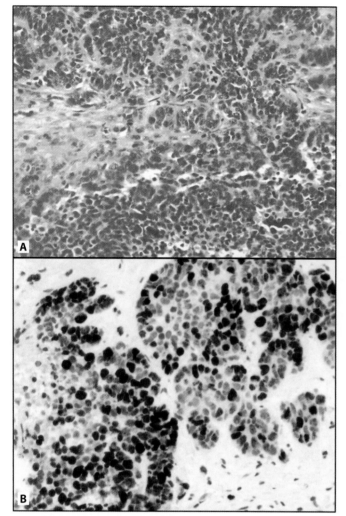

FIGURE 6-5. Poorly differentiated neuroendocrine carcinoma, small-cell carcinoma (World Health Organization grade 3). **A.** Hematoxylin and eosin stain showing frequent mitoses, apoptosis, and necrosis (original magnification ×100). **B.** Ki67 immunohistochemical stain showing a Ki67 index of approximately 70%.

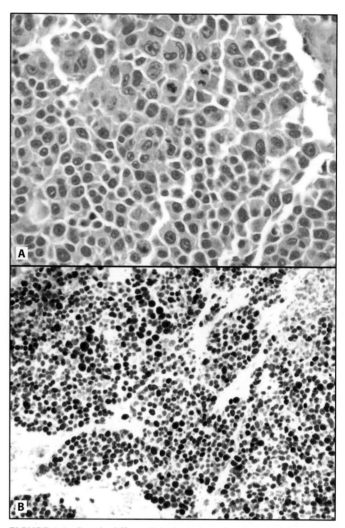

FIGURE 6-6. Poorly differentiated neuroendocrine carcinoma, large-cell neuroendocrine carcinoma (World Health Organization grade 3). **A.** Hematoxylin and eosin stain showing frequent mitoses and carcinoma cells with prominent nucleoli (original magnification ×400). **B.** Ki67 immunohistochemical stain showing a Ki67 index approaching 100% (original magnification ×100).

less than 20 mitoses/10 HPFs) (Figure 6-7). Based on the WHO criteria, these tumors would be classified as grade 3, high-grade NECs. Although they are more aggressive than grade 2–concordant NETs, studies have demonstrated that they are not as aggressive as true high-grade NECs. In addition, they respond differently to chemotherapy; Ki67 grade 3 tumors are resistant to platinum-based chemotherapy like most well-differentiated NETs, whereas true high-grade NECs are sensitive to chemotherapy. In such cases, the tumor should be reported as a well-differentiated NET but with the specific mitotic rate and Ki67 index. The findings also suggest that the cut points used in the ENETS/WHO classification need to be reassessed.

As described, intratumoral Ki67 heterogeneity is common in GI-NETs. When patients present with unresectable primary tumor or distant metastatic disease, a biopsy could be the only specimen for grading the tumors, which has the potential to miss higher-grade foci. Yang et al evaluated the effect of tumor heterogeneity on the assessment of the Ki67 index in well-differentiated NETs metastatic to the liver and found that grade 2 NETs would be misclassified as grade 1 in 65% of cases if only one biopsy was taken and in 52% of cases if three biopsies were taken.[30] Accurate identification of the higher-grade regions is important as studies have shown that the higher grade more accurately predicts the outcome in cases with heterogeneity. Therefore, multiple core biopsies are needed to better predict patient outcome.

Histologic Features of Well-Differentiated NETs

The GI-NETs grossly are firm tan to pale yellow nodules located just beneath the mucosal surface. The muscularis propria may be thickened in the area of the tumor, perhaps as a result of secretion of trophic factors by the tumor cells. Dense, fibrotic stroma associated with the tumor cells may

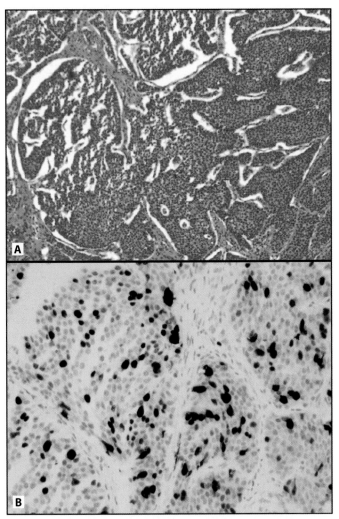

FIGURE 6-7. Well-differentiated neuroendocrine tumor with Ki67 greater than 20%. **A.** Hematoxylin and eosin stain showing a typical well-differentiated neuroendocrine carcinoma without frequent mitoses (original magnification ×100). **B.** Ki67 immunohistochemical stain showing a Ki67 index greater than 20% (original magnification ×200).

produce annular strictures, and mesenteric fibrosis may be seen in small-bowel NETs. Ischemic injury secondary to vascular sclerosis may also be seen in small-bowel tumors.[31] Multicentricity is common and is site related, with gastric and jejunoileal tumors (33%) more commonly multiple, whereas multiplicity is rare with colonic or appendiceal NETs. Molecular studies have shown that most multiple GI-NETs are independent primaries.[32]

Microscopically, most GI-NETs are readily recognizable as low-grade NETs. They are composed of solid nests, cords, trabeculae, and glands of relatively uniform cells with round-to-oval nuclei with finely granular chromatin and inconspicuous nucleoli. Less commonly, cystic, tubular, or angiomatoid patterns may be seen. The cytoplasm is generally pale, but in some cases, fine red granules are detectable (Figures 6-3, 6-4, and 6-7). Cytologic variants include

clear-cell NETs (generally found in the pancreas in patients with von Hippel–Lindau disease) and oncocytic and rhabdoid appearances. Large areas of tumor necrosis are uncommon and when present signify a higher-grade tumor, but punctate coagulative necrosis may be seen in larger low-grade tumors. Perineural and lymphovascular invasion are associated with more aggressive behavior[33] and are generally not seen in small low-grade tumors.

Histologic Features of Poorly Differentiated NECs

Poorly differentiated NECs are mainly located in the esophagus, ampulla of Vater, and large bowel. They include small-cell carcinoma (Figure 6-5) and large-cell NEC (Figure 6-6). Both carcinomas show high mitotic rates, prominent apoptosis, and frequent tumor necrosis. Small-cell carcinomas of the GI tract are mostly located in the esophagus and anorectal region and sometimes are associated with squamous cell carcinoma; large-cell NECs more commonly arise in the areas with glandular mucosa and are frequently associated with an adenocarcinoma component. If both neuroendocrine and adenocarcinoma components each comprise at least 30% of the tumor, mixed adenoneuroendocrine carcinoma (MANEC) should be designated.[29]

The morphology of GI small-cell carcinoma is similar to its lung counterpart. The carcinoma cells are small with scant cytoplasm, an oval-to-fusiform nucleus, and granular chromatin. A component of larger cells with more cytoplasm (intermediate cells) can be seen in some GI small-cell carcinoma. They express chromogranin A, synaptophysin, and CD56, but immunohistochemical labeling can be inconsistent and patchy. Large-cell NECs are composed of round-to-oval cells containing moderate-to-abundant cytoplasm and nuclei with evident nucleoli and vesicular chromatin. Large-cell NECs express chromogranin and synaptophysin. Expression of at least one of the neuroendocrine markers is required to diagnose large-cell NEC.[24]

Precursor Lesions

Endocrine cell hyperplasia is most commonly seen in the GI tract in the stomach in the setting of hypergastrinemia and chronic atrophic gastritis[3,10,34–36](see also Chapter 17). The WHO 2010 classification divides hyperplastic lesions of the gastric neuroendocrine system into simple, linear, and nodular patterns. A diagnosis of dysplasia is made when there are features of enlarging or fusing micronodules, microinvasion, or newly formed stroma. The lesion is classified as microcarcinoid when the nodules are larger than 0.5 mm but less than 0.5 cm or invade the submucosa but less than 0.5 cm, and carcinoid when the size is 0.5 cm or greater.[29] Duodenal gastrin- or somatostatin-producing cells undergo a similar hyperplasia in patients with multiple endocrine neoplasia type 1 (MEN 1) syndrome.[36] Gastrin- or somatostatin-producing lesions in the duodenum and measuring larger than 300 or 400 μm, respectively, are classified as GI-NETs as loss of heterozygosity (LOH) at the *MEN1* gene locus is detected in these lesions but not in hyperplastic gastrin and somatostatin cells.[37] Although the appendix, ileum, and rectum are common locations for GI-NETs, endocrine cell hyperplasia and dysplastic lesions are rarely encountered in these sites, and in general, sporadic NETs lack identifiable precursor lesions. Neuroendocrine cell hyperplasia and multiple GI-NETs have been reported in the setting of ulcerative colitis[38] and Crohn disease and are associated with epithelial dysplastic changes in some cases.[39]

Staging

The ENETS first proposed staging criteria for primary GI-NETs in 2006 and 2007; a T category is determined by tumor size, depth of invasion, and extent of local invasion. The N category is determined based on the absence (N0) or the presence of involved lymph nodes (N1).[27,28] Like other GI malignancies, the tumors with distant metastasis are designated as M1. The AJCC in 2010 adopted the ENETS staging system but with some modifications (Table 6-4).[40] All poorly differentiated NECs are staged as adenocarcinoma of their corresponding sites.

Differential Diagnosis

Distant metastasis is common for GEP-NETs, especially intestinal and pancreatic NETs. Immunohistochemical stains for neuroendocrine markers, mainly chromogranin A and synaptophysin, can be used to differentiate them from other epithelial malignancies. Lung and pancreatic NETs are the main differential diagnoses for GI-NETs. Lung primary carcinoids always express thyroid transcription factor 1 (TTF1), whereas well-differentiated GI-NETs do not.[41,42] However, poorly differentiated NETs of the gut may express TTF-1. Intestinal markers, including caudal type homeobox 2 (CDX2) and cadherin 17 (CDH17), are expressed by most GI-NETs but are not expressed by lung carcinoid tumors.[41,42] However, a small portion of pancreatic NETs express CDX2 or CDH17.[43] Some pancreatic biomarkers, including islet 1 (ISL-1), pancreaticoduodenal homeobox 1 (PDX-1) gene product, and paired box gene 8 (PAX8), can be also expressed by GI-NETs and lung carcinoid tumors.[41,44–47] ISL-1 expression is frequently found in well- and poorly differentiated neuroendocrine neoplasms of extrapancreatic origin, including colorectal and duodenal NETs. PAX8 is expressed by the majority of rectal NETs. In addition, PDX-1 expression is observed in some duodenal NETs (Table 6-5).

■ CELL OF ORIGIN AND MOLECULAR GENETICS

Well-differentiated GI-NETS arise as a result of molecular events in progenitor cells that are "neuroendocrine committed" but not necessarily terminally differentiated.[48] This concept helps explain why certain NETs are more homogeneous, with a dominant hormonal secretory pattern reflecting that of normal neuroendocrine cells in the location where they arise, and others secrete multiple hormones or lack apparent hormonal functionality. For instance, ECL cell NETs arise almost exclusively in the stomach, paralleling the

normal distribution of ECL cells.[10,34,35] Although GI-NETs are derived from epithelial stem cells of the gut, investigations of the neoplastic progression for these tumors have shown that they do not share the same molecular alterations as GI adenocarcinomas and infrequently show microsatellite instability or abnormalities of Wnt signaling.[2] In addition, biologically they are very different. Compared to GI adenocarcinomas, most GI-NETs display a relatively slower growth pattern and a more indolent disease course. On the other hand, it has been suggested that poorly differentiated NECs arise from multipotent stem cells, which may be the origin of GI adenocarcinomas.[49] It is likely that poorly differentiated NECs or MANECs share the complex pathogenetic setting of the common GI adenocarcinomas.

Although only 5% to 10% of GI-NETs are linked to hereditary syndromes (generally autosomal dominantly inherited syndromes resulting from mutations in tumor suppressor genes; Table 6-6), such cases have afforded important insights into molecular pathways involved in NETs. For instance, the *MEN1* gene is mutated in up to 40% of sporadic upper GI and pancreatic NETs.[50] Molecular events appear to be different in GI-NETs arising in different sites, with foregut tumors often showing loss of 11q, the site of *MEN1*, in contrast to midgut and hindgut tumors, which often show losses on 18q.[13,51]

While our understanding of the genetic basis underlying pancreatic NETs has been greatly expanded recently, information on carcinogenetic mechanisms underlying GI-NETs is still limited. However, recent genetic studies of both small-intestinal and pancreatic NETs have demonstrated that most GEP-NETs display a relatively small number of genetic abnormalities.[52,53] In addition, we now know that the genetic bases underlying tumorigenesis of small-intestinal and pancreatic NETs are different. *MEN1*, *DAXX/ARTX*, and genes in the phosphoinositide-3-kinase (PI3K)/mammalian target of rapamycin (mTOR) signaling pathway are frequently mutated in the pancreatic NET but are rarely mutated in small-intestinal NETs.[52–54] However, a recent whole-genomic sequencing study reported that alterations in several cancer-related pathways is common in small-intestinal NETs, which include the PI3K/Akt/mTOR signaling, the transforming growth factor β (TGF-β) pathway (through alterations in *SMAD* genes), and the *SRC* oncogene.[52] Recurrent somatic mutations and deletions in CDKN1B are present in approximately 10% of small-intestinal NETs.[54]

■ MANAGEMENT

Surgery is considered as a first-line treatment because it is the only treatment that may cure the patients with GI-NETs and NECs.[55,56] For patients with metastatic or unresectable disease, debulking surgery may be performed to reduce tumor burden and to control endocrinopathy or local symptoms. In addition, medical, radiological, and nuclear medicine strategies have been used for management of patients with advanced GI-NETs.[56–60] More recently, several biologic agents have been introduced to treat progressive GI-NETs.

TABLE 6-4. Comparison of ENETS and AJCC/UICC TNM staging system of gastrointestinal neuroendocrine tumors.

		ENETS	AJCC/UICC
Gastric neuroendocrine tumor			
T stage	Tis	In situ tumor/dysplasia (tumor size < 0.5 mm), confined to mucosa	Same as ENETS
	T1	Tumor invades LP or submucosa and is ≤ 1 cm in size	Same as ENETS
	T2	Tumor invades MP or subserosa or is > 1 cm	Tumor invades MP or > 1 cm in size
	T3	Tumor penetrates serosa	Tumor penetrates subserosa
	T4	Tumor invades adjacent organs or structures	Tumor invades serosa or other organs or adjacent structures
Small-intestinal neuroendocrine tumor			
T stage	T1	Tumor invades LP or submucosa and size is ≤ 1 cm (small-intestinal and ampullary tumor)	Tumor invades LP or submucosa and size ≤ 1 cm (small-intestinal tumor); tumor size ≤ 1 cm (ampullary tumor)
	T2	Tumor invades MP or size is > 1 cm (small-intestinal and ampullary tumor)	Tumor invades MP or size > 1 cm (small-intestinal tumor); tumor size > 1 cm (ampullary tumor)
	T3	Tumor invades subserosa/nonperitonealized tissues (jejunal/ileal tumor); tumor invades pancreas, retroperitoneum, or nonperitonealized tissues (ampullary/duodenal tumors)	Same as ENETS
	T4	Tumor invades serosa or other organs	Same as ENETS
Appendiceal neuroendocrine tumor			
T stage	T1	Tumor size ≤ 1 cm, invading submucosa and MP	Tumor size ≤ 2 cm
	T2	Tumor size > 1 cm but ≤ 2 cm, invading submucosa, MP, or minimally (up to 3 mm) invading subserosa/mesoappendix	Tumor size > 2 cm but ≤ 4 cm or with extension to the cecum
	T3	Tumor size > 2 cm or (> 3 mm) invasion of subserosa/mesoappendix	Tumor size > 4 cm or with extension to ileum
	T4	Tumor invades serosa/other organs	Tumor directly invades other adjacent organs or structures
Colorectal neuroendocrine tumor			
T stage	T1	Tumor invades LP or submucosa and size is ≤ 2 cm	Same as ENETS
	T2	Tumor invades MP or is > 2 cm with invasion of LP or submucosa	Same as ENETS
	T3	Tumor invades into subserosa or pericolic/perirectal soft tissue	Same as ENETS
	T4	Tumor invades peritoneum or other organs	Same as ENETS
NM stage for gastrointestinal neuroendocrine tumor (ENETS/AJCC/UICC)			
N stage	N0	No regional lymph node metastasis	
	N1	Regional lymph node metastasis	
M stage	Nx	Regional lymph node cannot be assessed	
	M0	No distant metastasis	
	M1	Distant metastasis	
	MX	Distant metastasis cannot be assessed	

Abbreviations: AJCC, American Joint Committee on Cancer; ENETS, European Neuroendocrine Tumor Society; LP, lamina propria; MP, muscularis propria; UICC, International Union Against Cancer.

Well-differentiated GI-NETs are generally resistant to cytotoxic chemotherapy, whereas treatment of poorly differentiated GI-NECs is similar to that of small-cell lung cancer. Studies on cisplatin and etoposide have shown a response rate of up to 67% in poorly differentiated GEP-NECs versus 7% in well-differentiated GI-NETs.[60,61] SSAs are considered to be the first-line medical therapy for well-differentiated GEP-NETs.[57,59,62,63] SSAs can be used to control hormonal secretion.[64] In addition, SSAs demonstrate antiproliferative efficacy, probably through activation of Gi-protein–coupled

TABLE 6-5. Markers for differential diagnosis of gastrointestinal neuroendocrine tumors.

	TTF-1	CDX2	CDH17	PAX8	ISL-1	PDX-1
Lung	+	–	Some +	Some +	Some +	Some +
Pancreas	–	Some +	Some +	+	+	+
Stomach	–	+	NA	Some +	Some+	NA
Duodenum	–	+	NA	+	+	+
Small intestine	–	+	+	–	Some+	–
Rectum	–	+	NA	+	+	–
Appendix	–	+	NA	Some +	Some +	Some +
GI NEC	+	+	NA	NA	+	NA

Abbreviations: GI NEC, gastrointestinal neuroendocrine carcinoma; ISL-1, islet 1; PDX-1, pancreaticoduodenal homeobox 1; Some +: positive in < 25% cases.

somatostatin receptor (SSTR) subtypes, mainly SSTR2, which is expressed by the majority of GI-NETs. Recent clinical trials have shown that radionuclide therapy with either ^{90}Y- or ^{177}Lu-labeled SSA (DOTATOC or DOTATATE) is a promising treatment option for patients with SSTR-expressing GEP-NETs.[57,59,62,64] While the mTOR inhibitor everolimus has been approved by the Food and Drug Administration (FDA) for treatment of advanced pancreatic NETs, the role of everolimus in the treatment of GI-NETs remains controversial.

SUMMARY

The GI-NETs are a heterogeneous group of neoplasms of the GI tract that have neuroendocrine differentiation. The genetic basis for GI-NETs remains largely unknown. While most GI-NETs are well-differentiated and slowly growing tumors, some are poorly differentiated and share similar biology with GI adenocarcinomas. Although the majority of GI-NETs have an indolent clinical course, patients with the disease frequently present at an advanced, unresectable stage, and medical therapy is needed to control symptoms and disease progression. A number of novel therapeutic approaches are being developed and show promising results.

REFERENCES

1. Plockinger U, Rindi G, Arnold R, et al. Guidelines for the diagnosis and treatment of neuroendocrine gastrointestinal tumours. A consensus statement on behalf of the European Neuroendocrine Tumour Society (ENETS). *Neuroendocrinology.* 2004;80:394–424.
2. Kloppel G, Rindi G, Anlauf M, Perren A, Komminoth P. Site-specific biology and pathology of gastroenteropancreatic neuroendocrine tumors. *Virchows Arch.* 2007;451(Suppl 1):S9–S27.
3. Solcia E, Vanoli A. Histogenesis and natural history of gut neuroendocrine tumors: present status. *Endocr Pathol.* 2014;25(2):165–170.
4. Williams ED, Sandler M. The classification of carcinoid tumours. *Lancet.* 1963;1:238–239.
5. Lawrence B, Gustafsson BI, Chan A, Svejda B, Kidd M, Modlin IM. The epidemiology of gastroenteropancreatic neuroendocrine tumors. *Endocrinol Metab Clin North Am.* 2011;40:1–18, vii.
6. Yao JC, Hassan M, Phan A, et al. One hundred years after "carcinoid": epidemiology of and prognostic factors for neuroendocrine tumors in 35,825 cases in the United States. *J Clin Oncol.* 2008;26:3063–3072.
7. Untch BR, Bonner KP, Roggin KK, et al. Pathologic grade and tumor size are associated with recurrence-free survival in patients with duodenal neuroendocrine tumors. *J Gastrointest Surg.* 2014;18:457–462; discussion 462–463.
8. Hauso O, Gustafsson BI, Kidd M, et al. Neuroendocrine tumor epidemiology: contrasting Norway and North America. *Cancer.* 2008;113:2655–2664.
9. Fraenkel M, Kim MK, Faggiano A, Valk GD. Epidemiology of gastroenteropancreatic neuroendocrine tumours. *Best Pract Res Clin Gastroenterol.* 2012;26:691–703.
10. Kidd M, Gustafsson B, Modlin IM. Gastric carcinoids (neuroendocrine neoplasms). *Gastroenterol Clin North Am.* 2013;42:381–397.
11. Mocellin S, Nitti D. Gastrointestinal carcinoid: epidemiological and survival evidence from a large population-based study (n = 25 531). *Ann Oncol.* 2013;24:3040–3044.
12. Li AF, Hsu CY, Li A, et al. A 35-year retrospective study of carcinoid tumors in Taiwan: differences in distribution with a high probability of associated second primary malignancies. *Cancer.* 2008;112:274–283.
13. Modlin IM, Kidd M, Latich I, Zikusoka MN, Shapiro MD. Current status of gastrointestinal carcinoids. *Gastroenterology.* 2005;128:1717–1751.
14. Mooney E. The flushing patient. *Int J Dermatol.* 1985;24:549–554.
15. Jacobs C. Neuroendocrine tumors a rare finding: part I. *Clin J Oncol Nurs.* 2009;13:21–23.
16. Frilling A, Akerstrom G, Falconi M, et al. Neuroendocrine tumor disease: an evolving landscape. *Endocr Relat Cancer.* 2012;19:R163–R185.
17. Habal N, Sims C, Bilchik AJ. Gastrointestinal carcinoid tumors and second primary malignancies. *J Surg Oncol.* 2000;75:310–316.
18. Kloppel G, Perren A, Heitz PU. The gastroenteropancreatic neuroendocrine cell system and its tumors: the WHO classification. *Annals N Y Acad Sci.* 2004;1014:13–27.
19. Hamilton SR, Aaltonen LA, eds. *World Health Organization Classification of Tumours. Pathology and Genetics of Tumours of the Digestive System.* Lyon, France: IARC Press; 2000.
20. Solcia E, Klöppel G, Sobin LH, eds. Histological typing of endocrine tumours. In: Solcia E, Klöppel G, Sobin LH, eds. *World Health Organization Edition. International Histological Classification of Endocrine Tumours.* New York, NY: Springer-Verlag; 2000;1-156.
21. Kloppel G. Classification and pathology of gastroenteropancreatic neuroendocrine neoplasms. *Endocr Relat Cancer.* 2011;18(Suppl 1):S1–S16.
22. Capelli P, Fassan M, Scarpa A. Pathology—grading and staging of GEP-NETs. *Best Pract Res Clin Gastroenterol.* 2012;26:705–717.
23. Klimstra DS. Pathology reporting of neuroendocrine tumors: essential elements for accurate diagnosis, classification, and staging. *Semin Oncol.* 2013;40:23–36.
24. Yang Z, Tang LH, Klimstra DS. Gastroenteropancreatic neuroendocrine neoplasms: historical context and current issues. *Semin Diagn Pathol.* 2013;30:186–196.

TABLE 6-6. Hereditary syndromes associated with GI-NETs.

Syndrome	Inheritance and prevalence	Gene	Gene product and function	GI-NETs	Major tumor sites
MEN type 1	Autosomal dominant; ~ 1:20,000 to 1:40,000	*MEN*; chromosome 11q13	Menin; controls cell growth and differentiation during development	Stomach and duodenum (gastrinomas); associated with Zollinger-Ellison syndrome; pancreas	Anterior pituitary, parathyroid, adrenal cortex, lung
Neurofibromatosis type 1	Autosomal dominant; ~ 1:4500	*NF1*; chromosome 17q11.2	Neurofibromin; tumor suppressor functions	1% of patients; usually duodenum/ampulla; express somatostatin but not associated with functional syndromes	Neurofibromas
Von Hippel–Lindau syndrome	Autosomal dominant; ~ 1:36,000	*VHL*, chromosome 3p25	VHL; multiple functions	Pancreatic NETs in 5% to 17%, usually non-functioning clear-cell tumors	Renal cell carcinoma, hemangioblastoma, pheochromocytoma
Tuberous sclerosis complex	Autosomal dominant; 1:10,000	*TSC1*, 9q34 *TSC2*, 16p13.3	Hamartin Tuberin Tumor suppressor functions	Pancreatic NETs (rare)	Hamartomatous lesions in brain, skin, eye, heart, lung, kidney

Abbreviations: GI-NET, gastrointestinal neuroendocrine tumor; MEN, multiple endocrine neoplasia.

25. College of American Pathologists. CAP Career & Life Preserver. http://www.cap.org/apps/cap.portal?_nfpb=true&_pageLabel=reference. Accessed on May 8, 2015.

26. Stephenson TJ, Cross SS, Chetty R. Standards and datasets for reporting cancers. The Royal College of Pathologists. 2012. http://www.rcpath.org/Resources/RCPath/Migrated%20Resources/Documents/G/G081_DatasetGIEndocrine_Sep12.pdf. Accessed on May 8, 2015.

27. Rindi G, Kloppel G, Alhman H, et al. TNM staging of foregut (neuro) endocrine tumors: a consensus proposal including a grading system. *Virchows Arch.* 2006;449:395–401.

28. Rindi G, Kloppel G, Couvelard A, et al. TNM staging of midgut and hindgut (neuro) endocrine tumors: a consensus proposal including a grading system. *Virchows Arch.* 2007;451:757–762.

29. Fred T. Bosman FC, Ralph H Hruban, Neil D Theise, ed. *WHO Classification of Tumours of the Digestive System.* 4th ed. Lyon, France: International Agency for Reasearch on Cancer (IARC); 2010.

30. Yang Z, Tang LH, Klimstra DS. Effect of tumor heterogeneity on the assessment of Ki67 labeling index in well-differentiated neuroendocrine tumors metastatic to the liver: implications for prognostic stratification. *Am J Surg Pathol.* 2011;35:853–860.

31. Qizilbash AH. Carcinoid tumors, vascular elastosis, and ischemic disease of the small intestine. *Dis Colon Rectum.* 1977;20:554–560.

32. Katona TM, Jones TD, Wang M, Abdul-Karim FW, Cummings OW, Cheng L. Molecular evidence for independent origin of multifocal neuroendocrine tumors of the enteropancreatic axis. *Cancer Res.* 2006;66:4936–4942.

33. Rorstad O. Prognostic indicators for carcinoid neuroendocrine tumors of the gastrointestinal tract. *J Surg Oncol.* 2005;89:151–160.

34. Mete O, Asa SL. Precursor lesions of endocrine system neoplasms. *Pathology.* 2013;45:316–330.

35. Crosby DA, Donohoe CL, Fitzgerald L, et al. Gastric neuroendocrine tumours. *Dig Surg.* 2012;29:331–348.

36. Kloppel G, Anlauf M, Perren A, Sipos B. Hyperplasia to neoplasia sequence of duodenal and pancreatic neuroendocrine diseases and pseudohyperplasia of the PP-cells in the pancreas. *Endocr Pathol.* 2014;25(2):181–185.

37. Anlauf M, Perren A, Henopp T, et al. Allelic deletion of the MEN1 gene in duodenal gastrin and somatostatin cell neoplasms and their precursor lesions. *Gut.* 2007;56:637–644.

38. Gledhill A, Hall PA, Cruse JP, Pollock DJ. Enteroendocrine cell hyperplasia, carcinoid tumours and adenocarcinoma in long-standing ulcerative colitis. *Histopathology.* 1986;10:501–508.

39. Sigel JE, Goldblum JR. Neuroendocrine neoplasms arising in inflammatory bowel disease: a report of 14 cases. *Mod Pathol.* 1998;11:537–542.

40. Edge S, Byrd DR, Compton CC, Fritz AG, Greene FL, Trotti A, eds. *AJCC Cancer Staging Handbook From the AJCC Cancer Staging Manual.* 7th ed. New York, NY: Springer; 2010.

41. Chan ES, Alexander J, Swanson PE, Jain D, Yeh MM. PDX-1, CDX-2, TTF-1, and CK7: a reliable immunohistochemical panel for pancreatic neuroendocrine neoplasms. *Am J Surg Pathol.* 2012;36:737–743.

42. Denby KS, Briones AJ, Bourne PA, et al. IMP3, NESP55, TTF-1 and CDX2 serve as an immunohistochemical panel in the distinction among small-cell carcinoma, gastrointestinal carcinoid, and pancreatic endocrine tumor metastasized to the liver. *Appl Immunohistochem Mol Morphol.* 2012;20:573–579.

43. Panarelli NC, Yantiss RK, Yeh MM, Liu Y, Chen YT. Tissue-specific cadherin CDH17 is a useful marker of gastrointestinal adenocarcinomas with higher sensitivity than CDX2. *Am J Clin Pathol.* 2012;138:211–222.

44. Hermann G, Konukiewitz B, Schmitt A, Perren A, Kloppel G. Hormonally defined pancreatic and duodenal neuroendocrine tumors differ in their transcription factor signatures: expression of ISL1, PDX1, NGN3, and CDX2. *Virchows Arch.* 2011;459:147–154.

45. Graham RP, Shrestha B, Caron BL, et al. Islet-1 is a sensitive but not entirely specific marker for pancreatic neuroendocrine neoplasms and their metastases. *Am J Surg Pathol.* 2013;37:399–405.

46. Agaimy A, Erlenbach-Wunsch K, Konukiewitz B, et al. ISL1 expression is not restricted to pancreatic well-differentiated neuroendocrine neoplasms, but is also commonly found in well and poorly differentiated neuroendocrine neoplasms of extrapancreatic origin. *Mod Pathol.* 2013;26:995–1003.

47. Koo J, Mertens RB, Mirocha JM, Wang HL, Dhall D. Value of Islet 1 and PAX8 in identifying metastatic neuroendocrine tumors of pancreatic origin. *Mod Pathol.* 2012;25:893–901.

48. Arnold CN, Sosnowski A, Schmitt-Graff A, Arnold R, Blum HE. Analysis of molecular pathways in sporadic neuroendocrine tumors of the gastro-entero-pancreatic system. *Int J Cancer.* 2007;120:2157–2164.

49. Sorbye H, Strosberg J, Baudin E, Klimstra DS, Yao JC. Gastroenteropancreatic high-grade neuroendocrine carcinoma. *Cancer.* 2014;120(18):2814–2823.

50. Grotzinger C. Tumour biology of gastroenteropancreatic neuroendocrine tumours. *Neuroendocrinology.* 2004;80(Suppl 1):8–11.

51. Perren A, Anlauf M, Komminoth P. Molecular profiles of gastroenteropancreatic endocrine tumors. *Virchows Arch.* 2007;451(Suppl 1):S39–S46.

52. Banck MS, Kanwar R, Kulkarni AA, et al. The genomic landscape of small intestine neuroendocrine tumors. *J Clin Invest.* 2013;123:2502–2508.

53. Jiao Y, Shi C, Edil BH, et al. DAXX/ATRX, MEN1, and mTOR pathway genes are frequently altered in pancreatic neuroendocrine tumors. *Science.* 2011;331:1199–1203.

54. Francis JM, Kiezun A, Ramos AH, et al. Somatic mutation of CDKN1B in small intestine neuroendocrine tumors. *Nat Genet.* 2013;45:1483–1486.

55. Knigge U, Hansen CP. Surgery for GEP-NETs. *Best Pract Res Clin Gastroenterol.* 2012;26:819–831.

56. Oberg K, Knigge U, Kwekkeboom D, Perren A. Neuroendocrine gastroentero-pancreatic tumors: ESMO clinical practice guidelines for diagnosis, treatment and follow-up. *Ann Oncol.* 2012;23(Suppl 7):vii124–130.

57. Pavel M, Baudin E, Couvelard A, et al. ENETS consensus guidelines for the management of patients with liver and other distant metastases from neuroendocrine neoplasms of foregut, midgut, hindgut, and unknown primary. *Neuroendocrinology.* 2012;95:157–176.

58. Costa FP, Gumz B, Pasche B. Selecting patients for cytotoxic therapies in gastroenteropancreatic neuroendocrine tumours. *Best Pract Res Clin Gastroenterol.* 2012;26:843–854.

59. Strosberg JR. Systemic treatment of gastroenteropancreatic neuroendocrine tumors (GEP-NETS): current approaches and future options. *Endocr Pract.* 2014;20:167–175.

60. Moertel CG, Kvols LK, O'Connell MJ, Rubin J. Treatment of neuroendocrine carcinomas with combined etoposide and cisplatin. Evidence of major therapeutic activity in the anaplastic variants of these neoplasms. *Cancer.* 1991;68:227–232.

61. Mitry E, Baudin E, Ducreux M, et al. Treatment of poorly differentiated neuroendocrine tumours with etoposide and cisplatin. *Br J Cancer.* 1999;81:1351–1355.

62. Castano JP, Sundin A, Maecke HR, et al. Gastrointestinal neuroendocrine tumors (NETs): new diagnostic and therapeutic challenges. *Cancer Metastasis Rev.* 2014;33(3):353–359.

63. Oberg K. Biotherapies for GEP-NETs. *Best Pract Res Clin Gastroenterol.* 2012;26:833–841.

64. Baudin E, Planchard D, Scoazec JY, et al. Intervention in gastroenteropancreatic neuroendocrine tumours. *Best Pract Res Clin Gastroenterol.* 2012;26:855–865.

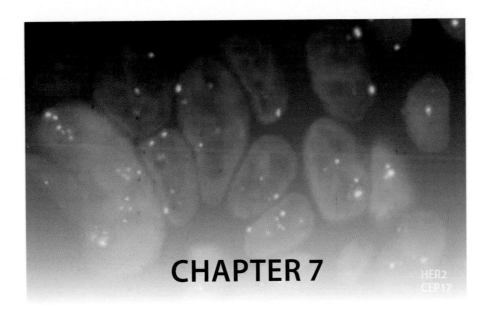

CHAPTER 7

Molecular and Other Ancillary Tests for GI Tumors

Nora Joseph and Shu-Yuan Xiao

INTRODUCTION

There has been increasing necessity for the surgical patholo-gist to be up to date on standard-of-care practices in molec-ular oncology, specifically familiarity with the significance and applicability of various biomarkers. With the boom in advanced capability to accurately and effectively discover novel mutations and variations in genetic sequence, there are limitless possibilities for future testing menus; how-ever, only a subset associated with treatment planning is currently in clinical use. Therefore, this chapter focuses on the most common and frequently requested molecular tests used for diagnostic, prognostic, or treatment purposes within gastrointestinal (GI) solid-tumor oncology. A quick reference for these markers is organized by methodology, specific tumor type, and cancer syndrome in Table 7-1. The following sections focus on tests most relevant to tumors of specific sites.

ESOPHAGEAL ADENOCARCINOMA

Most esophageal adenocarcinomas (EACs) arise in a back-ground of Barrett esophagus (BE). This specialized epithe-lium is prone to genetic alterations, such as amplification or overexpression of *EGFR*, *MET*, and *NFKB*. One member of the EGFR family, *ERBB2* (also known as *HER2*, *HER2/neu*) is amplified in approximately 25% of EACs and is believed to play an important role in driving cell proliferation and inhibiting apoptosis. Trastusumab, or Herceptin®, is a specific

monoclonal antibody targeting ERBB2 (HER2) that, when combined with conventional chemotherapy, has been shown to increase survival in patients with advanced disease.[1] Therefore, *ERBB2* (*HER2*) amplification is now routinely assessed in EAC and gastroesophageal junctional (GEJ) carci-noma for its therapeutic implications. The gene amplification can be detected directly by fluorescence in situ hybridiza-tion (FISH) and indirectly for protein overexpression by immunohistochemistry (IHC). IHC interpretation differs from breast carcinoma, and specific guidelines are described in detail in the gastric adenocarcinoma (GA) section next (and in Table 7-2).

GASTRIC ADENOCARCINOMA

Gastric adenocarcinomas most often arise in a background of chronic gastritis and are preceded by extensive intestinal metaplasia with dysplasia. A significant proportion of cases are related to *Helicobacter pylori* infection. GAs are aggres-sive tumors that have been historically difficult to treat. As the molecular landscape of GA unfolds, several distinct pathways have emerged, some with critical clinical signifi-cance. For example, *ERBB2* (*HER2*) amplification or overex-pression has been observed in 4%–36% of GAs. Accordingly, the small-molecule inhibitor trastusumab has become an integral addition to traditional fluoropyrimidine-based and platinum-based chemotherapy combinations. Other genes for receptor tyrosine kinases, such as *MET*, are amplified or overexpressed in approximately 5%–30% of GAs. MET

TABLE 7-1. Ancillary tests frequently performed for gastrointestinal tumors (GISTs).

A. By methodology

Immunohistochemistry (IHC)

ERBB2 (HER2)	Esophageal, gastrointestinal junctional, or gastric adenocarcinomas
E-cadherin (CDH1)	Hereditary gastric adenocarcinoma
SDHA, SDHB	Pediatric or Carney complex GISTs
MMRP	Lynch syndrome, sporadic microsatellite instability
MET	Metastatic gastric adenocarcinoma
p16	Anorectal squamous carcinoma
BRAF mutation specific	Colorectal carcinoma

PCR-based analysis

KIT/PDGFRA mutation	*GIST*
MSI	Lynch syndrome, sporadic microsatellite instability
KRAS	Colorectal adenocarcinoma
BRAF	Colorectal adenocarcinoma
HPV screening for high risk serotypes	Anorectal squamous carcinoma
E6/E7 oncotype mRNA	Anorectal squamous carcinoma
CDH1 mutation	Hereditary gastric adenocarcinoma

Hybridization (ISH)

ERBB2 (HER2) amplification	Esophageal, gastrointestinal junctional, or gastric adenocarcinomas
DNA methylation alterations (*MLH1* promoter methylation)	Microsatellite instability
HPV	Anorectal squamous carcinoma
ALK	
EGFR	

B. By tumor

Esophageal and gastroesophageal junctional adenocarcinoma	IHC: ERBB2
	FISH: *ERBB2* amplification
Gastric adenocarcinoma	IHC: ERBB2
	FISH for *ERBB2* amplification IHC: E-cadherin
	CDH1 (E-cadherin) germline mutation for hereditary diffuse-type gastric adenocarcinoma
Colorectal adenocarcinoma	IHC: MMR protein expression
	PCR: MSI markers
	MLH1 hypermethylation
	KRAS mutation
	BRAF mutation
	Mutational analysis for suspected Lynch tumor
Anorectal squamous cell carcinoma	IHC: p16
	PCR: HPV serotypes
	ISH: HPV integrated DNA
	RT-PCR: HPV E6/E7 mRNA
GI stromal tumor (GIST)	*KIT* with reflex to *PDGFRA*
	SDHA, SDHB in pediatric or Carney complex GISTs
Clear-cell sarcoma-like tumor of gastrointestinal tract (GNET)	

TABLE 7-1. Ancillary tests frequently performed for gastrointestinal tumors (GISTs) *(Continued)*

C. By syndrome	
Lynch syndrome	IHC for MMR proteins: MLH1, MSH2, MSH6, PMS2
	PCR: MSI
	Mutational analysis of MMR genes
Familial adenomatous polyposis (*APC*)	*APC, MUTYH*
Familial GIST syndrome	*KIT, PDGFRA* mutations
Carney-Stratakis syndrome	IHC: succinate dehydrogenase subunits A, B, C, D, E
	Mutation: *SDHA, SDHB*

Abbreviations: FISH, fluorescence in situ hybridization; HPV, human papilloma virus; ISH, in situ hybridization; MMR, mismatch repair; MMRP, mismatch repair protein; mRNA, messenger RNA; MSI, microsatellite instability; PCR, polymerase chain reaction; RT-PCR, reverse transcriptase polymerase chain reaction; SDH, succinate dehydrogenase.

shares similar downstream pathways as ERBB2 (HER2), and targeted small-molecule inhibitors to downregulate *MET* are currently in use to treat patients with metastatic GA.[2] Testing for *ERBB2* (*HER2*) amplification has become routine for advanced GAs. Quantification for MET protein expression is also gaining acceptance in oncologic practice in treatment of GAs.[2,3] IHC interpretation of ERBB2 (HER2) protein expression in gastric and GEJ carcinomas and EAC differs significantly from breast carcinoma.[1] The main differences are the result of significant intratumoral heterogeneity. Therefore, the criteria for a positive IHC result do not rely on complete membranous circumferential expression, and the percentage of positive tumor cells is not considered in biopsy specimens.[4,5] Table 7-2 outlines the guideline for interpretation of ERBB2 IHC results as used by the Trastuzumab for Gastric Cancer (ToGA) trial group; Figures 7-1 and 7-2 are representative images. In brief, the ToGA trial recommendations state that if the IHC results show 2+ or equivocal staining, FISH analysis is recommended to assess gene amplification. However, FISH is not recommended for tumors displaying 0–1+ IHC as all of these cases were proven not to be amplified by subsequent FISH analysis. Tumors with

3+ staining are also not recommended for FISH as these cases showed 100% *ERBB2* amplification by FISH.

A specific subset of diffuse GAs is the hereditary type, caused by germline mutations in the epithelial cadherin *CDH1* gene,[6] leading to loss or dysfunction of the E-cadherin protein. The loss can be detected by immunostaining. It is important to identify these patients due to significant implications for early prevention and treatment for relatives, who are at increased risk for developing GA.

A small percentage of patients with Lynch syndrome develop GA, and many GAs display evidence of mismatch repair (MMR) defects. However, clinical studies to assess such alterations are not routinely performed for GA. Please refer to the next section on colorectal adenocarcinoma section (CRC) for further details on Lynch syndrome.

■ COLORECTAL ADENOCARCINOMAS

At the tissue and cellular levels, CRC is considered a single type of malignancy. At the molecular level, however, CRCs develop through molecular abnormalities involving one of at least three main pathways: the tumor-suppressing gene *APC*

TABLE 7-2. Interpretation of immunohistochemistry (IHC) for ERBB2 (HER2) in gastric, gastroesophageal junctional, and esophageal adenocarcinoma.[a]

IHC interpretation surgical specimen	IHC interpretation biopsy specimen	Score and classification
No staining or membranous reactivity in < 10% of tumor cells	Complete absence of reactivity in tumor cells	0/negative
Faint or barely perceptible membranous reactivity in > 10% of tumor cells; cells show partial membranous staining at high magnification (×40)	Tumor cell cluster (5 or more cells) with faint membranous reactivity regardless of percentage of tumor cells stained	1+/negative
Weak-to-moderate complete, basolateral, or lateral membranous reactivity in > 10% of tumor cells	Tumor cell cluster with weak-to-moderate complete, basolateral, or lateral membranous reactivity regardless of percentage of tumor cells stained	2+/equivocal
Strong complete, basolateral, or lateral membranous reactivity in > 10% of tumor cells visible at low magnification	Tumor cell cluster with strong, complete, basolateral, or lateral membranous reactivity regardless of percentage of tumor cells stained	3+/positive

[a]Data from Ruschoff et al. HER2 diagnostics in gastric cancer-guideline validation and development of standardized immunohistochemical testing. *Virchows Arch.* 2010;457(3):299–307.[4]

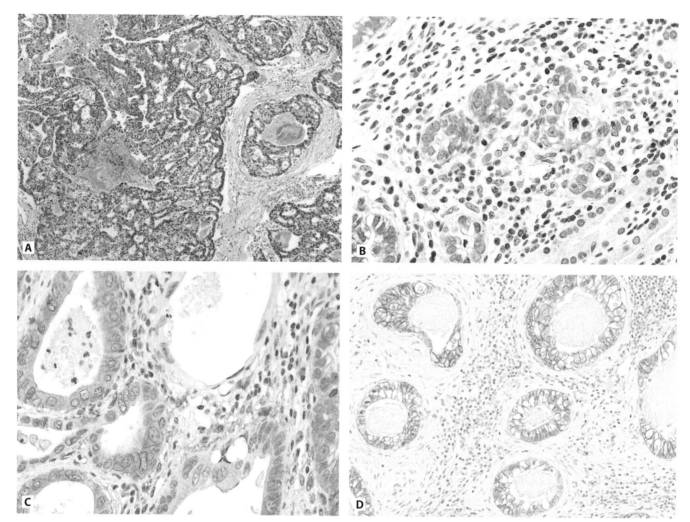

FIGURE 7-1. ERBB2 expression of a gastric adenocarcinoma detected by immunostaining. **A.** Invasive adenocarcinoma, with necrosis, H&E staining. **B.** Immunostain for Her2neu, 1+ (negative). **C.** 2+ staining (equivocal). **D.** 3+ staining (positive).

mutation, the hereditary microsatellite instability pathway (Lynch syndrome), and the serrated pathway (aberrant cytosine-guanosine island methylation). Many other gene products in cell signaling are also involved, which may affect the

FIGURE 7-2. *ERBB2* amplification by FISH.

tumor response to treatment. In current practice, only a few of these are included as part of standard-of-care molecular testing of CRC, including *KRAS*, *BRAF*, MSI, and so on (see Table 7-1). Other genes that may have clinical relevance for CRC treatment and prognosis, such *PI3K*, *PTEN*, and *AKT*, which encodes proteins in the PI3K pathway, are more appropriately covered in detail by texts focusing on molecular pathology.

KRAS Mutation Analysis

Anti-EGFR small molecules (such as erlotinib) and monoclonal antibodies (such as cetuximab or panitumumab) are the currently available targeted therapy agents for metastatic CRC. Overexpression of EGFR occurs in approximately 80% of CRC; however, less than 1% harbor *EGFR* somatic mutations. Therefore, testing for EGFR overexpression or mutational status is not part of a current diagnostic or therapeutic algorithm. On the other hand, KRAS, downstream of EGFR, can be activated constitutively due to gain-of-function *KRAS* mutations that render anti-EGFR treatment ineffective. Only patients with tumors lacking *KRAS* mutations (wild-type status) are deemed appropriate to receive anti-EGFR treatment.

As for indications for *KRAS* mutational analysis, it had been advocated that all CRCs be tested at resection. However, this "universal" approach does not benefit all patients and incurs unnecessary cost. Currently, testing is recommended for locally advanced (stage III or high-risk stage II cases) and metastatic colorectal carcinomas. This allows information to be available when further systematic treatment is needed. For *KRAS* wild-type CRC, *BRAF* mutational status should be assessed (see next topic).

BRAF Mutation Analysis

BRAF mutation is present in about 10% of all CRCs. RAF is a cytoplasmic kinase downstream of RAS and is part of the MAPK (mitogen-activated protein kinase) pathway. The majority of mutations in *BRAF* are point mutations, particularly at nucleotide 1799 in exon 15, T1799A resulting in V600E (valine-to–glutamic acid substitution). The V600E substitution is within the kinase domain and results in constitutive kinase activation. These mutations are most often present in tumors that are microsatellite instable due to hypermethylation of promoter regions of an MMR gene (see the section on MSI for further details).

BRAF and *KRAS* mutations are mutually exclusive in CRC. EGFR-based therapies are also ineffective in these *BRAF*-mutated cases. In addition, CRCs with *BRAF* mutations are associated with a relatively worse prognosis, regardless of treatment status.

Another rationale for testing for *BRAF* mutations is based on the phenomenon that although *BRAF* mutation maybe seen in sporadic tumors with MSI, it is not seen in Lynch syndrome cases.[7] For tumors with MSI-H or with loss of MLH1 expression, positivity for *BRAF* mutation indicates a sporadic CRC, and germline mutation analysis for the MMR gene can be avoided.

Microsatellite Instability

The function of the DNA MMR system is to replace mismatched bases with the correct ones immediately following DNA replication. Defects in the MMR process lead to a permissive environment for tumorigenesis. The hereditary form of MMR defects underlies the familial cancer syndrome, Lynch syndrome, also known as hereditary nonpolyposis colorectal carcinoma (HNPCC). The detectable phenotypic changes are reflected in the specific regions of DNA termed *microsatellite* sequences, which are comprised of 1–6 nucleotide repeats. These repeat areas of the genome are prone to errors due to slippage of the DNA replication machinery. The term *microsatellite instability* thus refers to expansion or contraction of the length of these repeats due to an ineffective DNA repair mechanism.

Microsatellite instability is observed in approximately 15% of all CRCs, including 12%–13% in sporadic cases as a result of hypermethylation of the promoter region of one MMR gene, *MLH1*, and 2%–3% in patients with Lynch syndrome. The last is underlined by a germline mutation mostly occurring in one of the four MMR genes: *MLH1, MSH2, MSH6,* or *PMS2.* Evidence of MSI is detected by two different methodologies: (1) IHC to assess expression of MMR proteins (MMRPs; Table 7-3, Figure 7-3)[8,9] and (2) multiplex polymerase chain reaction (PCR) and fragment analysis to detect size variation in microsatellite target sequences (Figure 7-4). For IHC, there is considerable staining variability in both the normal and the neoplastic components in a tissue section. Thus, interpretation involves critical evaluation of staining in both the neoplastic and the nonneoplastic internal controls (lymphocytes or adjacent nonneoplastic epithelium). Effective MMR will show nuclear expression of MMRPs in proliferating cells. Loss of expression of one or more of these proteins indicates a defect in the MMR gene. Normally, two proteins form a functional heterodimer; loss of one protein in the pair creates an unstable heterodimer, which may lead to loss of a detectable partner. PMS2 pairs with MLH1 exclusively, but MLH1 may dimerize with protein partners other than PMS2. As a result, loss of MLH1 leads to non-detection of PMS2 as well, but not vice versa. Similarly, loss of MSH2 leads to non-detection of MSH6. Thus, some investigators propose that, for screening purposes, only 2 of the MMRPs are tested (PMS2 and MSH6). Therefore, mutations in MMR genes can often be inferred from the pattern of protein expression among the four MMRPs (Table 7-3).

Polymerase chain reaction is performed to assess MSI phenotype in the predetermined target regions of DNA. The length variability within the repeats correlates to a loss of

TABLE 7-3. Interpretation of immunohistochemistry (IHC) for DNA mismatch repair proteins.

Gene/protein	Heterodimer	Expected positive IHC staining pattern
MLH1	PMS2	Gene mutation is associated with loss of both MLH1 and PMS2 protein expression.
PMS2	MLH1	Variable. Gene mutation can show loss of both PMS2 and MLH1 protein expression as well as isolated loss of PMS2 due to heterodimer formation of MLH1 with other proteins.
MSH2	MSH6	Gene mutation is associated with loss of both MSH2 and MSH6 protein expression.
MSH6	MSH2	Variable. Gene mutation can show loss of both MSH6 and MSH2 or isolated loss of MSH6 due to heterodimer formation of MSH2 with other proteins.

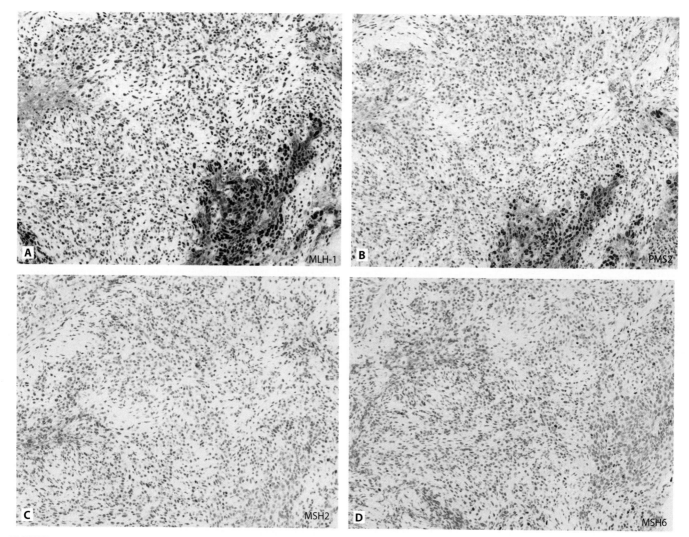

FIGURE 7-3. Immunostaining for MMRPs in a poorly differentiated invasive colonic adenocarcinoma. **A** and **B.** Intact expression of MLH1 and PMS2 (nuclear staining). **C** and **D.** Loss of expression of MSH2 and MSH6, respectively, in tumor cells. Note the positive staining in the background nonneoplastic inflammatory cell nuclei.

ability to repair DNA mismatches and possibly mutation in an MMR gene and is assessed by comparing tumor microsatellite DNA to the adjacent nonneoplastic microsatellite DNA; increases and decreases in the number of repeats are examined (Figure 7-4). A tumor is considered highly unstable, or MSI-H, if two or more of the commonly tested repeats show a change. If none of the designated repeats shows variability, the tumor is defined as microsatellite stable or MSS. Instability in 1 mononucleotide repeat may indicate underlying MMR; therefore, a diagnosis of indeterminate is rendered.

It is important to recognize that 10%–13% of sporadic tumors can also show MSI in which both alleles are lost due to either somatic mutation or epigenetic silencing. In this situation, two tests can help differentiate sporadic and Lynch-associated tumors: (1) *BRAF* mutation Val600Glu (V600E), seen in approximately 50% of sporadic MSI-H tumors, and (2) *MLH1* methylation; both are rarely seen in Lynch syndrome.

Several criteria or guidelines had been developed for selecting patients to undergo tests for MSI status. For practical purposes more relevant to the pathologist, the revised Bethesda criteria[10] were recommended (Table 7-4).[11] Factors included in the criteria are patient age at cancer diagnosis, high-risk family history, multiple tumors, and a battery of histopathologic features that are considered sensitive markers for MSI-H CRC.[12,13] These features include (1) mucinous or signet ring component, (2) medullary component, (3) prominent intratumoral lymphocytic infiltration, and (4) a Crohn-like inflammatory reaction.

Although this guideline is considered easy to use and has high sensitivity, it has been realized that an oversight regarding the age for testing may lead to missed cases. The summary states that for a patient 60 years of age, presence of one of these "MSI"-type histologic features should prompt testing. But, it was clearly stated that the age cutoff was arbitrary and not a consensus.[10] Understandably, using the age

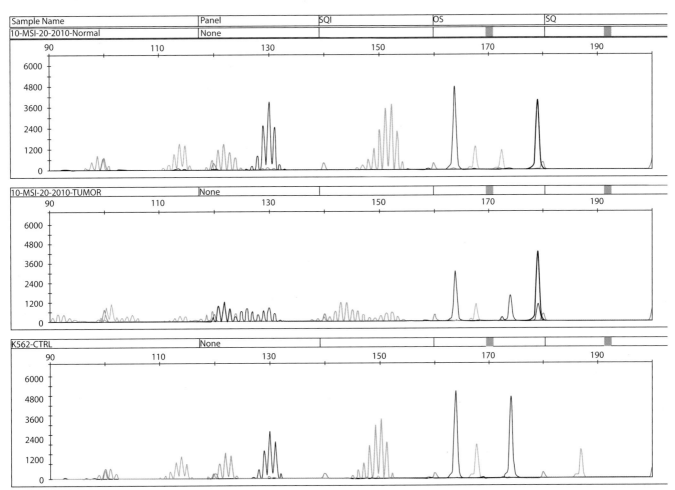

FIGURE 7-4. MSI-H status by fluorescent PCR. Composite electropherogram showing variation in product sizes in tumor sample compared to normal. (Used with permission of Dr. Loren Joseph.)

of 60 years as a cutoff will lead to missed cases. Naturally, in recent years, several studies showed that a significant portion of patients with MSI-H or Lynch syndrome failed to meet this testing criterion. Therefore, it was recommended that all patients newly diagnosed with CRC undergo screening testing for MSI.[14–16] This universal testing has been implemented in most healthcare settings. Others, however, recognize that the evidence in support of this approach is not sufficient to justify the marked addition in costs to the health care system. Furthermore, there has been inconsistency in test algorithms and in disposition of test results.[17]

TABLE 7-4. Revised Bethesda criteria to stratify patients for microsatellite instability testing.
Less than 50 years old at the time of diagnosis
Tumor histology including tumor-infiltrating lymphocytes, Crohn-like lymphoid reaction, mucinous/signet ring cell morphology, or medullary features
Presence of colon or other Lynch-associated tumors in the individual or family members

It must also be recognized that in the studies supporting universal testing, diligent effort in case definition may be lacking. For example, it was not clear in the population studies[14] if all the tumor specimens from different regional hospitals were examined by the study pathologist for histologic features of MSI. On another hand, a recent expert panel recommended no screening test for patients 72 years or older, but in one of the studies, both cases that did not meet the revised Bethesda guidelines involved individuals older than 72 years of age,[16] making the "missed" cases insignificant. Most recent studies have shown that if the histologic features were used regardless of patient age, virtually all potential cases of Lynch syndrome would have been "captured" for MSI testing.[17]

This being said, based on published data as well as our own experience, following the revised Bethesda guidelines does miss a significant portion of sporadic MSI-H cases. However, the intention of the guideline is to "capture" patients who potentially have Lynch syndrome, not the ones with sporadic MSI-H.

Another argument in favor of universal MSI testing is that, beyond identifying patients with Lynch syndrome, MSI status also has prognostic value. It is believed that patients with MSI-H tumors have better stage-specific and progression-free survival and show no benefit from 5-fluorouracil (5-FU) therapy.[18] Later studies have not uniformly confirmed this finding. A more recent National Cancer Institute (NCI) collaborative study showed no difference in either treatment response or survival in regard to MSI status.[19]

On the other hand, it should be recognized that intact expression of the MMRPs by IHC does not completely exclude Lynch syndrome, as 5%–8% of Lynch families carry a missense mutation (particularly *MLH1*), producing a defective but antigenically intact protein.

Currently, in our practice, we perform IHC testing for MMRPs if the patient meets the revised Bethesda criteria or if tumors exhibit MSI-type histology regardless of age. In following this approach, we hope to identify potential probands, possibly leading to meaningful follow-up genetic counseling or testing while also preventing wasteful spending. Due to the prevailing trend of universal testing, we also perform this test at the clinician's request.

Human Papilloma Virus

Rarely, squamous carcinoma may be encountered in the rectum. Human papilloma virus (HPV) is known to be associated with squamous cell carcinomas of the anogenital region (see the next section) and of the uterine cervix and the oropharynx. It is also associated with rectal squamous carcinoma.[20] When a diagnosis of squamous cell carcinoma is made from a rectal mass, p16 immunostaining should be performed (see next section). This is partly based on the difficulty in distinguishing between distal rectal tumor and tumors arising from the anal canal. In addition, low copy numbers of HPV 16, 18, and other types of HPV had been identified even in CRC.[21] The significance of these findings has not been determined, and no test for HPV is currently recommended for adenocarcinoma.

◼ ANAL SQUAMOUS CELL CARCINOMA

Squamous cell carcinoma arising in the anorectal region is often preceded by anal intraepithelial neoplasia (AIN), which has increased in incidence in patients infected with human immunodeficiency virus (HIV) treated with highly active antiretroviral therapy (HAART).[22] AIN is classified as AIN I, II, and III. AIN I is considered a low-grade lesion, and AIN II and III are considered high grade. The cytology terminology LSIL (low-grade squamous intraepithelial lesion) correlates with AIN I, and HSIL (high-grade intraepithelial lesion) correlates with AINII/III on histology. The molecular underpinnings of these lesions are HPV infections. HPV is classified into low- and high-risk serotypes. The low-risk group, including serotypes 6, 11, 13, 32, is associated with pre-malignant lesions, and the high-risk group, including serotypes 16, 18, 45, 58, and others, is associated with high-grade dysplasia and invasive squamous carcinoma. Detection and typing of HPV status have been recommended as an ancillary test to assist diagnosis of AIN in cytology

specimens.[23,24] In addition, some studies have suggested improved survival and response to combined chemoradiation treatment in HPV-positive squamous carcinomas as compared to HPV-negative ones.[25,26]

Direct identification of HPV can be accomplished using one or a combination of DNA PCR, reverse transcriptase PCR (RT-PCR) for E6/E7 messenger RNA (mRNA), in situ hybridization (ISH) for integrated viral DNA, and others.[27] It was shown that infection by high-risk (particularly serotypes 16 and 18) HPV often leads to overexpression of the cell cycle regular p16 protein (encoded by *INK4A*) due to inactivation of the RB protein, which can be reliably detected by immunostaining.[28,29] Therefore, in recent years, this last method was proposed as a surrogate marker for HPV status.[28–34] Overexpression as detected by IHC has been shown to correlate with high-grade dysplasia. It must be recognized that IHC for p16 tends to have high sensitivity and relatively lower specificity, as compared to direct detection of viral sequence.[35] A positive IHC result is defined as the presence of diffuse/continuous staining in more than one-third of tumor cells. For reference, the different staining patterns are illustrated in Figure 7-5.

◼ GASTROINTESTINAL STROMAL TUMOR

The gastrointestinal stromal tumors (GISTs) are discussed in detail in Chapter 5. The majority of GISTs (about 80%) harbor activating mutations in the *KIT* gene encoding a tyrosine kinase, while a minor population contain *PDGFRA* mutations encoding a related kinase. The mutations that occur in these two genes are mutually exclusive, with both resulting in constitutively active proteins. The presence of mutations in either *KIT* or *PDGFRA* essentially confirms the diagnosis of GIST; however, it is important to note that a small portion of GISTs lack mutations in either gene.

The discovery that Gleevec®, a small-molecule inhibitor, has efficacy in the treatment of advanced GIST has made testing for molecular alterations in GISTs mandatory. *KIT* mutation most commonly occurs in exon 11, with 10% in exon 9 and a minority in exons 13 and 17. Genotype/phenotype correlations have been shown to be clinically significant, with tumors harboring exon 11 mutations having a better response to Gleevec at a lower dose and tumors with exon 9 mutations requiring twice the dosage to achieve significant increases in progression-free survival time.[36,37] Interestingly, all of the mutations in PDGFRA, including the most common, D842V, create a protein product that is resistant to Gleevec. For pre-surgery treatment and for those with high-risk features after resection, *KIT* mutational analysis is routinely required. For *KIT* wild-type tumors, a *PDGFRA* mutation is necessary.

In recent years, much progress had been made in identifying genetic abnormalities involved in syndromic GIST, particularly the Carney-Stratakis syndrome (paragangliomas and GIST), in which there is a germline mutation in a succinate dehydrogenase (SDH) subunit gene.[38–41] Therefore,

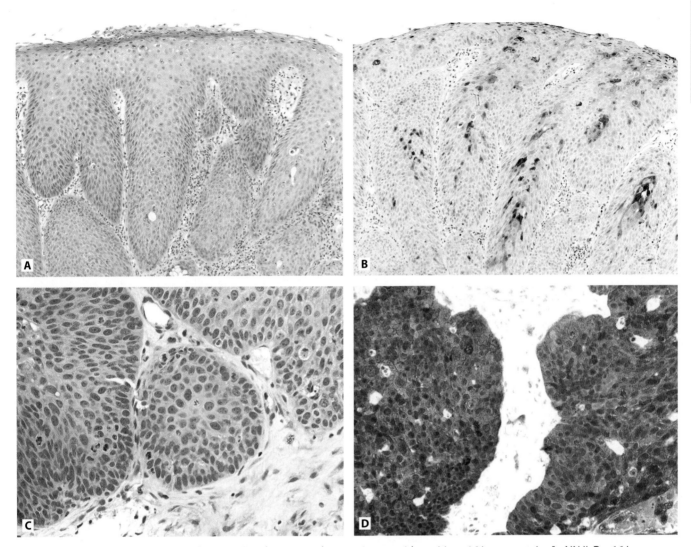

FIGURE 7-5. Anal intraepithelial neoplasia (AIN) and invasive adenocarcinoma with positive p16 immunostain. **A.** AIN II. **B.** p16 immuno-histochemistry. **C.** Anal squamous carcinoma, hematoxylin and eosin (H&E) stain. **D.** Anal squamous carcinoma with diffuse strong-positive stain for p16.

for multiple GISTs or pediatric GIST, testing to rule out SDH deficiency should be performed with immunostains, and mutational analysis for the gene corresponding to the SDH subunit should be performed in cases found to be deficient by IHC[41,42] (Tables 7-1B and C).

▪ CLEAR-CELL SARCOMA-LIKE TUMORS OF THE GI TRACT

Clear-cell sarcomas are rarely seen in the GI tract and have similar features to melanomas. However, they are genetically distinct from melanomas as they lack *BRAF* mutations and are often characterized by the recurrent translocation t(12;22)(q13;q12) that results in the fusion of the *EWS* and *ATF1* genes. Clear-cell sarcoma-like tumors of the GI tract have also been reported to have a distinct translocation that results in the fusion of *EWS* with a different, but related, partner *CREB1*.[43] These unique translocations can be identified either through FISH or targeted PCR analysis (Table 7-1B).

▪ INHERITED CANCER SYNDROMES

Lynch Syndrome (Hereditary Nonpolyposis Colorectal Cancer)

As discussed, Lynch syndrome results from one germline mutation and one acquired mutation or epigenetic silencing of one of four MMR genes: *MLH1, PMS2, MSH2,* and *MSH6.* Lynch syndrome accounts for approximately 3% of all colorectal carcinomas and is also associated with the development of extracolonic tumors, including those of the endometrium, stomach, ovary, ureters, brain, small bowel, hepatobiliary tract, pancreas, and skin. Ancillary tests are discussed in the colorectal tumor section (Table 7-1C).

Familial Adenomatous Polyposis

Patients with germline mutations in the *APC* gene can develop hundreds of colorectal adenomas, often starting in the teenage years. These patients with familial adenomatous polyposis (FAP) can also develop extracolonic polyps, cutaneous lesions, desmoid tumors, osteomas, and dental abnormalities. The attenuated form of FAP (aFAP) has a less-severe phenotype with fewer adenomas; it presents later in life and secondary to different genetic aberrations. *Gardner syndrome* is a variant of FAP with *APC* mutations specifically associated with supernumerary teeth, osteomas, cutaneous fibromas, or epithelial cysts. *Turcot syndrome* can be secondary to either mutations in *APC* or mutations in MMR genes (HNPCC). Turcot syndrome related to *APC* mutations is associated with an increased risk of colorectal cancer as well as medulloblastoma (Table 7-1C).

MUTYH-Associated Polyposis

Patients with *MUTYH*-associated polyposis (MAP) present with a similar phenotype as patients with AFAP. However, mutations are discovered in the base excision repair gene *MUTYH* (Table 7-1C).

Familial GIST Syndromes

Familial GIST syndromes are discussed in more detail in Chapter 5. Germline mutations have been seen in *KIT* and *PDGFRA* in patients with isolated GISTs.[44-47] In GIST syndromes such as Carney-Stratakis syndrome (paragangliomas and GIST), germline mutations in *SDH* are reported with high frequency, particularly those involving subunit B.[38-41] Chromosomal losses harboring *SDH* have been associated with Carney's triad (paragangliomas, GISTs, and pulmonary chondromas)[48] (Table 7-1C).

In addition, patients with neurofibromatosis I have increased risk for multiple GISTs.

■ REFERENCES

1. Bang YJ, Van Cutsem E, Feyereislova A, et al. Trastuzumab in combination with chemotherapy versus chemotherapy alone for treatment of HER2-positive advanced gastric or gastro-oesophageal junction cancer (ToGA): a phase 3, open-label, randomised controlled trial. *Lancet.* 2010 28;376(9742):687–697. PMID: 20728210.

2. Catenacci DV, Henderson L, Xiao SY, et al. Durable complete response of metastatic gastric cancer with anti-Met therapy followed by resistance at recurrence. *Cancer Discov.* 2011;1(7):573–579. PMID: 22389872. PMCID: 3289149.

3. Catenacci DV, Liao WL, Thyparambil S, et al. Absolute quantitation of Met using mass spectrometry for clinical application: assay precision, stability, and correlation with MET gene amplification in FFPE Tumor tissue. *PloS One.* 2014;9(7):e100586. PMID: 24983965. PMCID: 4077664.

4. Ruschoff J, Dietel M, Baretton G, et al. HER2 diagnostics in gastric cancer-guideline validation and development of standardized immunohistochemical testing. *Virchows Arch.* 2010;457(3):299–307. PMID: 20665045. PMCID: 2933810.

5. Ruschoff J, Hanna W, Bilous M, et al. HER2 testing in gastric cancer: a practical approach. *Mod. Pathol.* 2012;25(5):637–650. PMID: 22222640.

6. Kaurah P, MacMillan A, Boyd N, et al. Founder and recurrent CDH1 mutations in families with hereditary diffuse gastric cancer. *JAMA.* 2007;297(21):2360–2372. PMID: 17545690.

7. Domingo E, Niessen RC, Oliveira C, et al. *BRAF*-V600E is not involved in the colorectal tumorigenesis of HNPCC in patients with functional MLH1 and MSH2 genes. *Oncogene.* 2005;24(24):3995–3998. PMID: 15782118.

8. Chiaravalli AM, Furlan D, Facco C, et al. Immunohistochemical pattern of hMSH2/hMLH1 in familial and sporadic colorectal, gastric, endometrial and ovarian carcinomas with instability in microsatellite sequences. *Virchows Arch.* 2001;438(1):39–48. PMID: 11213834.

9. de Leeuw WJ, Dierssen J, Vasen HF, et al. Prediction of a mismatch repair gene defect by microsatellite instability and immunohistochemical analysis in endometrial tumours from HNPCC patients. *J Pathol.* 2000;192(3):328–335. PMID: 11054716.

10. Umar A, Boland CR, Terdiman JP, et al. Revised Bethesda guidelines for hereditary nonpolyposis colorectal cancer (Lynch syndrome) and microsatellite instability. *J Natl Cancer Inst.* 2004;96(4):261–268. PMID: 14970275. PMCID: 2933058.

11. Jenkins MA, Hayashi S, O'Shea AM, et al. Pathology features in Bethesda guidelines predict colorectal cancer microsatellite instability: a population-based study. *Gastroenterology.* 2007;133(1):48–56. PMID: 17631130.

12. Greenson JK, Bonner JD, Ben-Yzhak O, et al. Phenotype of microsatellite unstable colorectal carcinomas: well-differentiated and focally mucinous tumors and the absence of dirty necrosis correlate with microsatellite instability. *Am J Surg Pathol.* 2003;27(5):563–570. PMID: 12717242.

13. Greenson JK, Huang SC, Herron C, et al. Pathologic predictors of microsatellite instability in colorectal cancer. *Am J Surg Pathol.* 2009;33(1):126–133. PMID: 18830122. PMCID: 3500028.

14. Hampel H, Frankel WL, Martin E, et al. Screening for the Lynch syndrome (hereditary nonpolyposis colorectal cancer). *N Engl J Med.* 2005;352(18):1851–1860. PMID: 15872200.

15. Hampel H, Frankel WL, Martin E, et al. Feasibility of screening for Lynch syndrome among patients with colorectal cancer. *J Clin Oncol.* 2008;26(35):5783–5788. PMID: 18809606.

16. Perez-Carbonell L, Ruiz-Ponte C, Guarinos C, et al. Comparison between universal molecular screening for Lynch syndrome and revised Bethesda guidelines in a large population-based cohort of patients with colorectal cancer. *Gut.* 2012;61(6):865–872. PMID: 21868491.

17. Hartman DJ, Brand RE, Hu H, et al. Lynch syndrome-associated colorectal carcinoma: frequent involvement of the left colon and rectum and late-onset presentation supports a universal screening approach. *Hum Pathol.* 2013;44(11):2518–2528. PMID: 24034859.

18. Parc Y, Gueroult S, Mourra N, et al. Prognostic significance of microsatellite instability determined by immunohistochemical staining of MSH2 and MLH1 in sporadic T3N0M0 colon cancer. *Gut.* 2004;53(3):371–375. PMID: 14960518. PMCID: 1773950.

19. Kim GP, Colangelo LH, Wieand HS, et al. Prognostic and predictive roles of high-degree microsatellite instability in colon cancer: a National Cancer Institute–National Surgical Adjuvant Breast and Bowel Project Collaborative Study. *J Clin Oncol.* 2007;25(7):767–772. PMID: 17228023.

20. Kong CS, Welton ML, Longacre TA. Role of human papillomavirus in squamous cell metaplasia-dysplasia-carcinoma of the rectum. *Am J Surg Pathol.* 2007;31(6):919–925. PMID: 17527081.

21. Bodaghi S, Yamanegi K, Xiao SY, Da Costa M, Palefsky JM, Zheng ZM. Colorectal papillomavirus infection in patients with colorectal cancer. *Clin Cancer Res.* 2005;11(8):2862–2867. PMID: 15837733.

22. Palefsky JM, Holly EA, Efirdc JT, et al. Anal intraepithelial neoplasia in the highly active antiretroviral therapy era among HIV-positive men who have sex with men. *AIDS.* 2005;19(13):1407–1414. PMID: 16103772.

23. Pineda CE, Welton ML. Management of anal squamous intraepithelial lesions. *Clin Colon Rectal Surg.* 2009;22(2):94–101. PMID: 20436833. PMCID: 2780238.

24. Etienney I, Vuong S, Si-Mohamed A, et al. Value of cytologic Papanicolaou smears and polymerase chain reaction screening for human papillomavirus DNA in detecting anal intraepithelial neoplasia: comparison with histology of a surgical sample. *Cancer.* 2012;118(24):6031–6038. PMID: 22674290.

25. Kim S, Jary M, Mansi L, et al. DCF (docetaxel, cisplatin and 5-fluorouracil) chemotherapy is a promising treatment for recurrent advanced squamous cell anal carcinoma. *Ann Oncol.* 2013;24(12):3045–3050. PMID: 24114858.

26. Yhim HY, Lee NR, Song EK, et al. The prognostic significance of tumor human papillomavirus status for patients with anal squamous cell carcinoma treated with combined chemoradiotherapy. *Int J Cancer.* 2011;129(7):1752–1760. PMID: 21128253.

27. Jordan RC, Lingen MW, Perez-Ordonez B, et al. Validation of methods for oropharyngeal cancer HPV status determination in US cooperative group trials. *Am J Surg Pathol.* 2012;36(7):945–954. PMID: 22743284.

28. Lu DW, El-Mofty SK, Wang HL. Expression of p16, Rb, and p53 proteins in squamous cell carcinomas of the anorectal region harboring human papillomavirus DNA. *Mod. Pathol.* 2003;16(7):692–699. PMID: 12861066.

29. Walts AE, Lechago J, Bose S. P16 and Ki67 immunostaining is a useful adjunct in the assessment of biopsies for HPV-associated anal intraepithelial neoplasia. *Am J Surg Pathol.* 2006;30(7):795–801. PMID: 16819320.

30. Bernard JE, Butler MO, Sandweiss L, Weidner N. Anal intraepithelial neoplasia: correlation of grade with p16INK4a immunohistochemistry and HPV in situ hybridization. *Appl Immunohistochem Mol Morphol.* 2008;16(3):215–20. PMID: 18301250.

31. Duncan LD, Winkler M, Carlson ER, Heidel RE, Kang E, Webb D. p16 immunohistochemistry can be used to detect human papillomavirus in oral cavity squamous cell carcinoma. *J Oral Maxillofac Surg.* 2013;71(8):1367–1375. PMID: 23642549.

32. Sayed K, Korourian S, Ellison DA, et al. Diagnosing cervical biopsies in adolescents: the use of p16 immunohistochemistry to improve reliability and reproducibility. *J Lower Genital Tract Dis.* 2007;11(3):141–146. PMID: 17596758.

33. Thomas J, Primeaux T. Is p16 immunohistochemistry a more cost-effective method for identification of human papilloma virus-associated head and neck squamous cell carcinoma? *Ann Diagn Pathol.* 2012;16(2):91–99. PMID: 22197546.

34. Winters R, Trotman W, Adamson CS, et al. Screening for human papillomavirus in basaloid squamous carcinoma: utility of p16(INK4a), CISH, and PCR. *Int J Surg Pathol.* 2011;19(3):309–314. PMID: 20798066.

35. Bussu F, Sali M, Gallus R, et al. Human papillomavirus (HPV) infection in squamous cell carcinomas arising from the oropharynx: detection of HPV DNA and p16 immunohistochemistry as diagnostic and prognostic indicators—a pilot study. *Int J Radiat Oncol Biol Phys.* 2014;89(5):1115–1120. PMID: 25035216.

36. Heinrich MC, Corless CL, Demetri GD, et al. Kinase mutations and imatinib response in patients with metastatic gastrointestinal stromal tumor. *J Clin Oncol.* 2003;21(23):4342–4349. PMID: 14645423.

37. Zhi X, Zhou X, Wang W, Xu Z. Practical role of mutation analysis for imatinib treatment in patients with advanced gastrointestinal stromal tumors: a meta-analysis. *PloS One.* 2013;8(11):e79275. PMID: 24223922. PMCID: 3817038.

38. Pasini B, McWhinney SR, Bei T, et al. Clinical and molecular genetics of patients with the Carney-Stratakis syndrome and germline mutations of the genes coding for the succinate dehydrogenase subunits SDHB, SDHC, and SDHD. *Eur J Hum Genet.* 2008;16(1):79–88. PMID: 17667967.

39. Janeway KA, Kim SY, Lodish M, et al. Defects in succinate dehydrogenase in gastrointestinal stromal tumors lacking KIT and PDGFRA mutations. *Proc Natl Acad Sci U S A.* 2011;108(1):314–318. PMID: 21173220.

40. Miettinen M, Wang ZF, Sarlomo-Rikala M, Osuch C, Rutkowski P, Lasota J. Succinate dehydrogenase-deficient GISTs: a clinicopathologic, immunohistochemical, and molecular genetic study of 66 gastric GISTs with predilection to young age. *Am J Surg Pathol.* 2011;35(11):1712–1721. PMID: 21997692.

41. Celestino R, Lima J, Faustino A, et al. A novel germline SDHB mutation in a gastrointestinal stromal tumor patient without bona fide features of the Carney-Stratakis dyad. *Fam Cancer.* 2012;11(2):189–194. PMID: 22160509.

42. Miettinen M, Killian JK, Wang ZF, et al. Immunohistochemical loss of succinate dehydrogenase subunit A (SDHA) in gastrointestinal stromal tumors (GISTs) signals SDHA germline mutation. *Am J Surg Pathol.* 2013;37(2):234–240. PMID: 23282968.

43. Antonescu CR, Nafa K, Segal NH, Dal Cin P, Ladanyi M. EWS-CREB1: a recurrent variant fusion in clear cell sarcoma—association with gastrointestinal location and absence of melanocytic differentiation. *Clin Cancer Res.* 2006;12(18):5356–5362. PMID: 17000668.

44. Carballo M, Roig I, Aguilar F, et al. Novel c-KIT germline mutation in a family with gastrointestinal stromal tumors and cutaneous hyperpigmentation. *Am J Med Genet A.* 2005;132(4):361–364. PMID: 15742474.

45. Kim HJ, Lim SJ, Park K, Yuh YJ, Jang SJ, Choi J. Multiple gastrointestinal stromal tumors with a germline c-kit mutation. *Pathol Int.* 2005;55(10):655–659. PMID: 16185297.

46. Agaimy A, Dirnhofer S, Wunsch PH, Terracciano LM, Tornillo L, Bihl MP. Multiple sporadic gastrointestinal stromal tumors (GISTs) of the proximal stomach are caused by different somatic KIT mutations suggesting a field effect. *Am J Surg Pathol.* 2008;32(10):1553–1559. PMID: 18724245.

47. Thalheimer A, Schlemmer M, Bueter M, et al. Familial gastrointestinal stromal tumors caused by the novel KIT exon 17 germline mutation N822Y. *Am J Surg Pathol.* 2008;32(10):1560–1565. PMID: 18724244.

48. Matyakhina L, Bei TA, McWhinney SR, et al. Genetics of carney triad: recurrent losses at chromosome 1 but lack of germline mutations in genes associated with paragangliomas and gastrointestinal stromal tumors. *J Clin Endocrinol Metab.* 2007;92(8):2938–2943. PMID: 17535989.

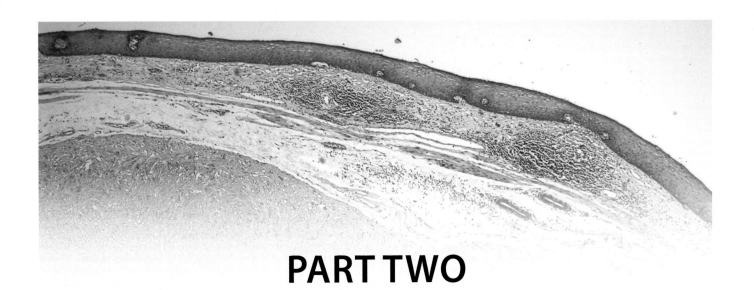

PART TWO

ESOPHAGUS

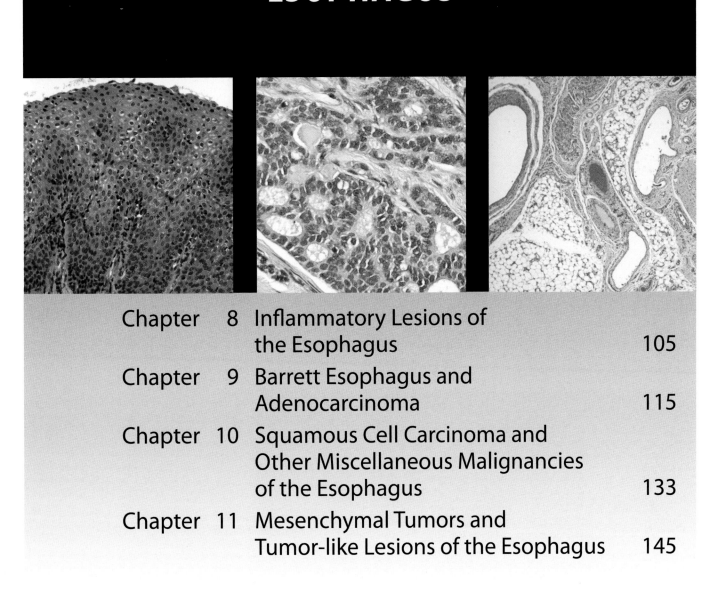

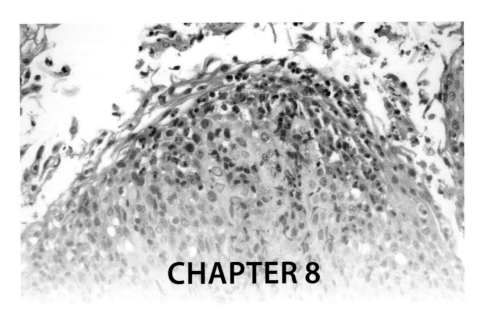

CHAPTER 8

Inflammatory Lesions of the Esophagus

INTRODUCTION

The most commonly encountered disorder in esophageal biopsies is active or erosive esophagitis. Inflammation of esophageal mucosa becomes histologically visible only when there is abnormal inflammatory cell infiltration and degenerative changes of the squamous epithelium. There are many causes, including infectious, reflux, eosinophilic, and so on (Table 8-1). The common histologic hallmarks of active esophagitis are centered on the squamous epithelium, including inflammatory cellular infiltration, intercellular edema (spongiosis), and reactive changes in the basal zone (basal zone hyperplasia) (Figure 8-1). These changes occur in response to environmental or abnormal immune-mediated injuries. When severe, overt erosion or ulcer may be evident (Figure 8-2).

In addition to these common histologic features, unique microscopic changes may be exhibited by different etiologic types of esophagitis, such as infectious esophagitis, reflux esophagitis (RE), eosinophilic esophagitis (EoE), drug-induced esophagitis, and immune-related esophagitis (Table 8-1). Some of these may have a location distribution that is more or less specific. A pragmatic approach can be recognized based on these factors to facilitate a differential diagnosis; these approaches are discussed in this chapter.

INFECTIOUS ESOPHAGITIS

Infectious esophagitis occurs mostly in immune-compromised patients, but immune-competent individuals can be affected as well. These types of esophagitis usually manifest histologically as erosive esophagitis, with neutrophilic infiltration as the key component (Figure 8-2), causing injury to and reactive changes of the squamous epithelium. The common agents are listed in Table 8-1. Among these, fungal infection, most commonly by candida, may be identified on sections stained with hematoxylin and eosin (H&E), particularly in severe cases when abundant fungal elements are present (Figure 8-3), which are highlighted by Gomori methenamine silver (GMS) stain (Figure 8-3). In mild cases, when fungal elements are scarce, GMS or periodic acid–Schiff (PAS) stain is necessary to ensure identification.

Both herpes simplex virus (HSV) and cytomegalovirus (CMV) esophagitis give rise to characteristic virus-induced cytopathic changes or viral inclusion bodies. In most cases, these are sufficiently characteristic to allow for diagnosis of herpes viral esophagitis (Figure 8-4) or CMV esophagitis (Figure 8-5) on H&E slides (Figures 8-4 and 8-5), with specific immunostains sometimes used to confirm atypical findings. In addition, while herpes virus mainly causes epithelial lesions, CMV esophagitis more often is accompanied by ulceration, with the viral inclusion bodies usually identified in the reactive stromal cells (Figure 8-5).

In practice, when a microscopic picture of active neutrophilic esophagitis is encountered, care should be exercised to identify fungal elements and cytopathic changes of viral infection in both the epithelial and the stromal cells. If negative, special stains (GMS or PAS) should be performed for fungal organisms and immunostains for HSV or CMV, particularly in patients with immunosuppression or who are immune compromised. As described in the following

TABLE 8-1. Types of esophagitis.
Erosive esophagitis due to an infection
HSV
CMV
Candida and other fungi
Reflux esophagitis
Eosinophilic esophagitis
Immune-mediated esophagitis
Lichenoid esophagitis
Lymphocytic esophagitis
Crohn disease
GVHD
Drug-induced esophagitis
Pill esophagitis, such as from bisphosphonate (alendronate)
NSAIDs
Sloughing esophagitis, such as from certain antibiotics (doxycycline, tetracycline)
Potassium chloride (most cases fatal)
Radiation esophagitis
Chemical esophagitis
Lye

Abbreviations: CMV, cytomegalovirus; GVHD, graft-versus-host disease; HSV, herpes simplex virus; NSAID, nonsteroidal anti-inflammatory drug.

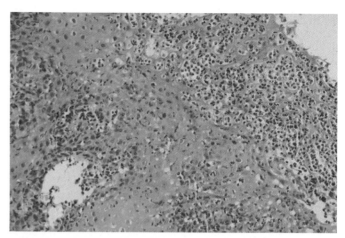

FIGURE 8-2. Active erosive esophagitis. The superficial zone is replaced by necrotic debris. The remaining squamous epithelium exhibits active esophagitis with neutrophilic infiltration.

section, severe RE occasionally manifests as erosive esophagitis with neutrophilic infiltration as well and should be considered when the these special studies are negative. Although infectious esophagitis may affect the upper and midesophagus, RE is mostly limited to the distal esophagus.

FIGURE 8-1. Active esophagitis. There is prominent spongiosis (widening of intercellular spaces), reactive hyperplasia of the basal zone, and eosinophilic infiltration (not in the field). The rete papillae are also elongated.

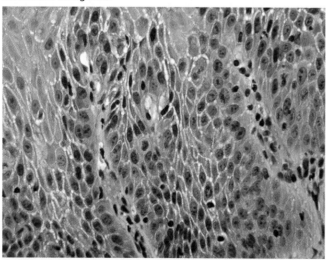

Patients with acquired immunodeficiency syndrome (AIDS) are prone to all the forms of infectious esophagitis mentioned. In addition, mycobacterial esophagitis and parasitic esophagitis may occur in this patient population. Among these types, CMV is relatively a more frequent cause of esophagitis in patients with AIDS and is often associated with ulcers, fistulas, or strictures.[1–4] Clinically, esophagitis in these patients is more frequently associated with severe chest pain because many cases are due to CMV. Therefore, an immunostain for CMV should be performed when typical inclusion bodies cannot be identified.

Other infectious etiologies are not discussed here as they are rare and not frequently associated with mucosal lesions.

REFLUX ESOPHAGITIS

Gastroesophageal reflux disease (GERD) induces inflammation of the affected squamous mucosa, most frequently of the distal esophagus. This may be the most common diagnosis rendered for esophageal biopsies in modern society. Histologically, most cases exhibit mild infiltration of the squamous epithelium by eosinophils, accompanied by mild reactive changes of the squamous cells and intercellular edema (spongiosis) (Figures 8-1 and 8-6). Often, the biopsies are obtained from the gastroesophageal junctional mucosa and contain squamous and cardia-type mucosa, both of which show inflammatory cellular infiltration (Figure 8-7). Another feature that is appreciated in well-oriented sections is the thickened basal zone and elongated lamina propria papillae (*rete papillae*), in addition to eosinophilic infiltration (Figure 8-8). In biopsies with RE, the intraepithelial eosinophilic (IEE) infiltrations range from rare to numerous (Figure 8-8). Furthermore, in severe cases, there can be neutrophilic infiltration as well, which may or may not be accompanied by mucosal erosion or ulceration. In these cases, an infectious etiology should be ruled out by

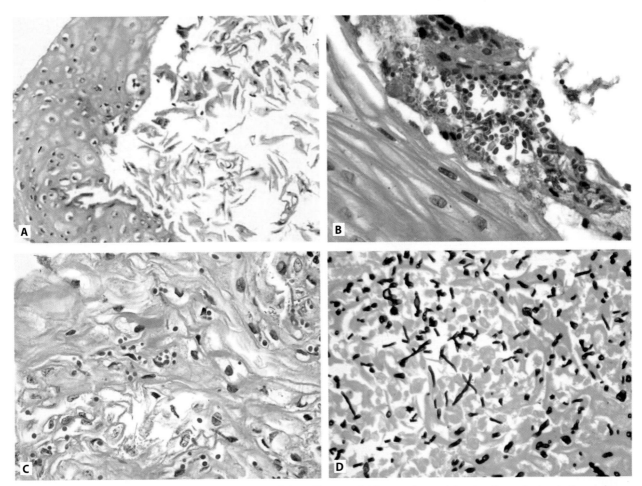

FIGURE 8-3. Candida esophagitis. **A.** Intraepithelial neutrophilic infiltration. **B.** Yeast and pseudohyphae form clusters in the surface necrotic debris. **C.** Same organisms in degenerative squamous epithelium. **D.** GMS stain.

special studies as described previously. Similarly, when IEEs are markedly increased, a distinction from EoE is necessary (Table 8-2) (see the next section).

EOSINOPHILIC ESOPHAGITIS

Eosinophilic esophagitis (EoE) is an emerging disease, described and increasingly recognized only during the last decade.[5-8] It is associated with feeding disorders, vomiting, reflux symptoms, and abdominal pain in children and dysphagia and food impactions in adults.[9,10] The underlying pathology is characterized by infiltration of the esophageal epithelium by eosinophils, similar to that of RE. However, treatments for reflux disease are ineffective. It was recognized that these cases represented a different disease (rather than RE), underlined by esophageal allergy to various food components. However, unlike classic immediate reaction to an allergen as mediated by immunoglobulin (Ig) E, EoE is associated with an altered immune response, characterized by a combination of IgE-mediated and non–IgE-mediated mechanisms.[11,12]

Histologically, when inflammation is characterized by prominent IEE infiltration, the possibility of EoE should be considered (Figures 8-9 and 8-10). Similar to, but more severe than, most biopsies of RE, EoE histologically exhibits marked reactive changes of both basal and top-zone epithelia, elongation of lamina propria papilla, and IEEs (Figure 8-10). This can be accompanied by superficial erosion (Figure 8-11A), eosinophilic degranulation (Figure 8-11B), or parakeratosis (Figure 8-11C).

It had been previously claimed that histologically it is not possible to distinguish between RE and EoE in any single case due to overlap in histologic abnormalities, and the final diagnosis can only be established after a course of trial treatment, for instance, if the patient exhibited persistent esophageal eosinophilia after receiving a proton pump inhibitor for 4–6 weeks. This is partly caused by a histologic diagnosis guideline that determined a high-power field (HPF) with 15 IEEs as the threshold.[13] Although for a minority of patients this may be the case, for many patients with EoE before treatment, the density of IEEs is remarkably much higher. In combination with additional microscopic

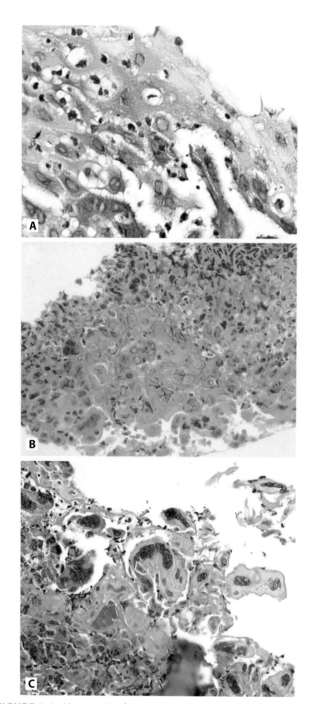

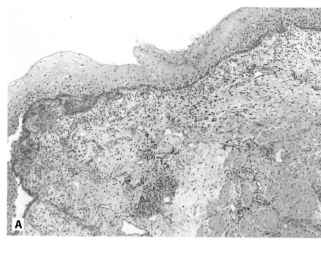

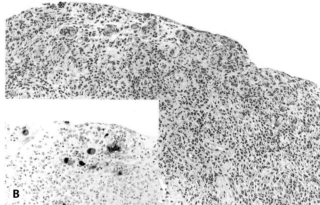

FIGURE 8-5. Cytomegalovirus (CMV) esophagitis. **A.** Mucosa adjacent to an ulcer has unremarkable epithelium, overlying edematous and inflamed lamina propria, with reactive vascular hyperplasia. **B.** Granulation tissue of the ulcer bed contains numerous large giant cells with meganuclei, characteristic of CMV inclusion bodies. Insert: immunostain for CMV.

FIGURE 8-4. Herpes simplex virus esophagitis. **A.** Epithelial cells contain pale blue nuclear inclusions. **B.** Infected epithelial cells transformed to multinucleated giant cells; the nuclei show ground glass appearance with chromatin pushed to periphery. **C.** Sometimes, the viral inclusion bodies are more basophilic.

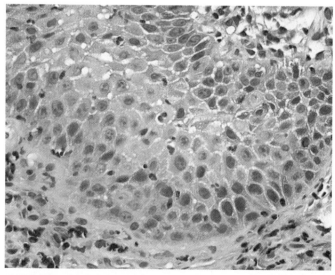

FIGURE 8-6. Reflex esophagitis with spongiosis and intraepithelial eosinophilic infiltration.

features (Figure 8-11), as well as disease distribution, the diagnosis can be established without a "treatment trial."

Biopsies from treated EoE can be difficult to distinguish from those for RE due to reduced severity of histologic changes. However, clinical history shall resolve this dilemma.

It is worth noting that attempts to define an IEE count cutoff number for the distinction between EoE and RE

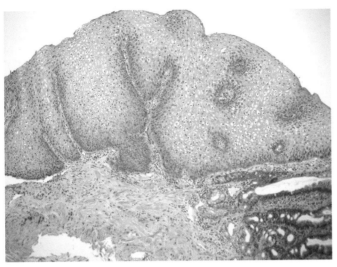

FIGURE 8-7. Reflux esophagitis. Gastroesophageal junctional mucosa with infiltration by mixed inflammatory cells.

TABLE 8-2. Features helpful in differentiating between reflux esophagitis and eosinophilic esophagitis.

Reflux esophagitis

- Abnormalities usually limited to the distal esophagus (lower one-third)
- Degree of eosinophil infiltration usually milder (occasional or a few IEEs seen except in most severe cases)
- Accompanying biopsies of the gastric cardia usually contain eosinophils as well

Eosinophilic esophagitis

- Eosinophilic infiltration involving the midesophagus or upper esophagus, sometimes more severe than that in the distal esophagus
- Dense IEE: can be as high as or more than 50 per HPF in untreated patients
- Eosinophilia more prominent in the superficial layer of the epithelium
- Prominent eosinophil degranulation
- Eosinophilic microabscesses
- Accompanying cardia biopsy usually lacks eosinophils

Abbreviations: HPF, high-power field; IEE, intraepithelial eosinophil.

have not been successful. As discussed, there are overlaps between RE and EoE among some patients, for whom the correct diagnosis can be reached only based on careful evaluation of a combination of histologic parameters with clinical correlation. For example, an IEE count of more than 20 per HPF, midesophageal involvement, and accentuation of IEEs in the superficial epithelial layer favor the diagnosis of EoE, particularly in a child or young patient. Similarly, when a higher IEE count is noted in the midesophagus than in the lower esophagus, the diagnosis of RE is less likely (Table 8-2).

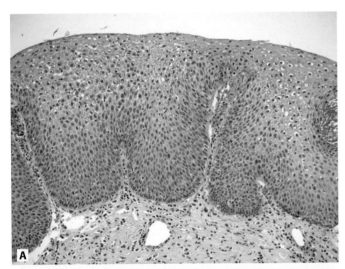

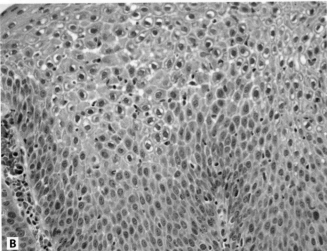

FIGURE 8-8. Chronic reflux esophagitis. In this view, the lamina propria papillae are markedly elongated due to hypertrophy of the squamous epithelium (**A**) which contains many intraepithelial eosinophils (**B**).

FIGURE 8-9. Eosinophilic esophagitis. Marked reactive change of the squamous epithelium, which contains many eosinophils; increased thickness of the basal zone; and elongation of the lamina propria papillae.

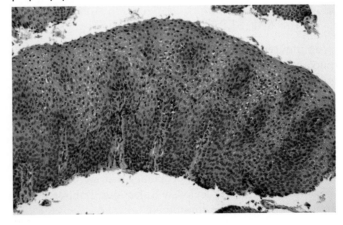

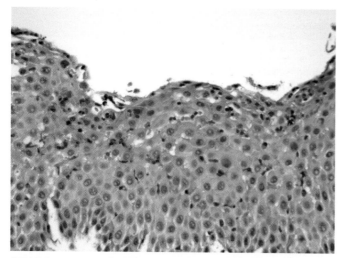

FIGURE 8-10. Eosinophilic esophagitis with superficial eosinophilia.

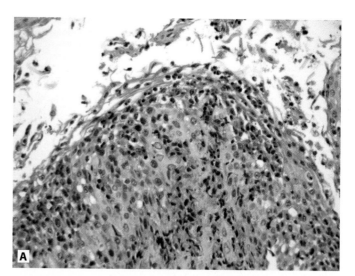

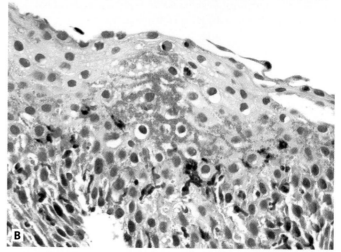

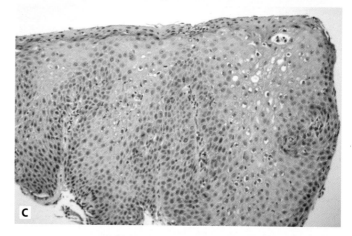

FIGURE 8-11. Eosinophilic esophagitis. **A.** Superficial erosion. **B.** Degranulation. **C.** Parakeratosis.

Counting IEEs in esophageal biopsies is a useful approach but usually unnecessary when the diagnosis is evidently RE. It is more useful for monitoring disease activity or response to treatment in EoE. This information should always be provided for biopsies for this purpose. Personally, I prefer counting per HPF up to 50 IEE; there are no data to suggest that comparison of higher counts has implications in current clinical practice settings.

Other features, such as intercellular edema (spongiosis) or thickening of the basal zone (basal hyperplasia), are helpful in substantiating the diagnosis of active and chronic esophagitis but are not so important in the distinction between RE and EoE.

The clinical significance of correctly distinguishing this disease from RE is related to specific treatment of EoE, including removing food or air allergens, basic essential diet, and systemic or ingestation of topical steroids.[14-16]

It should be noted that IEE infiltration is also associated with parasitic infestation (not further discussed), as well as drug-induced esophagitis (discussed next).

■ DRUG-INDUCED ESOPHAGITIS AND OTHER THERAPY-RELATED ESOPHAGITIS

Drug-induced or pill esophagitis refers to any esophageal mucosa injury due to prolonged local exposure to one of some hundred types of medicinal pills,[17] which may be represented by the cases caused by alendronate.[18-20] This occurs when a pill dissolves in the esophagus rather than quickly passing through and dissolving in the stomach. Most examples of pill esophagitis show patchy-to-severe epithelial cell damage or degeneration, with or without inflammatory infiltration. When a biopsy exhibits abnormalities that are unusual for the entities described previously (infectious, EoE, or RE), a drug etiology should be considered.

Alendronate Sodium (Fosamax)

Ingestion of Fosamax® for osteoporosis is a known cause of erosive esophagitis or ulcer in some patients. The histologic abnormalities were well described by Abraham et al.,[21] including polarizable crystalline foreign material,

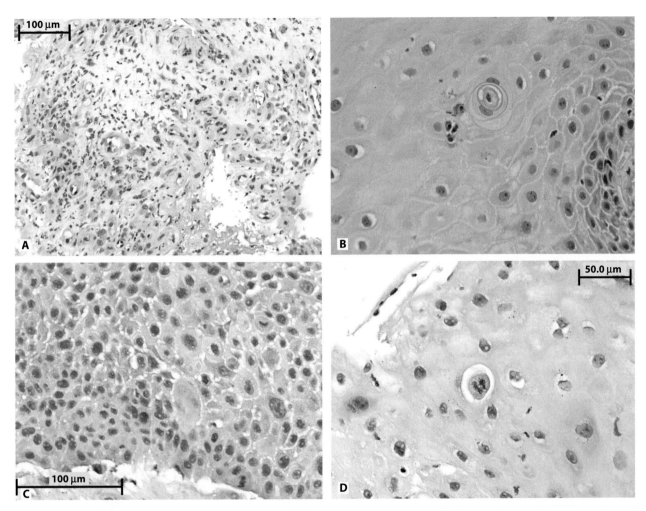

FIGURE 8-12. Pill esophagitis due to alendronate. **A.** Ulcer granulation tissue. **B.** Adjacent epithelium contains active inflammation with eosinophils. **C.** Large bizarre-appearing multinucleated degenerative cell. **D.** Dyskeratotic cells.

multinucleated giant cells, in addition to the common feature of inflamed granulation tissue of any ulcer base (Figure 8-12A). Adjacent squamous epithelium typically shows active inflammation and a reactive appearance with enlarged, hyperchromatic nuclei. In addition, large, "bizarre" squamous epithelial cells (Figure 8-12C) and scattered dyskeratotic squamous cells, either individually or in a cluster (Figure 8-12D),[20] have been observed, two findings not well described in previous reports.

Doxycycline

Esophagitis due to ingestion of doxycycline or similar antibiotics is well known.[22-24] This usually occurs in the middle third of the esophagus.[24] Severe cases can have superficial necrosis, causing erosion or ulcer (Figure 8-13). One of the unique features is the presence of ring-shaped blood vessel degeneration,[25] similar to what was observed in doxycycline-induced gastropathy.[26,27]

FIGURE 8-13. Drug-induced esophagitis showing ulceration or superficial necrosis.

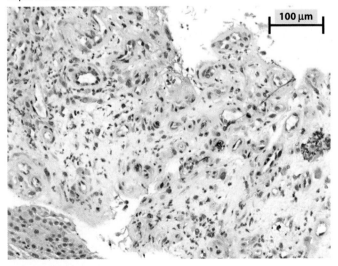

Nonsteroidal Anti-inflammatory Drugs

Like other medications that cause pill esophagitis, nonsteroidal anti-inflammatory drugs (NSAIDs) cause nonspecific inflammation of the esophageal mucosa in some patients, sometimes with erosion, ulcer,[28,29] or stricture.[30] NSAID-induced esophagitis may be superimposed on existing RE. There are no unique histologic features, and the diagnosis relies on clinical correlation.

Kayexalate

Kayexalate® (sodium polystyrene sulfonate) in sorbitol is a cation exchange resin for treatment of hyperkalemia. Occasionally, it can cause upper gastrointestinal damage, including ulcer or erosion, from the characteristic Kayexalate crystals.[31]

Radiation-Induced Esophagitis

Nearly half of patients who receive thoracic radiation therapy for lung cancer develop significant damage to esophageal mucosa, ranging from inflammatory infiltration to ulcer or stricture.[32,33] Histologically, the abnormalities of the squamous epithelium may be similar to that of severe reflux; some cases may exhibit degenerative change or necrosis involving the superficial squamous layer (Figure 8-14). As the findings are largely nonspecific, treatment history will help determine this etiology of esophagitis.

■ IMMUNE-RELATED ESOPHAGITIS

Graft-Versus-Host Disease

Esophagogastroduodenoscopy (EGD) biopsies are frequently performed to evaluate for graft-versus-host disease (GVHD) in recipients of stem cell transplants. Although the esophagus is less frequently affected compared to other segments of the gastrointestinal tract, in more severe cases, significant active inflammation can be identified in esophageal mucosa. These changes

FIGURE 8-14. Radiation-induced esophagitis. In this example of erosive esophagitis related to thoracic radiation therapy, there is marked parakeratosis, with marked neutrophilic infiltration, including intraepithelial microabscesses. The most superficial cells also exhibit reactive nuclear atypia.

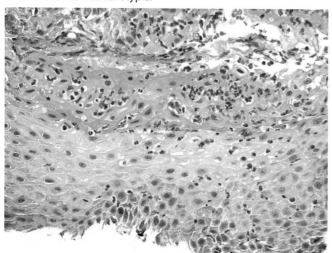

range from nonspecific lymphocyte-dominant inflammatory infiltration, apoptosis of the basal zone, desquamation, and ulceration with granulation tissues (see Chapter 2).

Lichenoid Esophagitis

Rarely, patients with lichen planus of the skin and oral cavity may have esophageal symptoms, and biopsy may show significant esophagitis.[34] Included may be prominent lymphocytic infiltration along the epithelial-stromal junction and degeneration of the basal epithelium and individual squamous cells (Civatte bodies) (Figure 8-15), a pattern similar to lichen planus of the skin.

Lymphocytic Esophagitis

Lymphocytes are often observed in the squamous epithelium of the esophagus in patients without esophageal symptoms and thus are considered as a component of normal epithelium. It was proposed recently that prominent lymphocytic infiltration represents a pathologic condition termed *lymphocytic esophagitis* (LE).[35] These studies defined the diagnosis purely

FIGURE 8-15. Lichenoid esophagitis. **A.** Band-line lymphocytic infiltration involving the basal zone, accompanied by spongiosis. **B.** Civatte body.

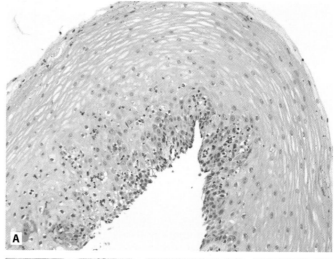

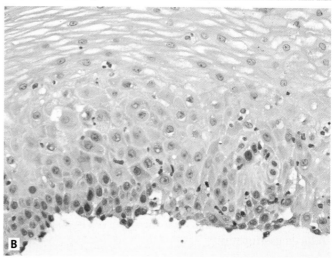

on histologic grounds, and cases recognized by this diagnosis included a mixture of diseases, such as reflux, Crohn disease, celiac disease, and *Helicobacter pylori* gastritis in normal individuals.[35-37] Therefore, it is reasonable to consider LE a histopathologic pattern rather than an independent disease and its use as a diagnostic term is not encouraged. As a recent large study showed,[38] at institutions where this diagnostic term is routinely used, the number of cases has increased dramatically. Follow-up has showed no long-term consequence except for those with other chronic diseases, such as Crohn disease.

Currently, LE cases are indicated by the presence of more than 50 intraepithelial lymphocytes/HPF and less than 1 granulocyte/50 intraepithelial lymphocytes.[37,39]

Esophagitis Due to Crohn Disease

Around 10% of patients with Crohn disease have esophageal involvement. As discussed in Chapter 4 and this chapter, esophagitis in these patients manifests as a spectrum of histologic changes, including inflammation mainly of lymphocytes,[36,37,39] granulomatous esophagitis, and more severely, ulcer.

■ SUMMARY

The basic histologic pattern of active esophagitis consists of injury and reactive changes of the epithelium (basal zone hyperplasia, spongiosis) and inflammatory cellular infiltration. If neutrophilic infiltration is noted, an infectious etiology should be considered and worked up. Careful examination of the H&E-stained section should yield most of these patterns (cytopathic changes characteristic of HSV or CMV, fungal yeasts, and pseudohyphae). However, due to the insensitivity intrinsic to this approach, a special stain (GMS) for a fungal element and immunostains for viral antigens are always warranted in this situation. If these stains are negative, other types of esophagitis, such as pill esophagitis, should be ruled out. Neutrophilic infiltration may also be seen in some cases of severe RE. In biopsies with prominent eosinophilic infiltration, a distinction can be made based on the pattern and distribution of the infiltration and endoscopic findings.

To facilitate initial differential consideration, some microscopic features, when present, are considered usefully unique to each entity discussed; these are listed in Table 8-3.

TABLE 8-3. Histologic features of drug-induced (pill) esophagitis and radiation-induced esophagitis.

Bisphosphonate (alendronate): individual dyskeratotic cells, multinucleated giant squamous cells
Antibiotics (doxycycline, tetracycline, etc): superficial necrosis
Nonsteroidal anti-inflammatory drugs: usually nonspecific active esophagitis
Chemotherapy: degenerative change, clinical history
Radiation-induced esophagitis: usually the proximal esophagus, superficial necrosis, parakeratosis, may be superimposed with candida esophagitis

■ REFERENCES

1. Blick G, Garton T, Hopkins U, LaGravinese L. Successful use of cidofovir in treating AIDS-related cytomegalovirus retinitis, encephalitis, and esophagitis. *J Acquir Immune Defic Syndr Hum Retrovirol.* 1997;15(1):84–85. PMID: 9215660.
2. Cirillo NW, Lyon DT, Schuller AM. Tracheoesophageal fistula complicating herpes esophagitis in AIDS. *Am J Gastroenterol.* 1993;88(4):587–589. PMID: 8470643.
3. Theise ND, Rotterdam H, Dieterich D. Cytomegalovirus esophagitis in AIDS: diagnosis by endoscopic biopsy. *Am J Gastroenterol.* 1991;86(9):1123–1126. PMID: 1652884.
4. Wilcox CM. Esophageal strictures complicating ulcerative esophagitis in patients with AIDS. *Am J Gastroenterol.* 1999;94(2):339–343. PMID: 10022626.
5. Liacouras CA, Markowitz JE. Eosinophilic esophagitis: a subset of eosinophilic gastroenteritis. *Curr Gastroenterol Rep.* 1999;1(3):253–258. PMID: 10980958.
6. Markowitz JE, Liacouras CA. Eosinophilic esophagitis. *Gastroenterol Clin North Am.* 2003;32(3):949–966. PMID: 14562583.
7. Munitiz V, Martinez de Haro LF, Ortiz A, et al. Primary eosinophilic esophagitis. *Dis Esophagus.* 2003;16(2):165–168. PMID: 12823222.
8. Liacouras CA, Ruchelli E. Eosinophilic esophagitis. *Curr Opin Pediatr.* 2004;16(5):560–566. PMID: 15367851.
9. Sgouros SN, Bergele C, Mantides A. Eosinophilic esophagitis in adults: a systematic review. *Eur J Gastroenterol Hepatol.* 2006;18(2):211–217. PMID: 16394804.
10. Ferguson DD, Foxx-Orenstein AE. Eosinophilic esophagitis: an update. *Dis Esophagus.* 2007;20(1):2–8. PMID: 17227302.
11. Weinbrand-Goichberg J, Segal I, Ovadia A, Levine A, Dalal I. Eosinophilic esophagitis: an immune-mediated esophageal disease. *Immunol Res.* 2013;56(2–3):249–260. PMID: 23579771.
12. Merves J, Muir A, Modayur Chandramouleeswaran P, Cianferoni A, Wang ML, Spergel JM. Eosinophilic esophagitis. *Ann Allergy Asthma Immunol.* 2014;112(5):397–403. PMID: 24566295.
13. Bohm M, Richter JE. Treatment of eosinophilic esophagitis: overview, current limitations, and future direction. *Am J Gastroenterol.* 2008;103(10):2635–2644; quiz 45. PMID: 18721234.
14. Almansa C, Devault KR, Achem SR. A comprehensive review of eosinophilic esophagitis in adults. *J Clin Gastroenterol.* 2011;45(8):658–664. PMID: 21836470.
15. Liacouras CA, Furuta GT, Hirano I, et al. Eosinophilic esophagitis: updated consensus recommendations for children and adults. *J Allergy Clin Immunol.* 2011;128(1):3–20 e6; quiz 1–2. PMID: 21477849.
16. Stewart MJ, Shaffer E, Urbanski SJ, Beck PL, Storr MA. The association between celiac disease and eosinophilic esophagitis in children and adults. *BMC Gastroenterol.* 2013;13:96. PMID: 23721294. PMCID: PMC3682941.
17. Kikendall JW. Pill esophagitis. *J Clin Gastroenterol.* 1999;28(4):298–305. PMID: 10372925.
18. Castell DO. "Pill esophagitis"—the case of alendronate. *N Engl J Med.* 1996;335(14):1058–1059. PMID: 8793934.
19. Rimmer DE, Rawls DE. Improper alendronate administration and a case of pill esophagitis. *Am J Gastroenterol.* 1996;91(12):2648–2649. PMID: 8947013.
20. Gomez V, Xiao SY. Alendronate-induced esophagitis in an elderly woman. *Int J Clin Exp Pathol.* 2009;2(2):200–203. PMID: 19079657.
21. Abraham SC, Cruz-Correa M, Lee LA, Yardley JH, Wu TT. Alendronate-associated esophageal injury: pathologic and endoscopic features. *Mod Pathol.* 1999;12(12):1152–1157. PMID: 10619269.
22. Amendola MA, Spera TD. Doxycycline-induced esophagitis. *JAMA.* 1985;253(7):1009–1011. PMID: 3968824.
23. Banisaeed N, Truding RM, Chang CH. Tetracycline-induced spongiotic esophagitis: a new endoscopic and histopathologic finding. *Gastrointest Endosc.* 2003;58(2):292–294. PMID: 12872108.
24. Kadayifci A, Gulsen MT, Koruk M, Savas MC. Doxycycline-induced pill esophagitis. *Dis Esophagus.* 2004;17(2):168–171. PMID: 15230733.

25. Medlicott SA, Ma M, Misra T, Dupre MP. Vascular wall degeneration in doxycycline-related esophagitis. *Am J Surg Pathol.* 2013;37(7):1114–1115. PMID: 23759934.

26. Xiao SY, Zhao L, Hart J, Semrad CE. Doxycycline-induced gastric and esophageal mucosal injuries with vascular degeneration. *Am J Surg Pathol.* 2013;37(7):1115–1116. PMID: 23759935.

27. Xiao SY, Zhao L, Hart J, Semrad CE. Gastric mucosal necrosis with vascular degeneration induced by doxycycline. *Am J Surg Pathol.* 2013;37(2):259–263. PMID: 23060354.

28. Yasuda H, Yamada M, Endo Y, Inoue K, Yoshiba M. Acute necrotizing esophagitis: role of nonsteroidal anti-inflammatory drugs. *J Gastroenterol.* 2006;41(3):193–197. PMID: 16699852.

29. Zografos GN, Georgiadou D, Thomas D, Kaltsas G, Digalakis M. Drug-induced esophagitis. *Dis Esophagus.* 2009;22(8):633–637. PMID: 19392845.

30. El-Serag HB, Sonnenberg A. Association of esophagitis and esophageal strictures with diseases treated with nonsteroidal anti-inflammatory drugs. *Am J Gastroenterol.* 1997;92(1):52–56. PMID: 8995937.

31. Abraham SC, Bhagavan BS, Lee LA, Rashid A, Wu TT. Upper gastrointestinal tract injury in patients receiving kayexalate (sodium polystyrene sulfonate) in sorbitol: clinical, endoscopic, and histopathologic findings. *Am J Surg Pathol.* 2001;25(5):637–644. PMID: 11342776.

32. Newburger PE, Cassady JR, Jaffe N. Esophagitis due to adriamycin and radiation therapy for childhood malignancy. *Cancer.* 1978;42(2):417–423. PMID: 98227.

33. Soffer EE, Mitros F, Doornbos JF, Friedland J, Launspach J, Summers RW. Morphology and pathology of radiation-induced esophagitis. Double-blind study of naproxen vs placebo for prevention of radiation injury. *Dig Dis Sci.* 1994;39(3):655–660. PMID: 8131705.

34. Abraham SC, Ravich WJ, Anhalt GJ, Yardley JH, Wu TT. Esophageal lichen planus: case report and review of the literature. *Am J Surg Pathol.* 2000;24(12):1678–1682. PMID: 11117791.

35. Rubio CA, Sjodahl K, Lagergren J. Lymphocytic esophagitis: a histologic subset of chronic esophagitis. *Am J Clin Pathol.* 2006;125(3):432–437. PMID: 16613348.

36. Purdy JK, Appelman HD, Golembeski CP, McKenna BJ. Lymphocytic esophagitis: a chronic or recurring pattern of esophagitis resembling allergic contact dermatitis. *Am J Clin Pathol.* 2008;130(4):508–513. PMID: 18794041.

37. Ebach DR, Vanderheyden AD, Ellison JM, Jensen CS. Lymphocytic esophagitis: a possible manifestation of pediatric upper gastrointestinal Crohn's disease. *Inflamm Bowel Dis.* 2011;17(1):45–49. PMID: 20848529.

38. Cohen S, Saxena A, Waljee AK, et al. Lymphocytic esophagitis: a diagnosis of increasing frequency. *J Clin Gastroenterol.* 2012;46(10):828–832. PMID: 22751335. PMCID: 3465631.

39. Sutton LM, Heintz DD, Patel AS, Weinberg AG. Lymphocytic esophagitis in children. *Inflamm Bowel Dis.* 2014;20(8):1324–1328. PMID: 24983984.

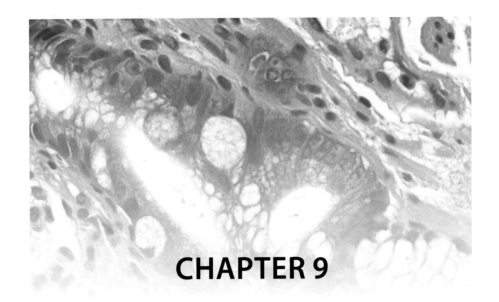

CHAPTER 9

Barrett Esophagus and Adenocarcinoma

Giovanni De Petris and David E. Fleischer

■ INTRODUCTION

Barrett esophagus (BE) is a preneoplastic condition caused by gastroesophageal reflux disease (GERD) and is characterized by the replacement of the squamous epithelium by columnar mucosa (columnar-lined esophagus, CLE), appearing velvety red to pink at macroscopic examination (Figure 9-1). BE is classified as long (>3 cm), short (1–3 cm), and ultrashort (<1 cm) according to the length of CLE between the squamocolumnar junction (SCJ) and the esophagogastric junction (EGJ). Long-segment BE is associated with a higher risk of adenocarcinoma[1] of the esophagus (ACA) than short or ultrashort BE. It should be appreciated that it is not possible for the endoscopist to distinguish ultrashort BE from an irregular Z-line. The American College of Gastroenterology (ACG) states that the diagnosis of BE can be made with any length of CLE that can be recognized at endoscopy and is confirmed to have intestinal metaplasia (IM) on biopsy.[2]

Barrett esophagus is increasing in frequency in Western countries, likely because of increased obesity, and is reported in approximately 10% of patients with GERD. The prevalence varies from 1.3% to 1.9% of the general population of China and Italy[3-6] to the higher value of 5.6% in the United States.[7,8]

Barrett esophagus is the only recognized precursor of adenocarcinoma in the esophagus, a neoplasia that has increased 300% to 500% over the last 30 to 40 years,[9] with poor response to treatment in an advanced stage but eminently treatable in its early stages. A study by Sharma et al[10] (Table 9-1) indicated an incidence of 0.5% of ACA in BE. More

recently, lower incidences of 0.12%–0.2% were reported in European countries,[11,12] raising questions on the need of surveillance for the prevention of adenocarcinoma in patients in which dysplasia is absent.

Dysplasia is the best-known marker for ACA risk stratification in BE. High-grade dysplasia (HGD) remains the best predictor of the development of ACA: 14% of patients with focal HGD developed cancer after 3 years vs 56% in cases of diffuse HGD.[13]

The histological diagnosis of dysplasia remains challenging; in addition, the use of novel endoscopic ablative and resection techniques poses new demands on the pathologist. The role of the correlation with endoscopic findings and awareness of the limits and pitfalls of pathological examination are central in the assessment of BE by pathologists. The main issues for the pathologist facing BE are: identification of IM, identification of the organ of origin of biopsy tissue (is it the esophagus?), identification and assessment of dysplasia, awareness of his or her role in local treatment of neoplasia, and knowledge of cancer staging.

■ INTESTINAL METAPLASIA

Intestinal metaplasia is defined by the presence of goblet cells. Goblet cells (GCs) are characterized by a small basal nucleus indented by a large mucin globule occupying the cytoplasm; the cytoplasm is filled by a globule of acidic mucin (Alcian blue stain positive at pH 2.5). Even in a routine (hematoxylin and eosin, H&E) stained section, the GCs

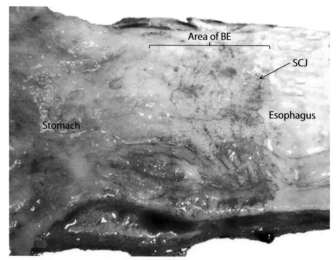

FIGURE 9-1. Resection specimen in a case of Barrett esophagus (BE). The red, velvety BE mucosa (salmon-color mucosa) contrasts with the pink squamous mucosa. SCJ indicates the squamocolumnar junction, now away from the esophagogastric junction.

FIGURE 9-2. Goblet cells are best identified by virtue of their shape (goblet-like appearance with the stem toward the basal lamina), their acidic basophilic/blue-appearing mucin even on hematoxylin-eosin stain, and the lateral displacement they impose on adjacent cells.

TABLE 9-1. Incidence of adenocarcinoma in Barrett esophagus.[a]			
Diagnosis	*Prevalence*	*Incident*	*Incidence (per year)*
N	1376	618	—
LGD	7.3%	16.1%	4.3%
HGD	3%	3.5%	0.9%
ACA detection	6.6%	1.9%	0.5%

ACA, adenocarcinoma; HGD, high-grade dysplasia; LGD, low-grade dysplasia; N, number of subjects.

[a]Data from Sharma P, Falk GW, Weston AP, et al. Dysplasia and cancer in a large multicenter cohort of patients with Barrett's esophagus. *Clin Gastroenterol Hepatol.* 2006;4(5):566–572.[10]

have a blue hue (Figure 9-2). The adjacent epithelial cells can have intestinal/enterocyte-like features with absorptive phenotype and typical brush border of enterocytes that are PAS (periodic acid–Schiff) positive (complete IM) or have a foveolar mucin phenotype with neutral (PAS-positive) mucin in the cytoplasm (incomplete IM) (Figure 9-3). In BE, the IM is usually of the incomplete type.

Both the frequency with which GCs are observed and their density increase proportionally with the length of BE. However, the density of GCs seems to be unrelated to risk of progression to adenocarcinoma.[14]

FIGURE 9-3. The two types of intestinal metaplasia in Barrett esophagus, complete and incomplete, are shown. Incomplete IM is much more common. (**A**) Incomplete IM: The columnar cells (arrowhead) are at least partially secretory and contain acidic sialomucins or sulfomucins (blue after Alcian blue pH2.5). In complete IM, the columnar cells (arrow) are absorptive and contain neutral mucins (**B**) (red after periodic acid–Schiff stain).

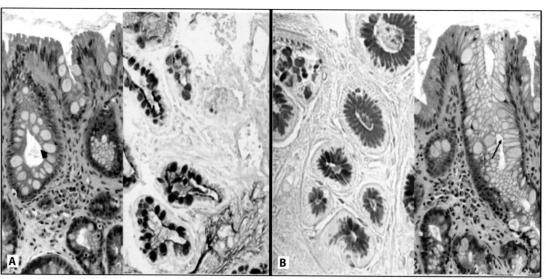

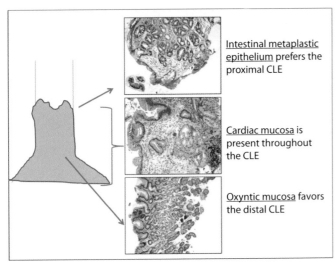

FIGURE 9-4. Distribution of the subtypes of columnar mucosa in CLE. Suggested is lack of randomness, with preferential proximal location of intestinalized mucosa, presence of cardiac subtype throughout, and preferential distal location for the oxyntic subtype.

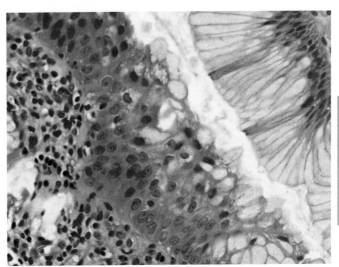

FIGURE 9-5. Multilayer epithelium (shown on the left) shows features of mixed columnar and squamous epithelium. Presence of ME would suggest origin from the esophagus proper rather than the cardia. ME is also considered a strong marker of reflux.

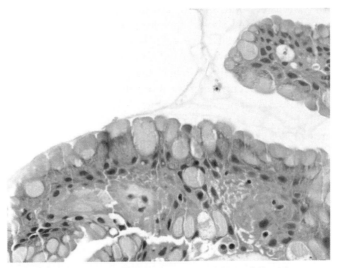

FIGURE 9-6. Pseudogoblet cells are one of the pitfalls in the diagnosis of Barrett esophagus. They do not stain for acidic mucins (blue) with Alcian blue pH 2.5 and often are lined up close to each other in short clusters.

Barrett esophagus columnar mucosa is morphologically heterogeneous (ie, not made exclusively of intestinalized [with GCs] epithelium) since it may also include cardiac and oxyntocardiac glands. Several authors maintained that a zonation of the types of glands exists along the CLE: The cardiac mucosa is distributed evenly along the metaplastic portion of the esophagus, while oxyntic mucosa is more common distally and the intestinalized mucosa is more abundant proximally[15,16] (Figure 9-4). Such an arrangement was not confirmed by others, which suggested instead a random distribution of the mucosae subtypes throughout the CLE.[17] Pancreatic acinar metaplasia, commonly seen in normal gastroesophageal junctional (GEJ), can also be seen in BE where it remains irrelevant.

Multilayer epithelium (ME) (defined as 4–8 layers of cells in which the suprabasal layers are made of columnar mucous cells and the basal cells are flattened and squamoid) (Figure 9-5) is the recent term used to describe a type of epithelium from the GEJ. It consists of both squamous and columnar epithelium (as indicated by morphology and expression of villin, cytokeratins of squamous epithelia, MUC2, CDX2).[18-20] The superficial cells display positive Alcian blue pH 2.5 stain for acidic mucin and resemble GCs but lack cytoplasmic distension. The prevalence of ME is low; although ME is thought to be a strong indicator of reflux disease, ME is currently considered an unlikely precursor of BE.[21]

Differing from native mucosa, the metaplastic epithelium of BE has reduced synaptophysin-positive endocrine cells.[22]

Cells can be mistaken for GCs because of their shape (eg, GC-shaped cells with light pink cytoplasm but without acidic mucin, also known as pseudo-GCs; Figure 9-6) or because of Alcian blue stain reactivity in the cytoplasm (columnar cells with acidic mucin, also known as tall blue columnar cells; metaplastic Alcian blue–positive cells of Offner[23]). The clinical impact of these mimickers is nil unless they are confused with GCs.[24] Finally, the pathologist may face biopsies of IM from inlet patch epithelium. The significance of inlet patch IM is unknown at this time.[25]

PROBLEMS WITH THE DEFINITION OF BARRETT ESOPHAGUS

The ACG definition of BE requires IM: This is not accepted worldwide. The British and Japanese gastroenterologists, for example, do not require the demonstration of GCs. The British Society of Gastroenterology defines BE as metaplastic columnar epithelium clearly visible endoscopically (more than or at

TABLE 9-2. Relation between number of biopsies and detection of intestinal metaplasia (IM) in columnar-lined esophagus.[a]

Number of biopsies per endoscopy	Mean percentage of detection of IM
1–4	34.6
5–8	67.9
9–12	74.1
13–16	71.4
>16	100

Note the significant increase in detection between 1–4 and 5–8 biopsies ($p < .001$) and lack of significant increase by taking more biopsies unless more than 16 are obtained.

[a]Reproduced with permission from Harrison R, Perry I, Haddadin W, et al. Detection of intestinal metaplasia in Barrett's esophagus: an observational comparator study suggests the need for a minimum of eight biopsies. *Am J Gastroenterol.* 2007;102(6):1154–1161.[27]

TABLE 9-3. An example of a formatted report of Barrett esophagus as suggested by the British Gastroenterological Association.[a]

Level/centimeter	*34*
Number of biopsies	2
Squamous mucosa (Y/N)	N
Glandular mucosa (Y/N)	Y
Native esophageal structures (Y/N)	N
Intestinal metaplasia (Y/N)	Y
Glandular dysplasia	
Indefinite (Y/N)	
Low grade(Y/N)	Y
High grade (Y/N)	
Intramucosal cancer(Y/N)	N
Invasive cancer(Y/N)	N
p53 overexpression (Y/N, equivocal, not performed)	Not performed
Highest grade of inflammation (none, mild, moderate, severe)	None

N, no; Y, yes.

[a]Adapted with permission from Fitzgerald RC, di Pietro M, Ragunath K, et al. British Society of Gastroenterology guidelines on the diagnosis and management of Barrett's oesophagus. *Gut.* 2014;63(1):7–42.[26]

least equal to 1 cm in length) above the GEJ, without the need for the presence of GCs at histologic examination (in other words, the importance of histology is merely corroborative).[26]

The reasons for these different definitions are multiple. An obvious reason is that the absence of GCs may be due to sampling bias and should therefore be downplayed. Some investigators suggested that eight H&E-stained biopsies are the minimum number needed to adequately detect IM[27] (Table 9-2); with this approach, the percentage of patients without GCs decreased from more than 50% to less than 10% in the 5-year period of the study.[28] Alcian blue/PAS stain contributes to a change of diagnosis from GCs absent to GCs present in a minority of cases (only in 5.4% in the series of Harrison et al[27]). There is controversy regarding the risk of carcinoma in absence of GCs.[29-31]

In support of the non-requirement of GCs for the diagnosis of BE, some investigators have shown that columnar mucosa without GCs can have intestinal differentiation, as evidenced by immunohistochemical markers such as CDX2, villin, and MUC2, and by similar molecular and DNA content abnormalities in mucosa with and without GCs.[30,31] In addition, there is lack of correlation between density of GCs and risk of adenocarcinoma or HGD.[14] Similarly, mitochondrial RNA (miRNA) dysregulation was found in both nonintestinalized and intestinalized columnar metaplasia.[32] A study from Germany and Japan[33] showed that 70% of small (<2 cm) early adenocarcinomas resected by endoscopic mucosal resection (EMR) arose in cardiac or oxyntic mucosa rather than intestinal-type mucosa. Follow-up studies have shown similar rates of progression to dysplasia or malignancy in mucosa with or without IM.[28] The possibility of sampling bias was significant in these studies as they were based, and depended, on the extent of the initial (index) sampling/biopsies.

Support for the ACG criteria derives from studies with abundant biopsy sampling that showed progression to dysplasia and malignancy only when GCs were present.[34,35] The study of Westerhoff also showed that short-segment BE without GCs remained without GCs at follow-up, suggesting that many short-segment BE cases without GCs may actually represent proximal stomach.[26]

The Prague classification[36] defines columnar metaplasia with a purely endoscopic grading system utilizing maximum extent [M] and length of complete circumferential involvement of esophagus [C] by columnar epithelium. The proponents of the Prague scoring system hope that this approach, based on more reproducible parameters, will allow easier comparison of studies across the world.

The surgical pathologist faced with this array of issues may benefit from the use of a formatted report for evaluating CLE biopsies. An example is provided in the 2014 guidelines of the British Society of Gastroenterology[26] (Table 9-3).

■ IDENTIFICATION OF THE ORGAN OF ORIGIN OF THE COLUMNAR MUCOSA: ARE WE IN THE ESOPHAGUS?

Diagnosis of BE requires that the biopsies originate in the esophagus. Doubts regarding the location of the EGJ due to an irregular Z-line will prompt the endoscopist to obtain a biopsy. The pathologist may then have to distinguish IM of the cardia from true BE. IM may develop in the proximal stomach and is indeed common in patients with an abnormal Z-line (up to 30% of cases). This is significant as 86 patients with IM of the EGJ followed for a median interval of 8 years failed to develop a single case of carcinoma).[37,38] The issue of the tissue origin may be solved when esophageal structures such as submucosal glands or their ducts are present (Figure 9-7). Some additional morphological features found in biopsies of the esophagus with CLE are squamous islands within glandular mucosa, glands covered by squamous

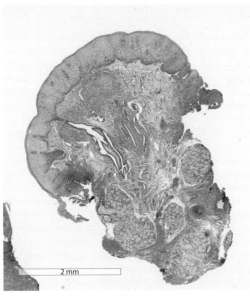

FIGURE 9-7. Endoscopic mucosal resection specimen with clearly visible submucosal glands and their ducts.

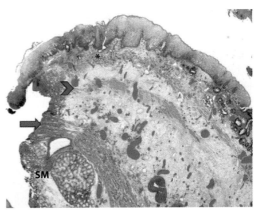

FIGURE 9-9. Triple muscularis mucosae (MM). Only the deepest layer, indicated by an arrow, is the true MM; the others (the most superficial MM indicated by the asterisk, the second MM indicated by the arrowhead) represent a structural reactive change induced by chronic injury, similar to duplicated MM in inflammatory bowel diseases. Notice the submucosal gland (SM) in the true submucosa. The spaces between the duplicated superficial MMs are duplicated lamina propria.

epithelium (buried glands, BGs), and hybrid glands (glands in which IM is limited to the superficial aspect of otherwise cardiac-type mucinous glands) (Figure 9-8).[39]

Microscopic changes characteristic of esophagus, but visible only in resection specimens are: duplicated muscularis mucosae (MM) and palisade vessels. Duplication of MM is common (Figure 9-9).[40] Palisade vessels (veins > 100 μm in size in and above the true MM) are a recently recognized marker of esophageal origin in CLE seen in the distal esophagus.[41]

The endoscopic criteria used to identify the GEJ are the proximal end of the gastric longitudinal folds[9] in lightly insufflated stomach and the distal limit of the visible lower esophageal longitudinal palisading veins[42] (Figure 9-10). In a person suffering from esophagitis, ulcers, or hiatal hernia, these landmarks may be obscured. The critical endoscopic identification of the EGJ can be arduous. It is necessary, therefore, that the endoscopist provides the pathologist with the best possible information regarding where the biopsies were obtained (including a picture of the area). Biopsies of the stomach just distal to what is thought to be the EGJ and from the distal stomach are needed so that comparisons can be performed. Isolated IM of the EGJ (metaplasia absent in the biopsies of the stomach) is likely to be secondary to GERD.

FIGURE 9-8. Two hybrid glands are shown. They have a mucinous base and intestinal metaplasia in the upper portions (left in the picture). Hybrid glands are a marker of the esophageal origin of the biopsy.

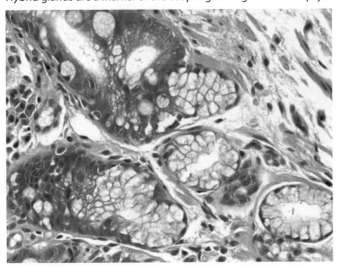

FIGURE 9-10. Palisade vessels in distal esophagus. Their abrupt disappearance in the distal aspect of the picture marks the EGJ. They are more commonly utilized for the identification of the EGJ in Japan than in the United States.

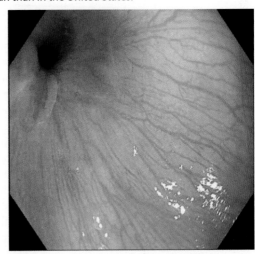

ASSESSMENT OF DYSPLASIA

The Endoscopy of Dysplasia

Patients with BE undergo endoscopic surveillance for detection of dysplasia or carcinoma. Dysplasia in BE either is imperceptible under routine white light endoscopic technique or may appear as an area of erythema or velvety change or as a nodule, polyp, plaque, or ulcer. The presence of dysplastic endoscopically visible nodules is associated with an increased probability of metachronous and synchronous adenocarcinoma. It is also well known that ulcerated lesions in BE have a high risk of association with HGD or adenocarcinoma and require follow-up (15 of 21 ulcerated HGDs demonstrated invasive adenocarcinoma at follow-up[43,44]). Complete reassessment of patients diagnosed with "invisible" HGD showed that expert endoscopic assessment (utilizing advanced endoscopic techniques) reveals HGD in 80% of cases.[45]

Dysplasia often is multifocal. Biopsies are obtained randomly or with a standardized protocol. Detection of prevalent dysplasia in a group of patients with an annual systematic biopsy approach was 13 times higher than in a group using an annual random biopsy approach for surveillance.[46]

More recent studies showed that intensive and demanding protocols, such as the Seattle protocol (4 quadrant biopsies every 1 cm and biopsies of visible lesions), do not predict more reliably the detection of cancer at the time of esophagectomy than a less-intensive surveillance protocol in BE with HGD.[47] New endoscopic techniques have been able to increase the diagnostic yield for the detection of dysplastic lesions[48] or decrease the number of biopsies needed.[49] The new techniques have different goals: detection of an area of abnormality (high-definition white light, autofluorescence) or tissue characterization of an abnormal area (narrow-band imaging, chromoendoscopy, and confocal laser endomicroscopy). They are rather promising and effective and are increasingly utilized to refine the examination of the esophagus.

The Histology of Dysplasia

Dysplasia is neoplastic epithelium confined within the basement membrane of the mucosa from which it arose. The Riddel classification of dysplasia (originally used in inflammatory bowel disease) is widely accepted in BE. The categories of this classification are indefinite for dysplasia (IND), low-grade dysplasia (LGD), and HGD. Patients with HGD are at a higher risk of developing adenocarcinoma; the incidence is estimated to be around 6% per year.[50] Two patterns of dysplasia are well described in BE: adenomatous and non-adenomatous or foveolar type. The first is better studied and known. Other dysplasia types, such as traditional serrated adenoma-type dysplasia,[51] are rarely seen in CLE.

Cytological and architectural features are used to diagnose and grade dysplasia. There are no definitive features of dysplasia and no definitive criteria to separate the subtypes of dysplasia (as stated eloquently by Shepherd et al in *Morson and Dawson Gastrointestinal Pathology*[52]); we therefore provide the guidelines shared by experts and repeatedly presented in the literature that are routinely used in practice.

TABLE 9-4. Variability in diagnosis of dysplasia.

Diagnosis	K statistics of Montgomery et al. study[48]
Negative	K:0.58
InD	K:0.15
LGD	K:0.32
HGD/ACA	K:0.65
Value of K	*Quality of agreement*
≤0.20	Poor
0.21–0.40	Fair
0.41–0.60	Moderate
0.61–0.80	Good
0.81–1.0	Very good

Abbreviations: ACA, adenocarcinoma; HGD, high-grade dysplasia; InD, indefinite for dysplasia; LGD, low-grade dysplasia; K, kappa value measuring the normed difference between the rate of agreement observed vs the rate of agreement expected by chance expressed between 0 and 1, with 0 indicating agreement if diagnosis were assigned at random and 1 when raters agree on every case

Data from Bertani H, Frazzoni M, Dabizzi E, et al. Improved detection of incident dysplasia by probe-based confocal laser endomicroscopy in a Barrett's esophagus surveillance program. *Dig Dis Sci.* 2013;58(1):188–193.

The agreement among observers in the diagnosis of dysplasia can be expressed numerically by the K statistic as, for example, in the well-known study of Montgomery et al[44] (Table 9-4). It is clear from that study that, at the lower end of the spectrum (indefinite, low grade), there is at best only fair agreement in the diagnosis.

Barrett esophagus mucosa negative for dysplasia is characterized by epithelium with minimal but detectable cytological atypia and normal or near-normal architecture. Intestinalized mucosa does display normally hyperchromatic, enlarged, penicillate nuclei. Regenerative changes will occur with inflammation or ulceration of BE mucosa. In markedly reactive epithelium, considerable atypia and a mild degree of architectural distortion can appear; the distinction from dysplasia in these situations can be challenging.

The cytological features that are helpful in the distinction of regenerative changes vs dysplasia are listed in Table 9-5. Surface maturation is a hallmark of nondysplastic epithelia; it is expressed in the table as an increase in cytoplasmic mucin and decrease of nuclear stratification toward the surface of the mucosa. The abrupt transition between dysplastic and nondysplastic epithelium is a useful marker of the presence of dysplasia (Figure 9-11).

A difficult distinction is that between dysplasia vs taxane-induced atypia in CLE.[53] Taxanes are chemotherapy drugs used to treat breast, lung, and esophageal cancers; the best known among them is paclitaxel. At therapeutic dosages and soon after injection (1 to 3 days), they can cause polymerization of the mitotic spindle microtubules, which will settle as a central cluster surrounded by dispersed chromatin, forming pseudoring mitoses in the proliferative compartment of the glands. Together with marked apoptosis

TABLE 9-5. Features helpful in the distinction of reactive changes from adenomatous dysplasia.

Features	Reactive epithelium	Adenomatous dysplasia
Smooth nuclear membranes	+	−
Normal N/C ratio	+	−
Normal mitoses	+	−
Prominent nucleoli	Possible	Common (in ACA)
Nuclear pleomorphism	−	+
Loss of cell polarity	−	+
High N/C ratio	−	+
Frequent GCs	+	−
Increase in cytoplasmic mucin toward the surface of the mucosa	+	−
Decrease in nuclear stratification toward the surface of the mucosa	+	−
Gradual transition from atypia to normal cells	+	−

ACA, adenocarcinoma; GC, goblet cell; N/C, nucleustocytoplasm.

the lack of nuclear pleomorphism and hyperchromasia are signs that favor taxane-induced atypia over BE-induced dysplasia (Figure 9-12). Of course, the clinical context is paramount for the differential diagnosis. The CLE is hardly the only portion of the intestines affected by taxane-induced atypia; similar changes can be seen in the gallbladder, colon, and stomach.

Indefinite for Dysplasia

When the changes are insufficient for a diagnosis of dysplasia but dysplasia cannot be excluded, then a diagnosis of

IND is rendered (Figure 9-13). This diagnosis is a practical way to indicate a transitional situation that follow-up biopsies should clarify. Historically, negative answers to the questions

1. Is this epithelium clearly reactive or clearly benign? and
2. Is this epithelium unequivocally neoplastic?

have been the trigger for the diagnosis of IND. Diligent use of deeper sections and the application of the criteria listed in Table 9-5 can help in the differential diagnosis. Immunohistochemical markers are discussed further in the paragraphs on dysplasia. From a practical point of view, when a gastroenterologist is confronted with a diagnosis of IND, it is typical to place the patient on a proton pump inhibitor (PPI) drug to reduce inflammation and to repeat the endoscopy in 6–8 weeks.

Adenomatous Low-Grade Dysplasia

The problem of the scarce reproducibility of the diagnosis of LGD is exemplified by several studies. In a study of 147 cases diagnosed with LGD by community pathologists,[54] the expert after review agreed with the diagnosis in only 22 cases; 110 were considered negative, 14 indefinite, and 1 HGD. Eight cases of the LGD group diagnosed by the expert evolved into HGD or adenocarcinoma, as did 2 of the cases considered negative by the expert (therefore the refrain often heard that LGD is over-diagnosed and under-estimated).

The cytological and architectural changes of LGD are: enlarged hyperchromatic and stratified nuclei with extension of these changes to the surface (loss of maturation). Nuclear polarity is preserved; severe nuclear pleomorphism is absent. It is significant that the nuclei remain generally confined to the basal half of the cells because in HGD they have an irregular distribution in the basal and the upper half of the cells.

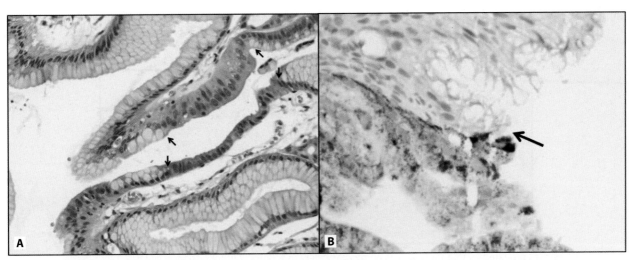

FIGURE 9-11. Adenomatous dysplasia. **A.** The arrows mark the abrupt transition between dysplasia and normal epithelium; notice the lack of mucin in dysplasia and the focally stratified arrangement of nuclei, with few nuclei in the upper half of the cytoplasm. **B.** Alpha-methylacyl-CoA-racemase (AMACR) immunostain also shows an abrupt stop at the arrow where dysplasia terminates. Reactive changes would have a gradual change of the atypia into normal-appearing epithelium.

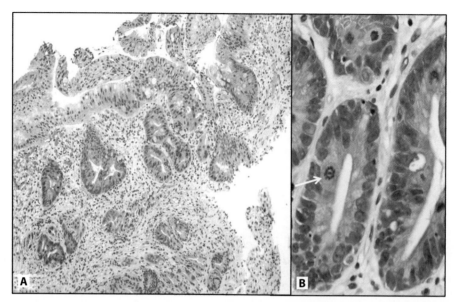

FIGURE 9-12. Taxane effect in Barrett esophagus. **A.** The area of glandular atypia is darker, but the surface appears spared. **B.** A central chromatin bar is clearly seen in one mitotic figure (white arrow) with pseudoring mitosis appearance. Not every mitosis will display this change. Notice also the increased apoptosis in the glands.

The glands affected are not crowded (Figure 9-14). A useful list of the features distinguishing LGD from HGD is given in Table 9-6.[55,56] The loss of maturation toward the surface epithelium has been considered a helpful and conceptually sound criterion for the diagnosis of dysplasia. An entity recently called basal crypt dysplasia (BCD) challenges that idea[57]: In BCD, cytological atypia sufficient for the diagnosis of LGD or HGD is limited to deep glands that stand out as markedly different from adjacent crypts. The lesion has an adenomatous look (Figure 9-15) with stratified nuclei and nuclear pleomorphism that distinguish it from reactive crypt changes. Aneuploidy and abnormal p53 and Ki-67 immunolabeling are identified in BCD. Currently, in these cases some experts would issue a diagnosis of IND or of "basal cell atypia warranting follow-up" similar to cases of IND. Finally, it is worthwhile to note that in the presence of significant inflammation, the diagnosis of BCD should not be rendered.

Adenomatous High-Grade Dysplasia

The histological features of adenomatous HGD (Figure 9-16) are presented briefly in Table 9-6. HGD can be diagnosed regardless of the presence of inflammation. It should in fact be recalled that HGD and intramucosal adenocarcinoma (IMC) tend to attract polymorphonuclear leukocytes.

Can the Morphology of HGD in the Biopsy Predict the Presence of Concurrent Adenocarcinoma? Zhu et al[58] classified HGD as "regular" or "suspicious" for associated carcinoma. Five clues were found that made HGD suspicious for associated carcinoma: cribriform/solid growth, dilated

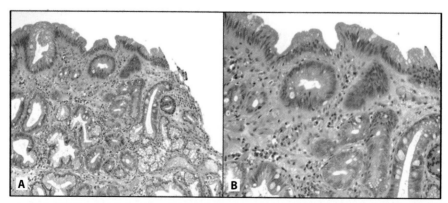

FIGURE 9-13. Diagnoses provided by four pathologists on this case were as follows: 2 indefinite for dysplasia, 1 low-grade dysplasia, 1 Barrett esophagus (number is the number of pathologists). **A.** The vicinity of intestinalized glands to cardiac-type glands makes the first stand out. **B.** It appears that the atypia of the glands (stratification of nuclei, hyperchromatism, and architectural disarray) is not clearly dysplastic and likely it merges smoothly with adjacent mucosa. A diagnosis of indefinite for dysplasia was issued.

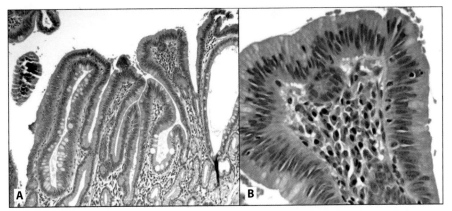

FIGURE 9-14. Typical adenomatous low-grade dysplasia of Barrett esophagus. The adenoma-like features are clear-cut; the architecture is not severely altered (**A**), and involvement of the surface (**B**) is clearly seen. Note the loss of goblet cells in the low-grade dysplasia and its abrupt ending.

TABLE 9-6. Low-grade vs high-grade dysplasia in Barrett esophagus.[a]

Feature	Low grade	High grade
Cytology		
Nuclear pleomorphism	–	+
Nuclear distribution	Basal half	Haphazard
Irregular nuclear contour	+	++
Increased nucleus-to-cytoplasm ratio	+	++
Hyperchromasia	+	++
Mitosis	+	+
Atypical mitosis	±	++
Full-thickness nuclear stratification	–	+
Loss of cell polarity	–	+
Large nucleoli	–	+
Multiple nucleoli	±	±
Fewer goblet cells	+	++
Architecture		
Parallelism of crypts and crypt shape	Generally well preserved	Lost
Crypts branching, budding, crowding	–	++
Villiform surface	–	±
Intraluminal papillae or ridges	–	±

[a]Adapted with permission from Odze RD. Diagnosis and grading of dysplasia in Barrett's oesophagus. *J Clin Pathol.* 2006;59(10):1029–1038.[56]

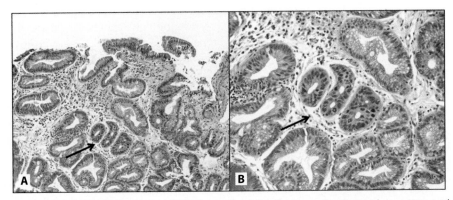

FIGURE 9-15. Basal crypt dysplasia (BCD). **A.** The focus of BCD is readily visible for its nuclear hyperchromatism and density (arrows in A and B indicate the area of BCD). Notice how the surface is unremarkable. **B.** A higher magnification of the same area shows changes indistinguishable from low-grade dysplasia. Variability in the diagnoses of these cases is to be expected. (Used with permission of Dr. Thomas Smyrk, Mayo Clinic, Rochester, MN.)

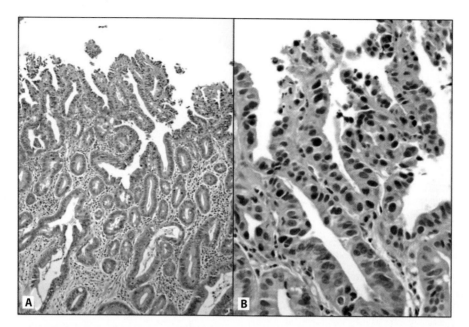

FIGURE 9-16. High-grade dysplasia (HGD) in Barrett esophagus (**A**) (higher magnification in **B**) shows marked nuclear pleomorphism, haphazard positioning of nuclei that have lost their perpendicular arrangement, marked architectural distortion. The area in **A** is completely involved by HGD. Superficial epithelium with HGD is in **B**.

glands with necrotic debris, ulcerated HGD, polymorpho-nucleates in HGD, and "invasion" of squamous epithelium by HGD (Figure 9-17). The impact of these factors in finding invasive adenocarcinoma (T1 or more) at esophagectomy was as follows: No factors present meant no cancer was found; presence of one factor was associated with cancer in 39% of cases; two, three, and four factors present were associated, respectively, in 83%, 87%, and 88% of cases with cancer; invasion into overlying squamous epithelium was always associated with adenocarcinoma.

FIGURE 9-17. Markedly atypical dysplastic glands of high-grade dysplasia in squamous epithelium appear "destructive" of it. This finding was always associated with adenocarcinoma in the study of Zhu et al.[68] Adenocarcinoma was present in this case also.

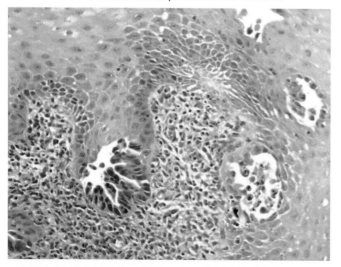

Nonadenomatous Foveolar Dysplasia

Although less recognized, nonadenomatous foveolar dysplasia may actually be more frequent than previously acknowledged[59–61] (prevalence: 15% of patients with Barrett dysplasia[61]). Adenomatous dysplasia is defined by stratified and elongated nuclei, by the presence of GCs and Paneth cells, and by relatively sizable glands, well distinct from each other at least in LGD. Foveolar dysplasia is instead paler overall but with glands closer to each other and smaller than those of adenomatous dysplasia, without GCs or Paneth cells. Foveolar dysplasia cells are cuboidal to columnar, with pale pink cytoplasm, high N/C (nucleus-to-cytoplasm) ratio, and basal round/oval and irregular nuclei with open chromatin (Figure 9-18); stratification of nuclei is often absent with a monolayer of nuclei seen in some cases. Foveolar dysplasia may occasionally mature superficially and displays its most marked abnormalities in the neck of the glands. Foveolar dysplasia has generally abundant mucin in epithelium that resembles gastric foveolar epithelium and that correspondingly expresses gastric foveolar immunophenotype (MUC5ac and MUC6 are positive). Intestinal adenomatous dysplasia has obviously an intestinal immunophenotype (CDX2 and CD10 are expressed).[59]

The differential diagnosis of low-grade foveolar dysplasia from reactive cardiac mucosa should be based on the architectural features as underlined by Patil et al.[62] Crowded glands with full-thickness atypia and lack of villiform appearance are hallmarks of foveolar dysplasia (Table 9-7). In high-grade foveolar dysplasia, the surface can become villiform, the architecture is more irregular, the cytoplasm is more eosinophilic, the nucleoli are prominent.

Foveolar dysplasia is frequently associated with adenomatous dysplasia. In that case the adenomatous dysplasia is

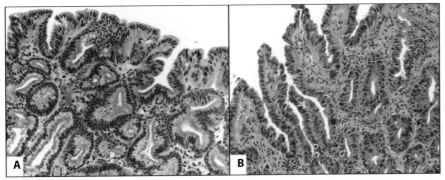

FIGURE 9-18. Foveolar type dysplasia: (**A**) low grade; (**B**) high grade. Abundant pale mucin is in the cytoplasm in **A**, reminiscent of foveolar-type epithelium, typical of low-grade foveolar dysplasia. The nuclear grade and loss of polarity, the villiform appearance, and the eosinophilic cytoplasm determine the diagnosis of high-grade foveolar dysplasia in **B**. (Used with permission of Dr. Ana Bennett, Cleveland Clinic, Cleveland, OH.)

TABLE 9-7. Features useful in the distinction of reactive cardia from low-grade foveolar dysplasia.[a]

Feature	Reactive cardia	Foveolar dysplasia
Villiform mucosa surface	+	−
Superficial atypia	+	−
Full-thickness atypia	−	+
Crowded glands	−	+

[a]Data from Patil DT, Bennett AE, Mahajan D, et al. Distinguishing Barrett gastric foveolar dysplasia from reactive cardiac mucosa in gastroesophageal reflux disease. *Hum Pathol.* 2013;44(6):1146–1153.[46]

frequently HGD, as shown by the presence of HGD in 77% of the cases with adenomatous dysplasia associated with foveolar dysplasia in a report by Rucker-Schmidt et al.[63]

What Are the Consequences of the Diagnosis of Dysplasia in Barrett Esophagus?

The histological diagnosis of dysplasia remains central in therapy decisions. The guidelines of the American Gastroenterology Association (AGA) and American Society for Gastrointestinal Endoscopy (ASGE) are shown in Table 9-8. A diagnosis of LGD means follow-up for the patient, while HGD always prompts therapeutic intervention to remove the area with HGD. The role of the pathologist has become more challenging, however, as compelling data from a recent trial comparing radio-frequency ablation (RFA) vs endoscopic

surveillance in LGD indicated a marked benefit with RFA: The progression to HGD/adenocarcinoma was reduced from 26.5% in controls to 1.5% after ablation of LGD.[64] The many unknowns regarding LGD natural history, the still-unsettled risk stratification of LGD, the imperfect results of the endoscopic surveillance, and the cost of repeated follow-up have convinced several experts to currently be in favor of treating LGD with RFA.

Review of the Diagnosis of Dysplasia by a Second Experienced Gastrointestinal Pathologist

Community pathologists clearly see the usefulness of the review of cases suspicious for dysplasia in BE by an expert gastrointestinal pathologist because diagnosis of dysplasia has the characteristics of an "art." A cogent argument in favor of review could be the evidence that agreement of pathologists on the diagnosis of LGD in the majority, but not all (eg, see results of the study of Wani in Table 9-9), of the studies indicated a higher risk of progression of LGD[65] (Table 9-9). It is strongly advised that an LGD diagnosis be confirmed by a second gastrointestinal pathologist as it remains "the best tissue biomarker for the assessment of cancer risk."[26] On the other end of the spectrum is the differential diagnosis of HGD with adenocarcinoma. A study by Stolte and Benicke[66] indicated that expert review of HGD is justified as follow-up of cases in which HGD was upgraded to adenocarcinoma by an expert pathologist confirmed the presence of adenocarcinoma in 86.8% of cases at the resection (see also EMR discussion that follows).

TABLE 9-8. Therapy and follow-up guidelines after diagnosis of dysplasia in Barrett esophagus.

	BE	InD and LGD	HGD
AGA guidelines, 2011	Endoscopic eradication via RFA, EMR, PDT could be an option	If LGD confirmed, could consider endoscopic eradication via EMR, RFA, PDT	Endoscopic eradication via RFA, EMR, PDT[a]
ASGE guidelines, 2012	Nondysplastic: no surveillance or ablation. If endoscopic surveillance: every 3–5 years	Surveillance every year or EMR or ablation	Endoscopic eradication via RFA, EMR, PDT[a]

Abbreviations: AGA, American Gastroenterological Association; ASGE, American Society for Gastrointestinal Endoscopy; EMR, endoscopic mucosal resection; HGD, high-grade dysplasia; LGD, low-grade dysplasia; PDT, photodynamic therapy; RFA, radio-frequency ablation.

[a]Strong evidence suggests that EMR-based histological staging should precede ablative therapies as correct staging may not be provided by biopsies alone.

TABLE 9-9. Progression of LGD to ACA or HGD.[a]

Author	No. of cases	No. of experts agree	Progression to HGD or ACA
Odze	77	3	31.8%
Skacel	25	2	41%
		3	80%
Montgomery	15	Majority (>6/12)	47%
Wani	41	2	0.84%/year
Wani	88	1 local pathologist	0.94%/year

Abbreviations: ACA, adenocarcinoma; HGD, high-grade dysplasia; LGD, low-grade dysplasia.

[a]Data from *Am J Gastroenterol* 2007;102:483; *Am J Gastroenterol* 200;95:382; *Hum Pathol* 2001;32:370; *Gastroenterology* 2011;141:1179. The difference in progression between local pathologist diagnosis and 2 expert pathologists' agreed diagnosis in the study of Wani was not statistically significant.

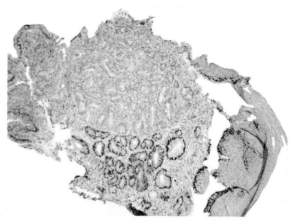

FIGURE 9-19. P53 immunostain is entirely negative in a round area of dysplasia in the center of the biopsy. This aberrant loss of expression of p53 should not be misinterpreted as benign or "normal" as it may instead indicate a higher risk of neoplastic progression.[77]

Are p53, α-Methylacyl-CoA-Racemase, or Other Markers Useful?

"Not conclusively" is the short answer for whether p53, α-methylacyl-CoA-racemase (AMACR), or other markers are useful; they can at best support the diagnosis of dysplasia. The diagnosis of dysplasia is currently entirely based on sections stained with H&E. The main objection to the studies of possible markers of dysplasia is that the gold standard diagnosis of dysplasia is histological and has been shown to be prone to variable interpretation. The best known of several molecules utilized to aid in the diagnosis of dysplasia is p53; p53 is expressed normally (weak expression or 1+) in the nuclei of a subset of proliferating cells (best seen in the esophagus in the basal cells of the squamous epithelium and, less numerously, in the crypt epithelium). Positivity is defined by stronger expression (overexpression) in the lesional area than in the surrounding "control" epithelium. Overexpression of p53 antigen at immunohistochemical examination is due to mutations in the p53 gene that stabilize p53 protein. In 30% of cases, however, there is no concordance between p53 gene mutation and immunohistochemical overexpression.

We know that nuclear overexpression of p53 increases as dysplasia grade increases; it is seen in 70%–90% of adenocarcinoma, 50%–70% of HGD, 30%–50% of LGD, and 10%–30% of IND; a few cases (5%) are considered negative[67] (false positive), indicating lack of specificity. Truncating p53 gene mutations or epigenetic silencing can cause protein inactivation and complete lack of expression of p53; this pattern may be equally good or better at predicting progression of dysplasia to higher-grade dysplasia or adenocarcinoma[68] (Figure 9-19).

AMACR is present in mitochondria and peroxisomes (explaining the granular quality of the cytoplasmic stain in the positive cases) (Figure 9-11). It is a stain specific for HGD and adenocarcinoma, but the percentage of staining in the spectrum BE-dysplasia-adenocarcinoma is highly variable among the studies. AMACR is not better than histology in prediction of progression in LGD.[69]

Multiple-antibody immunostains have also been tested. In van Dekken et al's study of the spectrum of pathology spanning from BE to adenocarcinoma of EGFR (epidermal growth factor receptor), Her-2-neu (Her2), MYC, CDKN2A(p16), SMAD4, MET, cyclin D1, β-catenin, and p53 were utilized. Significant results were the positivity of β-catenin in LGD vs BE and of cyclin D1 and p53 in LGD vs HGD; however, only 25% of the LGD cases had β-catenin, and HGD expression of cyclin D1 was seen in only 45% of cases.[70] The use of Her2 testing to modulate therapy for advanced adenocarcinoma of the esophagus is known. The Her2 oncogene is amplified with an increase in expression along the neoplastic progression, with occasional reports of positivity even in GERD and BE. The pathologist should therefore remember that non–adenocarcinoma tissue such as dysplasia can also show immunoreactivity for Her2. The role of Her2 positivity as a predictor of progression of dysplasia to adenocarcinoma is suggested but not confirmed.[71]

Ablative Therapy Effect and Buried Glands

Ablative therapy (eg, electrothermal coagulation, argon beam coagulation, RFA, cryoablation, photodynamic therapy) for early neoplastic changes in BE implies destruction via endoscopic probes of the neoplastic tissue. It works by heating or freezing the tissue to the point of vaporization or coagulation of the tissue proteins. Ablative therapy causes an initially acute and chronic inflammatory response and reactive epithelial changes followed by fibrosis of the lamina propria and alterations of the MM, including duplication. Post-ablation intraepithelial eosinophilia (>5 eosinophils/high power field) is a phenomenon noted in 16% of patients after ablation and can persist for more than a year. The significance of the phenomenon is unclear, but it should be remembered not to confuse it with eosinophilic esophagitis.[72]

Reepithelialization of BE by squamous epithelium (Figure 9-20) can occur spontaneously, after ablation therapies, after biopsy and PPI therapy. Reepithelialization by

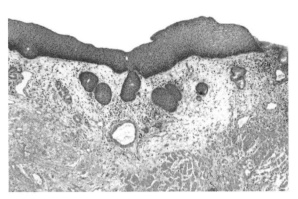

FIGURE 9-20. Reepithelialization in Barrett esophagus often shows a round island of squamous epithelium in the lamina propria related to the ducts of submucosal glands. Buried glands are also present in this case.

squamous epithelium can be seen as squamous islands of squamous epithelium or as entirely replaced columnar epithelium. Reepithelialization may be associated with underlying, concealed, buried metaplastic (or not) glands or even adenocarcinoma invisible to conventional endoscopy. BGs, however, are commonly seen also in untreated BE: After ablative treatment, their frequency actually decreases from 25%, for example, in a control untreated group to 5% after treatment.[73]

While RFA is successful (approximately 80% success rate with complete return to squamous mucosa), in some cases RFA cannot eradicate dysplasia; subsquamous HGD or even invasive adenocarcinoma, not visible endoscopically, can develop. Rates of dysplasia can increase over time after RFA.

Buried glands are detected more often after photoablation (14.2% of patients) than RFA (0.9% of patients, and, of note, much more commonly near the EGJ)[74]; these data, however, suffer because of the notoriously low rate of detection of lamina propria in biopsies of the esophagus (only 25.2%–37% of biopsies have lamina propria).[75] The importance of BGs remains unclear, and it is uncertain if routine random biopsies of neosquamous epithelium are useful. Although there are no current guidelines regarding biopsy protocols after ablative therapy, most commonly follow-up endoscopies are performed to look for residual disease as well as BGs, especially near the EGJ.

Recent studies have found pre-tumorigenic mutations (eg, p53 or CDKN2A gene mutations) in both post-ablation squamous epithelium and in submucosal glands and BGs. Persistence of mutations in residual glands may progress to adenocarcinoma, suggesting that mutation-free epithelium is perhaps the best goal of the therapy and that surveillance should persist if pre-tumorigenic mutations are detected. This is clearly a hypothesis to be tested in future studies.[76]

New techniques, such as optical coherence tomography (OCT), are utilized to detect BGs but have so far shown poor image quality and inability to identify IM. If large areas of BGs are present, they likely reach the surface,

making the search for significant foci of CLE after therapy less challenging.

The lack of a surface mucosa makes interpretation of dysplasia in BGs more difficult because the useful criterion of the lack of maturation toward the surface in dysplasia cannot be ascertained. A p53 immunostain may be helpful in these cases, but it is suggested that caution should be exercised: diagnosis of IND is the most reasonable one in the case of uncertainty.

ADENOCARCINOMA IN BARRETT ESOPHAGUS

Barrett esophagus increases the risk of adenocarcinoma 30-fold, and such risk is augmented with the length of BE: Adenocarcinoma prevalence in long-segment BE is 23% vs 9% in shorter-segment BE.[77] The spectrum of microscopic appearances of adenocarcinoma of the esophagus in BE includes tubular, papillary patterns primarily. Signet-ring cell, mucinous, adenosquamous carcinoma, and especially adenoid cystic, mucoepidermoid carcinoma and adenocarcinoma of submucosal glands, choriocarcinoma, and hepatoid carcinoma are much less common. Our goal here is to focus on the early stages of BE-associated adenocarcinoma. A more comprehensive subclassification scheme for early adenocarcinoma (Figure 9-21) useful for determining prognosis and selecting treatment divides mucosal tumors into three types based on the depth of invasion: M1 is limited to the epithelial layer, M2 invades the lamina propria, M3 invades into but not through the MM. M1 tumors correspond to the Tis stage in the AJCC stage definition, while both M2 and M3 tumors would be considered T1a lesions. Tumors invading the submucosa are subclassified as follows: SM1 penetrates the shallowest one-third of the submucosa (<500 μm), SM2 penetrates into the intermediate one-third of the submucosa, and SM3 penetrates the deepest one-third of the submucosa. All of these subcategories would be considered T1b disease according to the AJCC stage definitions.

FIGURE 9-21. Staging of early adenocarcinoma of the esophagus (see text for discussion). Notice how only penetration beyond the true MM, and not into the space between duplicated MM, is classified as T1b.

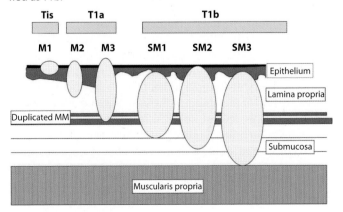

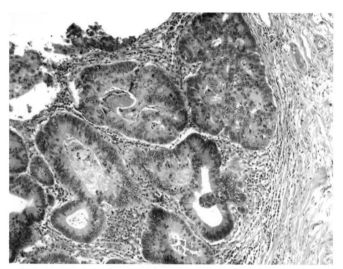

FIGURE 9-22. Highly atypical glands with intraluminal protrusions, fusion of adjacent glands, back-to-back growth of intramucosal adenocarcinoma. Notice the muscularis mucosae on the right and the lack of desmoplasia.

Intramucosal adenocarcinoma can metastasize to lymph nodes (LNs) in 0%–8% of cases, while submucosal invasion is associated with a marked increase in LN metastases: 21% in invasion of superficial submucosa and 56% in invasion of the deep submucosa.[78] Given the detectable risk of LN metastases in IMC, it is important to differentiate HGD from IMC. Architectural features linked to the neoplastic proliferation attempt to create new glands (abortive and angulated gland formation, cribriforming glands, single-cell infiltration, back-to-back glands, gland-in-gland appearance) (Figure 9-22) support the diagnosis of IMC.[56]

Patil et al,[79] in addition to the work of Zhu et al previously reported,[58] have confirmed and provided additional criteria to suspect concurrent adenocarcinoma in biopsies: Single infiltrating cells, dilated glands with necrotic debris in their lumen, invasion of squamous epithelium, and pagetoid spread of cancer cells are markers of malignancy. Pagetoid spread of tumor cells in particular is seen only in adenocarcinoma and not in HGD; however, it is an uncommon finding.[80] Finally, the pathologist should be aware that, in tangential sections, the bottom of distorted glands may appear as isolated or atypical infiltrating cells, and that upward splaying of MM may entrap dysplastic glands. Glandular dysplastic cysts may be particularly difficult to interpret; in favor of the diagnosis of cystic glands of adenocarcinoma are the presence of luminal necrotic debris and the contact of the stroma of the lamina propria with luminal contents secondary to the necrosis of a portion of the lining epithelium. Stromal desmoplasia is not seen or is, at best, focal in IMC and is considered a clue of invasion into submucosa if diffuse. Mucosal necrosis is also considered a clue that invasive adenocarcinoma into the submucosa might be present. The presence of dysplastic glands in MM cannot be taken as a sign of invasion in MM or in the submucosa because BE often has duplicated MM, in which case the true MM is the deepest one. While perhaps redundant, it is nonetheless worthwhile to say that the distinction of IMC from submucosal adenocarcinoma is occasionally impossible in biopsies. The pathologist should then not shy away from stating explicitly his or her uncertainty in that regard. The distinction between HGD and IMC is not as critical, however, given the invariable follow-up of imaging studies and therapeutic approach with endoscopic resection that such diagnoses incite and that will allow a more definitive classification.

Endoscopic Mucosal Resection

A seismic shift has occurred with regard to the treatment of HGD and T1a adenocarcinoma. The use of esophagectomy for the treatment of HGD and IMC, with its intrinsic significant mortality and morbidity, has been replaced by EMR (or endoscopic submucosal dissection mainly in Japan) followed by endoscopic ablation. The risk of morbidity and mortality due to esophagectomy is in fact higher than the risk of LN metastasis due to IMC.[81] Esophagectomy is generally preferred for lesions that invade the submucosa (SM1, SM2, and SM3 tumors).

Some studies have suggested that EMR may be appropriate for cancers that penetrate into the superficial submucosal (SM1 tumors with submucosal penetration < 500 μm). The reason EMR may be an option for SM1 penetrating tumors is that these lesions may have a low risk of positive LNs, provided that they do not show poorly differentiated cancer or lymphovascular invasion (LVI). However, most centers consider SM1 tumors to be an indication for surgery and reserve EMR for those patients who are considered to be at high surgical risk.

The EMR specimen should be pinned and fixed in formalin. The tissue should then be inked to mark the margins (lateral and deep) and serially sectioned, taking care to cut in a way that will obtain sections perpendicular to any visible lesion (Figure 9-23). The tumor size, histology, grade, extent of tumor penetration, lateral and deep margins, completeness of resection, and lymphatic and vascular involvement should be reported.

FIGURE 9-23. Suggested approach to the sectioning of the EMR specimen.

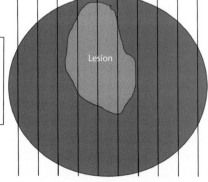

Pin and stretch gently.
Fix in formalin.
Photograph.
Ink margins.
Cut 2-mm parallel sections perpendicular to lesion if visible.
Lateral end sections of a small EMR are submitted en face.

Lesion

Lymphovascular invasion is the best predictor of LN metastases in pT1 adenocarcinoma.[82] High histologic tumor grade is also a risk factor that predicts LN metastases and local recurrence.[83] Piecemeal EMR tumor removal is associated with a higher risk of local recurrences.[83]

Endoscopic mucosal resection not only is used for therapeutic purposes but also is the most accurate staging technique for early BE-associated neoplasia. Ultrasound endoscopy is inadequate for the purpose of staging early adenocarcinoma. Biopsies also have significant limitations: In a study by Mino-Kenudson et al,[84] the grade of neoplasia of the biopsies appeared underreported in 21% of cases and overreported in 16% of cases. A systematic review showed that a change in diagnosis occurred in cases of HGD or adenocarcinoma after EMR in approximately 25% of the patients, with both upstaging and downstaging reported.[85] The degree of pathologist interobserver variability is decreased by EMR compared to biopsy evaluation certainly because of larger size and less distortion of the tissue and of the reliable assessment of the MM, submucosa (88% of EMRs have submucosa vs 1.5% of biopsies[86]), and margins of excision.

The previous observations are important: They indicate the central role of histological diagnosis based on EMR before ablative therapies are implemented because a significant percentage of cases might have been understaged by biopsies alone. Negative margins in cases of HGD treated with EMR that underwent a follow-up esophagectomy predicted absence of residual disease at the EMR site at esophagectomy.[87] A positive deep EMR margin is instead considered a therapeutic failure.

Duplicated Muscularis Mucosae

The issue of duplicated, or even triplicated, MM is of particular importance for the pathologist examining EMR specimens. In case of duplicated MM, the deepest layer of muscle represents the true MM. Duplicated MM is frequent; it is seen in approximately 79% of esophagectomy specimens and up to 95% of EMR specimens[21] if even focal duplication is considered. The assessment of MM is complicated not only by the focality of the finding of duplicated MM but also by the common detection of variations, including thickened single-layer MM and splaying of MM into lamina propria. Furthermore, the deep layer (true MM) is absent in superficial EMR specimens, with the obvious risk of overstaging adenocarcinoma.

Smoothelin is a protein expressed only in fully differentiated smooth muscle cells. Immunohistochemical reactivity to smoothelin antibody in BE is weaker in the neo-MM (superficially placed) than in the true MM. Comparison of the stains of the layers of MM is therefore necessary in case of the use of smoothelin to distinguish between MM layers, but this is a task possible only in a subgroup of EMRs or esophagectomies, not in biopsies.[88]

Invasion in the stroma between the layers of duplicated MM (or, in other words, invasion of the second lamina propria created by a duplicated MM) has no impact in LN metastatic rate when compared to invasion of true lamina propria, while invasion in submucosa below the duplicated MM has the expected significantly higher number of LN metastases.[82,89] How can pathologists recognize the true submucosa in an esophagus with duplicated MM? Three helpful morphological clues typical of submucosa are the presence of submucosal glands, of thick-walled muscular arterioles, and of diffuse desmoplasia in the case of involvement by adenocarcinoma.

Submucosal glands point to the submucosa layer, but they are not always present; the alteration of the architecture of the EMR tissues due to curling and contractions can make it difficult to assess submucosal glands for this purpose. The soft tissue between the layers of duplicated MM is similar to lamina propria, with small delicate vessels, while the true submucosa has thick-walled muscular arteries that can be easily identified.[90] Finally, diffuse desmoplasia is considered suggestive of submucosal invasion in case of carcinoma, but a definitive study on this aspect is lacking, and in our experience, it is not uncommon to see focal desmoplasia in intramucosal adenocarcinoma (Figure 9-24).

■ REFERENCES

1. Frazzoni M, Manno M, De Micheli E, Savarino V. Pathophysiological characteristics of the various forms of gastro-oesophageal reflux disease. Spectrum disease or distinct phenotypic presentations? *Dig Liver Dis*. 2006;38(9):643–648. PMID: 16627016.

2. Wang KK, Sampliner RE. Updated guidelines 2008 for the diagnosis, surveillance and therapy of Barrett's esophagus. *Am J Gastroenterol*. 2008;103(3):788–797. PMID: 18341497.

3. Ronkainen J, Aro P, Storskrubb T, et al. Prevalence of Barrett's esophagus in the general population: an endoscopic study. *Gastroenterology*. 2005;129(6):1825–1831. PMID: 16344051.

4. Spechler SJ, Fitzgerald RC, Prasad GA, Wang KK. History, molecular mechanisms, and endoscopic treatment of Barrett's esophagus. *Gastroenterology*. 2010;138(3):854–869. PMID: 20080098. PMCID: 2853870.

5. Zagari RM, Fuccio L, Wallander MA, et al. Gastro-oesophageal reflux symptoms, oesophagitis and Barrett's oesophagus in the general population: the Loiano-Monghidoro study. *Gut*. 2008;57(10):1354–1359. PMID: 18424568.

6. Zou D, He J, Ma X, et al. Epidemiology of symptom-defined gastroesophageal reflux disease and reflux esophagitis: the systematic investigation of gastrointestinal diseases in China (SILC). *Scand J Gastroenterol*. 2011;46(2):133–141. PMID: 20955088.

7. Hayeck TJ, Kong CY, Spechler SJ, Gazelle GS, Hur C. The prevalence of Barrett's esophagus in the US: estimates from a simulation model confirmed by SEER data. *Dis Esophagus*. 2010;23(6):451–457. PMID: 20353441. PMCID: 2896446.

8. Musana AK, Resnick JM, Torbey CF, Mukesh BN, Greenlee RT. Barrett's esophagus: incidence and prevalence estimates in a rural Mid-Western population. *Am J Gastroenterol*. 2008;103(3):516–524. PMID: 17970839.

9. Sharma P, McQuaid K, Dent J, et al. A critical review of the diagnosis and management of Barrett's esophagus: the AGA Chicago Workshop. *Gastroenterology*. 2004;127(1):310–330. PMID: 15236196.

10. Sharma P, Falk GW, Weston AP, Reker D, Johnston M, Sampliner RE. Dysplasia and cancer in a large multicenter cohort of patients with Barrett's esophagus. *Clin Gastroenterol Hepatol*. 2006;4(5):566–572. PMID: 16630761.

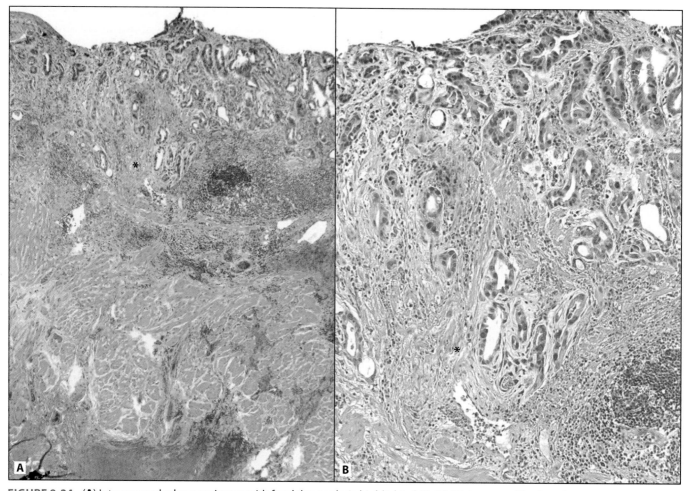

FIGURE 9-24. (**A**) Intramucosal adenocarcinoma with focal desmoplasia highlighted (*). (**B**) Higher magnification view.

11. Hvid-Jensen F, Pedersen L, Drewes AM, Sorensen HT, Funch-Jensen P. Incidence of adenocarcinoma among patients with Barrett's esophagus. *N Engl J Med.* 2011;365(15):1375–1383. PMID: 21995385.

12. Bhat S, Coleman HG, Yousef F, et al. Risk of malignant progression in Barrett's esophagus patients: results from a large population-based study. *J Natl Cancer Inst.* 2011;103(13):1049–1057. PMID: 21680910. PMCID: 3632011.

13. Buttar NS, Wang KK, Sebo TJ, et al. Extent of high-grade dysplasia in Barrett's esophagus correlates with risk of adenocarcinoma. *Gastroenterology.* 2001;120(7):1630–1639. PMID: 11375945.

14. Bansal A, McGregor DH, Anand O, Singh M, Rao D, Cherian R, et al. Presence or absence of intestinal metaplasia but not its burden is associated with prevalent high-grade dysplasia and cancer in Barrett's esophagus. *Dis Esophagus.* 2014;27(8):751–756. PMID: 24165297.

15. Chandrasoma PT, Der R, Dalton P, et al. Distribution and significance of epithelial types in columnar-lined esophagus. *Am J Surg Pathol.* 2001;25(9):1188–1193. PMID: 11688579.

16. Paull A, Trier JS, Dalton MD, Camp RC, Loeb P, Goyal RK. The histologic spectrum of Barrett's esophagus. *N Engl J Med.* 1976;295(9):476–480. PMID: 940579.

17. Theodorou D, Ayazi S, DeMeester SR, et al. Intraluminal pH and goblet cell density in Barrett's esophagus. *J Gastrointest Surg.* 2012;16(3):469–474. PMID: 22095525.

18. Glickman JN, Spechler SJ, Souza RF, Lunsford T, Lee E, Odze RD. Multilayered epithelium in mucosal biopsy specimens from the gastroesophageal junction region is a histologic marker of gastroesophageal reflux disease. *Am J Surg Pathol.* 2009;33(6):818–825. PMID: 19295405.

19. Takubo K. Squamous metaplasia with reserve cell hyperplasia in the esophagogastric junction zone. *Acta Pathol Jpn.* 1981;31(3):349–59. PMID: 7270146.

20. Takubo K, Vieth M, Honma N, et al. Ciliated surface in the esophagogastric junction zone: a precursor of Barrett's mucosa or ciliated pseudostratified metaplasia? *Am J Surg Pathol.* 2005;29(2):211–217. PMID: 15644778.

21. Appelman HD, Streutker C, Vieth M, et al. The esophageal mucosa and submucosa: immunohistology in GERD and Barrett's esophagus. *Ann N Y Acad Sci.* 2013;1300:144–165. PMID: 24117640.

22. Rubio CA, Kaufeldt A. Paucity of synaptophysin-expressing cells in Barrett's mucosa. *Histopathology.* 2013;63(2):208–216. PMID: 23763443.

23. Offner FA, Lewin KJ, Weinstein WM. Metaplastic columnar cells in Barrett's esophagus: a common and neglected cell type. *Hum Pathol.* 1996;27(9):885–889. PMID: 8816881.

24. Younes M, Ertan A, Ergun G, et al. Goblet cell mimickers in esophageal biopsies are not associated with an increased risk for dysplasia. *Arch Pathol Lab Med.* 2007;131(4):571–575. PMID: 17425386.

25. Chong VH. Clinical significance of heterotopic gastric mucosal patch of the proximal esophagus. *World J Gastroenterol.* 2013;19(3):331–338. PMID: 23372354. PMCID: 3554816.

26. Fitzgerald RC, di Pietro M, Ragunath K, et al. British Society of Gastroenterology guidelines on the diagnosis and management of Barrett's oesophagus. *Gut.* 2014;63(1):7–42. PMID: 24165758.

27. Harrison R, Perry I, Haddadin W, et al. Detection of intestinal metaplasia in Barrett's esophagus: an observational comparator study suggests the need for a minimum of eight biopsies. *Am J Gastroenterol.* 2007;102(6):1154–1161. PMID: 17433019.

28. Gatenby PA, Ramus JR, Caygill CP, Shepherd NA, Watson A. Relevance of the detection of intestinal metaplasia in non-dysplastic columnar-lined oesophagus. *Scand J Gastroenterol.* 2008;43(5):524–530. PMID: 18415743.

29. Chaves P, Cruz C, Dias Pereira A, et al. Gastric and intestinal differentiation in Barrett's metaplasia and associated adenocarcinoma. *Dis Esophagus.* 2005;18(6):383–387. PMID: 16336609.

30. Hahn HP, Blount PL, Ayub K, et al. Intestinal differentiation in metaplastic, nongoblet columnar epithelium in the esophagus. *Am J Surg Pathol.* 2009;33(7):1006–1015. PMID: 19363439. PMCID: 2807916.

31. Liu W, Hahn H, Odze RD, Goyal RK. Metaplastic esophageal columnar epithelium without goblet cells shows DNA content abnormalities similar to goblet cell-containing epithelium. *Am J Gastroenterol.* 2009;104(4):816–824. PMID: 19293780. PMCID: 2722438.

32. Fassan M, Volinia S, Palatini J, et al. MicroRNA expression profiling in the histological subtypes of Barrett's metaplasia. *Clin Transl Gastroenterol.* 2013;4:e34. PMID: 23677165. PMCID: 3671360.

33. Takubo K, Aida J, Naomoto Y, et al. Cardiac rather than intestinal-type background in endoscopic resection specimens of minute Barrett adenocarcinoma. *Hum Pathol.* 2009;40(1):65–74. PMID: 18755496.

34. Chandrasoma P, Wijetunge S, DeMeester S, et al. Columnar-lined esophagus without intestinal metaplasia has no proven risk of adenocarcinoma. *Am J Surg Pathol.* 2012;36(1):1–7. PMID: 21959311.

35. Westerhoff M, Hovan L, Lee C, Hart J. Effects of dropping the requirement for goblet cells from the diagnosis of Barrett's esophagus. *Clin Gastroenterol Hepatol.* 2012;10(11):1232–1236. PMID: 22642957.

36. Sharma P, Dent J, Armstrong D, et al. The development and validation of an endoscopic grading system for Barrett's esophagus: the Prague C & M criteria. *Gastroenterology.* 2006;131(5):1392–1399. PMID: 17101315.

37. Jung KW, Talley NJ, Romero Y, et al. Epidemiology and natural history of intestinal metaplasia of the gastroesophageal junction and Barrett's esophagus: a population-based study. *Am J Gastroenterol.* 2011;106(8):1447–1455;quiz 1456. PMID: 21483461. PMCID: 3150349.

38. Spechler SJ. Intestinal metaplasia at the gastroesophageal junction. *Gastroenterology.* 2004;126(2):567–575. PMID: 14762793.

39. Srivastava A, Odze RD, Lauwers GY, Redston M, Antonioli DA, Glickman JN. Morphologic features are useful in distinguishing Barrett esophagus from carditis with intestinal metaplasia. *Am J Surg Pathol.* 2007;31(11):1733–1741. PMID: 18059231.

40. Nishimaki T, Holscher AH, Schuler M, Becker K, Muto T, Siewert JR. Chronic esophagitis and subsequent morphological changes of the esophageal mucosa in Barrett's esophagus: a histological study of esophagectomy specimens. *Surg Today.* 1994;24(3):203–209. PMID: 8003861.

41. Aida J, Vieth M, Ell C, et al. Palisade vessels as a new histologic marker of esophageal origin in ER specimens from columnar-lined esophagus. *Am J Surg Pathol.* 2011;35(8):1140–1145. PMID: 21716084.

42. Takubo K, Aida J, Sawabe M, et al. The normal anatomy around the oesophagogastric junction: a histopathologic view and its correlation with endoscopy. *Best Pract Res Clin Gastroenterol.* 2008;22(4):569–583. PMID: 18656817.

43. Montgomery E, Bronner MP, Goldblum JR, et al. Reproducibility of the diagnosis of dysplasia in Barrett esophagus: a reaffirmation. *Hum Pathol.* 2001;32(4):368–378. PMID: 11331953.

44. Montgomery E, Goldblum JR, Greenson JK, et al. Dysplasia as a predictive marker for invasive carcinoma in Barrett esophagus: a follow-up study based on 138 cases from a diagnostic variability study. *Hum Pathol.* 2001;32(4):379–388. PMID: 11331954.

45. Curvers WL, Alvarez Herrero L, Wallace MB, et al. Endoscopic trimodal imaging is more effective than standard endoscopy in identifying early-stage neoplasia in Barrett's esophagus. *Gastroenterology.* 2010;139(4):1106–1114. PMID: 20600033.

46. Abela JE, Going JJ, Mackenzie JF, McKernan M, O'Mahoney S, Stuart RC. Systematic four-quadrant biopsy detects Barrett's dysplasia in more patients than nonsystematic biopsy. *Am J Gastroenterol.* 2008;103(4):850–855. PMID: 18371135.

47. Kariv R, Plesec TP, Goldblum JR, et al. The Seattle protocol does not more reliably predict the detection of cancer at the time of esophagectomy than a less intensive surveillance protocol. *Clin Gastroenterol Hepatol.* 2009;7(6):653–658;quiz 606. PMID: 19264576.

48. Bertani H, Frazzoni M, Dabizzi E, et al. Improved detection of incident dysplasia by probe-based confocal laser endomicroscopy in a Barrett's esophagus surveillance program. *Dig Dis Sci.* 2013;58(1):188–193. PMID: 22875309.

49. Sharma P, Hawes RH, Bansal A, et al. Standard endoscopy with random biopsies versus narrow band imaging targeted biopsies in Barrett's oesophagus: a prospective, international, randomised controlled trial. *Gut.* 2013;62(1):15–21. PMID: 22315471.

50. Rastogi A, Puli S, El-Serag HB, Bansal A, Wani S, Sharma P. Incidence of esophageal adenocarcinoma in patients with Barrett's esophagus and high-grade dysplasia: a meta-analysis. *Gastrointest Endosc.* 2008;67(3):394–398. PMID: 18045592.

51. Rubio CA, Tanaka K, Befrits R. Traditional serrated adenoma in a patient with Barrett's esophagus. *Anticancer Res.* 2013;33(4):1743–1745. PMID: 23564826.

52. Shepherd NA, Warren BF, Williams GT, Greenson JK, Lauwers GY, Novelli MR, eds. *Morson and Dawson Gastrointestinal Pathology.* 5th ed. New York, NY: Wiley-Blackwell; 2013.

53. De Petris G, Gatius Caldero S, Chen L, et al. Histopathological changes in the gastrointestinal tract due to drugs: an update for the surgical pathologist (part I of II). *Int J Surg Pathol.* 2014;22(2):120–128. PMID: 24021899.

54. Curvers WL, ten Kate FJ, Krishnadath KK, et al. Low-grade dysplasia in Barrett's esophagus: overdiagnosed and underestimated. *Am J Gastroenterol.* 2010;105(7):1523–1530. PMID: 20461069.

55. Flejou JF, Svrcek M. Barrett's oesophagus—a pathologist's view. *Histopathology.* 2007;50(1):3–14. PMID: 17204017.

56. Odze RD. Diagnosis and grading of dysplasia in Barrett's oesophagus. *J Clin Pathol.* 2006;59(10):1029–1038. PMID: 17021130. PMCID: 1861756.

57. Lomo LC, Blount PL, Sanchez CA, et al. Crypt dysplasia with surface maturation: a clinical, pathologic, and molecular study of a Barrett's esophagus cohort. *Am J Surg Pathol.* 2006;30(4):423–435. PMID: 16625087.

58. Zhu W, Appelman HD, Greenson JK, et al. A histologically defined subset of high-grade dysplasia in Barrett mucosa is predictive of associated carcinoma. *Am J Clin Pathol.* 2009;132(1):94–100. PMID: 19864239.

59. Khor TS, Alfaro EE, Ooi EM, et al. Divergent expression of MUC5AC, MUC6, MUC2, CD10, and CDX-2 in dysplasia and intramucosal adenocarcinomas with intestinal and foveolar morphology: is this evidence of distinct gastric and intestinal pathways to carcinogenesis in Barrett esophagus? *Am J Surg Pathol.* 2012;36(3):331–342. PMID: 22261707.

60. Brown IS, Whiteman DC, Lauwers GY. Foveolar type dysplasia in Barrett esophagus. *Mod Pathol.* 2010;23(6):834–843. PMID: 20228780.

61. Mahajan D, Bennett AE, Liu X, Bena J, Bronner MP. Grading of gastric foveolar-type dysplasia in Barrett's esophagus. *Mod Pathol.* 2010;23(1):1–11. PMID: 19838164.

62. Patil DT, Bennett AE, Mahajan D, Bronner MP. Distinguishing Barrett gastric foveolar dysplasia from reactive cardiac mucosa in gastroesophageal reflux disease. *Hum Pathol.* 2013;44(6):1146–1153. PMID: 23332925.

63. Rucker-Schmidt RL, Sanchez CA, Blount PL, et al. Nonadenomatous dysplasia in barrett esophagus: a clinical, pathologic, and DNA content flow cytometric study. *Am J Surg Pathol.* 2009;33(6):886–893. PMID: 19194279. PMCID: 2702161.

64. Phoa KN, van Vilsteren FG, Weusten BL, et al. Radiofrequency ablation vs endoscopic surveillance for patients with Barrett esophagus and low-grade dysplasia: a randomized clinical trial. *JAMA.* 2014; 311(12):1209–1217. PMID: 24668102.

65. Skacel M, Petras RE, Gramlich TL, Sigel JE, Richter JE, Goldblum JR. The diagnosis of low-grade dysplasia in Barrett's esophagus and its implications for disease progression. *Am J Gastroenterol.* 2000;95(12):3383–3387. PMID: 11151865.

66. Stolte M, Benicke J. Barrett's adenocarcinomas are frequently under-diagnosed as "high grade intraepithelial neoplasia." *Z Gastroenterol.* 2012;50(3):273–278. PMID: 22383282.

67. Younes M, Ertan A, Lechago LV, Somoano JR, Lechago J. p53 protein accumulation is a specific marker of malignant potential in Barrett's metaplasia. *Dig Dis Sci.* 1997;42(4):697–701. PMID: 9125634.

68. Kastelein F, Biermann K, Steyerberg EW, et al. Aberrant p53 protein expression is associated with an increased risk of neoplastic progression in patients with Barrett's oesophagus. *Gut.* 2013;62(12):1676–1683. PMID: 23256952.

69. Kastelein F, Biermann K, Steyerberg EW, et al. Value of alpha-methylacyl-CoA racemase immunochemistry for predicting neoplastic progression in Barrett's oesophagus. *Histopathology.* 2013;63(5):630–639. PMID: 24004067.

70. van Dekken H, Hop WCJ, Tilanus HW, et al. Immunohistochemical evaluation of a panel of tumor cell markers during malignant progression in Barrett esophagus. *Am J Clin Pathol.* 2008;130(5):745–753. PMID: ISI:000260188600010.

71. Rossi E, Grisanti S, Villanacci V, Della Casa D, Cengia P, Missale G, et al. HER-2 overexpression/amplification in Barrett's oesophagus predicts early transition from dysplasia to adenocarcinoma: a clinico-pathologic study. *J Cell Mol Med.* 2009;13(9B):3826–3833. PMID: 19292734.

72. Halsey KD, Arora M, Bulsiewicz WJ, et al. Eosinophilic infiltration of the esophagus following endoscopic ablation of Barrett's neoplasia. *Dis Esophagus.* 2013;26(2):113–116. PMID: 22394268.

73. Shaheen NJ, Sharma P, Overholt BF, et al. Radiofrequency ablation in Barrett's esophagus with dysplasia. *N Engl J Med.* 2009;360(22):2277–2288. PMID: 19474425.

74. Gray NA, Odze RD, Spechler SJ. Buried metaplasia after endoscopic ablation of Barrett's esophagus: a systematic review. *Am J Gastroenterol.* 2011;106(11):1899–1908;quiz 1909. PMID: 21826111. PMCID: 3254259.

75. Gupta N, Mathur SC, Dumot JA, et al. Adequacy of esophageal squamous mucosa specimens obtained during endoscopy: are standard biopsies sufficient for postablation surveillance in Barrett's esophagus? *Gastrointest Endosc.* 2012;75(1):11–18. PMID: 21907985.

76. Zeki SS, Haidry R, Graham TA, et al. Clonal selection and persistence in dysplastic Barrett's esophagus and intramucosal cancers after failed radiofrequency ablation. *Am J Gastroenterol.* 2013;108(10):1584–1592. PMID: 23939625.

77. Gopal DV, Lieberman DA, Magaret N, et al. Risk factors for dysplasia in patients with Barrett's esophagus (BE): results from a multicenter consortium. *Dig Dis Sci.* 2003;48(8):1537–1541. PMID: 12924649.

78. Holscher AH, Bollschweiler E, Schroder W, Metzger R, Gutschow C, Drebber U. Prognostic impact of upper, middle, and lower third mucosal or submucosal infiltration in early esophageal cancer. *Ann Surg.* 2011;254(5):802–807;discussion 807–808. PMID: 22042472.

79. Patil DT, Goldblum JR, Rybicki L, et al. Prediction of adenocarcinoma in esophagectomy specimens based upon analysis of preresection biopsies of Barrett esophagus with at least high-grade dysplasia: a comparison of 2 systems. *Am J Surg Pathol.* 2012;36(1):134–141. PMID: 22067333.

80. Abraham SC, Wang H, Wang KK, Wu TT. Paget cells in the esophagus: assessment of their histopathologic features and near-universal association with underlying esophageal adenocarcinoma. *Am J Surg Pathol.* 2008;32(7):1068–1074. PMID: 18496141.

81. Pouw RE, Bergman JJ. Endoscopic resection of early oesophageal and gastric neoplasia. *Best Pract Res Clin Gastroenterol.* 2008;22(5):929–943. PMID: 18790439.

82. Estrella JS, Hofstetter WL, Correa AM, et al. Duplicated muscularis mucosae invasion has similar risk of lymph node metastasis and recurrence-free survival as intramucosal esophageal adenocarcinoma. *Am J Surg Pathol.* 2011;35(7):1045–1053. PMID: 21602659.

83. Sgourakis G, Gockel I, Lang H. Endoscopic and surgical resection of T1a/T1b esophageal neoplasms: a systematic review. *World J Gastroenterol.* 2013;19(9):1424–1437. PMID: 23539431. PMCID: 3602502.

84. Mino-Kenudson M, Brugge WR, Puricelli WP, et al. Management of superficial Barrett's epithelium-related neoplasms by endoscopic mucosal resection: clinicopathologic analysis of 27 cases. *Am J Surg Pathol.* 2005;29(5):680–686. PMID: 15832094.

85. Sayana H, Wani SB, Keighley JD, et al. Endoscopic mucosal resection (EMR) as a diagnostic tool in Barrett's esophagus (Be) patients with high-grade dysplasia (HGD)and early esophageal adenocarcinoma (EAC): a systematic review. *Gastroenterology.* 2008;134(4):A724–A. PMID: ISI:000255101505282.

86. Wani S, Mathur SC, Curvers WL, et al. Greater interobserver agreement by endoscopic mucosal resection than biopsy samples in Barrett's dysplasia. *Clin Gastroenterol Hepatol.* 2010;8(9):783–788. PMID: 20472096.

87. Prasad GA, Buttar NS, Wongkeesong LM, et al. Significance of neoplastic involvement of margins obtained by endoscopic mucosal resection in Barrett's esophagus. *Am J Gastroenterol.* 2007;102(11):2380–2386. PMID: 17640326. PMCID: 2646408.

88. Faragalla HF, Marcon NE, Yousef GM, Streutker CJ. Immuno-histochemical staining for smoothelin in the duplicated versus the true muscularis mucosae of Barrett esophagus. *Am J Surg Pathol.* 2011;35(1):55–59. PMID: 21164287.

89. Abraham SC, Krasinskas AM, Correa AM, et al. Duplication of the muscularis mucosae in Barrett esophagus: an underrecognized feature and its implication for staging of adenocarcinoma. *Am J Surg Pathol.* 2007;31(11):1719–1725. PMID: 18059229.

90. Hahn HP, Shahsafaei A, Odze RD. Vascular and lymphatic properties of the superficial and deep lamina propria in Barrett esophagus. *Am J Surg Pathol.* 2008;32(10):1454–1461. PMID: 18685488.

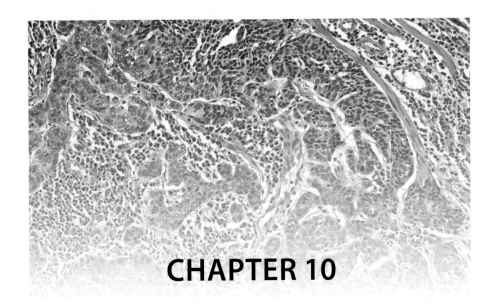

CHAPTER 10

Squamous Cell Carcinoma and Other Miscellaneous Malignancies of the Esophagus

Xiuli Liu

■ SQUAMOUS CELL CARCINOMA

Although the incidence has decreased in Western countries, squamous cell carcinoma (SCC) is still the most common malignancy of the esophagus worldwide. Many patients present at an advanced tumor stage and have a poor prognosis.[1-3] Alcohol and tobacco are the two major environmental cancer risk factors.[4,5] Human papilloma virus (HPV) infection may also play a role in the tumorigenesis.[6]

Histologically, esophageal SCC is similar to SCC of other sites and can be either keratinized (Figure 10-1) or nonkeratinized (Figure 10-2). The former exhibits cytoplasmic keratinization, keratin pearls, and intercellular bridges (desmosomes). SCC can be well, moderately, and poorly differentiated. Some of the poorly differentiated tumors exhibit no squamous features on hematoxylin and eosin (H&E) staining (Figure 10-3A), with considerable nuclear pleomorphism and mitotically activity. Table 10-1 lists histologic features of well-, moderately, poorly, and undifferentiated SCCs. It should be pointed out that despite all the seemingly characteristic features of SCC and adenocarcinomas, immunostains are almost always required for accurate distinction for poorly and undifferentiated carcinomas in biopsy, consisting of p40, p63, or cytokeratin (CK) 5/5 for squamous phenotype (Figures 10-3B, 10-3C) and MOC31 for adenocarcinoma phenotype, particularly when no precursor (dysplastic) lesions are evident.

While examining a biopsy for an esophageal squamous tumor, the pathologist may need to keep in mind several questions. First, is there invasion? An invasive component may be characterized by nests of or individual cells infiltrating a desmoplastic stroma (Figure 10-4). Occasionally, the tumor invades with a smooth pushing front, which is difficult to recognize as invasion on small biopsies. Second, is there sufficient material for grading the differentiation of the tumor? While examining resected surgical specimens, the relationship of the tumor to margins should be noted because the risk of local recurrence significantly increases with positive surgical margins. Lymphovascular invasion may also be present and should be specifically noted, as it is associated with shorter survival.[7]

Recognition of Squamous Dysplasia

Squamous cell carcinomas develop through a progression from premalignant or dysplastic precursor lesions. *Squamous dysplasia* is defined as neoplastic cells confined to the epithelium. We use a two-tier grading system for dysplasia: low-grade dysplasia (LGD) and high-grade dysplasia (HGD; including squamous carcinoma in situ). These correspond to the World Health Organization (WHO) classification scheme of low-grade intraepithelial neoplasia and high-grade intraepithelial neoplasia, respectively. The diagnoses of premalignant (dysplastic) lesions and early SCC (invading into the lamina propria) are clinically important as these can be properly treated with endoscopic mucosal resection.

Endoscopically, dysplastic squamous lesions may appear normal or as erythematous, friable, or irregular mucosa; some show erosion, plaque, or nodules. Mucosal staining

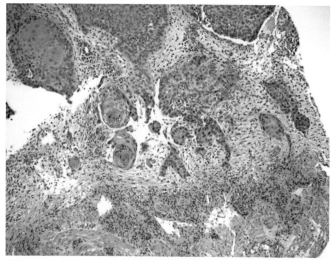

FIGURE 10-1. Invasive, esophageal squamous carcinoma with small nests of infiltrating cells with squamous differentiation, including keratinization.

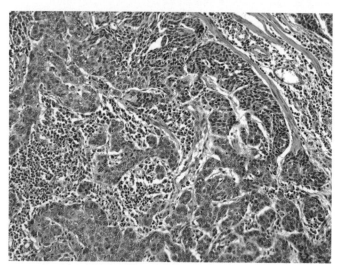

FIGURE 10-2. Invasive, poorly differentiated squamous cell carcinoma with sheets of tumor cells without keratinization.

TABLE 10-1. Histologic features of squamous cell carcinoma tumor grades.

Grade	Microscopic features
Well differentiated	Prominent keratinization and a minor component of nonkeratinizing basaloid cells; low mitotic count
Moderately differentiated	Keratinization ranging from parakeratotic to poorly keratinized areas without obvious pearl formation
Poorly differentiated	Predominantly basaloid cells forming nests with frequent necrosis but only small numbers of parakeratotic or keratinized cells
Undifferentiated	Nests and sheets of tumor cells lacking histologic features of squamous differentiation (often require immunostaining for p63, p40, or CK5/6)

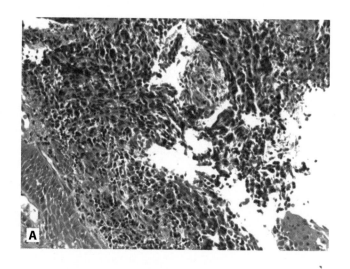

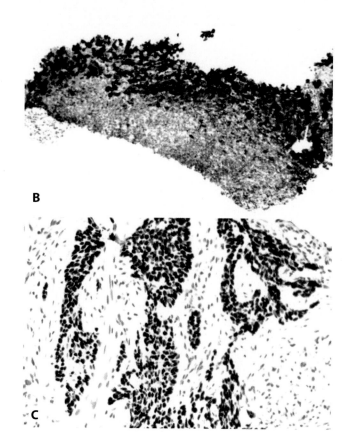

FIGURE 10-3. Poorly differentiated squamous carcinoma of the esophagus. There are sheets of tumor cells with hyperchromatic nuclei but no evident squamous differentiation (**A**). Immunohistochemistry: The tumor cells are positive for CK5/6 (**B**) and p63 (**C**), markers of squamous differentiation.

with Lugol iodine may be helpful to highlight dysplastic mucosa and increase the sensitivity of endoscopic surveillance in high-risk populations.[8] Histologically, squamous dysplasia includes a spectrum of architectural and cytologic abnormalities, such as nuclear hyperchromasia, pleomorphism, increased nucleus-to-cytoplasm (N/C) ratio, and

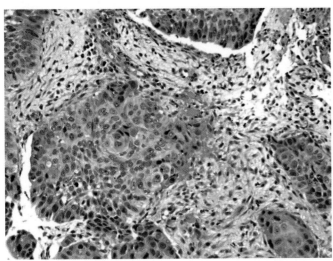

FIGURE 10-4. Invasive squamous cell carcinoma of the esophagus. Small nests infiltrate desmoplastic stroma.

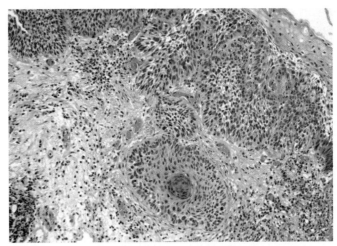

FIGURE 10-6. High-grade squamous dysplasia. Pleomorphic epithelial cells have a high nucleus-to-cytoplasm ratio and hyperchromatic nuclei. Loss of polarity is present focally. The high-grade dysplasia also involves a submucosal glandular duct.

increased mitotic figures (Figure 10-5). Architecturally, dysplastic cells show disorganization, with overlapping nuclei, loss of polarity, and lack of surface maturation (Figure 10-6).

Rarely, dysplasia is characterized by proliferation of disorganized large cells with normal or even lower-than-normal N/C ratio. However, these cells contain open irregular nuclei with a prominent single nucleolus or multiple nucleoli and with peripheral condensation of chromatin (Figure 10-7). In addition, the border of the epithelium abutting the lamina propria is often irregular with sharp, budding, or bulbous expansion of the epithelium, protruding into the lamina propria.

Squamous dysplasia should be distinguished from reactive changes associated with esophagitis (Figure 10-8A) or chemoradiation (Figure 10-8B). The most helpful features of dysplasia include nuclear pleomorphism, loss of polarity, nuclear overlapping/crowding, high N/C ratio, and abnormal mitoses (Table 10-2).

Low-grade dysplasia without a mass or associated carcinoma may be managed with continued surveillance and repeat biopsies.

VARIANTS OF SQUAMOUS CELL CARCINOMA

Basaloid Squamous Cell Carcinoma

Basaloid squamous cell carcinoma (BSCC), a morphologically and molecularly distinct variant, occurs rarely in the esophagus. Histologically, BSCC is characterized by variably-sized

FIGURE 10-7. High-grade squamous dysplasia. In this example, the dysplastic cells are characterized by marked pleomorphism with hyperchromatic nuclei but relatively normal nucleus-to-cytoplasm ratio.

FIGURE 10-5. High-grade squamous dysplasia. The epithelium is characterized by enlarged cells with a high nucleus-to-cytoplasm ratio and hyperchromatic nuclei. There is also nuclear overlapping.

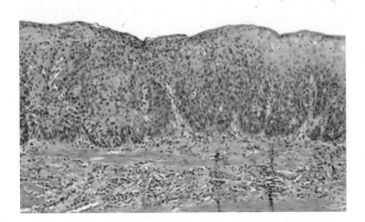

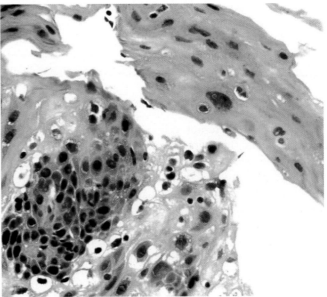

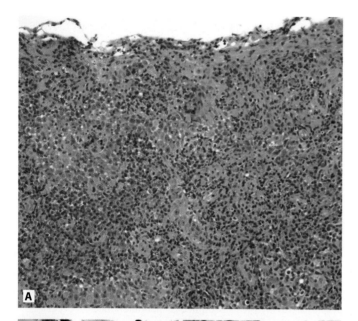

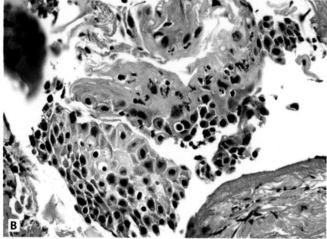

FIGURE 10-8. Reactive atypia of squamous epithelium. **A.** Ulcerated mucosa due to severe esophagitis. The squamous cells are relatively uniform, contain fine chromatin, and have a single prominent nucleolus. **B.** Atypia due to chemoradiation treatment. The patient received radiation for the treatment of an esophageal adenocarcinoma; the squamous epithelium shows enlarged and hyperchromatic nuclei. The maintained nucleus-to-cytoplasm ratio and "bubbling" cytoplasm in the context of recent chemoradiation therapy support a reactive change.

nests or sheets of tumor cells with scant cytoplasm and hyperchromatic, high-grade nuclei (Figure 10-9).[9,10] Abundant comedo-type tumor necrosis, brisk apoptotic activity, and high mitotic activity are common features. Areas of concomitant typical SCC, squamous dysplasia, or carcinoma in situ may be present.[11] BSCC is more aggressive than SCC in general, with rapid progression and a propensity for distant metastasis. Its histologic, immunocytochemical, and ultrastructural features correspond more to poorly differentiated SCC.[9]

TABLE 10-2. Features distinguishing squamous dysplasia from reactive squamous epithelium of the esophagus.

Features	Dysplasia	Reactive changes
Pleomorphism	++	–
Loss of polarity	++	–
Nuclear overlapping or crowding	++	–
Lack of surface maturation	++	±
High N/C ratio	++	±
Mitotic activity	+	+
Aberrant mitotic figures	±	–
Hyperchromasia	+	±
Chromatin	Coarse	Fine
Nucleolus	May be present	Usually present, but small
Inflammation	±	++

Note: ++, marked; +, mild; ±, minimal or may be present.

Verrucous Carcinoma and Carcinoma Cuniculatum

Verrucous carcinomas (VCs) lack overtly malignant cytologic features and exhibit a pushing growth border. The more recently described carcinoma cuniculatum is also a well-differentiated squamous carcinoma with unique macroscopic and histologic features.[12,13] Histologic diagnosis of these tumors is extremely difficult in biopsies, where tumor-stroma interface is limited, and thus demands closer clinico-radiographic-histologic correlation. Direct communication with the endoscopist is often necessary.

FIGURE 10-9. Basaloid squamous cell carcinoma of the esophagus. The lesion consists of small nests of small- to medium-size tumor cells.

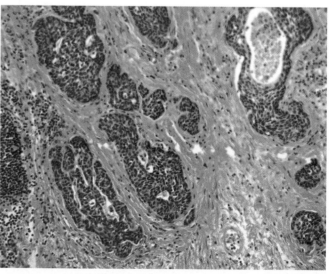

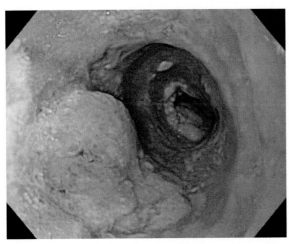

FIGURE 10-10. Verrucous carcinoma of the esophagus as a polypoid mass under endoscopic examination in a patient with chronic but progressive dysphagia.

Clinically, patients with VC and carcinoma cuniculatum usually present with chronic dysphagia.[12–15] Endoscopically or on gross examination, VC appears as an exophytically warty, papillary, spiked, or cauliflower-like mass (Figure 10-10). In contrast, carcinoma cuniculatum shows diffuse dipping of thickened mucosa (Figure 10-11). Endoscopic biopsies from these lesions usually include only the superficial portion and

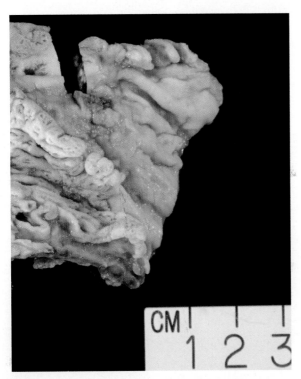

FIGURE 10-11. Carcinoma cuniculatum of the esophagus shows diffuse dipping of the thickened mucosa on macroscopic examination.

may only exhibit bland microscopic features, such as acanthosis, parakeratosis, and hyperkeratosis, with mixed inflammation. In some cases, due to the concurrent *Candida* infection, the biopsy may be simply indicated as "*Candida* esophagitis" (Figure 10-12). Attention to the clinical history of long-term dysphagia and the endoscopic finding of a mass/mural lesion should prompt a search for additional abnormalities that may be subtle. Identification of a set of histologic features is strongly suggestive of an abnormal squamous proliferation in the presence of long-term dysphagia and an esophageal mass. These features include hyperkeratosis, acanthosis, dyskeratosis, deep keratinization, keratin-filled cysts/furrows, koilocyte-like cells, intraepithelial neutrophils, intraepithelial neutrophilic microabscesses, and focal cytologic atypia[12,13] (Figure 10-13). In the proper clinical and endoscopic context, finding 7 or more of these features is highly suggestive of the diagnosis of carcinoma cuniculatum on mucosal biopsy in our experience.[13]

Spindle Cell Squamous Carcinoma

Spindle cell squamous carcinoma (SCSC) or carcinosarcoma usually occurs in the mid- or lower third of the esophagus as a polypoid mass (Figure 10-14A), sometimes with ulceration. Histologically, two tumor components are recognized—squamous and spindle cells (Figure 10-14B)—with a transition zone in between.[16] Unusual mesenchymal differentiation (muscle, bone, or cartilage) in the sarcoma-like areas may be observed. Immunohistochemically, the squamous cells are cytokeratin positive, and the spindle cells show variable expression of cytokeratin, vimentin, or smooth muscle actin.[16]

Diffusely Infiltrative Squamous Cell Carcinoma

Diffusely infiltrative SCC, as described in a recent report, is characterized by tumor cells infiltrating under non-neoplastic surface epithelium.[17] The subepithelial growth causes constriction and stenosis. The tumor is deeply invasive with extensive lymphovascular invasion. Endobronchial ultrasound-guided transbronchial needle aspiration (EBUS-TBNA) and biopsy are helpful in obtaining diagnostic material.[17]

Lymphoepithelial Carcinoma

Lymphoepithelial carcinoma is an undifferentiated carcinoma or poorly differentiated SCC, with prominent reactive lymphoplasmacytic infiltrates.[18] The histologic features are similar to those of the nasopharyngeal nonkeratinizing carcinoma, with rich lymphoplasmacytic infiltrates. The tumor cells are large, with marked nuclear atypia, hyperchromasia, and increased N/C ratio (Figure 10-15). There are frequent mitotic figures. The tumor cells show evidence of Epstein-Barr virus (EBV) infection, including EBV-encoded nuclear antigen 2 (EBNA2), EBV latent membrane protein 1

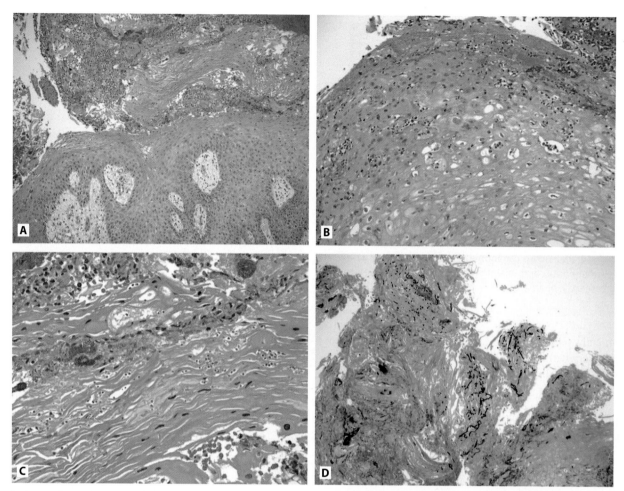

FIGURE 10-12. Carcinoma cuniculatum of the esophagus. **A** and **B.** Biopsies from verrucous carcinoma or carcinoma cuniculatum may only show hyperkeratosis and mixed inflammation. The presence of *Candida* species may lead to a diagnosis of *Candida* esophagitis in some cases (**C**, hematoxylin and eosin stain; **D**, Gomori methenamine silver stain).

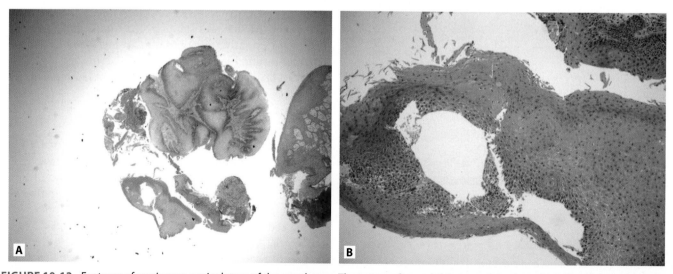

FIGURE 10-13. Features of carcinoma cuniculatum of the esophagus. The tumor often exhibits a combination of papillomatous or complex proliferation (**A**), hyperkeratosis (**A, B**), acanthosis, keratinization in the deep portion (**C**), invagination (**D**), keratin cyst (**E**), koilocyte-like cells (**F**), and neutrophilic inflammation. In some cases, mild cytological atypia may be seen.

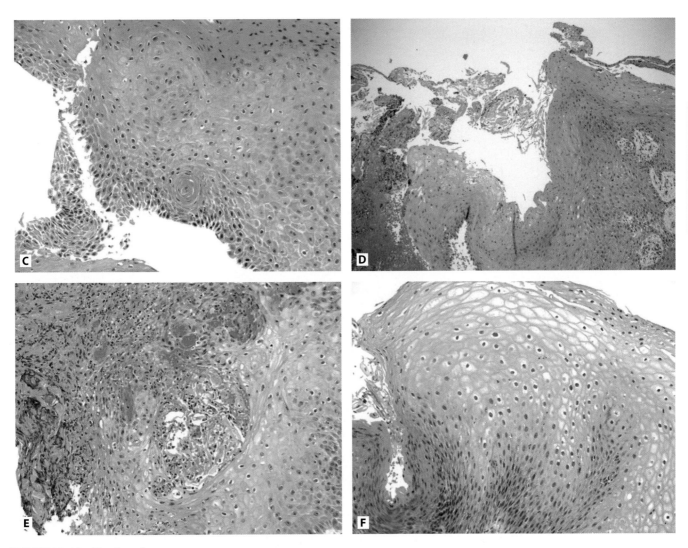

FIGURE 10-13. (*Continued*)

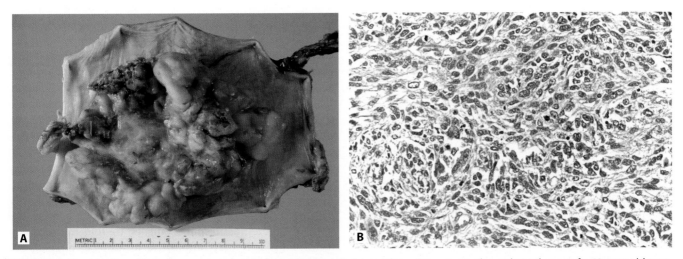

FIGURE 10-14. Spindle cell squamous carcinoma (carcinosarcoma). **A.** A large fungating mass in the mid esophagus of a 68-year-old man. **B.** The tumor is composed almost exclusively of spindle tumor cells, with marked nuclear atypia and high mitotic activity. Immunohistochemically, the tumor exhibits focal reactivity for cytokeratin CAM5.2 and AE1/3 (not shown). There is also focal reactivity for smooth muscle actin.

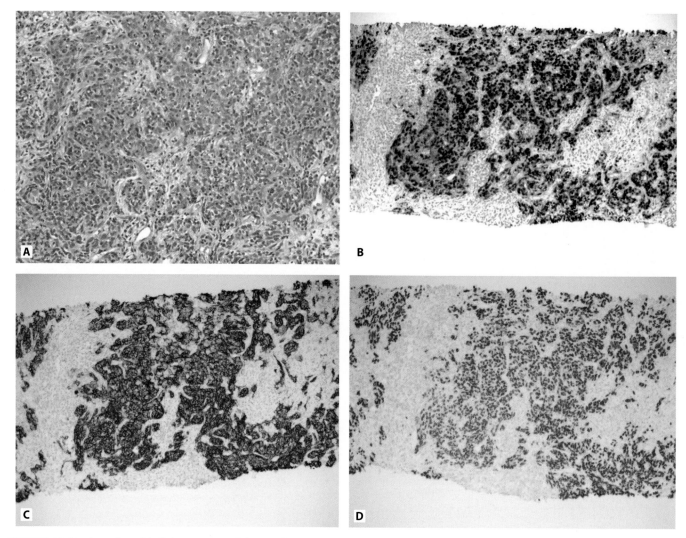

FIGURE 10-15. Lymphoepithelial carcinoma of the esophagus. The tumor consists of nests of cells with a high nucleus-to-cytoplasm ratio (**A**). There is marked lymphocytic infiltration. The tumor cells are positive for EBV infection (**B**, chromogenic in situ hybridization for EBV-encoded RNA) and are positive for CK5/6 and p63 (**C** and **D**, immunostains).

(LMP-1), and EBV-encoded RNAs (EBER) (Figure 10-15). The lymphoplasmacytic infiltrates include B and T cells, CD56-positive natural killer cells, as well as plasma cells.

Small-Cell Carcinoma

Small-cell carcinoma accounts for less than 5% of all esophageal malignancies.[19,20] It tends to occur in the middle-aged or elderly, in the mid- or distal esophagus.[20,21] Histologically, the tumor consists of small- to medium-size cells arranged in sheets, organoid nests, trabeculae, or cords. Tumor necrosis, brisk apoptotic activity, and high mitotic activity are the common findings. The tumor cells also exhibit significant nuclear "streaming" (a crush artifact) in biopsy material (Figure 10-16). The tumor cells contain only scant cytoplasm with extremely high N/C ratio. The nuclei are hyperchromatic or contain fine

chromatin and may mold over one another. The tumor cells may have inconspicuous nucleoli. Occasionally, SCC in situ or conventional SCC may be identified. Immunohistochemistry is required for diagnosis. Positive markers include synaptophysin (100%), CD56 (96%), chromogranin (69%), and p63 (50%).

The differential diagnosis for primary esophageal small-cell carcinoma includes a metastasis or direct extension from another sites, basaloid SCC, and lymphoma. Given the rarity of primary esophageal small-cell carcinoma and the proximity of the esophagus to the lung, the possibility of a pulmonary metastasis should always be excluded by clinical and imaging studies, as immunostain for thyroid transcription factor 1 (TTF-1) may be positive in esophageal small-cell carcinoma.[21] Identification of adjacent squamous dysplasia or SCC in situ favors a primary tumor.

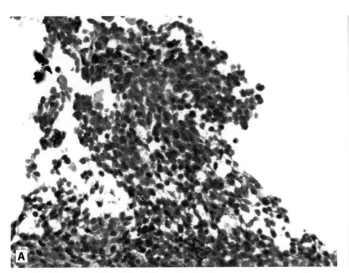

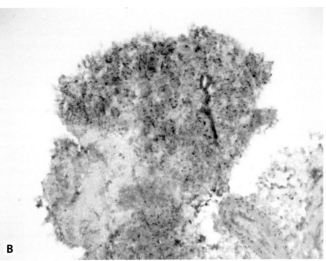

FIGURE 10-16. Small-cell carcinoma of the esophagus. **A.** A finely granular chromatin pattern suggests neuroendocrine differentiation. Single-cell necrosis is also present (not pictured). The tumor cells show immunoreactivity for chromogranin (**B**, immunostain).

■ OTHER MISCELLANEOUS MALIGNANCIES

Mucoepidermoid Carcinoma

Mucoepidermoid carcinoma accounts for less than 1% of the primary tumors of the esophagus.[22] Most tumors are located in the mid- and lower thirds of the esophagus.[22] Histologically, the tumor is characterized by the presence of an intimate mixture of mucinous, intermediate, and epidermoid cells (Figure 10-17). Preoperative diagnosis of mucoepidermoid carcinoma is difficult due to limited sampling, and most cases were misdiagnosed as SCC on biopsy.[22]

Choriocarcinoma

The extremely rare choriocarcinoma tumor affects adults of both genders, accompanied by elevated serum or urine levels of human chorionic gonadotropin (hCG). The tumor consists of two cell populations: mononuclear cells with

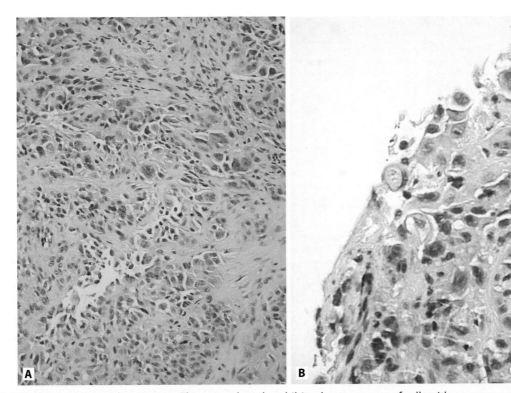

FIGURE 10-17. Mucoepidermoid carcinoma. This tumor largely exhibits sheets or nests of cells with squamous differentiation (**A**). However, rare cells with an intracellular mucin droplet are evident (**B**).

pale cytoplasm and bizarre giant cells. There may be extensive intratumoral hemorrhage. Immunohistochemically, the tumor cells are positive for hCG. Esophageal choriocarcinoma is highly aggressive, and the patients often die from the disease due to widespread hematogenous dissemination within a few months of presentation.[23]

Adenoid Cystic Carcinoma

True adenoid cystic carcinoma (ACC) of the esophagus is extremely rare, as many previously published series may have included cases that were basaloid SCC.[9] ACC of the esophagus shows three different growth patterns, similar to its counterpart in the salivary gland: cribriform, tubular, and solid[24] (Figure 10-18). Preoperative biopsy diagnosis of this tumor is difficult due to limited sampling and confusion with SCC.[24] Most ACCs of the esophagus are centered in the submucosa, suggesting a tumor origin from the submucosal mucus glands.

FIGURE 10-18. Esophageal ACC. **A.** Sheets and nests of tumor cells exhibit expansile or pushing growth. There is a focal cribriform component. **B.** Focally, the microcystic pattern can be prominent.

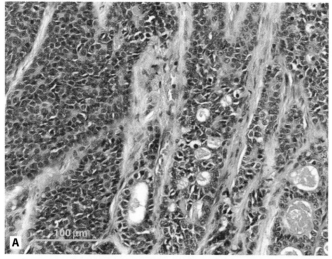

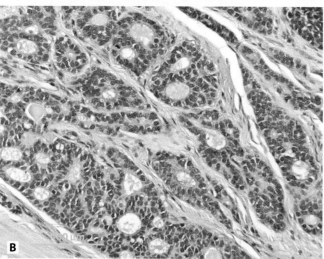

Melanoma

Melanoma of the esophagus is, again, extremely rare. It usually forms an exophytic polypoid mass. Microscopically, the tumor is composed of nests of loosely cohesive, large epithelioid-to-spindle cells with abundant granular cytoplasm and eccentric vesicular nuclei with prominent nucleoli, similar to melanomas in general. There may be cytoplasmic pigments and intranuclear cytoplasmic inclusions. An immunohistochemical panel consisting of cytokeratin, S-100, HMB45, and MART-1 may be required for reaching the diagnosis. Rarely, melanoma may show signet-ring cell morphology (Figure 10-19).[25] Findings of atypical junctional melanocytic activity, in situ melanoma, radial growth phase, melanocytosis, and mixed epithelioid and spindle cell morphology in the absence of a history of previous melanoma of other sites are useful features for distinguishing primary esophageal melanoma from a metastasis.[26]

■ REFERENCES

1. Trivers KF, Sabatino SA, Stewart SL. Trends in esophageal cancer incidence by histology, United States, 1998–2003. *Int J Cancer.* 2008; 123(6):1422–1428.
2. Ruol A, Castoro C, Portale G, et al. Trends in management and prognosis for esophageal cancer surgery: twenty five years of experience at a single institution. *Arch Surg.* 2009;144(3):247–254.
3. Worni M, Martin J, Gloor B, et al. Does surgery improve outcomes for esophageal squamous cell carcinoma? An analysis using the surveillance epidemiology and end results registry from 1998 to 2008. *J Am Coll Surg.* 2012;215:643–651.
4. Pandeya N, Olsen CM, Whiteman DC. Sex differences in the proportion of esophageal squamous cell carcinoma cases attributable to tobacco smoking and alcohol consumption. *Cancer Epidemiol.* 2013;37(5):579–584.
5. Shimizu Y, Kato M, Yamamoto J, et al. Histologic results of EMR for esophageal lesions diagnosed as high-grade intraepithelial squamous neoplasia by endoscopic biopsy. *Gastrointest Endosc.* 2006;63: 16–21.
6. Wang YF, Wang XS, Gao SG, et al. Clinical significance of combined detection of human papilloma virus infection and human telomerase RNA component gene amplification in patients with squamous cell carcinoma of the esophagus in northern China. *Eur J Med Res.* 2013;18:11.
7. Brücher BL, Stein HJ, Werner M, Siewert JR. Lymphatic vessel invasion is an independent prognostic factor in patients with primary resected tumor with esophageal squamous cell carcinoma. *Cancer.* 2001; 92(8):2228–2233.
8. Dawsey SM, Fleischer DE, Wang GQ, et al. Mucosal iodine staining improves endoscopic visualization of squamous dysplasia and squamous cell carcinoma of the esophagus in Linxian, China. *Cancer.* 1998;83:220–231.
9. Li TJ, Zhang YX, Wen J, et al. Basaloid squamous cell carcinoma of the esophagus with or without adenoid cystic features. *Arch Pathol Lab Med.* 2004;128(10):1124–1130.
10. Bellizzi AM, Woodford RL Moskaluk CA, et al. Basaloid squamous cell carcinoma of the esophagus: assessment for high-risk human papillomavirus and related molecular markers. *Am J Surg Pathol* 2009; 33:1608–14.
11. Sarbia M, Verreet P, Bittinger F, et al. Basaloid squamous cell carcinoma of the esophagus: diagnosis and prognosis. *Cancer.* 1997; 79(10):1871–1878.
12. Landau M, Goldblum JR, DeRoche T, et al. Esophageal carcinoma cuniculatum: report of 9 cases. *Am J Surg Pathol.* 2012;36:8–17.

13. Chen D, Goldblum JR, Landau M, et al. Semiquantitative histologic evaluation improves diagnosis of esophageal carcinoma cuniculatum on biopsy. *Mod Pathol.* 2013;26:806–815.

14. Sweetser S, Jacobs NL, Song LM. Endoscopic diagnosis and treatment of esophageal verrucous squamous cell cancer. *Dis Esophagus.* 2014;27(5):452–456.

15. Lagos AC, Marques IN, Reis JD, Neves BC. Verrucous carcinoma of the esophagus. *Rev Esp Enferm Dig.* 2012;104(8):443–435.

16. Handra-Luca A, Terris B, Couvelard A, et al. Spindle cell squamous carcinoma of the oesophagus: an analysis of 17 cases, with new immunohistochemical evidence for a clonal origin. *Histopathology.* 2001;39:125–132.

17. Usui A, Akutsu Y, Kano M, et al. Diffusely infiltrative squamous cell carcinoma of the esophagus presenting diagnostic difficult: report of a case. *Surg Today.* 2013;43:794–799.

18. Terada T. Epstein-Barr virus associated lymphoepithelial carcinoma of the esophagus. *Int J Clin Exp Med.* 2013;6:219–226.

19. Briggs JC, Ibrahim NBN. Oat cell carcinoma of the esophagus: a clinicopathologic study of 23 cases. *Histopathology.* 1983; 7:261–277.

20. Bennouna J, Bardet E, Deguiral P, et al. Small cell carcinoma of the esophagus: analysis of 10 cases and review of the published data. *Am J Clin Oncol.* 2000;23:455–459.

21. Huang Q, Wu H, Nie L, et al. Primary high-grade neuroendocrine carcinoma of the esophagus: a clinicopathologic and immunohistochemical study of 42 resection cases. *Am J Surg Pathol.* 2013; 37:467–483.

22. Chen S, Chen Y, Yang J, et al. Primary mucoepidermoid carcinoma of the esophagus. *J Thorac Oncol.* 2011;6:1426–1431.

23. Ishihara A, Mori T, Koono M. Diffuse pagetoid squamous cell carcinoma of the esophagus combined with choriocarcinoma and mucoepidermoid carcinoma: an autopsy case report. *Pathol Int.* 2002; 52:147–152.

24. Guo XF, Mao T, Gu ZT, et al. Adenoid cystic carcinoma of the esophagus: report of two cases and review of the Chinese literature. *Diagn Pathol.* 2012;7:179.

25. Grilliot MA, Goldblum JR, Liu X. Signet-ring cell melanoma of the gastroesophageal junction: a case report and literature review. *Arch Pathol Lab Med.* 2012;136:324–328.

26. Sanchez AA, Wu TT, Prieto VG, et al. Comparison of primary and metastatic malignant melanoma of the esophagus: clinicopathologic review of 10 cases. *Arch Pathol Lab Med.* 2008;132:1623–1629.

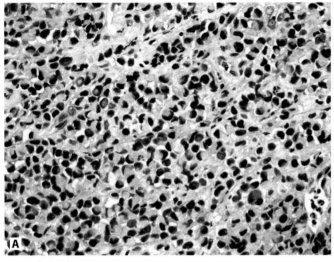

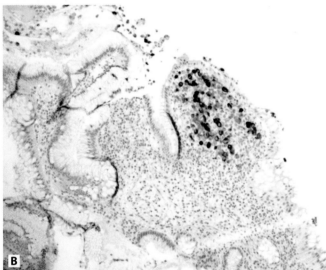

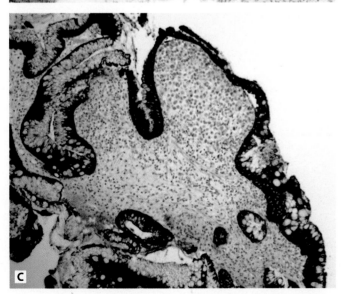

FIGURE 10-19. A melanoma at the gastroesophageal junction, with significant signet-ring cell morphology (**A**). Tumor cells are positive for HMB45 (**B**, immunostain) but negative for pancytokeratin (**C**, immunostain).

PART TWO

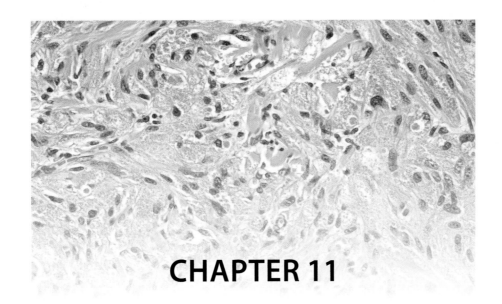

CHAPTER 11

Mesenchymal Tumors and Tumor-like Lesions of the Esophagus

■ INTRODUCTION

Subepithelial or submucosal nodules or masses of the esophagus are often biopsied for histologic diagnosis or endoscopically resected. The most frequently encountered diagnosis is leiomyoma; less common are gastrointestinal stromal tumors (GIST) and granular cell tumors. Other uncommon neoplastic or nonneoplastic nodules include benign cysts, giant fibrovascular polyps, ectopic tonsils, neurofibromas, inflammatory fibroid polyps, and leiomyosarcomas. Occasionally, a slow-growing mediastinal tumor may protrude into the esophageal lumen, mimicking an esophageal mesenchymal tumor and causing diagnostic difficulty. Most of the esophageal mesenchymal nodules or masses are not associated with diagnostic difficulties, as each has its unique gross and histologic features. However, histologic delineation of large spindle cell tumors may be difficult sometimes, particularly when sampling is limited, such as in needle biopsies guided by endoscopic ultrasound. As a result, a panel of immunostains is often necessary to reach a correct diagnosis.

■ LEIOMYOMA

Leiomyoma can be recognized by EUS based on the unique location, association with muscularis mucosa or muscularis propria, and texture of the tumor. It often presents as a well-circumscribed submucosal or intramuscular nodule or mass on gross examination or low-power microscopic view (Figure 11-1). It consists of bland spindle cells, but larger cells with granular cytoplasm or cytoplasmic clearing can be seen as well (Figure 11-2). Most tumors exhibit no mitotic figures.

Ultrasound-guided needle biopsies often yield fragments of spindle cell tumor, making definitive distinction from other spindle cell tumors of the esophagus difficult. Therefore, immunostains are necessary to confirm the diagnosis, with the tumor cells exhibiting diffuse positivity for smooth muscle actin (SMA) and desmin (Figure 11-3).

■ GASTROINTESTINAL STROMA TUMOR

The GISTs are discussed in detail in Chapter 5. In the esophagus, it is less common than leiomyoma.[1,2] An EUS-guided core biopsy makes it possible to obtain sufficient tissue not only for routine histologic evaluation but also for immunohistochemical markers. Furthermore, mutational analysis can be performed in some cases once a diagnosis of GIST is made.

The GISTs of the esophagus may present as a submucosal nodule or a mass with a smooth surface mucosal lining or a large polypoid, fungating mass with irregular surface (Figure 11-4). Microscopically, the tumor consists of slender spindle cells (as compared to shorter, plumper spindle cells of leiomyoma) with wavy nuclei (Figure 11-5). In contrast to its counterpart in the stomach, epithelioid morphology is rare. Depending on the aggressiveness, there may be rare-to-brisk mitosis (>10 per 50 high-power fields [HPF] in some cases). As discussed, the main differential diagnosis of esophageal GIST is leiomyoma. In our experience, a panel, including CD117, DOG-1 (discovered on GIST-1), desmin, SMA, and S100, is usually sufficient in sorting out the differential diagnosis among GIST, leiomyoma, granular cell tumor, and schwannoma (see Chapter 5).

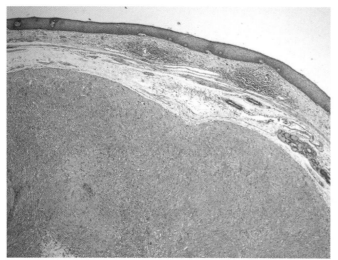

FIGURE 11-1. Leiomyoma. Low-power view of a well-circumscribed smooth muscle tumor in the submucosa, overlined by normal squamous mucosa. The tumor consists of bland spindle cells.

■ GRANULAR CELL TUMOR

Granular cell tumors are considered to originate with Schwann cell origin[3] and are benign with rare exceptions. Although most are solitary, multifocal tumors have been reported in up to 5% of cases.[3–5] Microscopically, most cases exhibit unique cytologic features, including large epithelioid cells with fine cytoplasmic granules and small nuclei (Figures 11-6 and 11-7), making diagnosis on sections stained with hematoxylin and eosin (H&E) fairly straightforward. Occasionally, the tumor cells may mimic plump smooth muscle cells, or strands of smooth muscle bundles

FIGURE 11-2. Leiomyoma. Here, the tumor cells are sectioned in cross or slanted fashion, giving rise to ovoid nuclear and focal cytoplasmic clearing. Large cytoplasmic eosinophilic "inclusions" are evident as well. These features mimic some examples of GISTs.

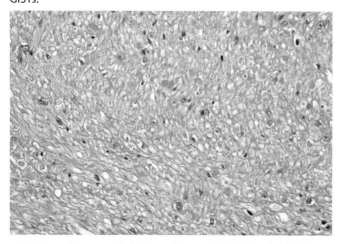

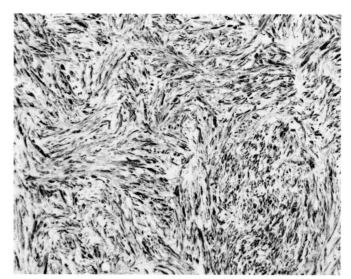

FIGURE 11-3. Leiomyoma immunoreactivity for desmin.

are intermixed in the tumor (Figures 11-8 and 11-10B). Distinction from leiomyoma thus requires immunostains, which demonstrate strong expression of CD68 (Figure 11-9) and S100 but are negative for muscular markers. Another differential diagnosis is squamous cell carcinoma; when a prominent epithelial hypertrophic reaction is present, it evidences the so-called pseudoepitheliomatous hyperplasia (Figure 11-10A).

FIGURE 11-4. A case of aggressive GIST of the esophagus exhibiting a large, fungating mass with irregular surface. Cut section (lower panel) demonstrates white-tan, fleshy appearance.

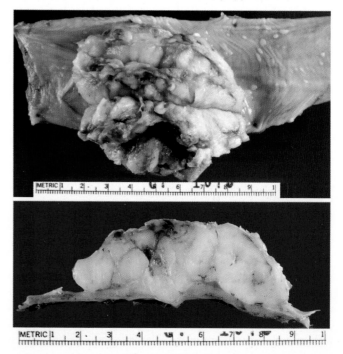

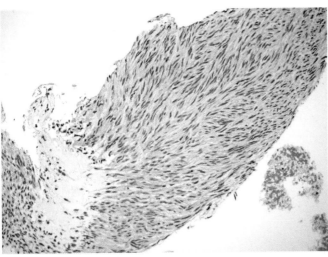

FIGURE 11-5. Esophageal GIST (needle biopsy guided by endoscopic ultrasound). Eosinophilic spindle cells with slender, long, curving nuclei. Focal degenerative change is evident.

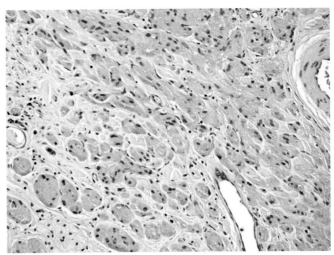

FIGURE 11-7. Granular cell tumor. Large epithelioid tumor cells with abundant cytoplasmic granules and small nuclei.

INFLAMMATORY FIBROID POLYP

The inflammatory fibroid stromal polyp is similar to that occurring in the stomach and consists of fibrovascular tissue infiltrated by mixed inflammatory cells, including eosinophils. There may be areas with myxoid change. Occasionally, immunostains are used to confirm the diagnosis in cases with atypical features. The fibroblasts show positive staining for CD34 and are negative for CD117 and smooth muscle markers.

GIANT FIBROVASCULAR POLYP

Giant fibrovascular polyps are large polypoid lesions with a smooth surface that protrude into the lumen of the esophagus. Rarely, these can extend and regurgitate into the oral

cavity or prolapse to the stomach. The patient presents with slowly worsening dysphagia or weight loss.[6-8] The same lesion has been recognized by many other names depending on the stage of lesional progression, including fibrovascular polyp, fibroma, fibrolipoma, fibromyxoma, lipoma, or giant prolapse polyp. Although a benign and likely nonneoplastic lesion, it rarely may cause death by asphyxia secondary to laryngeal obstruction.[7,9]

Endoscopically, the pedunculated polypoid masses are covered with a smooth lining of normal squamous mucosa (Figure 11-11). The cut surface reveals heterologous stromal components, including yellow adipose, white fibrous, or cystic areas (Figure 11-11). Some may consider this lesion a hamartomatous process, given these mostly normal

FIGURE 11-8. Granular cell tumor. Some cases may have focal prominent cytoplasmic granules with intermixed smooth muscle bundles.

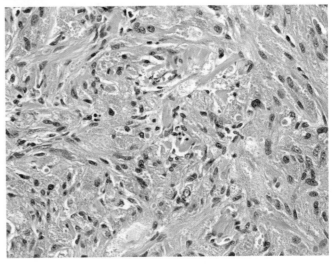

FIGURE 11-6. Granular cell tumor. Sheets of spindle cells with fine, eosinophilic granular cytoplasm.

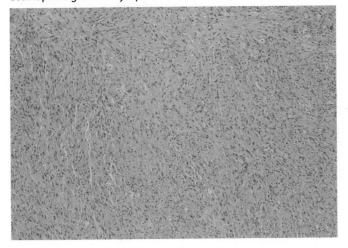

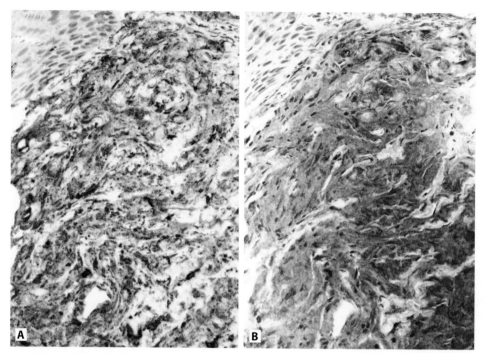

FIGURE 11-9. Granular cell tumor. Immunohistochemically, the tumor cells are strongly positive for CD68 (**A**) and S100 (**B**).

components of esophageal submucosa. Corresponding to the macroscopic appearance, histologic examination may reveal normal or hyperplastic squamous lining, adipose tissue, or fibrovascular proliferation (Figure 11-12). There is usually a lack of inflammatory infiltrate or cytologic atypia.

■ SCHWANNOMA

Primary esophageal schwannomas are extremely rare,[10–12] which include cases that show focal melanocytic features.[13] When large, a schwannoma of the mediastinum may protrude

FIGURE 11-10. Granular cell tumor. **A.** Marked pseudoepitheliomatous hyperplasia overlying the tumor. **B.** Strands of smooth muscle fibers intermixed with the tumor cells.

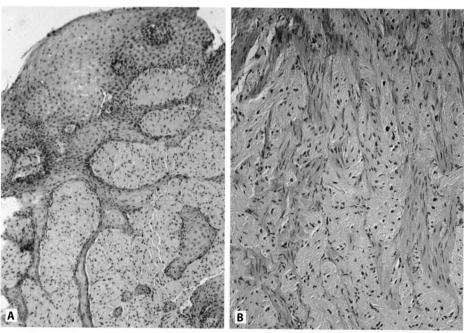

and the characteristic nuclear palisading (Figure 11-13). Occasional mitotic figures may be identified in some tumors (in contrast to neurofibroma). Because similar histologic features (spindle cell tumor with focal nuclear palisading) are not uncommon in GISTs, definitive differential diagnosis from the GISTs should rely on immunostains. Immunohistochemically, the tumor cells demonstrate strong staining for glial fibrillary acid protein (GFAP; Figure 11-13) and nuclear S100. If unsuspected, however, the tumor may be mistaken for a GIST or spindle cell carcinoma, as rare cases show aberrant cytokeratin AE1/3 expression immunohistochemically (Figure 11-13), and some cases of GIST (up to 5%) may show focal immunostaining for S100. In a biopsy, if the tumor cells demonstrate diffuse nuclear S100 reactivity, a diagnosis of schwannoma should be seriously considered. Other significant histologic features that strongly favor this diagnosis are fibrous capsule and lymphoid aggregates or follicles in the periphery of the tumor.

ECTOPIC TONSIL

Occasionally, a submucosal polyp or nodule may be endoscopically resected that includes large clusters of lymphoid follicles mixed with islands of mature squamous epithelium (Figures 11-14 and 11-15). These structures are well circumscribed and mimic normal tonsil. Even though it is easily recognized in well-oriented endoscopic mucosal resection (EMR) specimens, care should be taken not to mistake these structures for poorly differentiated squamous cell carcinoma in needle or mucosal biopsies.

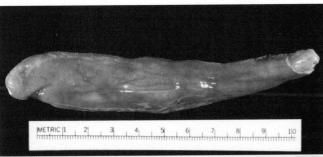
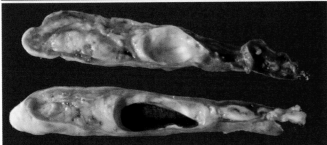

FIGURE 11-11. Giant fibrovascular polyp. A large, finger-like polyp with smooth surface was endoscopically resected from the esophageal mucosa. The surface appearance recapitulates normal esophageal mucosa. Lower panel shows the cut surface, with variegated, yellow-tan areas of fibroadipose tissue. A smooth-lined cyst is also present, which resulted from a dilation of a submucosal glandular duct.

into the esophageal lumen and present as an esophageal mass. The tumor exhibits morphologic features similar to its counterpart at other sites, with focal hypo- and hypercellular regions

FIGURE 11-12. Giant fibrovascular polyp. **A.** The polyp is lined by esophageal squamous epithelium, normal lamina propria, fibroadipose tissue, and smooth muscle bundles of the muscularis mucosa. There is a dilated glandular duct. **B.** Other areas of the polyp contain more abundant adipose tissue, mimicking a lipoma.

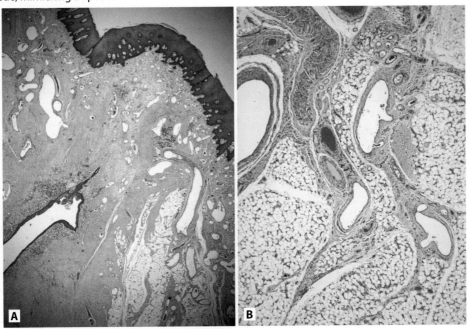

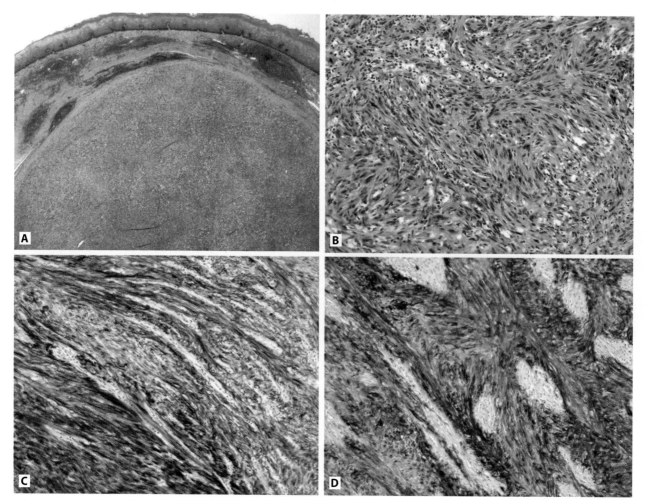

FIGURE 11-13. A mediastinal cellular schwannoma presenting as an esophageal tumor. **A.** Highly cellular but well-circumscribed tumor overlined by squamous mucosa and surrounded by prominent lymphoid follicles. **B.** On high-power view, the tumor cells are mostly spindle shape and exhibit cytologic atypia focally. **C.** The tumor cells exhibit aberrantly for cytokeratin AE1/3 (but negative for CAM 5.2, not shown). **D.** Tumor cells are strongly positive for glial fibrillary acid protein.

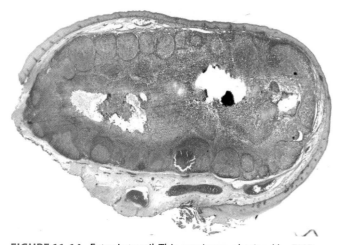

FIGURE 11-14. Ectopic tonsil. This specimen, obtained by EMR, demonstrates a well-circumscribed nodule of lymphoid tissue with reactive lymphoid follicles surrounding a central area of lympho-epithelial component.

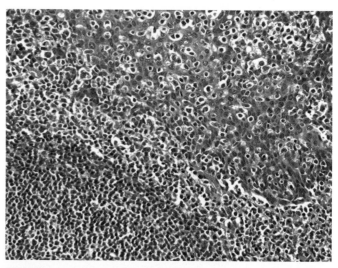

FIGURE 11-15. Ectopic tonsil. On higher-power view, the lympho-epithelial component contains both mature and basaloid squamous cells infiltrated by small lymphocytes.

REFERENCES

1. Gouveia AM, Pimenta AP, Lopes JM, et al. Esophageal GIST: therapeutic implications of an uncommon presentation of a rare tumor. *Dis Esophagus.* 2005;18(1):70–73. PMID: 15773848.

2. Miettinen M, Lasota J. Gastrointestinal stromal tumors: pathology and prognosis at different sites. *Semin Diagn Pathol.* 2006;23(2):70. PMID: S0740–2570(06)00143-2.

3. Lack EE, Worsham GF, Callihan MD, et al. Granular cell tumor: a clinicopathologic study of 110 patients. *J Surg Oncol.* 1980;13(4):301–316. PMID: 6246310.

4. John BK, Dang NC, Hussain SA, et al. Multifocal granular cell tumor presenting as an esophageal stricture. *J Gastrointest Cancer.* 2008;39(1–4):107–113. PMID: 19340612.

5. Mitomi H, Matsumoto Y, Mori A, et al. Multifocal granular cell tumors of the gastrointestinal tract: immunohistochemical findings compared with those of solitary tumors. *Pathol Int.* 2004;54(1):47–51. PMID: 14674995.

6. Lolley D, Razzuk MA, Urschel HC Jr. Giant fibrovascular polyp of the esophagus. *Ann Thorac Surg.* 1976;22(4):383–385. PMID: 984948.

7. Ramalho LN, Martin CC, Zerbini T. Sudden death caused by fibrovascular esophageal polyp: case report and study review. *Am J Foren Med Path.* 2010;31(1):103–105. PMID: 20010288.

8. Yu Z, Bane BL, Lee JY, et al. Cytogenetic and comparative genomic hybridization studies of an esophageal giant fibrovascular polyp: a case report. *Hum Pathol.* 2012;43(2):293–298. PMID: 21835434.

9. Carrick C, Collins KA, Lee CJ, Prahlow JA, Barnard JJ. Sudden death due to asphyxia by esophageal polyp: two case reports and review of asphyxial deaths. *Am J Foren Med Path.* 2005;26(3):275–281. PMID: 16121086.

10. Dutta R, Kumar A, Jindal T, Tanveer N. Concurrent benign schwannoma of oesophagus and posterior mediastinum. *Interact Cardiovasc Thorac Surg.* 2009;9(6):1032–1034. PMID: 19770133.

11. Eguchi T, Yoshida K, Kobayashi N, et al. Multiple schwannomas of the bilateral mediastinal vagus nerves. *Ann Thorac Surg.* 2011;91(4):1280–1281. PMID: 21440164.

12. Retrosi G, Nanni L, Ricci R, Manzoni C, Pintus C. Plexiform schwannoma of the esophagus in a child with neurofibromatosis type 2. *J Pediatr Surg.* 2009;44(7):1458–1461. PMID: 19573680.

13. Brown RM, Darnton SJ, Papadaki L, Antonakopoulos GN, Newman J. A primary tumour of the oesophagus with both melanocytic and schwannian differentiation. Melanocytic schwannoma or malignant melanoma? *J Clin Pathol.* 2002;55(4):318–320. PMID: 11919222. PMCID: PMC1769623.

PART TWO

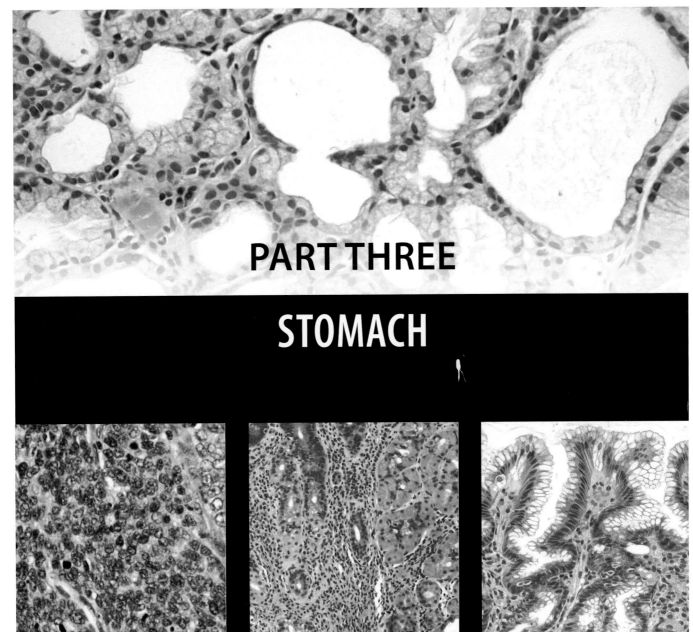

PART THREE

STOMACH

153

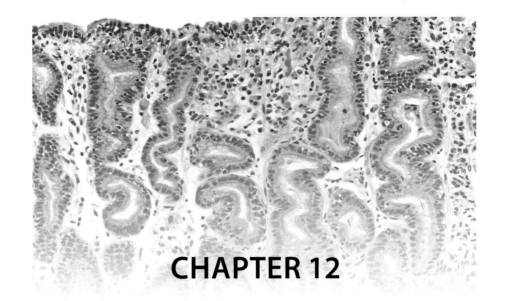

CHAPTER 12

Gastritis and Related Conditions

INTRODUCTION

Inflammation of the gastric mucosa assumes several different forms. Although all involve inflammatory cellular infiltration of the lamina propria, each form may have unique additional changes that correspond to the specific type of gastritis present and are therefore diagnostically useful. For example, diffuse fundic gland atrophy, often with intestinal metaplasia, points to autoimmune atrophic gastritis (AAG). On the other hand, if the main finding is lamina propria infiltration accompanied by superficial lymphoid follicles, *Helicobacter pylori* gastritis is the more likely diagnosis. Additional clinical history and ancillary tests will further help in reaching the correct diagnosis. Because the diagnosis of *H. pylori* is rather straightforward and its histologic features are well known, it is only briefly described.

ATROPHIC GASTRITIS AND PROLIFERATIVE ENDOCRINE CELL LESIONS

Although several types of chronic gastritis, including *H. pylori* gastritis and severe chronic graft-vs-host disease (GVHD), can lead to focal atrophy of the gastric mucosa, the term *atrophic gastritis* (AG) should be reserved for parietal cell antibody-associated autoimmune gastritis, which is often associated with *pernicious anemia* (Figure 12-1). The full version of the name, *autoimmune atrophic gastritis* or *chronic autoimmune gastritis* (CAG), may therefore be more appropriate (Table 12-1).

Autoimmune atrophic gastritis occurs mostly in elderly patients. The underlying pathogenesis is immune-mediated destruction, mainly of the parietal cell population but later affecting chief cells as well, which results in diffuse atrophy of gastric fundic glands and metaplasia (Figure 12-2). In addition to the parietal cell antibody, intrinsic factor antibody plays a role in the pathogenesis of this disease as well. Diagnostically, the intrinsic factor antibody is more specific than the parietal cell antibody but is less sensitive; detection of this antibody is virtually diagnostic of the disease. In well-developed, "classic" cases, the basic pathology is characterized by diffuse loss of gastric rugal folds and thinning or flattening of the gastric mucosa on gross or endoscopic examination (Figure 12-1); microscopically, there is plasma cell–predominant inflammation accompanied by fundic gland atrophy, with replacement by focal or diffuse intestinal metaplasia (Figure 12-2).

Microscopic Features of Classic Atrophic Gastritis

The primary lesion of AG involves the fundus and body. In all stages of the disease, the lamina propria contains a mixed inflammatory cellular infiltration, predominantly of plasma cells but accompanied by lymphocytes and sometimes eosinophils. There are various degrees of parietal cell loss, depending on the duration of the disease, leading to atrophy of the fundic glands (Figure 12-2). Neutrophilic infiltration of the glands and pits is not uncommon (pititis or activity) (Figure 12-3). Although focal or diffuse intestinal metaplasia is usually described as part of this atrophic process, it

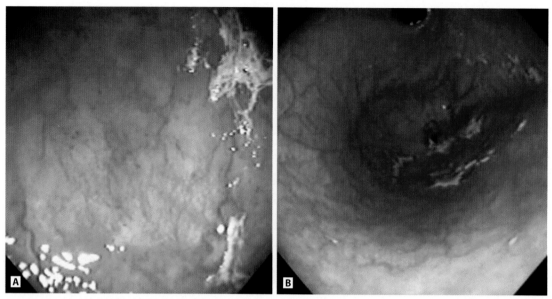

FIGURE 12-1. Atrophic gastritis. Endoscopic view of stomach body (**A**) and fundus (**B**) showing total loss of gastric rugal folds and thinning of the mucosa with a prominent submucosal vascular network.

should be noted that lost fundic glands are initially replaced by pyloric-type mucous glands (pyloric gland metaplasia) (Figure 12-2C). Sometimes this metaplastic process can be exuberant, leading to focal expansion of pyloric glands, giving rise to a pyloric gland adenoma (PGA) (see Chapter 14). It also must be emphasized that PGAs and intestinal metaplasia can progress through dysplasia and eventually to adenocarcinoma.

Gastric Low-Grade Neuroendocrine Tumors

One of the more common complications of AG is the development of hyperplasia of enterochromaffin-like (ECL) cells,[1] which are normally distributed in the gastric fundus and body, eventually resulting in endocrine tumors (Figure 12-2D). Gastric neuroendocrine tumors (NETs) are discussed in detail in Chapters 6 and 17. This section focuses on the so-called type 1 NET, which is associated with AG.

TABLE 12-1. Types of gastritis discussed in this chapter.
Atrophic gastritis
Gastritis caused by microorganisms
Gastritis in the setting of inflammatory bowel diseases
Other types of gastritis:
Acute hemorrhagic gastritis
Lymphocytic gastritis
Collagenous gastritis
Nonparietal cell antibody–associated autoimmune gastritis
Granulomatous gastritis

Atrophy of the normal fundic glands results in decreased production of hydrochloric acid, leading to hypochlorohydria or achlorhydria. Lack of negative feedback by gastric acid (which normally causes suppression of G-cell function) leads to hypersecretion of gastrin from these cells, resulting in G-cell hyperplasia in the gastric antral mucosa (Figure 12-4). The hypersecretion of gastrin leads to proliferation of endocrine cells (in particular, ECL cells) in the gastric body and fundus, which are spared from the immune-mediated damage; this pathway gives rise to ECL cell hyperplasia (Figure 12-2D) or small NETs (Figure 12-5). Evidently, because this process is initiated secondary to gastrin stimulation and is not a self-initiated clonal proliferation as in other types of endocrine tumors, type 1 NETs are often multifocal and smaller (less than 1 cm) and exhibit low proliferative activity (low Ki-67 index) (Figure 12-5). These tumors follow an indolent course, with low tumor-related mortality (less than 5% in 5 years). Based on this unique biology, treatment of type 1 gastric NETs is conservative. However, in hard-to control cases, antrectomy is performed to eliminate the stimulating factor for ECL cell proliferation.

Other Findings in the Setting of Atrophic Gastritis

The classical endoscopic appearance of AG is diffuse, uniform gastric gland atrophy (at least in the body and fundus) (Figure 12-1). However, early in the disease process, it is also common for the gastric mucosa to be described as appearing "multinodular" endoscopically. This finding has become more frequent with the popularity of proton pump inhibitor therapy. When biopsies are obtained from these nodular areas, they reveal focal fundic gland hypertrophy, which is referred to as parietal cell pseudohypertrophy[1];

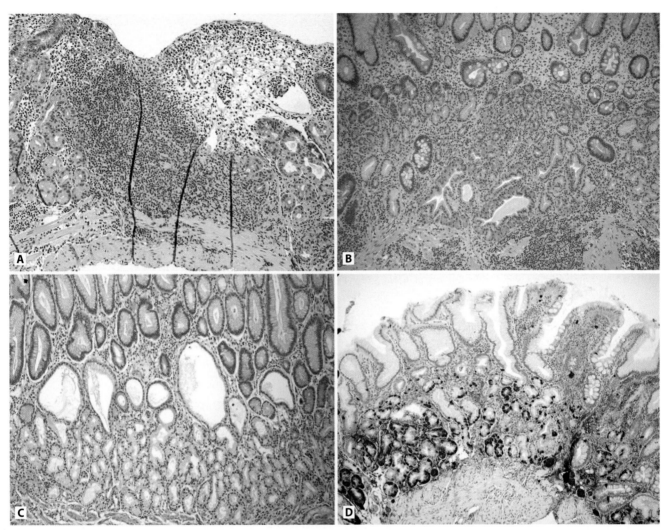

FIGURE 12-2. Atrophic gastritis. **A.** Loss of normal fundic glands. **B.** Gastric body mucosa completely replaced by antrum-type mucosa and intestinal metaplasia. **C.** Pyloric gland metaplasia: gastric fundic glands completely replaced by pyloric glands in the gastric body mucosa. **D.** Enterochromaffin-like (ECL) cell hyperplasia in atrophic gastric body mucosa (immunostain for chromogranin).

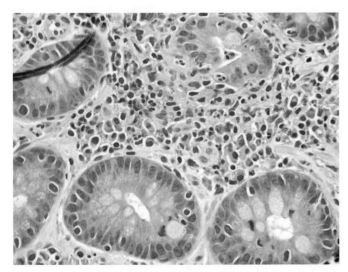

FIGURE 12-3. Atrophic gastritis with mild active inflammation characterized by pititis with neutrophils.

biopsies from the nonnodular regions show typical features of AG as described previously (Figure 12-6). The cause of this paradoxical change may be explained by uneven distribution of parietal cell sensitivity to the autoimmune injury. While some glands are affected and progress to atrophy, other glands or areas, stimulated by increased gastrin levels (discussed later in the chapter), exhibit parietal cell hyperplasia and focal nodular formation. Eventually, diffuse atrophy occurs.

A nodular endoscopic appearance may also be due to other factors, such as neuroendocrine cell tumors, as discussed previously. Another condition that causes a nodular pattern endoscopically is the development of a PGA. It should be reemphasized that AG is one of the most common background diseases in which PGAs occur.

In summary, to help understand and memorize the pathogenesis and the spectrum of AG pathology, a list of the key players or features is provided in Table 12-2.

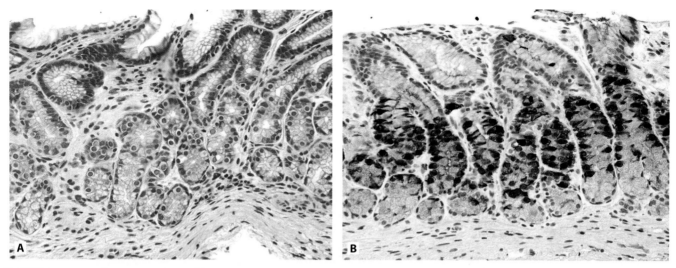

FIGURE 12-4. Antral mucosa with G-cell hyperplasia. **A.** Hematoxylin and eosin stain. **B.** Immunostain for gastrin.

INFECTIOUS GASTRITIS

Helicobacter pylori Gastritis

Helicobacter pylori gastritis is likely the most frequently encountered entity in daily practice; therefore, it does not require much description here. Some pathologists choose to perform an immunostain or special stain on all gastric antral biopsies to help identify *H. pylori* organisms. For those of us who order the immunostain only in selected cases, a few features can be used to trigger this additional test. One microscopic feature that is characteristic of *H. pylori* gastritis

TABLE 12-2. Key points associated with atrophic gastritis.
Parietal cell antibody and intrinsic factor antibody
Hypochlorhydria; achlorhydria
Pernicious anemia or iron-deficiency anemia
G-cell hyperplasia and hypergastrinemia
Enterochromaffin-like cell hyperplasia and type 1 gastric neuroendocrine tumor
Pyloric gland metaplasia and pyloric gland adenoma
Intestinal metaplasia

FIGURE 12-5. Type 1 gastric neuroendocrine tumor in atrophic gastritis. **A.** Irregular and nodular endocrine cell proliferation. **B.** The tumor exhibits a low Ki-67 index (Ki-67 immunostain).

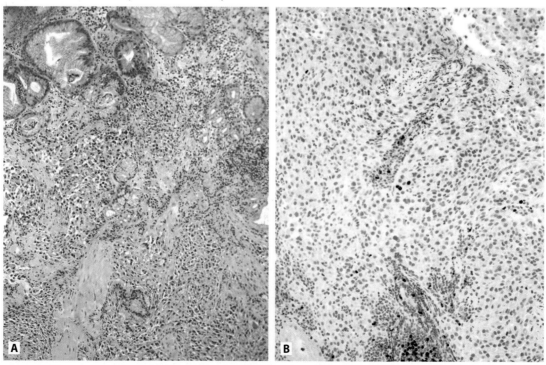

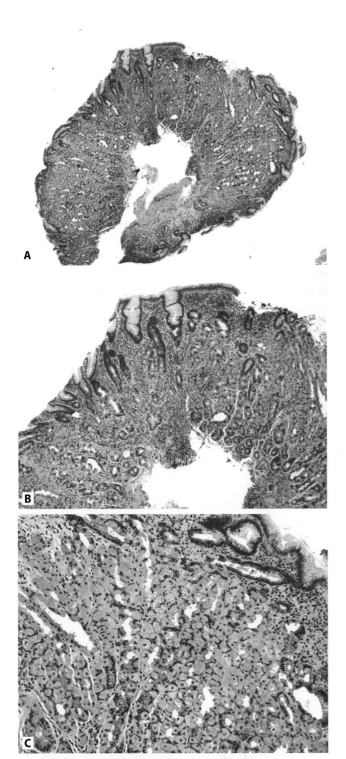

FIGURE 12-6. Atrophic gastritis: paradoxical parietal cell hypertrophy. The gastric body mucosa was described as multinodular endoscopically. **A.** At scanning power, there are alternating areas with fundic glands and those without (representing atrophy). **B.** Higher magnification demonstrates mixed inflammatory cellular infiltration in the superficial mucosa as well as in the atrophic areas. Note the lack of intestinal metaplasia. **C.** Plasma cells dominate the inflammation. In addition, there appears to be parietal cell hypertrophy, likely resulting from the effects of an increased gastrin level on the residual parietal cell population, which is also relatively less sensitive to the autoantibodies.

is superficial or more advanced lymphoplasmacytic infiltration of the mucosa, which is often accompanied by small or large superficial lymphoid follicles. Often, there is scattered-to-extensive activity in the form of neutrophilic infiltration of glands or pits. A careful search for *H. pylori* at high power is warranted in all gastric biopsies if gastritis is identified. If organisms cannot be identified with certainty, an immunostain should be performed. Sometimes, even if no activity is seen but the background inflammatory pattern suggests the diagnosis, the immunostain should be performed as well (Figure 12-7). In addition, bacterial forms similar to *H. pylori* but with an atypical appearance may be seen, often representing *Helicobacter heilmannii*. An immunostain for *H. pylori* will show these organisms as negative (Figure 12-8). Finally, if the clinical requisition specifically asks to rule out *H. pylori*, an immunostain should also be performed. Knowing that

FIGURE 12-7. A *Helicobacter pylori*–positive case with no activity. **A.** The antral mucosa exhibits inactive gastritis. **B.** An immunostain confirmed the diagnosis.

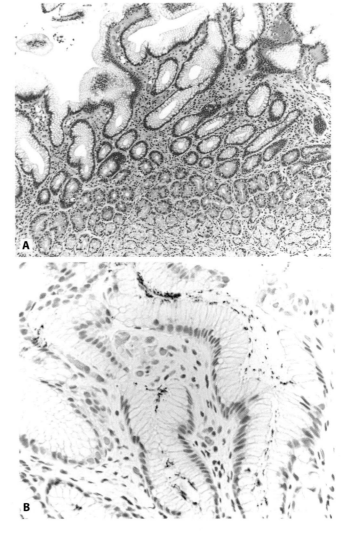

some pathologists may disagree with this approach, I prefer to follow this algorithm because it is not uncommon for *H. pylori* to be identified in an otherwise-atypical inflammatory pattern, and frequently the organisms simply do not present themselves on sections stained with hematoxylin and eosin (H&E) (Figure 12-7). Table 12-3 summarizes the conditions under which we perform immunohistochemistry for *H. pylori*.

As discussed in Chapter 15, *H. pylori* gastritis may be one of the most common underlying conditions for hyperplastic/inflammatory polyps. Therefore, when these polyps contain active inflammation, *H. pylori* should also be ruled out.

Cytomegalovirus Gastritis

Cytomegalovirus (CMV) infection or reactivation often occurs in the elderly or in immunosuppressed patients, including those who have undergone solid-organ or stem cell transplantation, are receiving chemotherapy, or have immunodeficiency disorders. Gastric mucosal involvement leads to a microscopic pattern of gastropathy (see Chapter 1) in most patients, in which inflammatory cellular infiltration

is not prominent.[2–5] In other patients, the infection presents with a microscopic pattern of gastritis (Figure 12-9).[6–10] The different pattern does not have implications for clinical management and is not related to patient outcome. In both CMV gastropathy and CMV gastritis, careful examination will likely reveal rare to frequent cytopathic changes such as CMV inclusion bodies (Figure 12-9), and an immunostain for CMV antigen can easily confirm the diagnosis.

TABLE 12-3. Algorithms for performing immunostaining for *Helicobacter pylori*.

Characteristic lymphoplasmacytic infiltration with activity (neutrophilic infiltration of epithelium)
Inactive gastritis, but with clinical history of *H. pylori* gastritis, status post treatment
Distinction between *H. pylori* and *H. heilmannii* when organisms are identified
Focal active gastritis in a patient with Crohn disease (to help distinguish between involvement by Crohn disease or *H. pylori* gastritis, as the latter may be common in patients with Crohn disease)[13]

FIGURE 12-8. Gastritis with *Helicobacter heilmannii*. The gastric biopsy exhibits changes similar to *H. pylori* gastritis (**A**), with bacilli resembling *H. pylori* (**B**). However, the immunostain was negative for *H. pylori* (**C**), and the organisms were highlighted by a Diff-Quick stain (**D**).

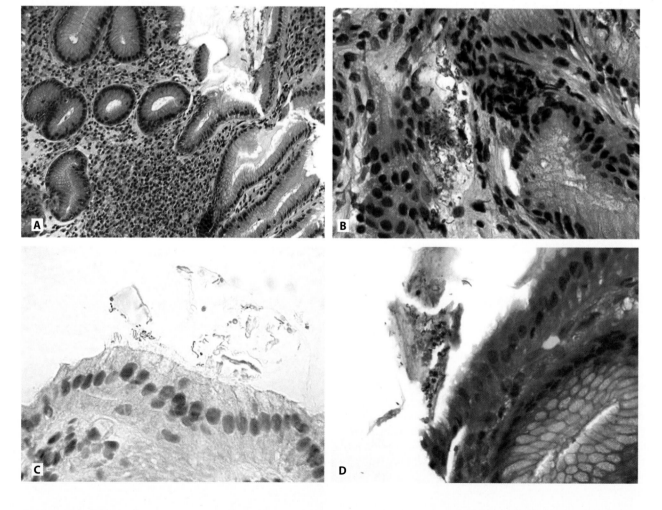

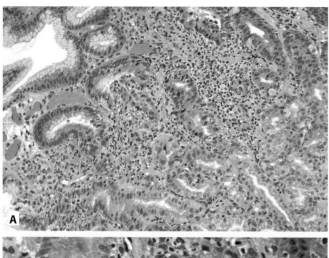

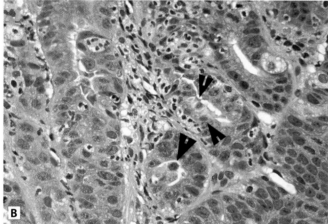

FIGURE 12-9. Cytomegaloviral (CMV) gastritis. **A.** Gastric body mucosa with mild inflammatory infiltration in the superficial lamina propria. **B.** Higher-power view reveals infiltration of the gastric glands by neutrophils. CMV inclusion bodies are evident in several epithelial cells (arrowheads). An immunostain confirmed the finding (not shown).

Fungal Gastritis

Systemic fungal infection such as by *Candida* and *Histoplasma* species may involve the stomach as well. Histoplasmosis causes granulomatous gastritis in addition to diffuse or focal lymphadenopathy. Occasionally, the gastric mucosa may exhibit multiple ulcers or appear diffusely thickened endoscopically, mimicking hypertrophic gastropathy.[11,12] Biopsies may reveal prominent mucosal or submucosal epithelioid granulomas, some with central necrosis. In practice, with microscopic findings of a granulomatous inflammation, special stains, including an acid-fast stain for mycobacteria and a Gomori methenamine silver (GMS) stain for fungus should be performed. However, these special stains are not sufficiently sensitive in detecting the organisms. Therefore, even though a histologic diagnosis of "granulomatous gastritis" without further characterization may be appropriate (Figure 12-10), it should be communicated to the clinician that an infectious etiology cannot be excluded based on tissue examination.

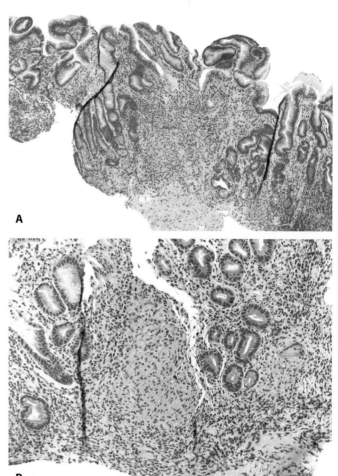

FIGURE 12-10. Chronic gastritis with granulomas from a patient with systemic lymphadenopathy. There are multiple epithelioid granulomas in a background of inflammatory cellular infiltration (**A**). Patchy activity is noted (**B**), as are occasional multinucleated giant cells (**B**). An acid-fast stain and a Gomori methenamine silver stain were negative for organisms. Serology was positive for histoplasma antibody.

■ OTHER FORMS OF GASTRITIS

Gastritis in the Setting of Inflammatory Bowel Diseases

Crohn disease involves the gastric mucosa in about 25%–33% of patients regardless of upper gastrointestinal symptoms.[13,14] This issue is discussed in more detail in Chapter 4. Some patients with ulcerative colitis who underwent total colectomy have subsequently developed severe extensive active gastritis and duodenitis (for details, see Chapter 19).[15,16] Early involvement by Crohn disease manifests as focally enhanced gastritis (FEG), which is characterized by focal accumulation of mixed inflammatory cells surrounding a single gland or group of glands in an otherwise-normal background. In contrast, *H. pylori* gastritis or autoimmune gastritis both exhibit diffuse inflammatory infiltration in lamina propria (Figure 12-11).

It must be emphasized that although suggestive of the diagnosis, the finding of FEG is not diagnostically specific

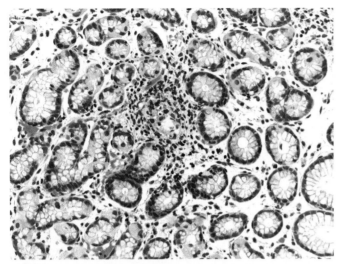

FIGURE 12-11. Focally enhanced gastritis in Crohn disease. The lamina propria is essentially normal except for a focus of mixed inflammatory infiltration damaging a gland.

for Crohn disease. Other clinicopathologic features of Crohn disease are required for the diagnosis. FEG was first described by Oberhuber[17] and was found to be more commonly associated with Crohn disease and as a helpful microscopic feature for making the diagnosis,[14,17,18] particularly among pediatric patients.[19-22] Other studies, however, have suggested that this feature has no specificity as it was seen with equal frequency in patients with ulcerative colitis.[23] However, it appears that the criteria used for FEG were less stringent in these later studies and the lesions described were less typical, hence lowering the correlation with Crohn disease. In my experience, unequivocal focal active gastritis that is negative for *H. pylori* in a patient with clinically suspected inflammatory bowel disease raises a high suspicion for Crohn disease in contrast to ulcerative colitis.[20-22]

Other than in the setting of inflammatory bowel disease, in a nonselected patient population, *H. pylori*–negative FEG has much less diagnostic value.

Acute Hemorrhagic Gastritis

Acute hemorrhagic gastritis, which is an acute onset, is associated with several potential causes, but is mainly due to acute stress-induced or chemically induced gastritis. The former usually occurs in intensive care unit patients (stress-induced gastric ulcers). The mechanism is unknown, but it is likely related to a combination of reduced blood supply to the superficial gastric mucosa, reduced epithelial protection, and acid exposure. Sources of chemically induced gastritis include alcohol, nonsteroidal anti-inflammatory drugs (NSAIDs), some antibiotics, and other commonly used drugs (see discussion in Chapters 1 and 13).

The endoscopic appearance of acute gastritis consists of diffuse mucosal hyperemia/erythema with erosions or ulcerations. Microscopically, fibrinoid necrosis may involve the most superficial layer of the lamina propria, along with focal or diffuse erosions. As a result of the compromised mucosal

barrier being exposed to the luminal environment, there may be recruitment of neutrophils to the site of injury, hence the term *gastritis*. Strictly speaking, these conditions are essentially a type of chemical gastropathy (discussed in Chapter 1), with neutrophilic infiltration as a secondary response to and not a primary cause of the gastric mucosal injury (Figure 12-12).

Lymphocytic Gastritis

Sometimes a gastric biopsy exhibits prominent intraepithelial lymphocytosis of the surface foveolar layer and gastric pits (Figure 12-13) in a background of mixed inflammatory cellular infiltration of the lamina propria; in this case, a histologic diagnosis of *lymphocytic gastritis* (LG) is rendered. Traditionally, this term was used to describe a special form of gastritis with the endoscopic appearance of mucosal

FIGURE 12-12. Acute gastritis. **A.** Antral mucosa with superficial necrosis and necrotic debris in the lumina of many "withered" glands. There is a patchy mild inflammatory infiltrate in the lamina propria. **B.** Focal neutrophilic infiltration of glands in a case of acute alcoholic gastritis (after binge drinking). Note the lack of significant infiltration in the lamina propria.

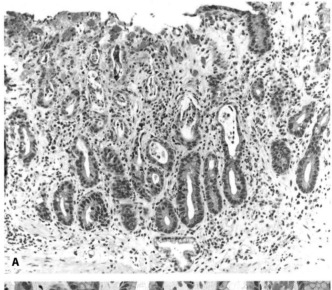

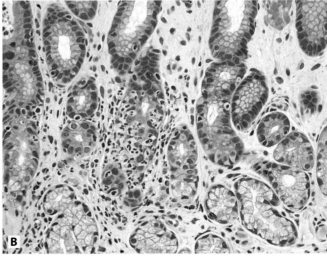

The following discussions are focused on increased IELs as a diffuse pattern; the finding should be seen in most, if not all, of the biopsy fragments uniformly. With the recognition of this pattern, a list of diseases should be "spontaneously" registered in one's mind as differential diagnoses (Table 12-4), as are individually discussed next.

Helicobacter pylori *Gastritis*

As mentioned, a patchy increase in IELs is often seen in *H. pylori* gastritis and is seldom a finding that should influence the diagnosis. In other cases, a significant and diffuse increase in IELs can be seen in biopsies that have features of *H. pylori* gastritis,[25,30–34] and such cases are thus diagnosed as *H. pylori*-associated LG. Microscopically, the gastric mucosa exhibits a marked increase in IELs. There is no universally agreed-on criteria for a normal IEL count, although 25 per 100 epithelial cells had been used as case inclusion criteria in clinical trials.[30–32] In practice, recognizing increased IELs is a gestalt process because when it occurs it is usually prominent.

After *H. pylori* gastritis is excluded, the diagnosis of LG should be made with a comment suggesting further clinical correlation regarding other potential etiologies or clinical entities.

Varioliform Lymphocytic Gastritis

Only rare patients with microscopic changes of LG have the VLG form of gastritis.[25,35,36] Grossly and endoscopically, VLG is characterized by thickened gastric folds, sometimes with superficial erosions, accompanied by multiple mucosal nodules. The endoscopic appearance closely resembles that of Ménétrier disease.[34,37–40] In fact, many patients have clinical presentations similar to Ménétrier disease as well, such as protein-losing gastropathy with low serum albumin.[34,40] The term *hypertrophic lymphocytic gastritis* (HLG) has been used by some to describe this condition.[40,41] Microscopically, most cases exhibit increased inflammatory cellular infiltration in the lamina propria and increased IELs, as described previously.

Lymphocytic Gastritis Associated with Celiac Disease

Lymphocytic gastritis associated with celiac disease is better known and more frequently encountered in practice than other types of LG.[24–29,42] In some instances, when this pattern is noted in gastric biopsies, examination of the duodenal biopsies (usually submitted at the same time) will reveal typical features of celiac disease (see Chapter 18) (Figure 12-14).

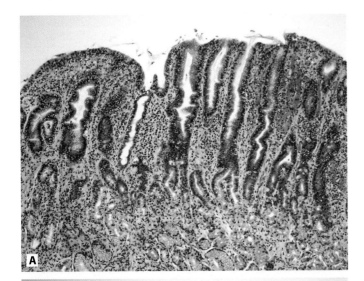

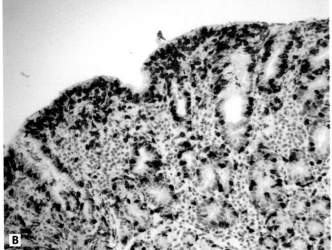

FIGURE 12-13. Lymphocytic gastritis. **A.** Marked intraepithelial lymphocytosis is evident. There is infiltration in the superficial lamina propria by lymphocytes and plasma cells as well. Endoscopically, the gastric mucosa appeared nodular (varioliform lymphocytic gastritis). **B.** An immunostain for CD8 highlights the cytotoxic T cells in the intraepithelial lymphocyte component.

nodularity; namely, *varioliform lymphocytic gastritis* (VLG), which is more frequently seen in children. However, similar microscopic changes can be seen in some patients with celiac disease[24–29] (see Chapter 18), microscopic colitis, or other forms of autoimmune enterocolitis (see Chapter 3). More recently, this finding has been described in patients with olmesartan-related mucosal injury. Therefore, the diagnosis of LG merely implies a unique microscopic pathologic pattern. To delineate the underlying associated disease, other clinical and pathologic information is necessary.

It should be noted that a focal increase in intraepithelial lymphocytes (IELs) may be seen in various gastric inflammatory or chemical injuries, including *H. pylori* gastritis and NSAID-induced gastropathy. However, in these conditions, the increase in IELs is usually mild and focal and does not need to be further considered in the differential diagnosis.

TABLE 12-4. Gastritis with increased intraepithelial lymphocytes.

Helicobacter pylori gastritis
Lymphocytic gastritis associated with celiac disease
Drug-induced gastritis
Lymphocytic gastritis associated with lymphocytic/collagenous colitis
Lymphocytic gastritis as part of a generalized autoimmune gastroenteropathy
Varioliform lymphocytic gastritis

PART THREE

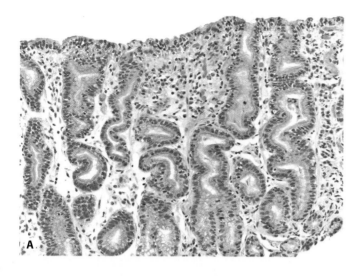

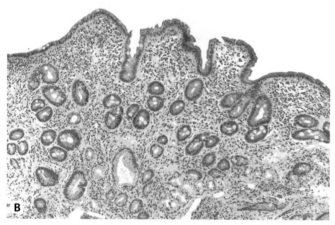

FIGURE 12-14. Lymphocytic gastritis associated with villous blunting duodenitis. **A.** The gastric antral mucosa exhibits foveolar hyperplasia and evident intraepithelial lymphocytosis, along with mild lamina propria infiltration. **B.** The duodenal mucosa exhibits moderate villous blunting and a mild increase in intraepithelial lymphocytes.

A correlation with available positive clinical history or positive serology, or a suggestion of such a correlation if this information is not available at the time of biopsy, is appropriate. In contrast to VLG, endoscopically the gastric mucosa may appear normal.

Lymphocytic Gastritis Associated with Microscopic Colitis

Occasionally, gastric biopsy findings from a patient are consistent with that of LG, and correlation with clinical history or concurrent colonoscopic biopsies may reveal lymphocytic or collagenous colitis microscopically.[25,43-47] Similar to colonoscopy, endoscopic findings will show an unremarkable gastric mucosal appearance.

Lymphocytic Gastritis Associated with Other Immune-Mediated Enterocolitis

Less well defined, and perhaps a diagnosis of heterogeneous diseases in itself, adult-onset autoimmune enterocolitis (or

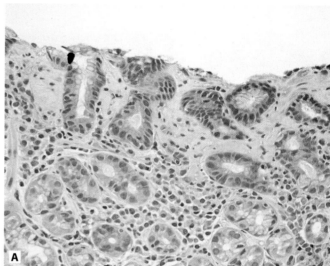

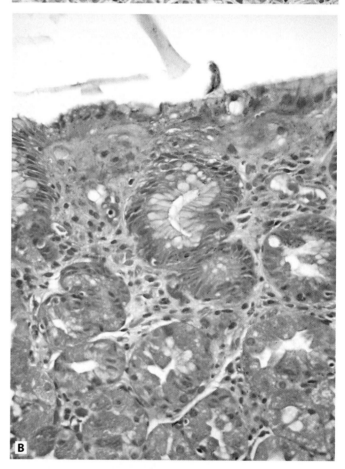

FIGURE 12-15. Collagenous gastritis of unknown etiology. **A.** Markedly thickened subepithelial collagen layer encroaching on the gastric pits, with surface foveolar epithelium lifted off. The lamina propria also contains a plasmacytic infiltrate. **B.** Masson trichrome stain highlighting the thickened collagen deposition.

diffuse lymphocytic gastroenterocolitis)[25,28] may have the concurrent finding of LG in the stomach. In such cases, careful evaluation may not reveal evidence of celiac disease (negative serology, no relationship with gluten sensitivity).

Other rare associations of LG include common variable immune deficiency (CVID), gastric lymphoma,[48,49] and gastric syphilis.[50]

Collagenous Gastritis

Collagenous gastritis is microscopically characterized by subepithelial band-like collagen deposition (Figure 12-15), in addition to an inflammatory pattern similar to that of LG.[51] It can occur in both children and adults, and in the former, mucosal nodularity is usually seen endoscopically.[47,52,53] Most of the adult patients have other associated autoimmune disorders, such as Hashimoto thyroiditis, celiac disease, collagenous sprue, or collagenous colitis.[47,52] Patients can present with anemia, abdominal pain or discomfort, chronic watery diarrhea,[52] or profound weight loss.[54] Long-term follow-up of some cases reveals an outcome similar to AG, with endocrine cell hyperplasia and intestinal metaplasia.[55] In addition, it has been increasingly recognized that Benicar® (olmesartan) may contribute to some cases of collagenous gastritis.

Non–Parietal Cell Antibody-Associated Autoimmune Gastritis

It is not uncommon to encounter cases that exhibit diffuse AG but have negative serologies for antiparietal cells or anti–intrinsic factor. Many of these cases are associated with a systemic autoimmune disorder, and these patients may have other types of autoantibodies as well.[56] Understandably, the diagnosis relies on a combination of these clinical features and the histologic findings. Since the recognition of increased IgG4+ plasma cells in a subset of autoimmune pancreatitis, there has been much interest in unifying chronic sclerosing inflammatory conditions of different sites with the common finding of increased IgG4+ plasma cells by immunostain. These conditions have been placed under the general category of "IgG4 sclerosing disease." Some authors proposed that autoimmune gastritis can be diagnosed based on increased IgG4+ plasma cells (Figures 12-16 and 12-17). However, this approach lacked sufficient specificity, and the clinical implications have not been established. It is likely that IgG4+ plasma cells merely represent a state of general

PART THREE

FIGURE 12-16. Anti–parietal cell antibody-negative autoimmune gastritis in a 34-year-old woman with anemia and abdominal discomfort. There was no significant drug history. Serologic tests revealed elevated immunoglobulin (Ig) G4, IgG3, and antinuclear antibodies. The gastric body appeared nodular endoscopically. **A.** Lymphoplasmacytic infiltration of the superficial lamina propria. **B.** Focal collagen deposition. **C.** Positive Masson trichome stain confirms the thickened collagen layer. **D.** Increased IgG4 plasma cells as part of the inflammatory infiltration.

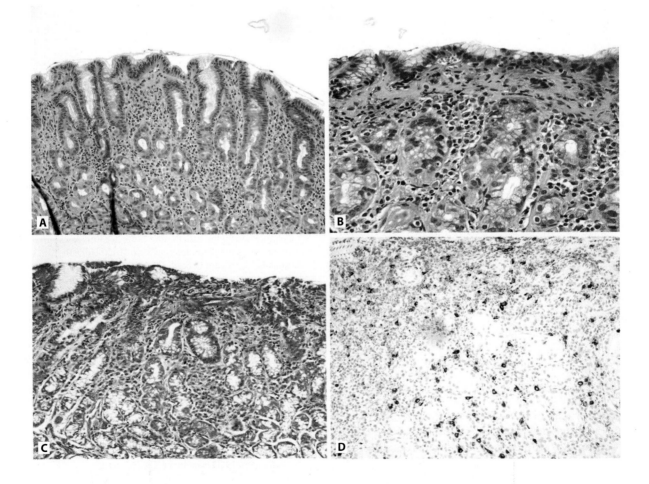

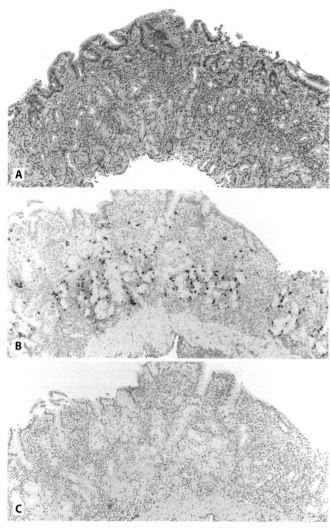

FIGURE 12-17. Same patient as in Figure 12-16. Two years after the diagnosis, the patient developed gastric body atrophy that was more prominent. **A.** The fundic glands are nearly replaced by pyloric glands. To confirm that the biopsy was taken from the gastric body, immunostains were performed and showed endocrine cell hyperplasia (**B**, chromogranin); the cells were negative for gastrin (**C**).

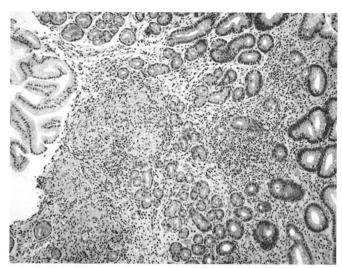

FIGURE 12-18. Granulomatous gastritis. The gastric biopsy demonstrates noncaseating epithelioid granulomas in a patient negative for Crohn disease and sarcoidosis. No infectious etiology was demonstrated.

chronic inflammation, and serum anti-IgG4 antibody is only one of many types of immunoglobulin subspecies associated with systemic autoimmune disorders. For example, sclerosing mesenteritis with and without increased IgG4+ plasma cells exhibited no difference in response to steroid treatment.

Granulomatous Gastritis

As discussed, both gastric involvement by Crohn disease and fungal gastritis can have epithelioid granulomas in gastric mucosal biopsies. In addition, sarcoidosis and several other conditions can exhibit gastric involvement. When an underlying cause cannot be identified, the diagnosis of granulomatous gastritis may be rendered (Figure 12-18). However, this may not be the final diagnosis in some patients; further clinical workup may still reveal a treatable cause, such as an infection.

■ REFERENCES

1. Torbenson M, Abraham SC, Boitnott J, Yardley JH, Wu TT. Auto-immune gastritis: distinct histological and immunohistochemical findings before complete loss of oxyntic glands. *Mod Pathol.* 2002;15(2):102–109. PMID: 11850538.
2. Cervoni J, Pico J, Fabre M, et al. Exudative gastropathy associated with cytomegalovirus infection after allogenic bone marrow transplantation [in French]. *Gastroenterol Clin Biol.* 1994;18(8–9):775–778.
3. Gilles I, Chevallier B, Gelez J, Gompel H, Lagardere B. Benign hypertrophic gastropathy associated with cytomegalovirus infection in children (letter) [in French]. *Presse Med.* 1994;23(4):182.
4. Eisenstat D, Griffiths A, Cutz E, Petric M, Drumm B. Acute cytomegalovirus infection in a child with Ménétrier's disease. *Gastroenterology.* 1995;109(2):592–595.
5. Xiao SY, Hart J. Marked gastric foveolar hyperplasia associated with active cytomegalovirus infection. *Am J Gastroenterol.* 2001;96(1):223–226. PMID: 11197257.
6. Khoshoo V, Alonzo E, Correa H, Levine S, Udall J Jr. Pathological case of the month. Ménétrier's disease with cytomegalovirus gastritis. *Arch Pediatr Adolesc Med.* 1994;148(6):611–612.
7. Nakazato Y, Toyoizumi S, Kinoshita F, Sugiura H, Iri H, Okubo K. Giant hypertrophic gastritis and acute hepatitis associated with cytomegalovirus infection. *Internal Med.* 1992;31(6):816–819.
8. Roussel M, Dupont C, Sidibe T, Andre C, Barbet P, Badoual J. Benign hypertrophic gastritis associated with cytomegalovirus infection [in French]. *Arch Fr Pediatr.* 1990;47(4):271–273.
9. Garcia F, Garau J, Sierra M, Marco V. Cytomegalovirus mononucleosis-associated antral gastritis simulating malignancy. *Arch Internal Med.* 1987;147(4):787–788.
10. Daniels JA, Lederman HM, Maitra A, Montgomery EA. Gastrointestinal tract pathology in patients with common variable immuno-deficiency (CVID): a clinicopathologic study and review. *Am J Surg Pathol.* 2007;31(12):1800–1812. PMID: 18043034.
11. Colaiacovo R, de Castro AC, Shiang C, Ganc RL, Ferrari AP Jr. Disseminated histoplasmosis: a rare cause of multiple ulcers in the gastrointestinal tract. *Endoscopy.* 2011;43(Suppl 2 UCTN):E216. PMID: 21590612.
12. Nudelman HL, Rakatansky H. Gastric histoplasmosis. A case report. *JAMA.* 1966;195(1):44–46. PMID: 5951831.

13. Annunziata ML, Caviglia R, Papparella LG, Cicala M. Upper gastrointestinal involvement of Crohn's disease: a prospective study on the role of upper endoscopy in the diagnostic work-up. *Dig Dis Sci.* 2012;57(6):1618–1623. PMID: 22350786.

14. Sonnenberg A, Melton SD, Genta RM. Frequent occurrence of gastritis and duodenitis in patients with inflammatory bowel disease. *Inflamm Bowel Dis.* 2011;17(1):39–44. PMID: 20848539.

15. Hori K, Ikeuchi H, Nakano H, et al. Gastroduodenitis associated with ulcerative colitis. *J Gastroenterol.* 2008;43(3):193–201. PMID: 18373161.

16. Ruuska T, Vaajalahti P, Arajarvi P, Maki M. Prospective evaluation of upper gastrointestinal mucosal lesions in children with ulcerative colitis and Crohn's disease. *J Pediatr Gastroenterol Nutr.* 1994;19(2):181–186. PMID: 7815240.

17. Oberhuber G, Puspok A, Oesterreicher C, et al. Focally enhanced gastritis: a frequent type of gastritis in patients with Crohn's disease. *Gastroenterology.* 1997;112(3):698–706. PMID: 9041230.

18. Danelius M, Ost A, Lapidus AB. Inflammatory bowel disease-related lesions in the duodenal and gastric mucosa. *Scand J Gastroenterol.* 2009;44(4):441–445. PMID: 19110988.

19. McHugh JB, Gopal P, Greenson JK. The clinical significance of focally enhanced gastritis in children. *Am J Surg Pathol.* 2013;37(2):295–299. PMID: 23108022.

20. Franks I. IBD: Focally enhanced gastritis could help in the diagnosis of paediatric IBD. *Nat Rev Gastroenterol Hepatol.* 2013;10(2):66. PMID: 23247508.

21. Roka K, Roma E, Stefanaki K, Panayotou I, Kopsidas G, Chouliaras G. The value of focally enhanced gastritis in the diagnosis of pediatric inflammatory bowel diseases. *J Crohns Colitis.* 2013;7(10):797–802. PMID: 23207168.

22. Ushiku T, Moran CJ, Lauwers GY. Focally enhanced gastritis in newly diagnosed pediatric inflammatory bowel disease. *Am J Surg Pathol.* 2013;37(12):1882–1888. PMID: 24121177.

23. Xin W, Greenson JK. The clinical significance of focally enhanced gastritis. *Am J Surg Pathol.* 2004;28(10):1347–1351. PMID: 15371951.

24. Diamanti A, Maino C, Niveloni S, et al. Characterization of gastric mucosal lesions in patients with celiac disease: a prospective controlled study. *Am J Gastroenterol.* 1999;94(5):1313–1319. PMID: 10235212.

25. Wu TT, Hamilton SR. Lymphocytic gastritis: association with etiology and topology. *Am J Surg Pathol.* 1999;23(2):153–158. PMID: 9989841.

26. Feeley KM, Heneghan MA, Stevens FM, McCarthy CF. Lymphocytic gastritis and coeliac disease: evidence of a positive association. *J Clin Pathol.* 1998;51(3):207–210. PMID: 9659261.

27. Niemela S, Karttunen T, Kerola T, Karttunen R. Ten year follow up study of lymphocytic gastritis: further evidence on *Helicobacter pylori* as a cause of lymphocytic gastritis and corpus gastritis. *J Clin Pathol.* 1995;48(12):1111–1116. PMID: 8567997.

28. Lynch DA, Sobala GM, Dixon MF, et al. Lymphocytic gastritis and associated small bowel disease: a diffuse lymphocytic gastroenteropathy? *J Clin Pathol.* 1995;48(10):939–945. PMID: 8537495.

29. De Giacomo C, Gianatti A, Negrini R, et al. Lymphocytic gastritis: a positive relationship with celiac disease. *J Pediatr.* 1994;124(1):57–62. PMID: 8283376.

30. Niemela S, Karttunen TJ, Kerola T. Treatment of *Helicobacter pylori* in patients with lymphocytic gastritis. *Hepato-Gastroenterology.* 2001;48(40):1176–1178. PMID: 11490827.

31. Muller H, Volkholz H, Stolte M. Healing of lymphocytic gastritis by eradication of *Helicobacter pylori*. *Digestion.* 2001;63(1):14–19. PMID: 11173895.

32. Hayat M, Arora DS, Dixon MF, Clark B, O'Mahony S. Effects of *Helicobacter pylori* eradication on the natural history of lymphocytic gastritis. *Gut.* 1999;45(4):495–498. PMID: 10486354.

33. Luzza F, Mancuso M, Imeneo M, et al. *Helicobacter pylori* infection in children with celiac disease: prevalence and clinicopathologic features. *J Pediatr Gastroenterol Nutr.* 1999;28(2):143–146. PMID: 9932844.

34. Groisman GM, George J, Berman D, Harpaz N. Resolution of protein-losing hypertrophic lymphocytic gastritis with therapeutic eradication of *Helicobacter pylori*. *Am J Gastroenterol.* 1994;89(9):1548–1551. PMID: 8079936.

35. Haot J, Jouret A, Willette M, Gossuin A, Mainguet P. Lymphocytic gastritis—prospective study of its relationship with varioliform gastritis. *Gut.* 1990;31(3):282–285. PMID: 2323590.

36. Haot J, Hamichi L, Wallez L, Mainguet P. Lymphocytic gastritis: a newly described entity: a retrospective endoscopic and histological study. *Gut.* 1988;29(9):1258–1264. PMID: 3198002.

37. Haot J, Bogomoletz WV, Jouret A, Mainguet P. Ménétrier's disease with lymphocytic gastritis: an unusual association with possible pathogenic implications. *Hum Pathol.* 1991;22(4):379–386. PMID: 2050372.

38. Ricci S, Bonucci A, Fabiani E, et al. Protein-losing gastroenteropathy (Ménétrier's disease) in childhood: a report of 3 cases [in Italian]. *Pediatr Med Chir.* 1996;18(3):269–273.

39. Johnson MI, Spark JI, Ambrose NS, Wyatt JI. Early gastric cancer in a patient with Ménétrier's disease, lymphocytic gastritis and *Helicobacter pylori*. *Eur J Gastroenterol Hepatol.* 1995;7(2):187–190. PMID: 7712313.

40. Wolfsen HC, Carpenter HA, Talley NJ. Ménétrier's disease: a form of hypertrophic gastropathy or gastritis? *Gastroenterology.* 1993;104(5):1310–1319. PMID: 8482445.

41. Amenomori M, Umemoto T, Kushima R, Hattori T. Spontaneous remission of hypertrophic lymphocytic gastritis associated with hypoproteinemia. *Intern Med.* 1998;37(12):1019–1022. PMID: 9932632.

42. Sirigu F, Dessi A, Usai P, Capeccioni S, Masia AM. A retrospective study on the incidence of lymphocytic gastritis in patients with *Helicobacter pylori* infection. *Riv Eur Sci Med Farmacol.* 1995;17(2–3):85–89. PMID: 8545561.

43. Koskela RM, Niemela SE, Lehtola JK, Bloigu RS, Karttunen TJ. Gastroduodenal mucosa in microscopic colitis. *Scand J Gastroenterol.* 2011;46(5):567–576. PMID: 21291294.

44. Verkarre V, Asnafi V, Lecomte T, et al. Refractory coeliac sprue is a diffuse gastrointestinal disease. *Gut.* 2003;52(2):205–211. PMID: 12524401.

45. Christ AD, Meier R, Bauerfeind P, Wegmann W, Gyr K. Simultaneous occurrence of lymphocytic gastritis and lymphocytic colitis with transition to collagenous colitis [in German]. *Schweiz MedWochenschr.* 1993;123(30):1487–1490. PMID: 8367708.

46. Maguire AA, Greenson JK, Lauwers GY, et al. Collagenous sprue: a clinicopathologic study of 12 cases. *Am J Surg Pathol.* 2009;33(10):1440–1449. PMID: 19641452.

47. Leung ST, Chandan VS, Murray JA, Wu TT. Collagenous gastritis: histopathologic features and association with other gastrointestinal diseases. *Am J Surg Pathol.* 2009;33(5):788–798. PMID: 19295410.

48. Miettinen A, Karttunen TJ, Alavaikko M. Lymphocytic gastritis and *Helicobacter pylori* infection in gastric lymphoma. *Gut.* 1995;37(4):471–476. PMID: 7489930.

49. Griffiths AP, Wyatt J, Jack AS, Dixon MF. Lymphocytic gastritis, gastric adenocarcinoma, and primary gastric lymphoma. *J Clin Pathol.* 1994;47(12):1123–1124. PMID: 7876391.

50. Long BW, Johnston JH, Wetzel W, Flowers RH 3rd, Haick A. Gastric syphilis: endoscopic and histological features mimicking lymphoma. *Am J Gastroenterol.* 1995;90(9):1504–1507. PMID: 7661178.

51. Colletti RB, Trainer TD. Collagenous gastritis. *Gastroenterology.* 1989;97(6):1552–1555. PMID: 2583419.

52. Lagorce-Pages C, Fabiani B, Bouvier R, Scoazec JY, Durand L, Flejou JF. Collagenous gastritis: a report of six cases. *Am J Surg Pathol.* 2001;25(9):1174–1179. PMID: 11688577.

53. O'Brien BH, McClymont K, Brown I. Collagenous ileitis: a study of 13 cases. *Am J Surg Pathol.* 2011;35(8):1151–1157. PMID: 21716082.

54. Wang HL, Shah AG, Yerian LM, Cohen RD, Hart J. Collagenous gastritis: an unusual association with profound weight loss. *Arch Pathol Lab Med.* 2004;128(2):229–232. PMID: 14736276.

55. Winslow JL, Trainer TD, Colletti RB. Collagenous gastritis: a long-term follow-up with the development of endocrine cell hyperplasia, intestinal metaplasia, and epithelial changes indeterminate for dysplasia. *Am J Clin Pathol.* 2001;116(5):753–758. PMID: 11710694.

56. Jevremovic D, Torbenson M, Murray JA, Burgart LJ, Abraham SC. Atrophic autoimmune pangastritis: a distinctive form of antral and fundic gastritis associated with systemic autoimmune disease. *Am J Surg Pathol.* 2006;30(11):1412–1419. PMID: 17063082.

PART THREE

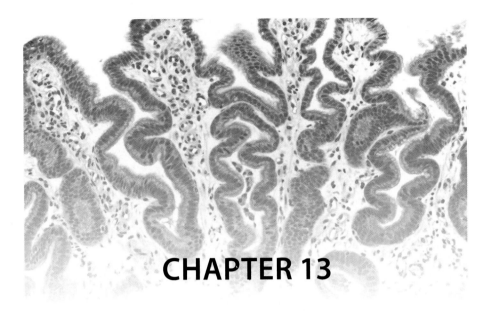

CHAPTER 13

Reactive (Chemical) Gastropathy

David Hernandez Gonzalo and Rish K. Pai

OVERVIEW

Reactive gastropathy (RG) refers to the constellation of microscopic changes caused by chemical injury to the gastric mucosa (Figure 13-1). It is the most commonly rendered diagnosis in gastric biopsies. Based on a large cohort of patients, the diagnosis of RG was rendered in 15.6% of patients undergoing upper endoscopy.[1] The incidence is increasing in part due to an aging population and the broad use of over-the-counter nonsteroidal anti-inflammatory drugs (NSAIDs).

In many cases, the histologic changes fit the toxic-ischemic injury pattern described in Chapter 1. Various mucosal abnormalities can be seen in this setting (Table 13-1), of which foveolar hyperplasia represents the most salient feature. However, these changes are neither sensitive nor specific for an underlying etiology and can be seen in many clinical settings. Reflux of duodenopancreatic contents into the stomach and aspirin/NSAIDs are recognized as the two main causes of RG. William Beaumont in 1833 realized the damaging effects of bile to the gastric mucosa after observing Alexis St. Martin's permanent open gastric fistula.[2] In the 1980s, Dixon et al used the term *reflux gastritis* for the histopathologic findings systematically noted in patients with increased bile acid concentrations in the stomach.[3] They assigned a cumulative reflux gastritis score with a range from 0 to 15. Scores of 10 or greater were thought to be characteristic of RG. More recently, the term *chemical gastritis* or *type C gastritis* was introduced after noticing that most of the "reflux gastritis" cases were indeed associated with long-term use of NSAIDs. There is still controversy among experts on whether the term RG should be favored over chemical gastropathy, but the choice of terminology is not considered crucial as much as the wider recognition of this histological entity. Although not used in daily practice, loss of membrane-associated mucin glycoprotein (MUC1) along with aberrant expression of secretory mucin glycoprotein MUC5AC in pyloric glands have been noted in RG.[4]

CLINICAL ASPECTS

The most common indications for upper endoscopy in patients found to have RG on biopsy are gastroesophageal reflux disease (GERD; 46%), epigastric pain (40%), dyspepsia (17%), and dysphagia (16%).[1] The endoscopic appearance varies from unremarkable gastric mucosa to patchy erythema, edema, erosions, or polypoid mucosal changes. Reddish streaks and bile may be present.[5] The changes are frequently confined to the gastric antrum but can be seen in the body and even cardiac mucosa to a lesser degree.

ETIOLOGY

Bile Reflux

Bile salts increase the permeability of gastric mucosa,[6] resulting in H+ ion back-diffusion, causing accelerated exfoliation of gastric surface epithelial cells and degranulation of mast cells.[7] Bile reflux occurs most commonly as a surgical

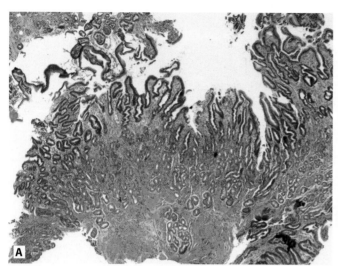
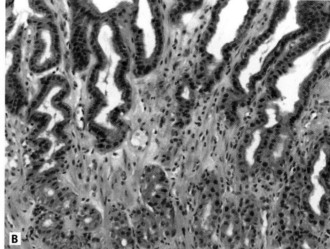

FIGURE 13-1. Reactive gastropathy. **A.** A biopsy of antral mucosa demonstrating foveolar hyperplasia characterized by tortuous foveolar pits imparting a "corkscrew" appearance. **B.** A higher-power view demonstrating a paucity of inflammatory cells and mild fibromuscular hyperplasia of the lamina propria. Note the presence of mucin depletion in the foveolar epithelium.

complication due to gastrectomy or gastric bypass surgery for morbid obesity. However, it may be present in normal individuals, in patients evaluated for GERD, secondary to pyloric sphincter abnormalities (eg, peptic ulcers). Clinically, it may not be easily demonstrated. Bile reflux has also been described post-cholecystectomy or post–ampullary sphincteroplasty due to unregulated and continuous flow of bile.[8]

Gastritis cystica polyposa, a polypoid lesion developed on the anastomotic gastric mucosa characterized by mucosal and submucosal cysts with foveolar hyperplasia, is also a form of RG. Its incidence has rapidly declined with the decrease of the Billroth II partial gastrectomy. Another long-term complication of the Billroth II procedure is gastric stump carcinomas, defined as carcinomas occurring in the gastric remnant at least 5 years after surgery. This is believed to be due to bile reflux-related dysplasia.[9]

Aspirin/NSAIDs

As carboxylic acids, aspirin and NSAIDs can be absorbed across the gastric mucosa and inhibit cyclooxygenase (COX) activity, blocking the production of prostaglandins. The effectiveness in inhibiting COX-1 and COX-2 and the potential to produce adverse effects vary among the different NSAIDs.[10] Short-term use of NSAIDs can produce subepithelial hemorrhage and erosion with fibrin aggregates and few neutrophils (Figure 13-2). Regenerative epithelial changes can be seen adjacent to the eroded areas. In patients on long-term NSAIDs, RG has been identified in 45% of the patients.[11]

FIGURE 13-2. Reactive gastropathy attributable to NSAIDs. The antral biopsy in this case demonstrates foveolar hyperplasia, mucin depletion, fibromuscular hyperplasia, and surface erosion. Erosions tend to be more common in reactive gastropathy due to NSAIDs.

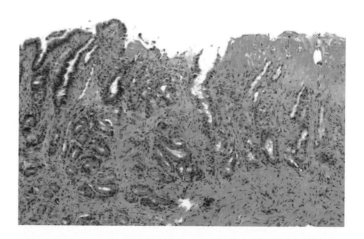

TABLE 13-1. Histologic features of reactive gastropathy.
Foveolar hyperplasia
Epithelial damage with small erosions
Mucous depletion of surface and pit epithelium
Villiform transformation
Prominent fibromuscular hyperplasia
Superficial edema
Congestion of superficial mucosal capillaries
Reactive nuclei with variable nuclear enlargement and hyperchromasia
Increased mitoses in transition zone
No or focal intestinal metaplasia
Paucity of inflammatory cells

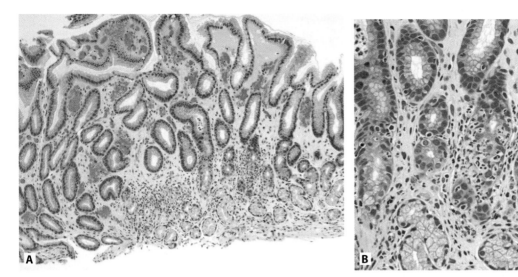

FIGURE 13-3. Alcohol gastropathy. **A.** Marked foveolar hyperplasia, mucosal hemorrhage, and foci of neutrophilic infiltration. **B.** High-power view of neutrophilic infiltration of gastric pits. Note the total lack of inflammatory cellular infiltration in the lamina propria. The term *alcohol gastritis* may be used diagnostically by some pathologists.

Alcohol

Sobala et al[10] noticed a trend toward an association with high alcohol intake and "chemical gastritis." The term *hemorrhagic gastritis* is frequently applied to the subepithelial hemorrhages seen endoscopically in alcoholic patients. The hemorrhage occurs primarily in the foveolar region.[12] Mucosal edema and foveolar hyperplasia can be noted in the adjacent nonhemorrhagic mucosa, and the inflammatory infiltrates are usually mild (Figure 13-3).

Iron Pill

In iron pill gastropathy, there is extracellular iron deposition with golden-brown crystals embedded in granulation tissue or entrapped in the superficial lamina propria (Figure 13-4). The crystals can also be identified in macrophages and other stromal cells and focally in epithelium and vessel walls. A Prussian blue stain can be useful when there is doubt regarding the nature of these deposits. Erosions and foveolar hyperplasia can be present. Of note, the epithelial changes in iron pill gastritis can be striking and mimic dysplasia.[13]

FIGURE 13-4. Iron pill gastritis. **A.** This biopsy of oxyntic/fundic mucosa demonstrates mild foveolar hyperplasia as well as attenuated surface epithelium. There is prominent deposition of golden-brown material within the lamina propria. **B.** A Prussian blue stain highlights these lamina propria deposits.

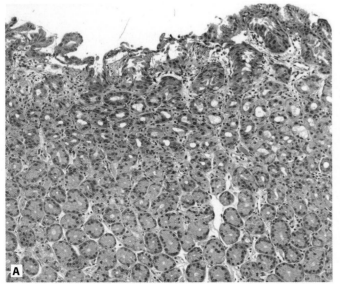
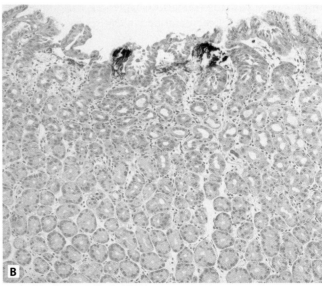

Kayexalate Resin Crystals

Kayexalate (sodium polystyrene sulfonate) in sorbitol used in hyperkalemia can induce damage to the upper gastrointestinal (GI) tract, including erosions and ulcerations.[14] The crystals display a mosaic pattern resembling fish scales. They are refractile, nonpolarizable, and basophilic on hematoxylin and eosin (H&E) stain. Acid-fast, periodic acid–Schiff (PAS)/Alcian blue, and Diff-Quick can be helpful in their identification.

Gastric Mucosal Calcinosis

Gastric mucosal calcinosis (GMC) is described in patients with organ transplantation or chronic renal failure who are taking aluminum-containing antacids or sucralfate.[15] The cyanophilic granular deposits consist of aluminum, phosphorus, calcium, and chlorine. They are present within the lamina propria beneath the surface epithelium at the tips of the foveolae surrounded by macrophages (Figure 13-5). These changes can be seen in association with foveolar hyperplasia, reactive epithelium, and lamina propria edema. Von Kossa stain highlights the presence of calcium deposits.

Colchicine

Colchicine, an alkaloid with antimitotic activity, is used to treat gout and many rheumatologic disorders. Patients with renal or liver failure are at risk for its toxicity. The morphologic features of colchicine toxicity include metaphase mitoses restricted to the neck region of gastric mucosa, epithelial pseudostratification with loss of polarity, and not infrequently abundant crypt apoptotic bodies. The changes are preferentially seen in duodenum and gastric antrum.[16]

Mycophenolate Mofetil

Mycophenolate mofetil (MMF) is an immunosuppressive drug used in patients with solid-organ transplant. Histologic changes include mild increase in apoptotic bodies, mimicking mainly grade 1 graft-vs-host disease (GVHD). The gastric mucosa can demonstrate features of RG, erosion, or chronic active gastritis (see also Chapter 2). Ballooning of the parietal cells has been described in this setting.[17]

Steroids

Steroids stimulate G-cell hyperplasia, producing an increase in acid production by parietal cells.[18] The literature on corticosteroids as an independent risk factor producing gastric damage is limited. Some studies have shown a two-fold increased risk of upper GI complications.[19] Patients using steroids concomitantly with high-dose NSAIDs have the highest risk of upper GI complications.

Doxycycline Gastropathy

Patients who are taking some oral antibiotics may develop abdominal pain or other upper GI symptoms. More recently, doxycycline, a tetracycline-like drug, has been found to induce severe gastropathy characterized by superficial epithelial loss, erosion, and microangiopathic changes in the

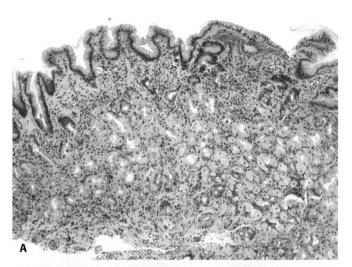

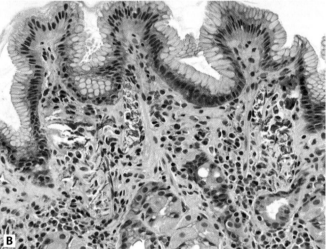

FIGURE 13-5. Gastric mucosal calcinosis in a 75-year-old female patient with end-stage renal disease. **A.** There is mild mixed inflammatory infiltrate in the superficial lamina propria, associated with mild fibrosis. **B.** High-power view demonstrates foci of "fractured" calcifications.

superficial lamina propria, including microthrombi (see Chapter 1). Discontinuation of the drug leads to both symptomatic and histologic resolution.[20,21]

Chemo-Radiotherapy–Induced Gastric Damage

Radiation often accompanies chemotherapy, so differentiating between both effects may not be feasible. Both can produce erosion/ulceration, ectatic capillary vessels, and stromal edema. Epithelial damage with minimal or no inflammation is typically noted. The cytoplasm demonstrates vacuolation and eosinophilic transformation. The nuclei are markedly enlarged and bizarre, without significant increase in nuclear-to-cytoplasmic (N/C) ratio. Prominent apoptosis and mitotic arrest with ring mitoses have been associated with the effect of taxanes.[22] In radiation-induced injury, the lamina propria becomes hyalinized, and there is more

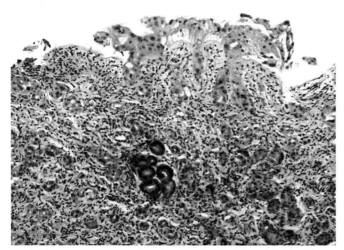

FIGURE 13-6. Radiation injury. There is loss of surface epithelium, epithelial flattening, and mucin depletion. The gastric pits and surface epithelial cells demonstrate marked reactive cytologic atypia. Note the hyalinized lamina propria with increased inflammatory infiltrate comprised mostly of lymphocytes and plasma cells.

arterial damage than with chemotherapy (Figure 13-6). Selective internal radiation with yttrium microspheres used for inoperable primary or metastatic liver tumors can be a cause of radiation gastritis as the microspheres can be lodged in the gastric circulation.[23]

MICROSCOPIC FEATURES

Foveolar Hyperplasia
Foveolar hyperplasia consists of an extension/elongation and tortuosity of the gastric pits as a reflection of an increased turnover of the foveolar cells, compensating the accelerated loss of surface epithelial cells. The luminal outlining adopts a serrated "corkscrew" appearance, and the surface mucosa may demonstrate a villiform configuration (Figures 13-1 and 13-2).

Mucin Depletion of Surface and Pit Epithelium
The foveolar cells show mucin depletion, adopting a cuboidal shape (normal foveolar cells are columnar), with cells having an increased N/C ratio. These areas are easily spotted at low-power magnification.

Nuclear Enlargement and Hyperchromasia
The nuclei of the foveolar cells demonstrate mild-to-moderate nuclear enlargement and become hyperchromatic. Nuclei tend to be centered within the cell (as opposed to basally located in normal foveolar epithelium), and a single nucleolus can commonly be noted.

Lamina Propria Edema and Congestion of Superficial Mucosal Capillaries
Lamina propria edema and congestion represent the histamine-mediated vascular component of the inflammatory response.

They have been found to be good predictors of an elevated bile acid level.[10] Edema is an occasional finding in patients on NSAIDs and can also be seen in active cases of *Helicobacter pylori* gastritis.

Paucity of Active and Chronic Inflammatory Cells
No or mild inflammation should be the rule for RG. Few lymphocytes can be noted sprinkled in the lamina propria, but finding small clusters or bands of lymphocytes or plasma cells in the superficial mucosa is indicative of chronic gastritis.[24] Neutrophils can be identified, generally restricted to the lamina propria without neutrophil-mediated epithelial injury except in areas with erosions or ulcerations (Figure 13-3).

Fibromuscular Replacement of the Lamina Propria
There is a proliferation of smooth muscle fibers in the interfoveolar lamina propria perpendicular to the surface epithelium secondary to release of platelet-derived growth factor (PDGF). This histologic finding is not specific and has been described in other entities, such as gastric antral vascular ectasia (GAVE). In addition, smooth muscle fibers are noted in the lamina propria of the gastric antrum, especially when some degree of prolapse into the pylorus is present.

Increased Mitoses
Due to the increased turnover, increased mitotic figures can be noted, mostly in the transition zone. Atypical mitotic figures should not be encountered in RG.

Other Features
Although not a feature classically described in RG, Rubio et al demonstrated the presence of foveolar cell vacuolization in patients with prior Billroth I and II gastrectomies.[25] Endocrine cell hyperplasia and parietal cell alterations are increasingly seen in conjunction with RG due to the fact that NSAIDs-mediated injury can be reduced by proton pump inhibitors (PPIs).

DIFFERENTIAL DIAGNOSIS

Helicobacter pylori Gastritis
Mild foveolar hyperplasia can be seen in cases of *H. pylori* gastritis as a consequence of the epithelial degeneration caused when the bacteria and their toxins interact with the surface cell membrane (Figure 13-7). However, marked foveolar hyperplasia may alert for a concomitant gastric chemical injury.[24] The pattern of injury is usually limited to the gastric antrum, although the vast use of PPIs leads to a decreased number of bacteria and shift from antrum to proximal stomach. Microscopically, diffuse chronic monocytic inflammation is identified. The presence of neutrophils is indicative of active infection, and large lymphoid follicles may develop. Immunohistochemical stain for *H. pylori* is favored over other special stains because it can identify small coccoid forms present in partially treated patients.[26]

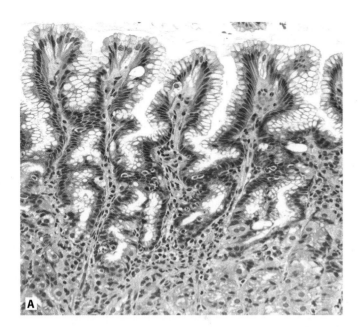

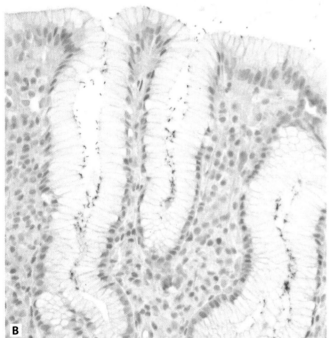

FIGURE 13-7. *Helicobacter pylori* gastritis. **A.** *H. pylori* gastritis can demonstrate mild foveolar hyperplasia. However, a lymphoplasmacytic infiltrate along with scattered foci of neutrophilic pititis are not usually seen in reactive gastropathy. **B.** Immunostain for *H. pylori* highlights numerous organisms.

Gastric Antral Vascular Ectasia

The GAVE entity is an uncommon cause of GI hemorrhage. Endoscopically, longitudinal rugal folds converging from the gastric antrum into the pylorus are identified that contain red mucosa stripes resembling the stripes on a watermelon. GAVE typically affects elderly women with iron deficiency anemia. Cirrhosis is present in 30% of cases, and GAVE has also been associated with autoimmune conditions.[27] Histologic examination reveals foveolar hyperplasia, marked vascular ectasia, intravascular fibrin thrombi, and fibromuscular proliferation (Figure 13-8). Endoscopic thermal ablation is the treatment of choice.

Portal Hypertensive Gastropathy

Similar to GAVE, portal hypertensive gastropathy (PHG) can also cause GI bleeding. Endoscopic findings are classically described as a "mosaic pattern" with or without red spots.[28] It is characterized by dilated large-caliber capillaries and dilated veins in the mucosa and submucosa (Figure 13-9). The vessels, unlike GAVE, lack fibrin thrombi. The changes may only be present in the submucosa, and a normal gastric biopsy

FIGURE 13-8. Gastric antral vascular ectasia (GAVE). **A.** GAVE often has all the histologic features characteristic of reactive gastropathy, including foveolar hyperplasia and fibromuscular hyperplasia of the lamina propria. **B.** GAVE is often characterized by the presence of fibrin thrombi within small lamina propria vessels, as seen in this example.

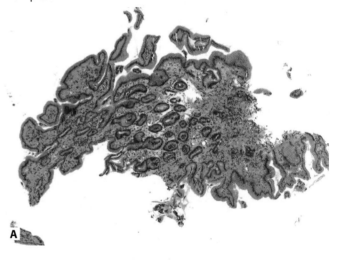

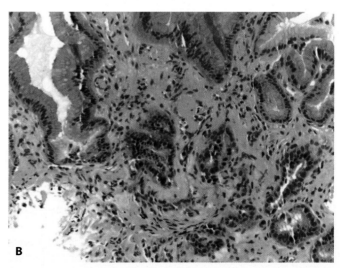

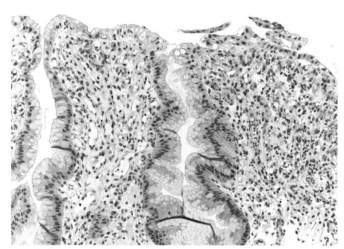

FIGURE 13-9. Portal hypertensive gastropathy. Foveolar hyperplasia in this entity is accompanied by capillary proliferation and dilation, mixed with mild or minimal inflammatory infiltration. There are no microthrombi.

does not therefore exclude PHG. In addition, the presence of capillary dilation in gastric mucosal biopsies may be seen in patients with and without portal hypertension.[27] Reduction of portal hypertension is the mainstay of treatment. GAVE and PHG may coexist in some patients.

Low-Grade Dysplasia

As opposed to RG, for which there is a gradual transition between the atypical and adjacent normal cells as well as the characteristic architectural configuration of foveolar hyperplasia (Figure 13-10), in dysplasia this transition tends to be sharp (Figure 13-11). Reparative changes in the vicinity of erosions and ulcers can be striking in RG and may resemble

FIGURE 13-10. Chemical gastropathy with marked reactive changes. The epithelial cells exhibit mucin depletion, rendering the impression of increased nuclear-to-cytoplasmic ratio; there are marked nuclear hyperchromasia and mitotic figures. However, the overall architecture of reactive foveolar hyperplasia is evident.

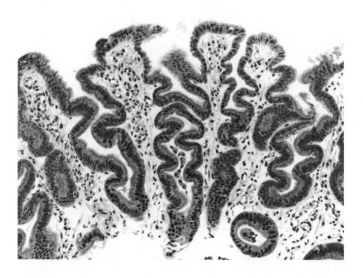

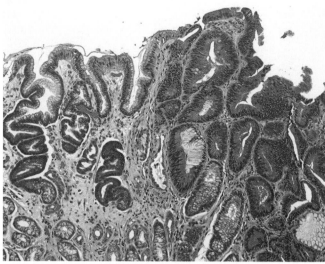

FIGURE 13-11. Low-grade dysplasia. Reactive gastropathy can sometimes mimic gastric dysplasia. In this example, an area of foveolar hyperplasia (left) is adjacent to an area of low-grade dysplasia (right). The area of dysplasia clearly has more nuclear enlargement, stratification, and hyperchromasia. Foveolar hyperplasia can also be seen adjacent to an ulcer or mass.

low-grade dysplasia (LGD). Intestinal metaplasia (mostly focal) or atrophy may develop in long-standing RG, but extensive intestinal metaplasia is more frequently seen in the background of chronic gastritis. Foci of intestinal metaplasia may also be concerning for adenomatous-type dysplasia (type 1), especially if there are superimposed reactive epithelial changes.[29] The cuboidal shape of the cells can be seen both in RG and in nonadenomatous gastric epithelial dysplasia (type 2 dysplasia), for which the nuclei are less stratified than in type 1.[30] The degree of architectural complexity is variable and might not be helpful in most instances in the differential diagnosis of RG vs LGD. Mitoses in RG tend to be limited to the transition zone, whereas in LGD they can be seen in the surface epithelium.

Ménétrier Disease

Ménétrier disease (MD) is a rare cause of gastric foveolar hyperplasia. It is a hypertrophic gastropathy characterized by giant gastric fundic folds, hypochlorhydria, protein loss, abdominal pain, and peripheral edema (see Chapter 14). The pathology diffusely affects the gastric body and results in marked thickening of the rugal folds. Histologically, there is marked foveolar hyperplasia; glandular tortuosity with cystic dilation and marked reduction in parietal cell number are invariably present (Figures 13-12 and 13-13).[31] Other frequent histologic findings include smooth muscle hyperplasia, edema, and prominent eosinophils or plasma cells in lamina propria. Full-thickness mucosal biopsy is recommended in MD because superficial biopsies might not be deep enough to reveal the presence of glandular atrophy or cystic dilation at the base.

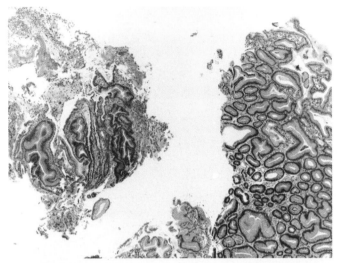

FIGURE 13-12. Ménétrier disease. The histologic features resemble reactive gastropathy and gastric hyperplastic polyps, with marked foveolar hyperplasia and edema. No normal fundic glands are present in this biopsy of the gastric body.

Hyperplastic Polyps and Hamartomatous Polyps

Hyperplastic polyps and hamartomatous polyps can demonstrate histologic findings present in RG, such as foveolar hyperplasia with mucin depletion, surface erosion, and edematous lamina propria (Figure 13-14). However, as opposed to RG and MD, hyperplastic polyps show a loss of parallelism of the glandular units with distortion of mucosal architecture.[32] Hyperplastic polyps and juvenile polyps do not show in general significant increase in lamina propria eosinophils as frequently is seen in MD.

FIGURE 13-13. Ménétrier disease. A higher-power view showing prominent foveolar hyperplasia and focally with epithelial reactive change due to erosions.

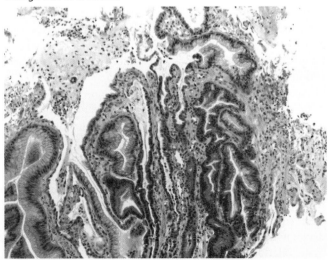

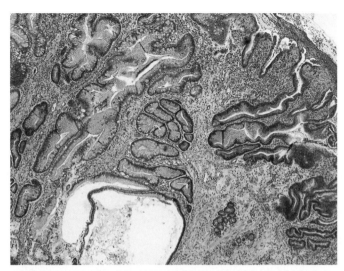

FIGURE 13-14. Hyperplastic polyps. Hyperplastic polyps are characterized by distorted, irregular, cystically dilated gastric pits lined by hyperplastic foveolar epithelium. Often, the lamina propria is edematous and inflamed. Erosions are common. The foveolar hyperplasia can mimic changes seen in reactive gastropathy; however, the marked edema and lamina propria inflammation along with the endoscopic appearance of a polyp differentiate the two diagnoses.

■ CONCLUSIONS

Reactive gastropathy is an increasingly common entity seen in gastric antral biopsies. Most RG is associated with either NSAIDs or bile reflux. The diagnosis relies on the pathologist, and it is based on the recognition of a group of histologic features for which foveolar hyperplasia should invariably be present for a definitive degree of certainty. RG may sometimes be overlooked by pathologists in their effort not to miss *H. pylori* gastritis, especially if the changes are not marked. The finding of focal intestinal metaplasia should not automatically prompt a diagnosis of chronic gastritis because it can be seen especially in the elderly population on long-standing NSAIDs therapy. Moderate-to-severe chronic inflammation in a gastric antral biopsy is not a feature of RG. However, concomitant prominent foveolar hyperplasia should raise the possibility of a chemical gastropathy component. Although RG is not a predictor for adverse effects such as bleeding or ulcer formation, recognizing this entity helps the clinician modify the patient's management by reducing/discontinuing NSAIDs treatment or by adding protective drugs, such as PPIs.

■ REFERENCES

1. Maguilnik I, Neumann WL, Sonnenberg A, Genta RM. Reactive gastropathy is associated with inflammatory conditions throughout the gastrointestinal tract. *Aliment Pharmacol Ther.* 2012;36:736–743.
2. Bensley EH. Alexis St. Martin. *CMAJ.* 1959;80(11):907–909. PMID: 13662949. PMCID: 1831067.
3. Dixon MF, O'Connor HJ, Axon AT, King RF, Johnston D. Reflux gastritis: distinct histopathological entity? *J Clin Pathol.* 1986;39:524–530.

4. Mino-Kenudson M, Tomita S, Lauwers GY. Mucin expression in reactive gastropathy: an immunohistochemical analysis. *Arch Pathol Lab Med.* 2007;131:86–90.

5. Chen T-S, Li AF-Y, Chang F-Y. Gastric reddish streaks in the intact stomach: endoscopic feature of reactive gastropathy. *Pathol Int.* 2010;60:298–304.

6. Bushnell L, Bjorkman D, McGreevy J. Ultrastructural changes in gastric epithelium caused by bile salt. *J Surg Res.* 1990;49:280–286.

7. Bechi P, Amorosi A, Mazzanti R, et al. Reflux-related gastric mucosal injury is associated with increased mucosal histamine content in humans. *Gastroenterology.* 1993;104:1057–1063.

8. Warshaw AL. Bile gastritis without prior gastric surgery: contributing role of cholecystectomy. *Am J Surg.* 1979;137:527–531.

9. Sinning C, Schaefer N, Standop J, Hirner A, Wolff M. Gastric stump carcinoma—epidemiology and current concepts in pathogenesis and treatment. *Eur J Surg Oncol.* 2007;33:133–139.

10. Sobala GM, O'Connor HJ, Dewar EP, King RF, Axon AT, Dixon MF. Bile reflux and intestinal metaplasia in gastric mucosa. *J Clin Pathol.* 1993;46:235–240.

11. Quinn CM, Bjarnason I, Price AB. Gastritis in patients on nonsteroidal anti-inflammatory drugs. *Histopathology.* 1993;23:341–348.

12. Laine L, Weinstein WM. Histology of alcoholic hemorrhagic "gastritis": a prospective evaluation. *Gastroenterology.* 1988;94:1254–1262.

13. Marginean EC, Bennick M, Cyczk J, Robert ME, Jain D. Gastric siderosis: patterns and significance. *Am J Surg Pathol.* 2006;30:514–520.

14. Abraham SC, Bhagavan BS, Lee LA, Rashid A, Wu TT. Upper gastrointestinal tract injury in patients receiving kayexalate (sodium polystyrene sulfonate) in sorbitol: clinical, endoscopic, and histopathologic findings. *Am J Surg Pathol.* 2001;25:637–644.

15. Greenson JK, Trinidad SB, Pfeil SA, et al. Gastric mucosal calcinosis. Calcified aluminum phosphate deposits secondary to aluminum-containing antacids or sucralfate therapy in organ transplant patients. *Am J Surg Pathol.* 1993;17:45–50.

16. Iacobuzio-Donahue CA, Lee EL, Abraham SC, Yardley JH, Wu TT. Colchicine toxicity: distinct morphologic findings in gastrointestinal biopsies. *Am J Surg Pathol.* 2001;25:1067–1073.

17. Nguyen T, Park JY, Scudiere JR, Montgomery E. Mycophenolic acid (Cellcept and Myofortic) induced injury of the upper GI tract. *Am J Surg Pathol.* 2009;33:1355–1363.

18. Delaney JP, Michel HM, Bonsack ME, Eisenberg MM, Dunn DH. Adrenal corticosteroids cause gastrin cell hyperplasia. *Gastroenterology.* 1979;76:913–916.

19. Hernández-Díaz S, Rodríguez LA. Steroids and risk of upper gastrointestinal complications. *Am J Epidemiol.* 2001;153:1089–1093.

20. Xiao SY, Zhao L, Hart J, Semrad CE. Gastric mucosal necrosis with vascular degeneration induced by doxycycline. *Am J Surg Pathol.* 2013;37(2):259–263. PMID: 23060354.

21. Xiao SY, Zhao L, Hart J, Semrad CE. Doxycycline-induced gastric and esophageal mucosal injuries with vascular degeneration. *Am J Surg Pathol.* 2013;37(7):1115–1116. PMID: 23759935.

22. Hruban RH, Yardley JH, Donehower RC, Boitnott JK. Taxol toxicity. Epithelial necrosis in the gastrointestinal tract associated with polymerized microtubule accumulation and mitotic arrest. *Cancer.* 1989;63:1944–1950.

23. Ogawa F, Mino-Kenudson M, Shimizu M, Ligato S, Lauwers GY. Gastroduodenitis associated with yttrium 90-microsphere selective internal radiation: an iatrogenic complication in need of recognition. *Arch Pathol Lab Med.* 2008;132:1734–1738.

24. Dixon M. The components of gastritis: histology and pathogenesis. In: Graham DY, Genta RM, Dixon MF, eds. *Gastritis.* Philadelphia, PA: Lippincott Williams & Williams; 1999:51–56.

25. Rubio CA, Slezak P. Foveolar cell vacuolization in operated stomachs. *Am J Surg Pathol.* 1988;12:773–776.

26. Montgomery E, Voltaggio L. Stomach. In: Biopsy interpretation of the gastrointestinal tract mucosa, Vol 1: Non-neoplastic, 2nd ed. Philadelphia, PA: Lippincott Williams & Williams; 2012:73.

27. Dulai GS, Jensen DM, Kovacs TOG, Gralnek IM, Jutabha R. Endoscopic treatment outcomes in watermelon stomach patients with and without portal hypertension. *Endoscopy.* 2004;36:68–72.

28. Misra SP, Dwivedi M, Misra V, et al. Endoscopic and histologic appearance of the gastric mucosa in patients with portal hypertension. *Gastrointest Endosc.* 1990;36:575–579.

29. DeNardi F, Riddell R. Gastropathy and gastritis. In: Graham DY, Genta RM, Dixon MF, eds. *Gastritis.* Philadelphia, PA: Lippincott Williams & Williams; 1999:125–146.

30. Srivastava A, Lauwers GY. Gastric epithelial dysplasia: the Western perspective. *Dig Liver Dis.* 2008;40:641–649.

31. Rich A, Toro TZ, Tanksley J, et al. Distinguishing Ménétrier's disease from its mimics. *Gut.* 2010;59:1617–1624.

32. Komorowski RA, Caya JG. Hyperplastic gastropathy. Clinicopathologic correlation. *Am J Surg Pathol.* 1991;15:577–585.

PART THREE

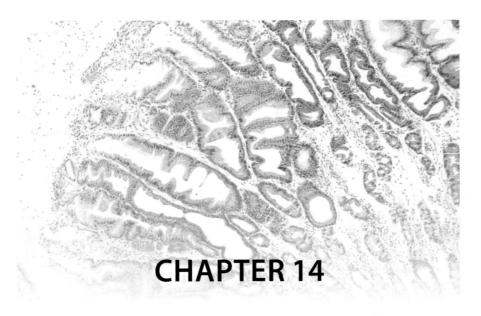

CHAPTER 14

Hypertrophic Gastropathy

Safia Nawazish Salaria and Mary Kay Washington

INTRODUCTION

The pathologic correlation to endoscopically observed "giant" or "thickened" gastric folds spans myriad pathologies that range from common reactive epithelial responses to rarer disorders. Definitive diagnoses require knowledge of the gastric mucosal compartment, which is hyperplastic, coupled with endoscopic and clinical findings and lab values. Superficial pinch forceps biopsies may be inadequate to evaluate thickened gastric folds given the histomorphologic overlap of gastric mucosal responses to a variety of injuries. For this reason, full-thickness sampling with a snare biopsy is encouraged.

An understanding of normal gastric body and antral mucosal histology is crucial for recognizing deviations and irregularities present in hypertrophic gastropathies. Mucin-secreting foveolar epithelium (also known as mucous neck cells) constitutes the superficial mucosal layer in all areas of the stomach and extends into the gastric pits. Gastric fundus and body glands contain parietal cells, chief cells, and endocrine cells (enterochromaffin-like [ECL] cells, somatostatin cells); pits are relatively short and occupy about one-quarter of the mucosa. In the gastric cardia and antrum, the pits occupy about one-half of the mucosal thickness. The deep mucosa in these areas is predominantly composed of mucin-secreting glands. Gastrin-secreting G cells are found only in the antrum, and scattered parietal cells are present, although chief cells are rare (Figure 14-1).

Gastric hypertrophic changes are observed in a variety of pathologic entities, including foveolar hyperplasia in response to an adjacent erosion/ulcer, nodular hyperplastic polyps, and hamartomatous syndromes. The hyperplasia maybe focal, as seen in solitary hyperplastic polyps, or diffuse; it may involve one compartment, such as the foveolar epithelium in Ménétrier disease, or all gastric glandular components, such as in hypersecretory hypertrophic gastritis (Table 14-1).

DIFFUSE HYPERPLASIAS

Ménétrier Disease

First described in 1888 by the eponymous Dr. Pierre Eugène Ménétrier, Ménétrier disease is a rare, acquired, premalignant, gastric body–centric, protein-losing gastropathy.[1] It is also known as hypoproteinemic hypertrophic gastropathy and giant hypertrophic gastritis.[2] Ménétrier disease has two distinct forms; the classic, chronic form is seen in adults (average age is 55 years) and has an unfavorable prognosis. A second form, associated with cytomegalovirus (CMV) infection and characterized by acute onset and spontaneous resolution, has been observed in the pediatric age group.[3]

Clinical Features

The classic form of Ménétrier disease shows a male predominance (3:1). Onset is insidious, and symptoms are primarily sequelae of hypoproteinemia and hypochlorhydria. Peripheral edema, epigastric pain, diarrhea, anemia, weight loss, and malnutrition are common at presentation. Laboratory values indicate hypoalbuminemia along with a

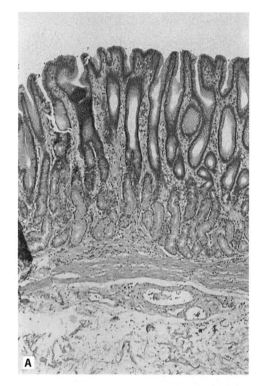

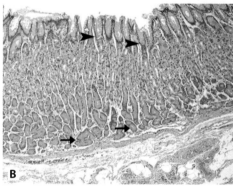

FIGURE 14-1. Normal gastric mucosa. **A.** Mucous-secreting glands deep in the mucosa are characteristic of the gastric antrum. **B.** Oxyntic mucosa of the gastric body, showing short gastric pits (arrowheads) and gastric glands with parietal and chief cells (arrows). Note the intact 4:1 gland-to-pit ratio.

TABLE 14-1. Morphologic approach to gastric mucosal hyperplasias.

Hyperplastic mucosal compartment	Differential diagnosis
Foveolar epithelium	Focal foveolar hyperplasia
	Hyperplastic polyp
	Hamartomatous polyp
	Ménétrier disease
Parietal cells	Zollinger-Ellison syndrome
All layers	Hypertrophic hypersecretory gastropathy

TABLE 14-2. Diagnostic features of Ménétrier disease in patients with chronic symptoms.

Clinical	Endoscopic	Histologic
↓ Serum albumin	Diffusely enlarged folds in corpus	Massive foveolar hyperplasia
Peripheral edema	↓ Gastric acidity	Decreased parietal cells
Normal serum gastrin	Increased mucin production	Maintenance of mucosal architecture

decrease in other proteins (eg, transferrin, immunoglobulins). Parietal cell loss leads to an increase in gastric pH; despite this, serum gastrin levels remain relatively normal (Table 14-2).

Ménétrier disease has also been associated with autoimmune conditions such as sclerosing cholangitis and ankylosing spondylitis, as well as with inflammatory bowel disease.[4,5]

Endoscopic Features

Ménétrier disease primarily affects the gastric body, only rarely involving the antrum as well. Convolutions of enlarged hypertrophic mucosal folds are reminiscent of cerebral gyri (Figure 14-2).

Gastric mucus is often viscous and has a neutral or alkaline pH (pH 4–7; normal gastric pH 1–3) due to the decreased number of parietal cells (Figure 14-3).

Microscopic Features

Full-thickness snare biopsies are essential for accurate evaluation of pathologic features.

FIGURE 14-2. Ménétrier disease with markedly thickened mucosal folds with notable sparing of the antrum (arrow).

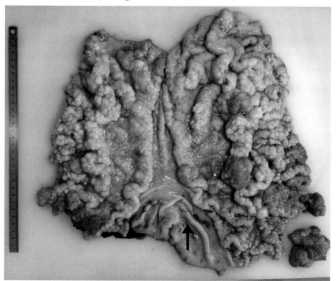

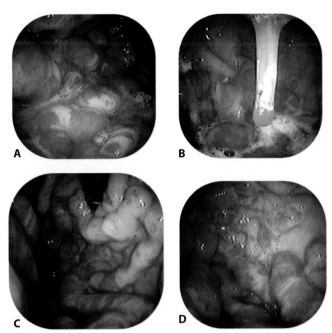

FIGURE 14-3. Endoscopic appearance of Ménétrier disease. **A.** Gastric body greater curvature. Thick, bright red folds with interspersed whitish areas; viscous light-green mucous pools are present between hypertrophic gastric folds. **B.** One of several hanging mucous strands in the gastric body. **C.** Turnaround view in the gastric body. The folds are grossly thickened even with full insufflation, and they surround the entry point of the endoscope in a serpentine pattern. **D.** Body/antral interface, greater curvature. The thick distal body folds taper off into a more normal antral mucosa (right).

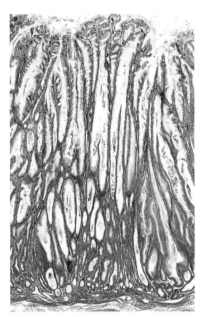

FIGURE 14-4. Ménétrier disease, low-power view showing elongated glands due to foveolar hyperplasia, with tortuous superficial glands with cystic dilation prominent in the deeper glands.

General The most striking feature of Ménétrier disease is massive hyperplasia of the foveolar compartment of the mucosa. Variable amounts of predominantly chronic inflammation with scattered clusters of eosinophils may be seen, and superficial erosion of the enlarged folds is common, although intestinal metaplasia and deep ulcers are not features of the disorder.

Foveolar Glands The gastric foveolar glands are markedly elongated and tortuous due to preferential hyperplasia of the foveolar epithelium, with relatively few parietal cells and chief cells. The deeper glands may be cystically dilated (Figure 14-4).

Oxyntic Glands In most cases of Ménétrier disease, there is a decrease in parietal cell mass. Overall atrophy of the oxyntic mucosa and replacement by extension of foveolar-type cells deep into the mucosa is a prominent feature. Scattered strands of smooth muscles intervening between mucous glands are often seen within the lamina propria (Figure 14-5).

Pathophysiology

Transforming growth factor α (TGF-α), a ligand that binds to epidermal growth factor receptor (EGFR) and is present in a number of other epithelia (eg, pancreas, breast, intestine, and

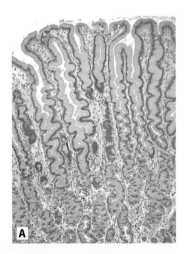

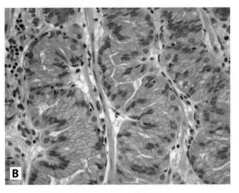

FIGURE 14-5. Ménétrier disease. **A.** Medium power shows gastric body with notably decreased oxyntic glands. **B.** Prominent strands of smooth muscle within the lamina propria.

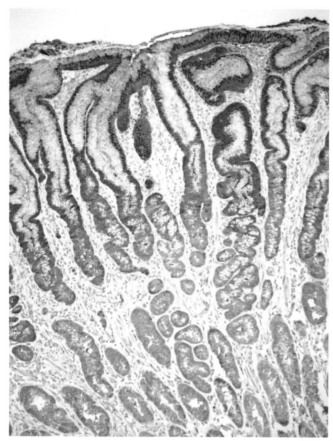

FIGURE 14-6. Transforming growth factor α (TGF-α) immunoreactivity in the gastric mucosa of a patient with Ménétrier disease.

liver) activates downstream signaling pathways that promote gastric epithelial repair and renewal while inhibiting acid secretion. More than 20 years ago, studies using mouse models with overexpression of TGF-α demonstrated a gastric phenotype of foveolar hyperplasia with decreased parietal cells analogous to histologic changes observed in human patients[6] with Ménétrier disease. Subsequently, TGF-α immunoreactivity has been demonstrated in the hyperplastic gastric mucosa of patients with Ménétrier disease[1,7,8] (Figure 14-6). As part of the normal response to injury in the gastric mucosa, TGF-α levels generally subside as the injury heals. However, this normal feedback loop appears to be disrupted in Ménétrier disease, which is characterized by sustained high levels of mucosal TGF-α. While the cause of this persistent overexpression of gastric mucosal TGF-α has not been elucidated in Ménétrier disease, it is possible that subclinical gastric injury may trigger appropriate TGF-α release and activation of downstream EGFR signaling. Ménétrier disease may result from a failure of the normal feedback loop.

Variants

Spontaneously Remitting Form　Cytomegalovirus and *Helicobacter pylori* infections have been associated with acute onset and spontaneous remission of Ménétrier disease. Although CMV-associated Ménétrier disease is more commonly reported in children older than 6 weeks, adults may also be affected[9] (also see Chapter 15, Figure 15-23). The principal envelope protein of CMV, glycoprotein B, serves as a ligand, binding to EGFR, leading to heterodimerization of EGFR with other cell surface receptors activating signaling pathways regulating cell proliferation.

Familial　Although the majority of Ménétrier disease cases appear to be acquired, there are reports of inherited Ménétrier disease transmitted in an autosomal dominant fashion and presenting with anemia rather than hypoproteinemia. Given the histologic overlap between Ménétrier disease and gastric polyposis syndromes and lack of increased TGF-α[10] by immunohistochemistry and reverse transcriptase polymerase chain reaction (RT-PCR) in the reported cases, the possibility that such cases represent uncharacterized forms of gastric polyposis should be considered.

Hypertrophic Lymphocytic Gastritis　Hypertrophic lymphocytic gastritis, like classic Ménétrier disease, often presents as giant mucosal folds in the gastric body with relative sparing of the antrum. It is characterized by diffuse and severe lymphocytic mucosal inflammation with prominent intraepithelial lymphocytosis. Studies comparing this entity to Ménétrier disease have concluded that it is best categorized within the spectrum of lymphocytic gastritis.[11]

Treatment and Prognosis

Ménétrier disease in adults is a chronic debilitating condition with a poor prognosis. Adult patients run an estimated 2%–15% lifetime risk of gastric cancer. Conversely, the disease is often self-limiting in children, with no increased predisposition to neoplasia reported. Gastrectomy remains the mainstay of treatment of the chronic form of the disease. The use of cetuximab, an EGFR ligand-binding antibody, has shown near-total histologic remission along with marked improvement of clinical symptoms in the research setting.[12-14] Results with other medical treatments, including steroids, octreotide, antibiotics, and nonsteroidal anti-inflammatory agents, have been inconsistent. Ultimately, most patients undergo gastrectomy due to lack of medical treatment options and the concern for increased risk of gastric neoplasia.

Hypertrophic Hypersecretory Gastropathy

Hypertrophic hypersecretory gastropathy is a rare acquired gastropathy defined as hyperplasia of all glandular compartments of the gastric body with hypersecretion of acid, pepsin, and mucoprotein. Much of the literature on this condition pre-dates the recognition of *Helicobacter pylori* gastritis, and it is possible that some cases represent polypoid gastritis due to infection with this organism.

Clinical Features

Abdominal pain, anorexia, and nausea are common clinical presenting symptoms. Laboratory tests demonstrating hypoalbuminemia and normal to slightly elevated serum gastrin are similar to those observed in Ménétrier disease.

Endoscopic Features

Hypertrophied gastric folds and "cobblestone" gastric body mucosa are seen endoscopically.[15,16] Distinct masses and tumors are uncommon. The gastric antral mucosa has been described as atrophic. Concomitant gastric and duodenal ulcers are common; reportedly, 70% of patients have documented peptic ulcer disease.[16]

Microscopic Features

Although clinical and endoscopic features of hypertrophic hypersecretory gastropathy overlap with Ménétrier disease, the histomorphology differs in that hyperplasia of both the foveolar epithelium and parietal cell compartments are seen. Cystically dilated gastric glands may also be seen (Figure 14-7).

Treatment and Prognosis

Hypertrophic hypersecretory gastropathy is an unremitting disease that is refractory to traditional antacid therapy. The progression and risk to gastric dysplasia and malignancy has not been well studied. Gastrectomy has been recommended in patients with chronic pain despite prolonged medical therapy.[17]

Zollinger-Ellison Syndrome

The characteristic triad of Zollinger-Ellison syndrome (ZES) is (1) ectopic gastrin secretion (gastrinoma), (2) increased gastric acid production, and (3) intractable peptic ulcer disease.

Clinical Features

Both males and females with ZES are affected equally, and it has been described in adults and children. Most patients are diagnosed between 20 and 50 years of age. Of these patients, 20%–60% have multiple endocrine neoplasia type 1 (MEN type 1). Patients often present with long-standing abdominal pain due to peptic ulcer disease from persistently elevated gastrin, leading to increased gastric acid output (up to five times normal). Diagnosis is often made by obtaining a fasting serum gastrin level in patients who are not taking proton pump inhibitors.[18]

The gastrinomas responsible for ZES are most frequently located in the "gastrinoma triangle" formed by the junction of the cystic and common bile ducts superiorly, the second and third portions of the duodenum laterally, and the neck of the pancreas medially. These tumors, however, have been described in many unusual sites, including lymph nodes, liver, heart, and even ovaries. Gastrinomas in ZES can be widely metastatic to the liver and lymph nodes.

Endoscopic Features

Imaging studies and endoscopy alike show diffuse thickening of gastric folds (Table 14-3). Hypertrophic gastric folds

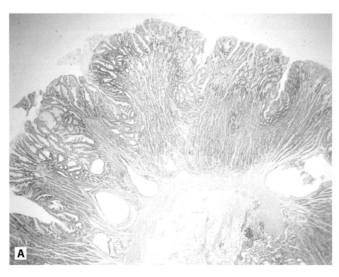

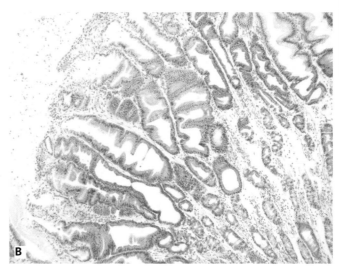

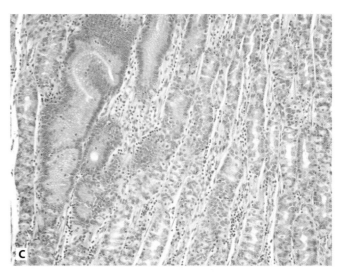

FIGURE 14-7. Hypertrophic hypersecretory gastropathy. **A.** Low-power image depicts giant gastric folds. Foveolar (**B**) and oxyntic glands (**C**) both show hypertrophy.

TABLE 14-3. Differential diagnosis of thickened gastric folds.

Condition	Location in stomach	Endoscopic features	Clinical findings	Pathologic feature
Ménétrier disease	Corpus; may also involve antrum	Cerebriform thickened folds	Nausea, vomiting, peripheral edema	Massive foveolar hyperplasia
Zollinger-Ellison syndrome	Corpus	Folds thickened up to 8 mm	Refractory peptic ulcer disease	Parietal cell hyperplasia
Hypertrophic hyperplastic gastropathy	Corpus	Diffuse cobblestone nodularity	Peptic ulcer disease	Hyperplasia of all glandular elements
Hyperplastic polyp	Antrum; also in corpus and cardia	Polyp(s), single or multiple	Associated with chronic atrophic gastritis	Foveolar hyperplasia with architectural disarray
Polypoid gastritis	Antrum and corpus	Nodularity	Epigastric pain	Chronic active gastritis with *Helicobacter pylori*
Polyposis syndrome	Antrum and corpus	Variable; diffuse nodular enlargement of gastric folds or discrete polyps	Juvenile polyposis, Peutz-Jaeger syndrome, other undefined polyposis syndrome	Features overlap with hyperplastic polyp
Gastritis cystica profunda/polyposa	Body and antrum; gastric remnant in operated stomach	Usually localized	Usually found in operated stomach	Entrapped cystic glands in submucosa or deeper layers
Lymphoma	Antrum and corpus	Thickened folds	Variable	Effacement of gastric mucosal architecture by neoplastic lymphoid infiltrate
Carcinoma	Antrum and corpus	Thickened folds	Variable	Infiltrating carcinoma, noncohesive type
Amyloidosis	Antrum and corpus	Thickened folds, hemorrhagic mucosa	Epigastric pain, dyspepsia	Acellular, amorphous eosinophilic material surrounds glands and vessels

can be up to 5 cm in size. Much of the hypertrophic changes are in the gastric fundus and body; the gastric antral mucosal thickness is often decreased. Erythema and inflammation of the esophagus, stomach, and duodenum are often noted. Multiple peptic ulcers can also be seen in these locations.

Microscopic Features

Gastric body mucosal thickening is present. The histologic hallmark of ZES is diffuse parietal cell hyperplasia and hypertrophy. Parietal cells extend to the base of the glands, in zones normally occupied by chief cells (Figure 14-8). In addition, prominent expansion of parietal cells into the gastric antrum is common. Nodular and linear ECL cell hyperplasia is a frequent finding in disease associated with MEN type 1 rather than sporadic ZES. The foveolar glands are unremarkable.

Treatment and Prognosis

The peptic symptoms and complications of ZES respond well to proton pump inhibitors.[19,20] Even patients with metastatic disease may have a relatively indolent course, although more aggressive disease occurs in a subset. The extent of liver metastases is an important factor influencing survival.[21,22] Intractable cases may be treated with gastric resection. Patients with localized disease are ideal candidates for partial resection of small intestinal or pancreatic gastrinomas.[23]

Association of ZES with MEN type 1 indicates a better prognosis than sporadic cases (80% vs 33% 5-year overall survival).[24]

Pseudo–Zollinger-Ellison Syndrome

Gastric acid hypersecretion related to vagal hyperactivity is the underlying etiology of pseudo-ZES in most cases.[25] Most patients are middle-aged Caucasian males with normal serum gastrin levels. A negative secretin stimulation test is useful in differentiating pseudo-ZES from ZES. Primary antral G-cell hyperplasia has been reported in some cases. Patients generally respond to proton pump inhibitor therapy.

▇ DISORDERS WITH FOCAL HYPERPLASIA

The disorders discussed next can present as solitary gastric polyps and are also discussed in Chapter 15 with emphasis on differential diagnosis.

Hyperplastic Polyps

Gastric hyperplastic polyps are among the most frequently encountered gastric epithelial polyps, having a prevalence of up to 70% relative to other polyps in some series.[26]

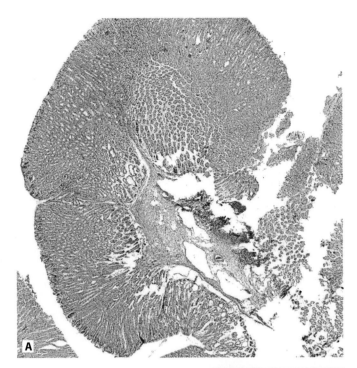

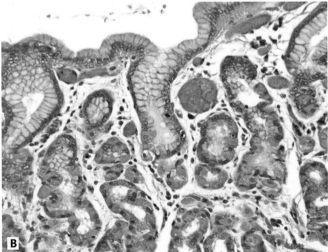

FIGURE 14-8. Zollinger-Ellison syndrome. **A.** Low-power view shows enlarged polypoid gastric folds with parietal cell expansion. **B.** In the high-power view, parietal cells are seen close to the surface.

Clinical Features

Hyperplastic polyps are seen in both males and females. In order of frequency, they are most common in the antrum, body, and cardia. These lesions are seen in all age groups but are most frequently diagnosed in the sixth and seventh decades. They are often incidental findings on endoscopy. Patients complain of vague symptoms (eg, abdominal pain, nausea, and dyspepsia). Larger polyps, however, can result in gastric outlet obstruction. The etiology of these lesions is not known; they are thought to be part of a regenerative response to mucosal insults.

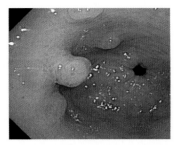

FIGURE 14-9. Gastric hyperplastic polyps. Protruding polyps with focal mucosal erythema are noted.

Endoscopic Features

Hyperplastic polyps show a variation in size, from a few millimeters to larger polyps of up to 8 cm. They can be solitary or multiple (20%). They are often broad-based sessile lesions with a lobulated, smooth, and glistening surface. Pedunculated polyps, however, can show areas of surface irregularity corresponding to ulcerations and erosions (Figure 14-9).

Microscopic Features

Hyperplastic polyps are almost always associated with some sort of pathology in the background gastric mucosa, including atrophic gastritis,[27] reactive gastropathy (chemical gastropathy), or any form of acute and chronic gastritis. The polyps comprise hyperplastic foveolar epithelium, with 15% of lesions microscopically demonstrating foci of intestinal metaplasia. The glands are deep, dilated, and tortuously embedded in an edematous stroma. Stromal lymphoid aggregates and a mixed population of inflammatory cells are frequently seen. In addition, larger hyperplastic polyps have strands of smooth muscle spindles scattered throughout the stroma,[28] which may be related to prolapse (Figure 14-10). These mucosal prolapse-related polyps show cystic dilation of gastric pits and involvement of the oxyntic and pyloric glands.[28]

Hyperplastic polyps often show areas of surface erosions and ulcerations with associated reactive changes. Rarely, hyperplastic polyps may contain focal dysplasia (also see Chapter 15).[29]

Prognosis and Treatment

Hyperplastic polyps are regarded as benign nonneoplastic lesions. The risk of neoplastic transformation in hyperplastic polyps is proportional to polyp size, with resection recommended for those measuring greater than 1.5 cm. Treatment recommendations include complete removal by either snare polypectomy or endoscopic mucosal resection and therapy for the background gastritis.[30]

Polyposis Syndromes

Syndromic gastric polyps are multiple and diffusely distributed, imparting a hypertrophic appearance to the stomach. Patients can present with symptoms that overlap with those seen in Ménétrier disease, making clinical and histologic distinction challenging.

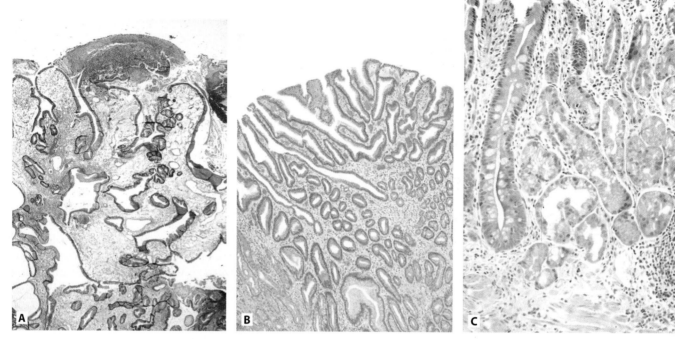

FIGURE 14-10. Gastric hyperplastic polyp. **A.** A low-power view demonstrates cystically dilated glands lined by foveolar-type epithelium embedded in edematous lamina propria. **B.** A closer look reveals a chronic inflammatory infiltrate within the lamina propria. **C.** The background mucosa associated with hyperplastic polyps is frequently abnormal. This example shows intestinal metaplasia occurring in a background of inactive gastritis.

Juvenile Polyposis Syndrome

Juvenile polyposis syndrome (JPS) is an autosomal dominant syndrome characterized by the development of gastrointestinal polyps, most commonly in the large intestine. While most colonic juvenile polyps are sporadic, germline mutations causing inactivation of either *BMPR1A* or *SMAD4* genes have been observed in 50% of patients with JPS.

Clinical Features   Males are affected more frequently than females. Patients with sporadic colonic juvenile polyps are diagnosed before they are 10 years old. Patients with JPS often present at a mean age of 9.5 years and have a family history of gastrointestinal polyps; the latter is included in the criteria for diagnosis in addition to criteria of more than five juvenile colonic polyps and the presence of extracolonic juvenile polyps. The number of gastrointestinal polyps in JPS cases can range from four to hundreds. *SMAD4* mutations, particularly nonsense mutations resulting in a stop codon (c. 1527 G>A) in exon 11 and a deletion of four base pairs in exon 9 at codon 415, have been associated with a severe gastric phenotype.[31] *SMAD4* mutations have also been noted in patients with JPS with concurrent hereditary hemorrhagic telangiectasias and other arteriovenous malformations.[32]

Endoscopic Features   Gastric juvenile polyps range in size from 1 cm to 5 cm. Endoscopically, they appear as smooth-surface, rounded sessile polyps. Surface erosions and associated reactive stromal changes may be seen in larger polyps.

Microscopic Features   Hyperplasia of the surface epithelium and areas of erosions with reactive changes are commonly seen microscopically in large polyps. Foveolar glands are often cystically dilated, suspended in edematous stroma. The lamina propria is often inflamed, with numerous small congested vessels.[33] Reactive atypia is not uncommon (Figure 14-11). Larger polyps (>1.0 cm) have been associated with dysplastic changes (nuclear enlargement, crowding, hyperchromasia, pseudostratification, increased mitoses, and prominent nucleoli).

Treatment and Prognosis   Juvenile polyposis syndrome is associated with an increased risk for both gastric (21% risk with gastric polyps) and colorectal carcinoma (17%–22% by 35 years with colorectal polyps). When possible, all polyps should be removed and reviewed for adenomatous changes. If no dysplasia is identified, yearly follow-up with upper and lower gastrointestinal endoscopy is recommended; subsequently, if no polyps are found, screening should occur every three years.[34,35] The presence of dysplasia or malignant changes may require surgical treatment.[35]

Cronkhite-Canada Syndrome

Cronkhite-Canada syndrome (CCS) is a rare nonhereditary syndrome affecting the gastrointestinal and integumentary systems.[36] The etiology is currently unknown, although an underlying dysregulation in immunity has been proposed.[37]

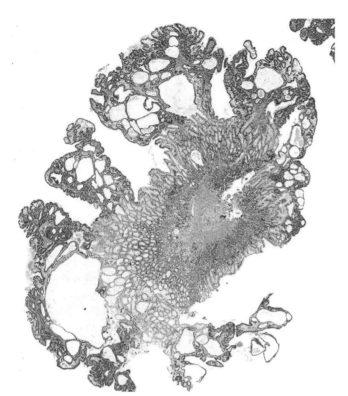

FIGURE 14-11. Gastric juvenile polyp, low power. The hyperplastic foveolar epithelium has a cap-like configuration, with intervening areas of less-thickened mucosa. Large dilated glands are prominent.

Clinical Features Males are more frequently affected by CCS than females. The disease usually presents in the fifth and sixth decades of life. Gastrointestinal manifestations include diffuse polyposis, which can be distributed throughout the gastrointestinal tract. Patients present with protein-losing enteropathy, weight loss, and anorexia. Lab tests demonstrate electrolyte imbalance, hypoproteinemia, and anemia. In addition, alopecia, cutaneous hyperpigmentation, and onychodystrophy are reported.[36] A diagnosis of CCS based on upper gastrointestinal biopsies alone is notoriously challenging, and a multidisciplinary approach is essential.

Endoscopic Features Apart from relative sparing of the esophagus, polyps can occur throughout the gastrointestinal tract and show diffuse mucosal involvement. Their gross appearance ranges from focal mucosal nodularity to larger proliferative lesions. Generalized gastric and duodenal mucosal edema is a common endoscopic finding.

Microscopic Features Gastric polyps of CCS are sessile. Microscopically, they share a number of histologic features with juvenile polyps, including large cystically dilated glands surrounded by edematous lamina propria. A mixed lamina propria inflammatory infiltrate with prominent eosinophils and eosinophilic cryptitis and crypt abscesses is a helpful finding in the upper gastrointestinal tract. Indeed, differentiating between these two syndromes on histologic grounds

alone can be challenging. Awareness of the clinical history, any accompanying ectodermal lesions, and sampling the background gastric mucosa, which shows edematous changes in CCS, will aid in distinguishing between CCS and JPS.[38] In addition, the duodenal mucosa in CCS has been described as edematous with villous effacement.[39]

Treatment and Prognosis Although nearly 15% of patients develop gastrointestinal malignancies, the true premalignant potential of CCS is not well established.[40] Some patients report spontaneous remission, while others can suffer potentially fatal CCS complications, including gastrointestinal bleeding, infections, and malnutrition.[37] The mortality from untreated CCS is as high as 60%. Treatment includes supportive, medical (antibiotics, steroids), and surgical options.

Peutz-Jeghers Syndrome

Peutz-Jeghers syndrome (PJS) is an autosomal dominant inherited syndrome of hamartomatous gastrointestinal polyps, and skin and mucosal pigmentation is the second most common polyposis syndrome after familial adenomatous polyposis (FAP).

Clinical Features Mutation of the serine/threonine kinase 11 (*STK11*) tumor suppressor gene is the underlying genetic basis of PJS; the disease can show variable or incomplete penetrance. It affects both genders and all races, with the average age of diagnosis in the second and third decades of life. Hamartomatous polyps occur throughout the gastrointestinal tract, most frequently in the small bowel. Patients also present clinically with distinctive skin and mucous membrane pigmentation; melanin deposits in the buccal mucosa are characteristic.

Endoscopic Features Endoscopically, gastric polyps can range from 0.1 to 8 cm in size; many are pedunculated. A diagnosis of PJS based solely on gastric polyps should use the following criteria: (1) family history of autosomal dominant inheritance, (2) aberrant pigmentation of the mucocutaneous surfaces, and (3) histologically confirmed PJS-associated polyps.[41]

Microscopic Features The PJS polyps are hamartomatous, classically described as hyperplastic mature epithelium divided by arborizing bands of smooth muscle imparting the classic "leaf-like" appearance. Interestingly, while this description fits most polyps, it is not the case for gastric PJS polyps. While exuberant clusters of dilated hyperplastic glands are a feature of gastric PJS polyps, microscopically strands of smooth muscles are less prominent.[33] This phenomenon often leads to misinterpretation of these lesions and hyperplastic polyps or Ménétrier disease (Figure 14-12). Knowledge of the clinical history and comparison with nongastric polyps can be beneficial, as diagnosis of PJS should not be based solely on gastric polyps.[42] Dysplastic change is not a common feature of these polyps.

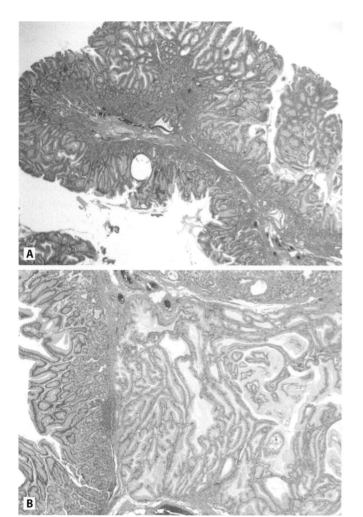

FIGURE 14-12. Gastric Peutz-Jeghers polyp. **A.** Exuberant proliferation of dilated gastric glands is seen. **B.** This example highlights smooth muscle bundles between hamartomatous glands.

Treatment and Prognosis Patients are at greatest risk for gastrointestinal neoplasms (colorectal, pancreas, gastric) but are also at significant risk for breast carcinoma. For treatment, proper management includes complete removal of the polyps along with active surveillance of high risk organs.[43]

Cowden Syndrome

Cowden syndrome is an autosomally dominant inherited hamartomatous condition characterized by numerous hamartomas of the gastrointestinal tract and extraintestinal sites (skin, breast, thyroid, gynecologic, oral cavity, central nervous system).

Clinical Features Males and females are equally affected, with a peak onset of disease in the fourth decade of life. Mutations in phosphatase and tensin homolog (PTEN) protein are noted in over one-half of patients with Cowden disease.

Endoscopic Features A unique endoscopic finding described in the esophagus is diffuse, "carpet-like" distribution of glycogenic acanthosis, which by some is considered

pathognomonic for Cowden syndrome.[44] Polyps are relatively small, with a predilection for the distal gastrointestinal tract, and are often numerous (>50).[45]

Microscopic Features Gastric polyps in Cowden syndrome are hamartomatous. They are often sessile and small, showing histomorphologic overlap with hyperplastic polyps or juvenile polyps.

Treatment and Prognosis There is a significant lifetime risk of development of breast carcinoma (85%–50%) and thyroid carcinoma (35%–10%). Current data are evolving to suggest that neoplasias of the colorectum and kidney along with melanoma are also increased in patients with *PTEN* mutations.[46] Close surveillance is recommended.

Gastric Adenocarcinoma and Proximal Polyposis of the Stomach

The autosomal dominant entity of gastric adenocarcinoma and proximal polyposis of the stomach (GAPPS) was first described[47] in 2011. It carries a high risk of gastric adenocarcinoma.

Clinical Features Limited studies have shown the probands are Caucasians of Canadian, Australian, and American descent. Clinically, the disease affects both genders, with a slight female predominance. The age of onset ranges from 10 to 77 years. There is an inverse relationship between GAPPS and *H. pylori* infection. Serum gastrin and progastrin levels are reportedly normal. Abnormalities in gastric acid homeostasis and Wnt signaling have been implicated as possible etiologies.

Endoscopic Features Florid gastric polyposis (often > 100) carpeting the proximal stomach with sparing of the esophagus, antrum, pylorus, and duodenum is described endoscopically, with most polyps 1.0 cm or less in size. Of note, patients did not have any associated colorectal polyposis.

Microscopic Features Gastric polyps in this syndrome are limited to the oxyntic mucosa gastric body and fundus and morphologically are fundic gland polyps with multiple foci of dysplasia. Occasional hyperplastic polyps and adenomatous polyps have also been described.

Seven of the total 55 patients with GAPPS studied in a cohort consisting of three families developed intestinal-type gastric adenocarcinoma.[47]

Treatment and Prognosis The earliest gastric cancer was noted in a 33-year-old patient. Management must include vigilant endoscopic surveillance; some patients eventually require gastrectomy.[47,48]

Gastritis Cystica Profunda/Polyposa

Gastritis cystica profunda/polyposa, an uncommon cause of hypertrophic gastropathy, is often seen in patients with prior gastric surgical procedures. It is associated with glandular herniation into the deeper layers of the gastric wall.

Clinical Features Gastritis cystica profunda/polyposa has been associated clinically with a history of gastroenterostomy with or without gastric resection. Historically, it has been noted in men who have undergone a Billroth I or Billroth II procedure. Deep displacement of glandular elements into the gastric wall or the formation of an exophytic component dictates whether the term *profunda* or *polyposa* is used, respectively. This condition is often associated with chronic bile reflux and likely represents a reactive proliferation of entrapped herniated mucosal elements. Exophytic masses can range in size from 0.5 to 7 cm, leading to gastric outlet obstruction.

Endoscopic Features Endoscopically, grossly apparent lesions are often centered on the stoma site and can be solitary sessile polyps or a protruding convergence of numerous smaller polyps.[49,50] The mucosal appearance can also be smooth or erythematous (Figure 14-13).

Microscopic Features Gastritis cystica profunda/polyposa lesions are akin to mucosal prolapse–related changes seen in the colon. Prior surgical site changes include lamina propria and submucosal inflammation, scarring, and fibrosis. Hyperplastic and regenerative changes in the surface foveolar epithelium are common microscopically. Cystically dilated pyloric-type glands maybe dispersed through all layers of the gastric wall, not just confined to the submucosa (Figure 14-14). These glands are often surrounded by splayed fibers of muscularis propria, mimicking invasive adenocarcinoma. However, the glands of gastritis cystica profunda/polyposa lack nuclear atypia and associated desmoplastic stroma typical of a neoplastic process.

Treatment and Prognosis Gastritis cystica profunda/polyposa has been associated with Ménétrier disease. Although it is not a pre-malignant condition, concurrent dysplasia and gastric stump adenocarcinomas are not infrequently seen in association.[49] Therapy consists of resection of obstructing masses, along with cancer surveillance.

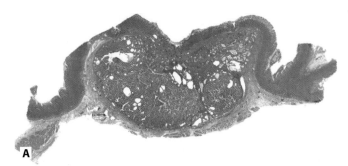

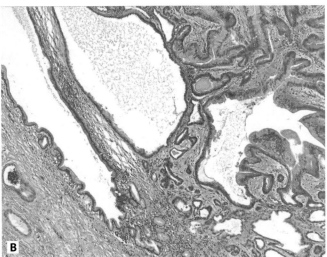

FIGURE 14-14. Gastritis cystica profunda/polyposa. **A.** A full-mount scan highlights invagination of dilated glands into the submucosa. **B.** At higher power, the herniated glands show prolapse-associated changes; such changes can be misinterpreted as an invasive adenocarcinoma.

OTHER CAUSES OF THICKENED GASTRIC FOLDS

Diffuse Gastric Carcinoma

Also known as discohesive carcinoma, linitis plastica, and signet-ring cell adenocarcinoma, the diffuse gastric carcinoma extensively infiltrating neoplastic process often involves the entire stomach, grossly mimicking hypertrophic gastropathy[51] (Figure 14-15) (see also Chapter 16). The lesional cells are arranged in small clusters or individually

FIGURE 14-13. Gastritis cystica profunda/polyposa. A gastrectomy specimen shows sessile polypoid folds in close proximity to a prior surgical site (arrow).

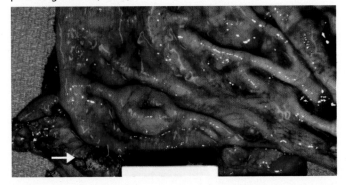

FIGURE 14-15. Diffuse gastric carcinoma. Diffusely thickened gastric folds are indistinguishable from other causes of hypertrophic gastropathy.

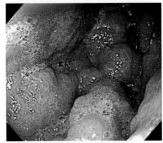

infiltrating throughout the gastric wall with rare foci of well-formed glands (Figure 14-16). Detecting gastric carcinomas arising in Ménétrier disease is particularly arduous given the difficulty in identifying localized lesions at endoscopy in a background of diffusely thickened mucosa. Cytokeratin immunohistochemical studies may help with diagnosis in problematic biopsies.

Gastric Lymphoma

Half of gastrointestinal lymphomas arise in the stomach, making it the most frequently affected extranodal site for such neoplasias. Diffuse large B-cell lymphoma and extranodal marginal zone lymphoma (EMZL) of mucosa-associated tissue are the two most common[52] subtypes.

The patient demographics of EMZL are shared with Ménétrier disease. As the neoplastic cells infiltrate the mucosa, diffuse thickening of the gastric folds is a common feature. Erosions and shallow ulcers may also be seen. Histologically, a lymphoproliferative process with submucosal or deeper involvement along with the absence of epithelial hyperplasia is an important feature distinguishing lymphomas from hypertrophic gastropathies (Figure 14-17).

Amyloidosis

The amyloidosis systemic condition can be acquired or hereditary. It is associated with both neoplastic diseases (eg, myeloma) or chronic inflammatory states, resulting in the deposition of insoluble protein throughout the body. Within the gastrointestinal tract, the small intestine is affected most frequently.

Amyloid deposition in the stomach is seen transmurally and can be patchy or diffuse. The latter deceptively reproduces the appearance of hypertrophic gastropathy.[53] Mucosal appearance can range from smooth to hemorrhagic. Amyloid deposits tend to envelope gastric glands and vasculature, imparting an acellular, thick, waxy appearance (Figure 14-18). Congo red stains imparting red/green birefringence under polarized light are easy diagnostic studies.

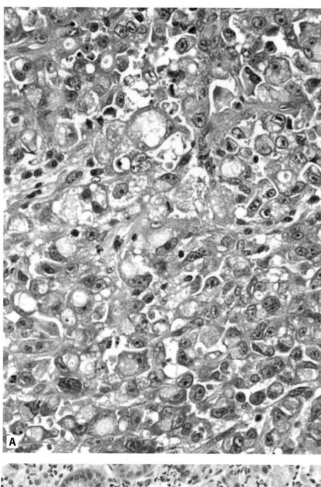

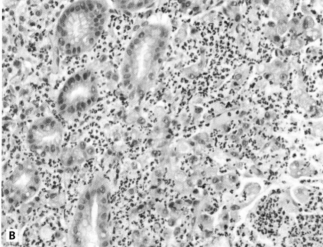

FIGURE 14-16. Diffuse gastric carcinoma. **A.** Poorly differentiated adenocarcinoma with signet-ring features is shown. **B.** Neoplastic cells infiltrate the mucosa.

FIGURE 14-17. Gastric lymphoma. Expansion of the lamina propria by atypical lymphocytes leads to mucosal thickening; note that the overlying surface epithelium is not hyperplastic.

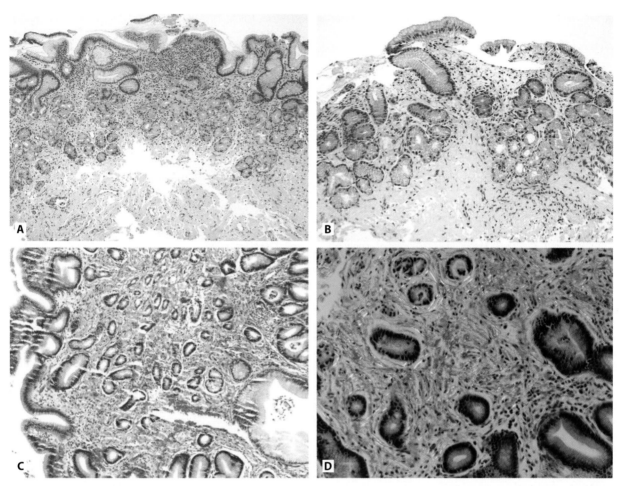

FIGURE 14-18. Gastric amyloidosis. **A.** Amyloid deposits in the mucosal and submuocosal compartments and around the blood vessels are seen. **B.** Amyloid deposits are characteristically amorphous, acellular, and eosinophilic in appearance. **C.** Light microscopy of Congo red histochemistry highlights salmon-colored amyloid deposits. **D.** Congo red examined by polarized microscopy reveals classic "apple green" birefringence of amyloid in the lamina propria. (Used with permission of Dr. Aatur Singhi, University of Pittsburgh Medical Center, and Dr. Michael Cruise, Cleveland Clinic.)

SUMMARY

Gastric hypertrophy can result from numerous systemic and localized processes, including both benign entities and neoplastic processes. A multidisciplinary approach encompassing awareness of the patient's clinical picture, endoscopic findings, and accurate interpretation of the histopathologic findings is essential in determining the etiology and thus guiding adequate treatment.

REFERENCES

1. Coffey RJ Jr, Tanksley J. Pierre Ménétrier and his disease. *Trans Am Clin Climatol Assoc.* 2012;123:126–133; discussion 133–134.
2. Scharschmidt BF. The natural history of hypertrophic gastrophy (Ménétrier's disease). Report of a case with 16 year follow-up and review of 120 cases from the literature. *Am J Med.* 1977;63(4):644–652.
3. Stamm B. Localized hyperplastic gastropathy of the mucous cell- and mixed cell-type (localized Ménétrier's disease): a report of 11 patients. *Am J Surg Pathol.* 1997;21(11):1334–1342.
4. Arthurs Y, Fielding JF. Ménétrier's disease in a patient with ileocolonic Crohn's disease. *Irish J Med Sci.* 1983;152(6):248–250.
5. Hemmings CT. Ménétrier's disease in a patient with ulcerative colitis: a case report and review of the literature. *Pathology.* 2007;39(2):282–283.
6. Dempsey PJ, Goldenring JR, Soroka CJ, et al. Possible role of transforming growth factor α in the pathogenesis of Ménétrier's disease: supportive evidence from humans and transgenic mice. *Gastroenterology.* 1992;103(12):1950–1963.
7. Coffey RJ, Romano M, Goldenring J. Roles for transforming growth factor-alpha in the stomach. *J Clin Gastroenterol.* 1995;21(Suppl 1): S36–S39.
8. Bluth RF, Carpenter HA, Pittelkow MR, Page DL, Coffey RJ. Immunolocalization of transforming growth factor-alpha in normal and diseased human gastric mucosa. *Hum Pathol.* 1995;26(12):1333–1340.
9. Xiao SY, Hart J. Marked gastric foveolar hyperplasia associated with active cytomegalovirus infection. *Am J Gastroenterol.* 2001;96(1): 223–226.
10. Strisciuglio C, Corleto VD, Brunetti-Pierri N, et al. Autosomal dominant Ménétrier-like disease. *J Pediatr Gastroenterol Nutr.* 2012;55(6):717–720.
11. Wolfsen HC, Carpenter HA, Talley NJ. Ménétrier's disease: a form of hypertrophic gastropathy or gastritis? *Gastroenterology.* 1993;104(5):1310–1319.
12. Burdick JS, Chung E, Tanner G, et al. Treatment of Ménétrier's disease with a monoclonal antibody against the epidermal growth factor receptor. *N Engl J Med.* 2000;343(23):1697–1701.

13. Settle SH, Washington K, Lind C, et al. Chronic treatment of Méné-trier's disease with Erbitux: clinical efficacy and insight into patho-physiology. *Clin Gastroenterol Hepatol.* 2005;3(7):654–659.

14. Fiske WH, Tanksley J, Nam KT, et al. Efficacy of cetuximab in the treatment of Ménétrier's disease. *Sci Transl Med.* 2009;1(8):8ra18.

15. Stempien SJ, Dagradi AE, Reingold IM, et al. Hypertrophic hyperse-cretory gastropathy. Analysis of 15 cases and a review of the pertinent literature. *Am J Dig Dis.* 1964;9:471–493.

16. Tan DT, Stempien SJ, Dagradi AE. The clinical spectrum of hypertro-phic hypersecretory gastropathy. Report of 50 patients. *Gastrointest Endosc.* 1971;18(2):69–73.

17. Byun J, Kwon S, Oh SY, et al. Laparoscopic management of hypertro-phic hypersecretory gastropathy with protein loss: a case report. *Asian J Endosc Surg.* 2014;7(1):48–51.

18. Rehfeld JF, Gingras M-H, Bardram L, Hilsted L, Goetze JP, Poitras P. The Zollinger-Ellison syndrome and mismeasurement of gastrin. *Gastroenterology.* 2011;140(5):1444–1453.

19. Wilcox CM, Seay T, Arcury JT, Mohnen J, Hirschowitz BI. Zollinger-Ellison syndrome: presentation, response to therapy, and outcome. *Dig Liver Dis.* 2011;43(6):439–443.

20. Wilcox CM, Seay T, Arcury J, Hirschowitz BI. Presentation, response to lansoprazole therapy, and outcome of Zollinger-Ellison syndrome-like gastric acid hypersecretors. *Scand J Gastroenterol.* 2011;46(3):277–280.

21. Weber HC, Venzon DJ, Lin J-T, et al. Determinants of metastatic rate and survival in patients with Zollinger-Ellison syndrome: a prospec-tive long-term study. *Gastroenterology.* 1995;108(6):1637–1649.

22. Yu F, Venzon DJ, Serrano J, et al. Prospective study of the clinical course, prognostic factors, causes of death, and survival in patients with long-standing Zollinger-Ellison syndrome. *J Clin Oncol.* 1999; 17(2):615–630.

23. Krampitz GW, Norton JA. Current management of the Zollinger-Ellison syndrome. *Adv Surg.* 2013;47:59–79.

24. O'Toole D, Delle Fave G, Jensen RT. Gastric and duodenal neuro-endocrine tumours. *Best Pract Res Clin Gastroenterol.* 2012;26(6): 719–735.

25. Tomaszewska R, Kedra B, Stachura J. Hypertrophic gastritis, primary diffuse G-cell hyperplasia and pancreatic metaplasia of the gastric mucosa (pseudo-Zollinger-Ellison syndrome)—case report. *Pol J Pathol.* 2000;51(1):51–54.

26. Carmack SW, Genta RM, Schuler CM, Saboorian MH. The current spectrum of gastric polyps: a 1-year national study of over 120,000 patients. *Am J Gastroenterol.* 2009;104(6):1524–1532.

27. Park JY, Cornish TC, Lam-Himlin D, Shi C, Montgomery E. Gastric lesions in patients with autoimmune metaplastic atrophic gastritis (AMAG) in a tertiary care setting. *The Am J Surg Pathol.* 2010;34(11): 1591–1598.

28. Gonzalez-Obeso E, Fujita H, Deshpande V, et al. Gastric hyperplastic polyps: a heterogeneous clinicopathologic group including a distinct subset best categorized as mucosal prolapse polyp. *Am J Surg Pathol.* 2011;35(5):670–677.

29. Raftopoulos SC, Efthymiou M, Streutker CJ, May GR. Education and imaging. Gastrointestinal: atypical hyperplastic gastric polyposis: a case report and brief review of the literature. *J Gastroenterol Hepatol.* 2011;26(11):1693.

30. Shaib YH, Rugge M, Graham DY, Genta RM. Management of gastric polyps: an endoscopy-based approach. *Clin Gastroenterol Hepatol.* 2013;11(11):1374–1384.

31. Pintiliciuc OG, Heresbach D, de-Lajarte-Thirouard AS, et al. Gastric involvement in juvenile polyposis associated with germline SMAD4 mutations: an entity characterized by a mixed hypertrophic and polypoid gastropathy. *Gastroenterol Clin Biol.* 2008;32(5 Pt 1):445–450.

32. O'Malley M, LaGuardia L, Kalady MF, et al. The prevalence of heredi-tary hemorrhagic telangiectasia in juvenile polyposis syndrome. *Dis Colon Rectum.* 2012;55(8):886–892.

33. Lam-Himlin D, Park JY, Cornish TC, Shi C, Montgomery E. Morpho-logic characterization of syndromic gastric polyps. *Am J Surg Pathol.* 2010;34(11):1656–1662.

34. Larsen Haidle J, Howe JR. Juvenile polyposis syndrome. In: Pagon RA, Adam MP, Ardinger HH, et al, eds. *GeneReviews(R).* Seattle, WA: University of Washington; 1993–2014.

35. Brosens LA, Langeveld D, van Hattem WA, Giardiello FM, Offer-haus GJ. Juvenile polyposis syndrome. *World J Gastroenterol.* 28 2011;17(44):4839–4844.

36. Cronkhite LW Jr, Canada WJ. Generalized gastrointestinal polyposis; an unusual syndrome of polyposis, pigmentation, alopecia and ony-chotrophia. *N Engl J Med.* 1955;252(24):1011–1015.

37. Sweetser S, Ahlquist DA, Osborn NK, et al. Clinicopathologic features and treatment outcomes in Cronkhite-Canada syndrome: support for autoimmunity. *Dig Dis Sci.* 2012;57(2):496–502.

38. Burke AP, Sobin LH. The pathology of Cronkhite-Canada pol-yps. A comparison to juvenile polyposis. *Am J Surg Pathol.* 1989; 13(11):940–946.

39. Bettington M, Brown IS, Kumarasinghe MP, de Boer B, Bettington A, Rosty C. The challenging diagnosis of Cronkhite-Canada syndrome in the upper gastrointestinal tract: a series of 7 cases with clinical follow-up. *Am J Surg Pathol.* 2014;38(2):215–223.

40. Sweetser S, Boardman LA. Cronkhite-Canada syndrome: an acquired condition of gastrointestinal polyposis and dermatologic abnormali-ties. *Gastroenterol Hepatol.* 2012;8(3):201–203.

41. Giardiello FM, Welsh SB, Hamilton SR, et al. Increased risk of cancer in the Peutz-Jeghers syndrome. *N Engl J Med.* 1987;316(24):1511–1514.

42. Keller JJ, Offerhaus GJ, Giardiello FM, Menko FH. Jan Peutz, Har-old Jeghers and a remarkable combination of polyposis and pig-mentation of the skin and mucous membranes. *Fam Cancer.* 2001; 1(3–4):181–185.

43. van Lier MG, Wagner A, Mathus-Vliegen EM, Kuipers EJ, Steyer-berg EW, van Leerdam ME. High cancer risk in Peutz-Jeghers syn-drome: a systematic review and surveillance recommendations. *Am J Gastroenterol.* 2010;105(6):1258–1264; author reply 1265.

44. Coriat R, Mozer M, Caux F, et al. Endoscopic findings in Cowden syndrome. *Endoscopy.* 2011;43(8):723–726.

45. Heald B, Mester J, Rybicki L, Orloff MS, Burke CA, Eng C. Fre-quent gastrointestinal polyps and colorectal adenocarcinomas in a prospective series of PTEN mutation carriers. *Gastroenterology.* 2010;139(6):1927–1933.

46. Tan MH, Mester JL, Ngeow J, Rybicki LA, Orloff MS, Eng C. Life-time cancer risks in individuals with germline PTEN mutations. *Clin Cancer Res.* 2012;18(2):400–407.

47. Worthley DL, Phillips KD, Wayte N, et al. Gastric adenocarcinoma and proximal polyposis of the stomach (GAPPS): a new autosomal dominant syndrome. *Gut.* 2012;61(5):774–779.

48. Carneiro F. Hereditary gastric cancer. *Pathologe.* 2012;33(Suppl 2): 231–234.

49. Deery S, Yates R, Hata J, Shi C, Parikh AA. Gastric adenocarcinoma associated with gastritis cystica profunda in an unoperated stomach. *Am Surg.* 2012;78(8):E379–E380.

50. Okada M, Iizuka Y, Oh K, Murayama H, Maekawa T. Gastritis cystica profunda presenting as giant gastric mucosal folds: the role of endo-scopic ultrasonography and mucosectomy in the diagnostic work-up. *Gastrointest Endosc.* 1994;40(5):640–644.

51. Mei M, Jingmei N, Zongming C, Mei J, Leimin S. Diffuse type gas-tric carcinoma presenting as giant gastric folds: lessons learned from six miss diagnosed cases. *Clin Res Hepatol Gastroenterol.* 2012;36(5):505–509.

52. O'Malley DP, Goldstein NS, Banks PM. The recognition and clas-sification of lymphoproliferative disorders of the gut. *Hum Pathol.* 2014;45(5):899–916.

53. Ebert EC, Nagar M. Gastrointestinal manifestations of amyloidosis. *Am J Gastroenterol.* 2008;103(3):776–787.

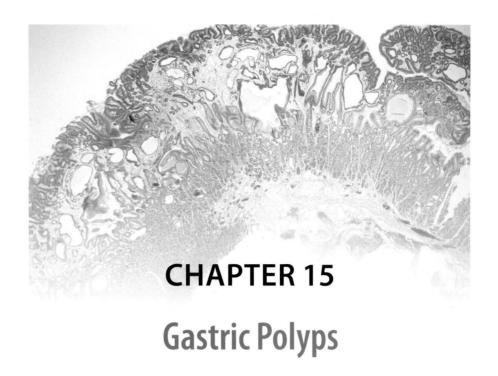

CHAPTER 15

Gastric Polyps

■ INTRODUCTION

Polyps of the stomach include inflammatory, hamarto-matous, and neoplastic types. It is important to accurately categorize a gastric polyp histologically because most are endoscopically indistinguishable from one another.

The commonly encountered polyps in the stomach include the fundic gland polyp (FGP), hyperplastic/inflam-matory polyp, pyloric gland adenoma (PGA), and gastric adenoma. All these are benign. Adenomatous transforma-tion may occur in the FGP and hyperplastic polyp. PGA may progress to well-differentiated adenocarcinoma.

■ FUNDIC GLAND POLYP

Fundic gland polyps are polypoid growths in the gastric fun-dus or body; they are microscopically characterized by a mix-ture of normal and dilated fundic glands (Figures 15-1 and 15-2). Most FGPs are sporadic, but increasingly more FGPs are encountered in association with use of proton pump inhibitors (PPIs). Multiple FGPs often occur in patients with familial adenomatous polyposis (FAP) syndrome; these have a high prevalence of dysplasia (Figure 15-3). FGPs and gastric hyperplastic polyps (GHPs; see next section) are the most common gastric polyps (there is no agreement regard-ing which of these two are more common).

Microscopic identification of FGPs is straightfor-ward; thus, the diagnosis is usually not difficult. The polyp consists of clusters of normal-appearing or hypertrophic

fundic glands, with a few or many interspersed dilated glands (Figures 15-1 and 15-2). The lining epithelium is often atten-uated, but many still retain the granular cytoplasm of parietal cells. On a biopsy specimen of an endoscopically recognized polyp, finding a single dilated fundic gland is considered suf-ficient for the diagnosis.

Occasionally, similar microscopic findings may be appre-ciated in a specimen not labeled as a polyp. These changes often result from extended PPI use. A diagnosis of gastric fundic gland hyperplasia may be rendered, with a comment suggesting correlation with possible PPI use (Figure 15-4). The changes often show prominence or hypertrophy of the fundic glands, with increased density of parietal cells com-pared to normal.

Dysplasia can occur in sporadic FGP (Figure 15-5). However, about 40% of FGPs occurring in FAP may have dysplasia (Figure 15-3).

■ GASTRIC HYPERPLASTIC POLYPS

The GHP type likely includes a group of entities that share a common microscopic appearance but have diverse underly-ing etiology and pathogenesis. The basic histologic feature is characterized by an overgrowth of the surface foveo-lar epithelium and the associated gastric pits (Figure 15-6) within an edematous and often-inflamed lamina propria (Figure 15-7). Therefore, the terms *hyperplastic polyp* and *inflammatory polyp* may be applied interchangeably in many cases (or simultaneously as *hyperplastic/inflammatory*

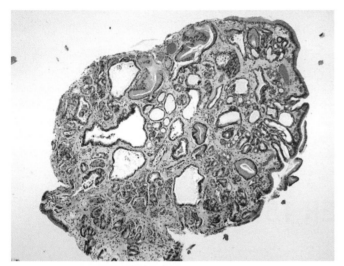

FIGURE 15-1. Fundic gland polyp.

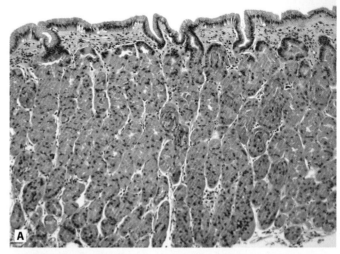

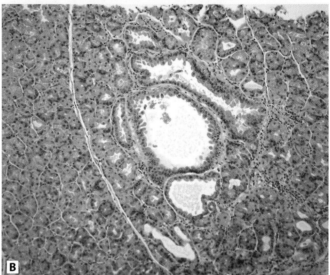

FIGURE 15-4. Fundic gland hypertrophy due to proton pump inhibitor effect. **A.** Fundic glands with increased parietal cell component. **B.** Occasional dilated fundic glands.

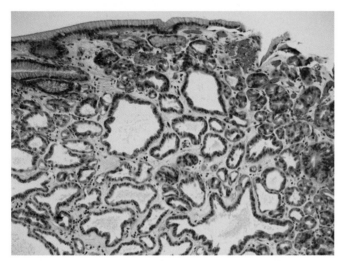

FIGURE 15-2. Fundic gland polyp, higher power. The dilated glands are lined by attenuated parietal cells and chief cells.

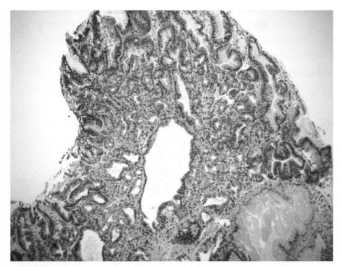

FIGURE 15-3. Fundic gland polyp with adenomatous change (low-grade dysplasia).

polyp, which I prefer). The reason to lump these two types of polyps together is due to the lack of criteria to distinguish them reproducibly. Many GHPs occur in a background of chronic *Helicobacter pylori* gastritis and occasionally contain the organisms identifiable either on a section stained with hematoxylin and eosin (H&E) or using immunostain. Some authors believe that at least a subset of the sporadic GHPs results from mucosal prolapse (see next section), a mechanism similar to prolapse polyps seen in the colon. In addition, several types of syndromic or hamartomatous polyps manifest as hyperplastic polyps when involving the stomach, such as juvenile polyps (JPs), Cronkhite-Canada syndrome (CCS) polyps, and Peutz-Jeghers (PJ) polyps (see separate discussion that follows). Distinction among these polyps can be made only on clinical grounds.

The GHPs are usually less than 1 cm in size, but larger polyps are not uncommon (therefore, size is not irrelevant

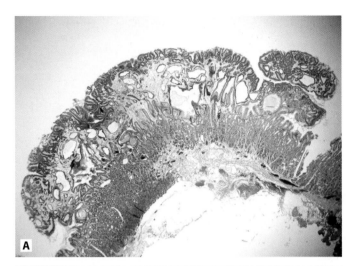

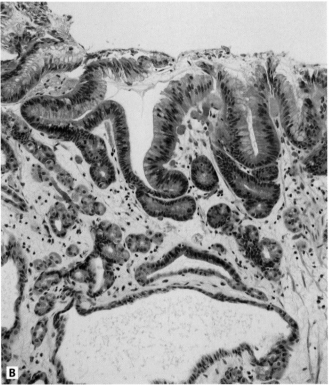

FIGURE 15-5. Low-grade dysplasia in a sporadic fundic gland polyp.

Gastric Mucosal Prolapse Polyp

The gastric mucosal prolapse polyps are rather large, usually located in the pylorus, and are characterized by marked cystic dilation (Figure 15-9). There is often retention of pyloric or fundic glands at the base of the polyp (Figure 15-9). Thick-wall blood vessels and muscularized stroma are also evident. As a "redundant" portion protruding from the mucosal surface, the polyp may be subject to mechanical damage from gastric contents, thus exhibiting surface erosion and a secondary inflammatory reaction. Purely based on morphologic grounds, it is indistinguishable from the usual hyperplastic polyp (when smaller) and a gastric PJ polyp (when larger).

Juvenile Polyp

Juvenile polyps occur in patients with a known history of juvenile polyposis, a syndrome with an underlying genetic abnormality of *SMAD4* (on chromosome 18) or BMPR1A (bone morphogenetic protein receptor type 1A). The gastric polyps are microscopically identical to the usual GHP, with hyperplasia of the foveolar zone and gastric pits, cystic dilation of glands, and lamina propria edema (Figure 15-10). Because gastric JPs usually occur in syndromic patients, dysplasia or adenocarcinoma may occur in these polyps (Figure 15-11). These foci may be a minor component within an otherwise-typical hyperplastic polyp. Therefore, careful microscopic scrutiny is warranted.

Cronkhite-Canada Syndrome Polyp

Gastric polyps occur as a part of the CCS generalized gastrointestinal polyposis, with hyperpigmentation, alopecia, and onychotrophia.[1] The etiology is unknown. Patients usually present with severe protein-losing gastroenteropathy that is associated with a mortality rate approaching 50%.[2-5] Involvement of the gastric mucosa may manifest endoscopically as multiple polyps, diffuse polypoid appearance, or prominent gastric folds. Histologically, CCS polyps closely resemble JPs or hyperplastic/inflammatory polyps, with dilated glands and lamina propria edema with mild inflammatory infiltration (Figure 15-12). This microscopic pattern is rather noncharacteristic in itself. If the possibility of this disease is not suspected, it is easy to miss or delay the diagnosis and instead make a diagnosis of foveolar hyperplasia or hyperplastic polyp. Another fact related to the diagnostic difficulty is that these patients nearly always present without a known syndromic background (unlike patients with juvenile polyposis or PJ syndrome) and with severe clinical symptoms of protein-losing enteropathy. The diagnostic focus is usually on the life-threatening abnormalities, and the "trivial" external abnormalities of pigmentation, hair loss, or nail dystrophy are usually not initially appreciated clinically. Often, these features are identified only after the pathologist suggests the diagnosis. As mentioned, histologically it is not possible to distinguish CCS polyps from GHP or JP. However, a biopsy taken from the intervening nonpolypoid gastric mucosa in

for their identification). Epithelial hyperplasia renders the microscopic findings of slightly or cystically dilated mucous glands, elongated gastric pits, and hyperplasia of the foveolar layer (Figure 15-6). The last often gives rise to the so-called corkscrew appearance (Figure 15-8). Another term, *polypoid foveolar hyperplasia* (PFH) was used by some authors, but the clinical significance of this last diagnosis and its distinction from GHP are not well defined.

Other polyps with similar microscopic appearances can be classified by recognizing some characteristic histologic clues and clinical background, as discussed next.

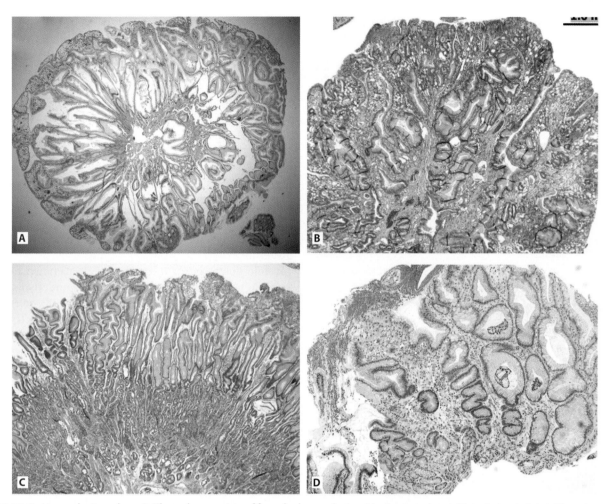

FIGURE 15-6. Hyperplastic polyps. **A.** The polyp consists of foveolar hyperplasia with elongated and dilated glands (pits). There is no inflammation. **B.** This polyp contains prominent capillary proliferation (resembling pyogenic granuloma). **C.** A hyperplastic polyp from the gastric body, with typical hyperplastic change overlying native fundic glands at the base. Note there is no fundic gland dilation as seen in a fundic gland polyp. **D.** At higher magnification, there is minimal lamina propria inflammation.

CCS reveals the same microscopic abnormalities of foveolar hyperplasia and edema. This feature is most helpful in reaching the correct diagnosis (Figure 15-12).

The diffuse involvement of gastric mucosa by marked foveolar hyperplasia accompanied by severe protein-losing gastropathy may raise the possibility of Ménétrier disease. Ménétrier disease, however, is characterized by diffuse, uniform hyperplasia of the gastric mucosa, with marked thickening of the rugal folds (see Chapter 14).

■ PEUTZ-JEGHERS POLYP

Patients with the PJ autosomal dominant (AD) hereditary polyposis syndrome usually have STK11/LKB1 gene mutation.[6] In addition to gastrointestinal polyps, patients present with skin and mucosal pigmentation and clubbed fingers and toes. Gastric polyps occur in patients who had previous or concurrent small-bowel and colon PJ polyps. Thus, the diagnosis is usually not challenging for gastric

polyp biopsies. Like PJ polyps of the small bowel and colon (Chapters 21 and 29, respectively), as a hamartomatous process, gastric PJ polyps consist of hyperplasia of different glandular components with arborizing smooth muscle fibers or bundles (Figure 15-13). The marked foveolar and mucous gland hyperplasia resembles that of hyperplastic polyps. However, lamina propria edema is usually not as prominent (Figure 15-13).

Patients with PJ polyposis have clearly increased risk for gastrointestinal carcinomas, as well as carcinomas of other sites, such as breast, testicular, and thyroid cancers and melanoma.[7–11]

■ PYLORIC GLAND ADENOMA

Pyloric gland adenomas may occur in the cardia, body, or antrum. They consist of tightly packed mucous glands of the pyloric type. The superficial foveolar layer may be normal or mildly hyperplastic. About one-third of PGAs arise in the

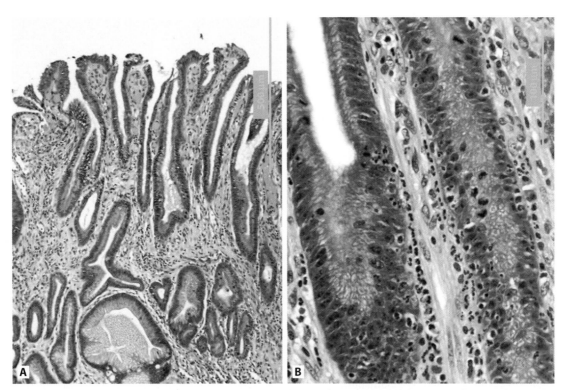

FIGURE 15-7. Inflammatory polyp. **A.** There is marked foveolar hyperplasia, inflammation infiltration, and fibrosis of the lamina propria. **B.** At higher magnification, neutrophilic infiltration and reactive epithelial changes are evident.

background of atrophic gastritis (see Chapter 12).[12] Other patients who have increased risk for PGA include those with FAP[13] or Lynch syndrome.[14] In traditional pathology texts, intestinal metaplasia has been listed as salient mucosal findings associated with diffuse atrophic gastritis. However, it is evident microscopically that atrophy of the normal gastric fundic mucosa with loss of parietal cells often is replaced by

FIGURE 15-8. Some hyperplastic polyps exhibit the "corkscrew"-like configuration in the superficial zone.

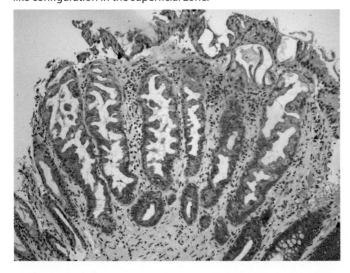

gastric pyloric-type glands (Figure 15-14). Focally increased proliferation of these pyloric glands thus gives rise to PGAs (Figure 15-15). More common are sporadic PGAs that occur without a background of atrophic gastritis; these can occur in the cardia or rarely **gastroesophagea**l junctional mucosa.[15,16]

In contrast to GHPs, PGAs are more frequently associated with dysplasia or progression to adenocarcinoma within the polyp, particularly in larger lesions. Therefore, it is imperative that the polyp be entirely processed for histology and carefully examined for foci of dysplasia or invasive component. The cytologic atypia may be subtle, but identifying the angulated growth pattern of the glands and invasion into the submucosa will help in reaching the correct diagnosis (Figure 15-16).

ADENOMATOUS POLYPS

Sporadic adenomas resembling their counterpart in the colon or small bowel are rare in the stomach, except for patients with chronic gastritis with intestinal metaplasia and patients with FAP. Most non–FAP-associated gastric adenomas likely represent discrete or polypoid dysplasia in the background of intestinal metaplasia.

Endoscopically, these are discrete polypoid or depressed lesions, exhibiting low- or high-grade dysplasia of the surface or glandular epithelium microscopically. Histologic recognition and diagnosis of gastric adenomas rely on the presence of intestinal-type adenomatous changes, similar to their counterpart in the colon or small bowel. Adenomas may

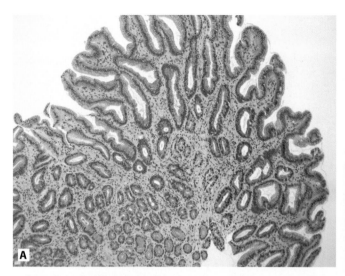

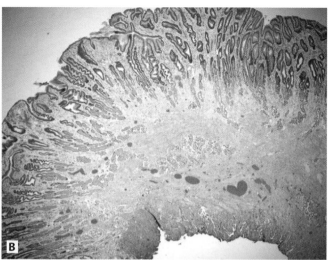

FIGURE 15-9. Prolapse polyp. **A.** This small prolapse polyp exhibits mild foveolar hyperplasia and early lamina propria fibrosis. **B.** A large antral prolapse polyp with exuberant foveolar hyperplasia (corkscrew-like configuration) as well as entrapment of pyloric mucous glands in proliferating fibromuscular bands toward the base.

exhibit predominantly a tubular, a papillary, or a mixed tubular-papillary configuration (Figure 15-17). The epithelium exhibits nuclear elongation, overlap (pseudostratification), and nuclear hyperchromasia. There is an increase in mitotic figures. Often, these changes are accompanied by mucin depletion.

As mentioned, other types of gastric polyps may undergo surface dysplasia, giving rise to a mixed microscopic appearance, such as in FGP (Figure 15-5) or a hyperplastic polyp (Figure 15-18). However, because hyperplastic polyps are often subject to inflammatory injury and exhibit marked reactive atypia, caution should be taken when making the diagnosis of dysplasia in these lesions (Figure 15-19).

One of the helpful features in favor of reactive atypia is that the changes are more prominent in the normal proliferative zone, with maturation toward the surface. There is also usually a gradual transition from the adjacent nonatypical area. In contrast, adenomatous change occurs abruptly.

■ GASTRITIS CYSTICA PROFUNDA

The gastritis cystica profunda (GCP) lesion is characterized endoscopically by irregular polypoid or nodular lesions, sometimes with ulceration. Microscopically, it consists of dilated or irregular glands focally extending to the submucosa.[17,18]

FIGURE 15-10. Juvenile polyp from a patient with juvenile polyposis syndrome. Foveolar hyperplasia, lamina propria edema, and inflammatory infiltration are seen. This example also shows a focal complex glandular configuration.

FIGURE 15-11. Juvenile polyp with intramucosal carcinoma. At higher magnification, a focal intramucosal invasive component is evident, showing irregular anastomosing glands with marked cytologic atypia.

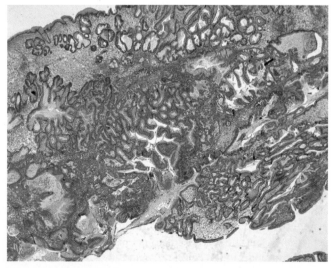

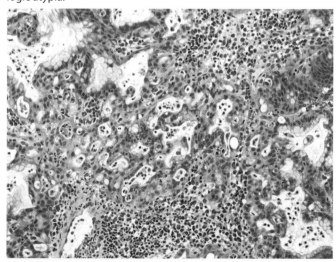

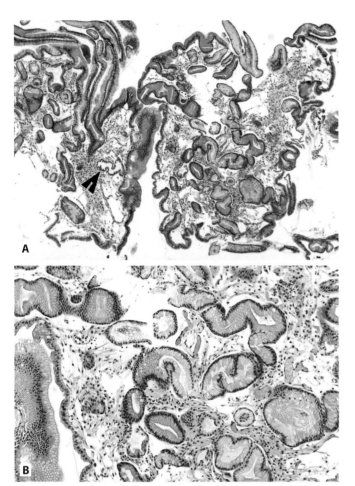

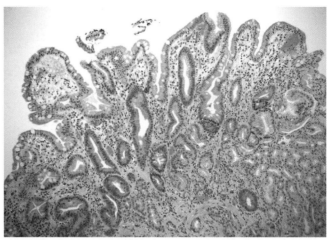

FIGURE 15-14. Pyloric gland metaplasia in atrophic gastritis. The gastric body has complete loss of normal fundic glands, replaced by pyloric-type mucous glands (lower right). Focal intestinal metaplasia is also evident.

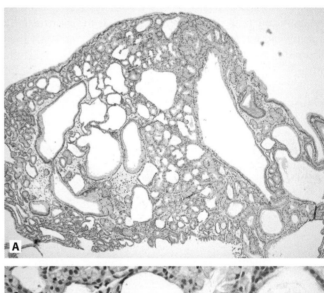

FIGURE 15-12. Cronkhite-Canada syndrome polyps. **A.** Two polyps in this view with marked lamina propria edema, large foveolar glands. Rare dilated fundic gland can be seen as well (arrowhead). **B.** Biopsy from nonpolypoid intervening mucosa showing similar microscopic pattern. There is mild lymphocytic infiltration.

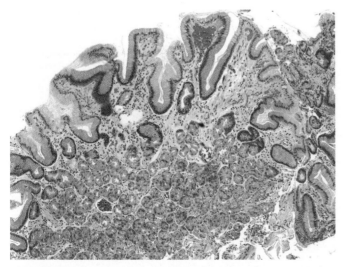

FIGURE 15-13. Gastric Peutz-Jeghers (PJ) polyp. This gastric polyp from a patient with small-bowel PJ polyps consists of hypertrophic glands and a foveolar layer, with patchy smooth muscle strands in lamina propria.

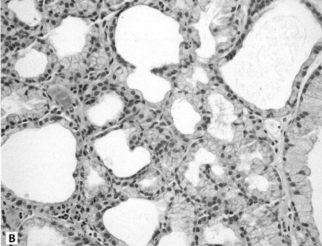

FIGURE 15-15. Pyloric gland adenoma. **A.** Tightly arranged pyloric-type glands with dilation. **B.** At higher magnification, the lining cells are bland and mucous type. There is minimal intervening lamina propria.

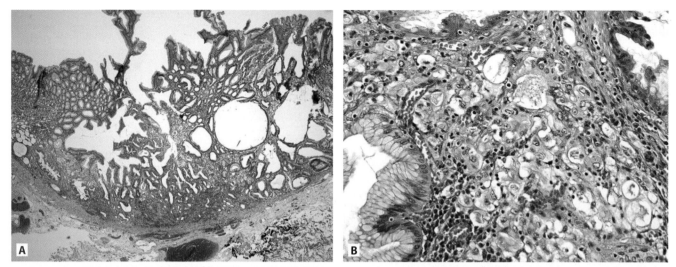

FIGURE 15-16. Pyloric gland adenoma with intramucosal carcinoma. **A.** Focal "consolidated" areas intervening among small as well as dilated glands, particularly toward the base of the mucosa. **B.** At higher magnification, these consolidated foci are occupied by clusters of epithelial cells infiltrating stroma.

A significant proportion of cases arises at the gastroenteric anastomosis (such as Billroth II gastrectomy), and some may occur during the repair process from repeated endoscopic procedures.[19] De novo cases without these histories also occur,[20] with some resulting from atrophy of ectopic pancreatic tissue with cystic dilation of remnant ducts (Figure 15-20).

The histologic hallmark of GCP is the misplaced glands in the submucosa (Figure 15-21), leading to confusion with invasive adenocarcinomas. In fact, some of these lesions highly resemble gastric carcinomas in radiographic appearance, making the histologic distinction critical. Fortunately, the benign, "entrapped" nature of these misplaced glands is

FIGURE 15-17. Gastric adenoma. **A.** Upper zone of this polyp exhibits adenomatous changes over mucous-type glands (tubular type). **B.** Adenoma with papillary configuration. **C.** The adenomatous change is characterized by elongated hyperchromatic nuclei and mucin depletion, similar to that in a typical intestinal tubular adenoma.

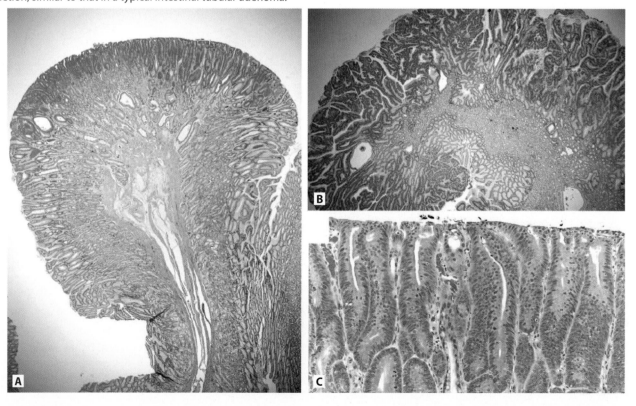

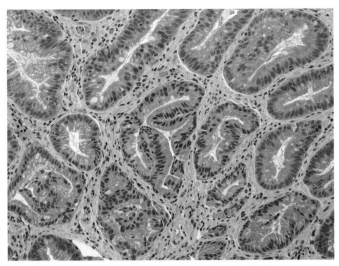

FIGURE 15-18. Hyperplastic polyp with adenomatous change.

characterized by an investing cuff of normal lamina propria, often associated with hemorrhage and hemosiderin deposit and without desmoplastic stromal reaction.

That said, adenocarcinoma can develop within a GCP lesion. Therefore, careful histologic examination is critical so that small foci of adenocarcinoma can be recognized. For cases with atypical-appearing glands, immunostains for p53 and Ki-67 may be helpful; if discrete foci of epithelial cells exhibit increased nuclear accumulation and high Ki-67 staining index, both are suggestive (but not diagnostic) of the dysplastic nature of the cells.

Gastric Neuroendocrine Tumors

The gastric neuroendocrine tumor (NET) lesions often manifest as a mucosal polyp and need to be included in the differential consideration of gastric polyps (Figure 15-22). These are discussed in Chapter 16.

FIGURE 15-19. Hyperplastic polyp with marked reactive atypia. The foveolar cells focally exhibit an increased nucleus-to-cytoplasm (N/C) ratio with nuclear hyperchromasia. However, gradual maturation toward the surface is evident. The increased N/C ratio is mainly due to mucin depletion and shrinkage of the cytoplasm.

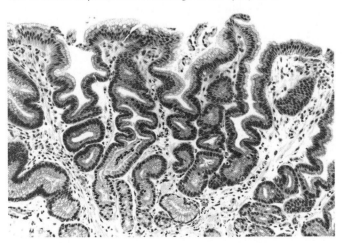

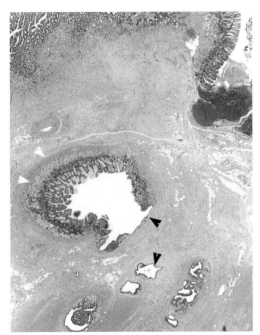

FIGURE 15-20. Gastritis cystica profunda from a pancreatic rest remnant. There are cystically dilated remnant ducts and acinar tissue.

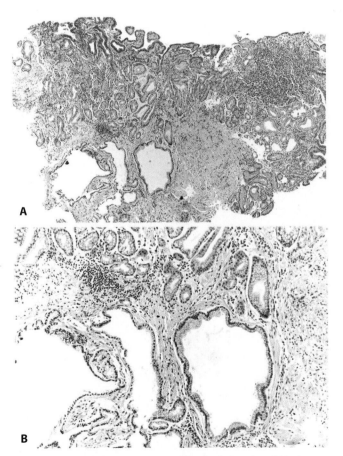

FIGURE 15-21. Gastritis cystica profunda. **A.** A polypoid lesion near a gastrojejunal anastomosis, with inflammatory infiltration, foveolar hyperplasia, and large dilated glands, focally extending into the muscular mucosa. **B.** At higher magnification, no desmoplastic reaction to the bland-appearing glands.

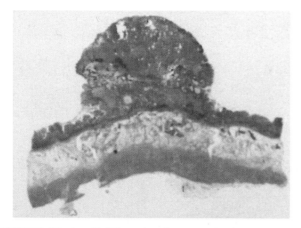

FIGURE 15-22. A well-differentiated neuroendocrine tumor as a gastric polyp.

Miscellaneous Polypoid Lesions

Many other pathologic processes involving the stomach may lead to focal polypoid lesions and should be kept in mind when forming differentials on microscopic examination, such as localized antrum-predominant Menetrier disease (Figure 15-23). Also, ectopic pancreatic tissue or

FIGURE 15-23. Localized Ménétrier polyps in an elderly patient. **A.** Endoscopic view of multilobular giant antral polyps, which microscopically resemble hyperplastic polyps. **B.** A cytomegalovirus inclusion body is evident in the stroma of the eroded area.

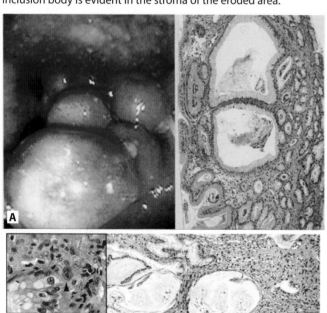

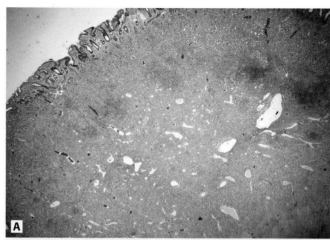

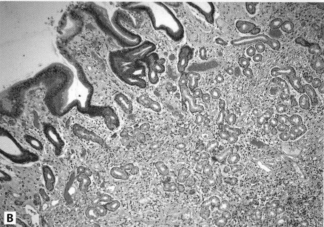

FIGURE 15-24. Inflammatory fibroid polyp. **A.** The polyp largely consists of fibrovascular proliferation, inflammatory infiltration, and lymphoid aggregates. The process involves both submucosa and mucosa. **B.** The intramucosal portion exhibits dense fibrous reaction, entrapping small native glands.

pancreatic acinar heterotopia are easily recognized on H&E sections. Similarly, an inflammatory fibroid polyp (IFP) can be recognized by the presence of exuberant stromal proliferation, with mixed inflammatory cellular infiltration, and relative lack of glandular epithelium (Figure 15-24). An IFP can involve both the submucosa and the mucosa. In addition, a small gastrointestinal stromal tumor or metastatic carcinoma may occasionally present as a small mucosal polyp.

■ SUMMARY

The two most common types of gastric polyp are GHPs and FGPs, which possess unique histologic features and are not difficult to recognize. PGAs also have characteristic features, namely, tightly arranged, uniform, pyloric-type mucous glands. Dysplasia can occur in FGPs; when identified, or in the case of a gastric adenoma (either PGA or intestinal type), the possibility of FAP should be ruled out. Several syndrome-related hamartomatous gastric polyps (such as JP and PJ polyps) histologically resemble hyperplastic polyps, and diagnosis should be considered within the proper clinical context. When encountered with multiple GHPs and hyperplastic polyps harboring dysplasia, the pathologist should raise the possibility of polyposis syndrome. Furthermore, patients with CCS usually have gastric biopsies for the first time without a prior known history of the syndrome. If the biopsy of polyps reveals hyperplastic/inflammatory features in a patient with symptoms of protein-losing enteropathy, the possibility of CCS should be indicated. Other less-common lesions include GCPs and IFPs. In addition, well-differentiated NETs may present as mucosa polyps. These are discussed in separate chapters.

■ REFERENCES

1. Cronkhite LW Jr, Canada WJ. Generalized gastrointestinal polyposis; an unusual syndrome of polyposis, pigmentation, alopecia and onychotrophia. *N Engl J Med.* 1955;252(24):1011–1015. PMID: 14383952.

2. Miyoshi M, Fujii H, Iwasa N, Nishitani T, Nishimura S. Two autopsy cases of diffuse gastrointestinal polyposis with ectodermal changes. Cronkhite-Canada syndrome. *Am J Gastroenterol.* 1975;64(5):357–364. PMID: 1211385.

3. Burke AP, Sobin LH. The pathology of Cronkhite-Canada polyps. A comparison to juvenile polyposis. *Am J Surg Pathol.* 1989;13(11):940–946. PMID: 2552848.

4. Murata I, Yoshikawa I, Endo M, et al. Cronkhite-Canada syndrome: report of two cases. *J Gastroenterol.* 2000;35(9):706–711. PMID: 11023043.

5. Bettington M, Brown IS, Kumarasinghe MP, de Boer B, Bettington A, Rosty C. The challenging diagnosis of Cronkhite-Canada syndrome in the upper gastrointestinal tract: a series of 7 cases with clinical follow-up. *Am J Surg Pathol.* 2014;38(2):215–223. PMID: 24418855.

6. Hemminki A, Markie D, Tomlinson I, et al. A serine/threonine kinase gene defective in Peutz-Jeghers syndrome. *Nature.* 1998;391(6663):184–187. PMID: 9428765.

7. Hizawa K, Iida M, Matsumoto T, Kohrogi N, Yao T, Fujishima M. Neoplastic transformation arising in Peutz-Jeghers polyposis. *Dis Colon Rectum.* 1993;36(10):953–957. PMID: 8404388.

8. Bignell GR, Barfoot R, Seal S, Collins N, Warren W, Stratton MR. Low frequency of somatic mutations in the LKB1/Peutz-Jeghers syndrome gene in sporadic breast cancer. *Cancer Res.* 1998;58(7):1384–1386. PMID: 9537235.

9. Churchman M, Dowling B, Tomlinson IP. Identification of a novel mRNA species of the LKB1/STK11 Peutz-Jeghers serine/threonine kinase. *DNA Seq.* 1999;10(4–5):255–261. PMID: 10727082.

10. Sato N, Rosty C, Jansen M, et al. STK11/LKB1 Peutz-Jeghers gene inactivation in intraductal papillary-mucinous neoplasms of the pancreas. *Am J Pathol.* 2001;159(6):2017–2022. PMID: 11733352.

11. Ryan MW, Cunningham S, Xiao SY. Maxillary sinus melanoma as the presenting feature of Carney complex. *Int J Pediatr Otorhinolaryngol.* 2008;72(3):405–408. PMID: 18082273.

12. Park JY, Cornish TC, Lam-Himlin D, Shi C, Montgomery E. Gastric lesions in patients with autoimmune metaplastic atrophic gastritis (AMAG) in a tertiary care setting. *Am J Surg Pathol.* 2010;34(11):1591–1598. PMID: 20975338.

13. Wood LDMDP, Salaria SNMD, Cruise MWMDP, Giardiello FMMD, Montgomery EAMD. Upper GI tract lesions in familial adenomatous polyposis (FAP): enrichment of pyloric gland adenomas and other gastric and duodenal neoplasms. *Am J Surg Pathol.* 2014;38(3):389–393.

14. Lee SE, Kang SY, Cho J, et al. Pyloric gland adenoma in Lynch syndrome. *Am J Surg Pathol.* 2014;38(6):784–792. PMID: 24518125. PMCID: 4014525.

15. Vieth M, Kushima R, Borchard F, Stolte M. Pyloric gland adenoma: a clinico-pathological analysis of 90 cases. *Virchows Arch.* 2003;442(4):317–321. PMID: 12715167.

16. Kushima R, Vieth M, Mukaisho K, et al. Pyloric gland adenoma arising in Barrett's esophagus with mucin immunohistochemical and molecular cytogenetic evaluation. *Virchows Arch.* 2005;446(5):537–541. PMID: 15838649.

17. Franzin G, Novelli P. Gastritis cystica profunda. *Histopathology.* 1981;5(5):535–547. PMID: 7286916.

18. Okada M, Iizuka Y, Oh K, Murayama H, Maekawa T. Gastritis cystica profunda presenting as giant gastric mucosal folds: the role of endoscopic ultrasonography and mucosectomy in the diagnostic work-up. *Gastrointest Endosc.* 1994;40(5):640–644. PMID: 7988836.

19. Greywoode G, Szuts A, Wang LM, Sgromo B, Chetty R. Iatrogenic deep epithelial misplacement ("gastritis cystica profunda") in a gastric foveolar-type adenoma after endoscopic manipulation: a diagnostic pitfall. *Am J Surg Pathol.* 2011;35(9):1419–1421. PMID: 21836475.

20. Bechade D, Desrame J, Algayres JP. Gastritis cystica profunda in a patient with no history of gastric surgery. *Endoscopy.* 2007;39(Suppl 1):E80–E81. PMID: 17440878.

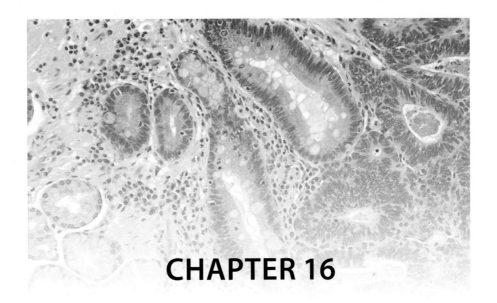

CHAPTER 16

Dysplasia and Adenocarcinoma

▣ INTRODUCTION

This chapter focuses on diagnosis and grading of dysplasia, morphologic variants of gastric adenocarcinomas, and practical aspects in examining gastric biopsy and resection specimens. Poorly differentiated gastric adenocarcinoma can be focal in mucosal distribution, causing diagnostic challenges in both endoscopic sampling and microscopic identification. It is important to recognize this unique and common pitfall to avoid missed diagnoses. Helpful histologic features to increase diagnostic sensitivity are discussed. Finally, an update on ancillary tests for gastric carcinomas is provided.

▣ DYSPLASIA

Dysplasia is the defining feature of gastric adenomas. It may also occur in other types of gastric polyps, including fundic gland polyps (FGPs), hyperplastic polyps, and pyloric gland adenoma (PGA). These polyps are described in greater detail in Chapter 15 but are briefly discussed here for completeness. Low- and high-grade dysplasias also develop in a subset of patients with long-term chronic gastritis with intestinal metaplasia in a nonpolypoid setting. Although intestinal-type adenocarcinomas arise in the background of intestinal metaplasia with dysplasia, no precursor lesions have been identified for a significant portion of other types of adenocarcinomas. In most cases of diffuse-type or signet-ring cell carcinoma, no dysplastic or in situ lesions could be identified. It has been reported that in situ signet-ring carcinoma

can be identified in patients with *CDH1* gene mutation, representing the precursor lesion for the related hereditary diffuse gastric cancer (HDGC).[1-3] However, there is lack of proven morphologic specificity for this finding, and further studies are needed.

▣ DYSPLASIA IN GASTRIC POLYPS

The pathologic features of gastric polyps are discussed in Chapter 15. Overall, small gastric polyps carry a low risk of malignant transformation in long-term follow-up studies, with the exception of adenomas and PGA.[4-6] For example, an FGP with dysplasia (Figure 16-1) is associated with only a negligible risk of malignant transformation,[7,8] although rare cases of adenocarcinoma arising from it have been reported.[9] Therefore, for patients with such polyps, endoscopic follow-up is sufficient. On the other hand, because FGP with dysplasia is common in patients with familial adenomatous polyposis (FAP),[10,11] its recognition may help uncover the underlying syndrome in some previously undiagnosed patients.

Adenomas of the stomach encompass at least 2 main categories: the usual intestinal type and PGA. In routine practice, the generic term *gastric adenoma* is applied to the former. These adenomas by definition harbor at least low-grade dysplasia, similar to that of colonic tubular adenoma (Figure 16-2). In contrast, PGA, despite the name, usually does not harbor dysplasia. Only a subset of PGAs undergoes

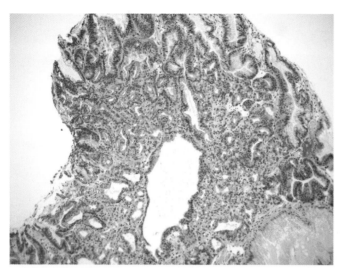

FIGURE 16-1. Dysplasia in a sporadic fundic gland polyp (FGP). The surface epithelium is replaced by atypical columnar cells with large, overlapping, hyperchromatic nuclei in a polyp otherwise typical of FGP.

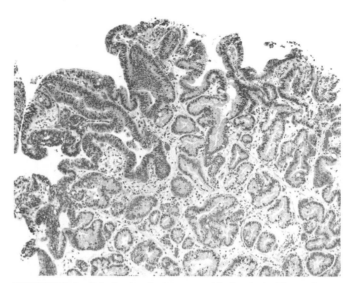

FIGURE 16-3. Pyloric gland adenoma with dysplasia. The surface epithelium is focally replaced by dysplastic cells; elongated atypical nuclei involve partial to full thickness of the epithelial cells.

low- or high-grade dysplasia (Figure 16-3). Some may harbor intramucosal carcinoma (see Chapter 15). Therefore, polypectomy with PGA should be histologically examined in its entirety, with careful orientation for assessment of margins.

Gastric hyperplastic polyps may undergo focal dysplasia, and adenocarcinoma may develop in rare cases.[12–15] Dysplastic foci in these polyps are histologically similar to the intestinal-type adenomatous changes (Figure 16-4).

Less commonly, gastric juvenile polyps (Figure 16-5) may develop dysplasia and even intramucosal carcinoma (see Chapter 15).

■ DYSPLASIA IN NONPOLYPOID SETTINGS

It is well known that focal or extensive dysplasia occurs in a subset of patients with long-standing chronic gastritis or atrophic gastritis with intestinal metaplasia, following an inflammation-metaplasia-dysplasia-carcinoma pathway (Figure 16-6). Adenocarcinoma of different stages, from carcinoma in situ to intramucosal carcinoma, superficial carcinoma, and deeply invasive carcinoma, may occur in this setting, with a pure or predominant intestinal morphology or phenotype. Occasionally, the spectrum of changes can be identified in a single microscopic field (Figure 16-7).

FIGURE 16-2. Gastric adenoma. The villous-type proliferation is lined by tall, columnar epithelial cells with nuclear hyperchromasia, overlapping, and elongation, resembling intestinal adenocarcinoma.

FIGURE 16-4. Gastric hyperplastic polyp (GHP) with low-grade dysplasia (adenomatous change). Note the cystically dilated foveolar glands of the GHP.

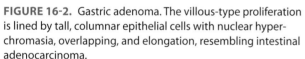

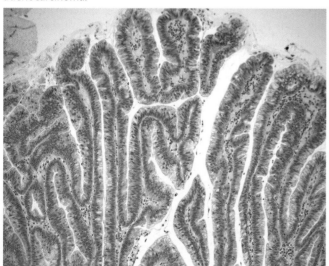

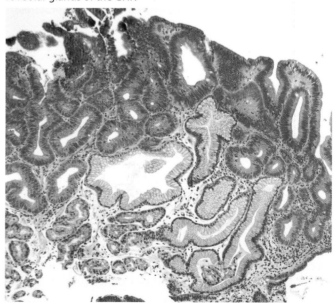

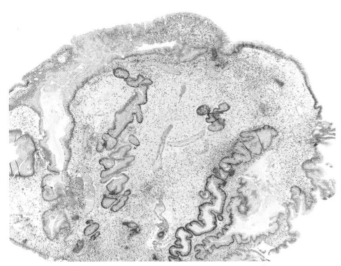

FIGURE 16-5. Gastric juvenile polyp. This patient had juvenile polyposis syndrome and was under endoscopic surveillance. This polyp was negative for dysplasia. However, a subsequent examination revealed a gastric juvenile polyp containing an intramucosal adenocarcinoma (see Chapter 15, Figures 15-10 and 15-11).

Rarely, the native gastric foveolar epithelium many also undergo dysplasia (Figure 16-8), which can progress to adenocarcinoma of the gastric type.

Dysplasia of gastric mucosa should be further classified as low or high grade. In general, for low-grade dysplastic lesions (Figure 16-9A), the risk of an associated high-grade dysplasia or invasive adenocarcinoma is low.[16–18] Annual surveillance repeatedly revealed low-grade dysplasia in many patients had no progression to high-grade dysplasia or carcinoma. Some authors found that the risk of progression was slightly increased if the patients were older, male, or had atrophic gastritis.[16] There has been a lack of consensus regarding how to best manage these patients. Some authors recognized a depressed endoscopic appearance, lesions larger than 1 cm, and surface erythema as risk factors that prompt endoscopic resection.[18]

FIGURE 16-6. Dysplasia arising in a patient with chronic gastritis and intestinal dysplasia. The hyperchromatic nuclei exhibit pseudostratification occupying the full thickness of the epithelium, making this a high-grade dysplasia (carcinoma in situ).

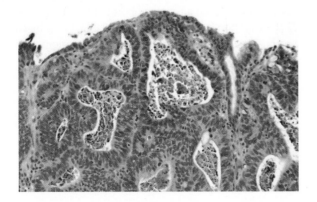

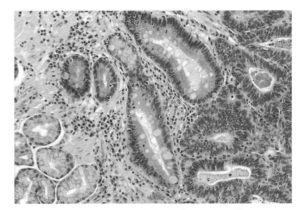

FIGURE 16-7. Native gastric glands (left), intestinal metaplasia (middle), and high-grade dysplasia (right) captured in a single microscopic field.

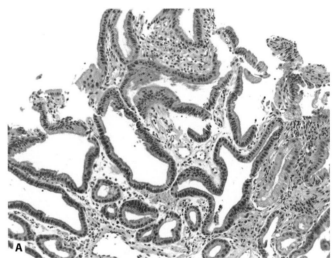

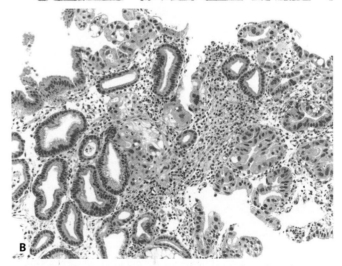

FIGURE 16-8. Gastric adenocarcinoma arising from foveolar-type dysplasia. There is lack of intestinal metaplasia. **A.** The background exhibits foveolar hyperplasia. **B.** The tumor lacks intestinal epithelial morphology. Although the biopsy is superficial and only revealed intramucosal invasion, the patient presented with liver metastasis.

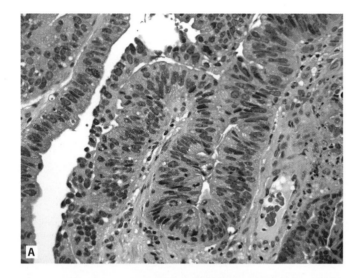

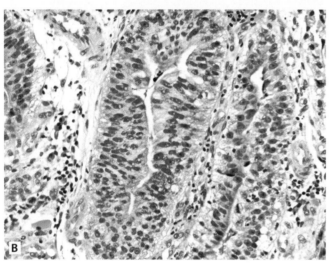

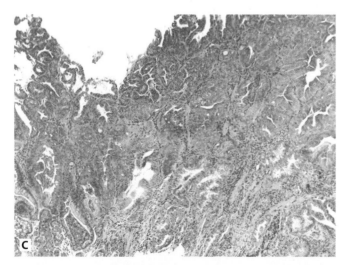

FIGURE 16-9. Grading of dysplasia. **A.** Low-grade dysplasia. The atypical nuclei occupy the basal aspect of the epithelium, maintaining the polarized appearance. **B.** High-grade dysplasia, with elongated atypical nuclei involving the full thickness of the epithelium. **C.** High-grade dysplasia, with complex architecture of the dysplastic gland.

For other lesions, annual endoscopic surveillance with rebiopsy is recommended. However, for patients with high-grade dysplasia, endoscopic mucosal resection (EMR), endoscopic submucosal dissection (ESD), or surgery is warranted due to its association with significant risk of adenocarcinoma.[17,19]

High-grade dysplasia is characterized by either enlarged/elongated atypical nuclei occupying the full thickness of the epithelium (Figure 16-9B) or architectural complexity, such as cribriform pattern (Figure 16-9C).

As mentioned, studies of prophylactic total gastrectomy suggested the presence of signet-ring cell carcinoma in situ,[1-3] in which individual or clusters of signet-ring cells are identified among benign cells of the gastric glands, particularly fundic-type glands. However, sufficient control cases were not included in these studies, making it difficult to evaluate the specificity of these cells that exhibit signet-ring cell morphology. Cells of similar morphology can be seen in other unselected gastric resections or biopsies without the associated risk for carcinoma (Figure 16-10). Therefore, in its current status, further studies are needed to validate the biological concept of signet-ring cell carcinoma in situ before reproducible diagnostic criteria can be developed and their significance understood. Otherwise, pathologists will face the obvious dilemma of whether to render the diagnosis of signet-ring cell carcinoma in situ in routine biopsies or resections performed for indications other than carcinoma.

ADENOCARCINOMA

Traditionally gastric adenocarcinomas were classified as intestinal, diffuse, or mixed type based on the histologic pattern of glandular formation.[20] Nevertheless, it is well known that many gland-forming carcinomas exhibit gastric epithelial morphology and thus should be considered gastric type. The Lauren and the World Health Organization (WHO) tumor classification systems rely on mixed criteria of phenotype (eg, intestinal) and histologic pattern (diffuse, tubular, etc.) and are in fact descriptive instead of taxonomic. Not all gland-forming tumors (ie, nondiffuse pattern) are of the intestinal phenotype, and some poorly differentiated carcinomas (eg, mucinous ones) may exhibit intestinal phenotype. In addition, there are other less-common types of primary gastric carcinomas, such as squamous, adenosquamous, hepatoid, lymphoepithelioma-like, and sarcomatoid. Primary choriocarcinoma also occurs rarely. From a practical point of view, until a more logical classification system becomes available it may be advisable to place individual cases, on thorough histologic examination, into one of the categories listed in Table 16-1.

The following descriptions are arranged by these histologic types:

Intestinal type: Most intestinal-type adenocarcinomas arise from a background of chronic gastritis with intestinal metaplasia and various degrees of dysplasia, and are well differentiated (Figure 16-11). However, larger tumors may consist of moderate to poorly differentiated

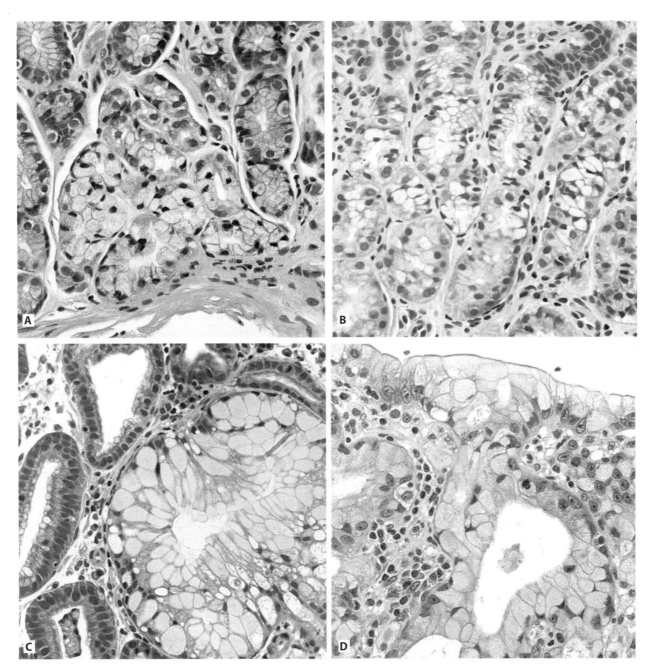

FIGURE 16-10. Examples of intra-epithelial cells that mimic signet ring cells. **A.** Mucinous cell change in gastric glands (otherwise normal stomach). **B.** Focal mucinous cell changes in biopsy from a patient with CDH1 mutation. **C.** Mucinous tumor cells focally forming glands in a biopsy with intramucosal carcinoma. **D.** Mucinous cells in gastric glands adjacent to a focus of signet ring cell carcinoma. Without context, these intraglandular mucinous cells all resemble signet ring cells and thus lack specificity as a diagnostic entity for "signet ring cell carcinoma in situ."

areas. Some diffuse poorly differentiated carcinomas may have a focal glandular formation of the intestinal type and may be labeled as mixed type. Intestinal-type carcinomas are more common in the distal stomach. Although not necessary for routine diagnosis, immunohistochemical stains reveal the tumor cells exhibit an intestinal profile, being positive for MUC2 and CK20 but negative for MUC5AC or MUC6. Occasionally, a tumor exhibiting a morphology not typical for

intestinal type can be found to be consistent with the latter immunohistochemically (Figure 16-12). Intestinal-type adenocarcinomas almost always arise from a dysplastic surface or glandular epithelium. In other words, they usually have precursor lesions adjacent to the invasive carcinoma.

Tubular type: These tumors often exhibit glandular or tubular formation (Figure 16-13A). Instead of typical intestinal adenomatous epithelium, the tubular epithelium exhibits

TABLE 16-1. Histologic types of gastric carcinomas.

Predominantly gland-forming gastric carcinomas

    Intestinal type

    Gastric tubular or papillary type

Predominantly non–gland-forming gastric carcinomas

    Diffuse type (poorly differentiated)

    Signet-ring cell carcinoma

    Mucinous carcinoma

    Medullary carcinoma (carcinoma with lymphoid stroma)

    Hepatoid adenocarcinoma

    Adenosquamous carcinoma

    Hereditary diffuse gastric carcinoma (HDGC)

Mixed adenoendocrine carcinoma

gastric foveolar (Figure 16-13B) or pyloric gland morphology: tall-to-cuboidal columnar cells with pale mucinous or fine granular cytoplasm (Figure 16-13C). Carcinomas arising from PGA also exhibit this morphology, consistent with their gastric gland origin (Figure 16-14). Some of the tumors can have a focal papillary configuration or be predominantly papillary (Figure 16-15). However, all these can be considered morphologic variants of gastric-type adenocarcinoma. Immunohistochemically, the epithelial cells exhibit reactivity for MUC5AC, MUC6, or CK7 but are negative for MUC2. Interestingly, a significant subset

FIGURE 16-11. Well-differentiated adenocarcinoma, intestinal type, arising in a background of intestinal metaplasia.

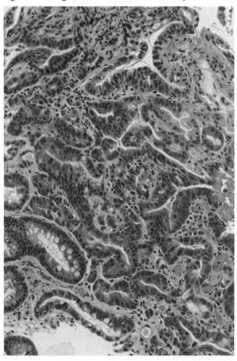

of small-bowel adenocarcinomas arising in Crohn disease also have this gastric phenotype, possibly related to pyloric gland metaplasia commonly seen in Crohn enteritis.[21]

Diffuse type: The tumors usually consist of solid sheets or clusters of mostly discohesive malignant cells infiltrating the lamina propria or beyond the mucosa, without forming glands. Some cases have various degrees of a signet-ring cell component (Figure 16-16) or mucinous component. When the latter components are prominent, the term *signet-ring cell carcinoma* or *mucinous carcinoma* is applied. In this regard, the diffuse type is a morphologically categorical, but not specific, tumor type. Furthermore, by default, the diffuse-type tumor is classified as a poorly differentiated carcinoma. A more significant aspect of this type is that these tumors, particularly signet-ring cell carcinomas, are often not associated with a dysplastic surface or glandular epithelium (Figure 16-17A). The lamina propria infiltration may be erroneously interpreted as merely inflammatory (with foamy macrophages, eg) at scanning magnification due to lack of the stromal desmoplastic reaction seen in most other invasive carcinomas (Figure 16-17B). Some diffuse, poorly differentiated carcinomas are more concentrated in the deeper mucosa, with minimal involvement of the superficial mucosa but with submucosa and wall invasion (Figure 16-18).

One possible explanation for the lack of in situ lesion in many diffuse-type gastric carcinomas is that diffuse or signet-ring cell carcinoma may arise from cells of endocrine origin because many tumor cells express synaptophysin or chromogranin A protein.[22]

Mucinous carcinoma. This histologic type is characterized by abundant mucin production and accumulation, with a relatively minor cellular component. Based on cytomorphology and histologic architecture, at least two subtypes can be distinguished. Tumors of the first subtype are characterized by strips of mucinous columnar cells (goblet cells) at the periphery of the mucin pools (Figure 16-19A), corresponding to well-differentiated or low-grade adenocarcinoma. The second subtype contains clusters of or individual tumor cells with prominent cytological atypia in mucin pools (Figure 16-19B). Sometimes the malignant cells exhibit features of signet-ring cells (Figure 16-19C). This type of tumor is poorly differentiated and thus high grade. In providing tumor grading, this distinction should be made if possible.

Medullary type (carcinoma with lymphoid stroma): Rare cases of diffuse carcinoma contain prominent lymphocytic infiltration, similar to medullary carcinoma of other sites (Figure 16-20A). Other terms used for this type of tumor are *carcinoma with lymphoid stroma* and *lymphoepithelioma-like carcinoma*. This tumor more frequently involves the proximal stomach or gastric stump. The tumor cells are large and often form syncytial sheets or nests (Figure 16-20B). This type was shown to be highly associated with the presence of Epstein-Barr virus

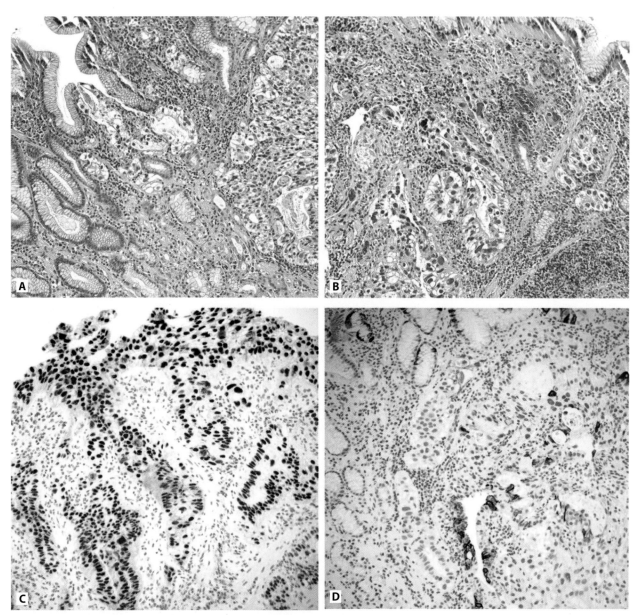

FIGURE 16-12. Gastric adenocarcinoma. This tumor presented as an angularis ulcer that lacked the usual intestinal-type morphology, and the adjacent nontumor glands are foveolar type (**A**, **B**). However, immunohistochemically there is diffuse nuclear expression of CDX-2 (**C**) and focal cytoplasmic staining for CK20 (**D**), indicating intestinal differentiation.

(EBV),[23] as EBV-encoded small RNA (EBER) can be readily identified in most cases of this morphologic type by in situ hybridization (Figure 16-21). Currently, a firm etiologic relationship has not been confirmed between medullary carcinoma and EBV. However, anecdotal evidence is not hard to find. For example, the tumor illustrated in Figure 16-22 is a typical medullary carcinoma containing a well-differentiated glandular component. Interestingly, nuclear accumulation of EBER is demonstrated not only in the medullary tumor cells but also in the glandular epithelium. Assuming the glandular component represents an earlier step in progression to the medullary morphology, this finding is thus suggestive of a causative relationship between EBV and medullary change.

Mixed adenoendocrine carcinoma (MAEC). In the WHO classification, this tumor is defined as a tumor with a mixed component in which both the glandular and endocrine components are malignant; the latter should independently qualify for neuroendocrine carcinoma (Figure 16-23). Occasionally, an otherwise-typical carcinoid (endocrine tumor, type I) may contain entrapped metaplastic intestinal glands (Figure 16-24A), which can be erroneously diagnosed as MAEC, particularly when the latter component exhibits reactive cytologic atypia and mitosis (Figure 16-24B). In some of these lesions, the herniation of the glandular component may be clearly identified in deeper sections (Figure 16-25). It is important not to over-identify these lesions as mixed

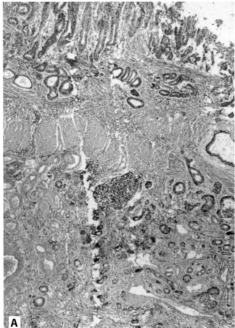

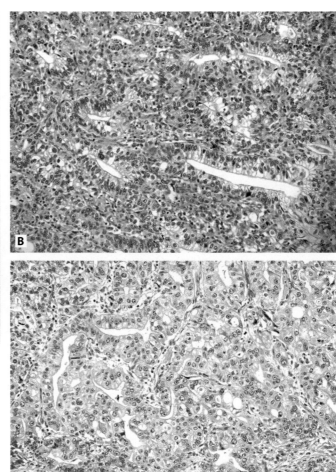

FIGURE 16-13. Tubular adenocarcinoma. **A.** This deeply invasive carcinoma consists of small, well-formed tubules, lined by cells similar to foveolar cells. There is no intestinal metaplasia in the background. **B.** Higher-power view of a tubular-type carcinoma, mainly consisting of dysplastic foveolar cells. **C.** A tubular-type carcinoma consisting mainly of pyloric gland epithelium. Note the small hyaline globules.

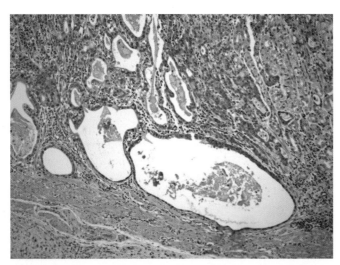

FIGURE 16-14. Tubular-type adenocarcinoma arising in a pyloric gland adenoma.

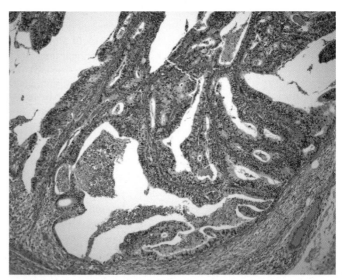

FIGURE 16-15. Papillary-type adenocarcinoma. Note tumor cells retained a gastric phenotype.

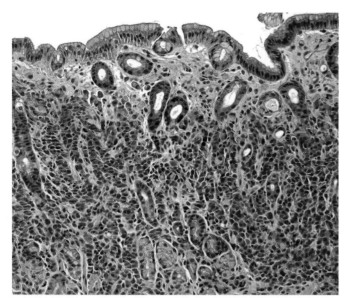

FIGURE 16-16. Diffuse-type gastric carcinoma. Sheets or cords of tumor cells with solid cytoplasm are present between normal and slightly reactive gastric antral glands. Despite the invasive carcinoma, there was no significant stroma reaction.

adenoendocrine carcinomas as this will lead to unnecessary surgery, while most patients with type I gastric carcinoids are managed by endoscopic resection and follow-up (see Chapters 6 and 17).

PRACTICAL ISSUES

There are several issues that pathologists face in daily practice when examining biopsy or resection specimens of the stomach. First, for prognostic and treatment purposes, gastric carcinomas are classified into intramucosal, superficial, and the rest (ie, deeply invasive). Second, to reiterate a famous pathologist's phrase, every pathologist who sees gastric biopsies had missed a diagnosis of gastric carcinoma. This reflects the challenges inherent in biopsy diagnosis of diffuse-type gastric adenocarcinoma, which deserve detailed discussion and recognition. Third, tumors of other sites may present or be discovered initially in gastric biopsies; many can be resolved if high alertness is maintained. Last, there are unique features that should be considered while examining gastric specimens resected for adenocarcinoma.

Superficial Gastric Carcinoma

Many early gastric carcinomas, despite being poorly differentiated (signet-ring carcinoma), are limited to the mucosa (Figure 16-26A). These tumors and those invading the submucosa are classified as superficial gastric carcinoma (Figure 16-26B). Even for intramucosal carcinomas, there is a risk of lymph node metastasis in 2%–3% of patients. Therefore, complete surgical resection of intramucosal carcinoma is the treatment of choice.

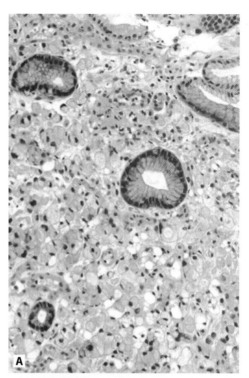

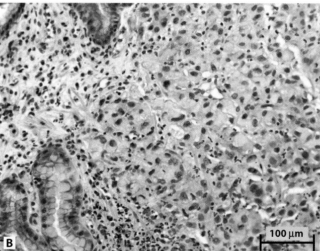

FIGURE 16-17. Signet-ring cell carcinoma. **A.** Note the tumor infiltrates among completely unremarkable foveolar glands. **B.** Diffuse-type gastric adenocarcinoma infiltrating the lamina propria without stromal reaction.

Challenges in Biopsy Diagnosis of Gastric Adenocarcinoma

Sampling Error

Two main factors may lead to inadequate sampling. The first relates to the fact that many early signet-ring cell carcinomas are small and have patchy distribution, often not easily identifiable endoscopically. Using data from mapping examinations of total gastrectomy specimens from CDH1 mutation carriers, it was estimated that to avoid missing a single focus of small signet-ring cell carcinoma in a patient with known

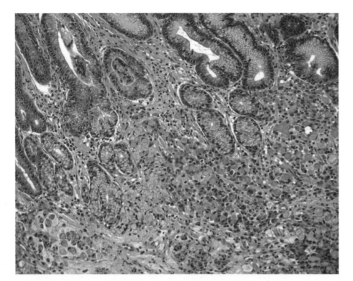

FIGURE 16-18. A signet-ring cell carcinoma infiltrating the deeper portion of the mucosa, sparing the superficial mucosa.

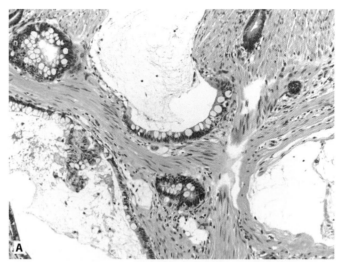

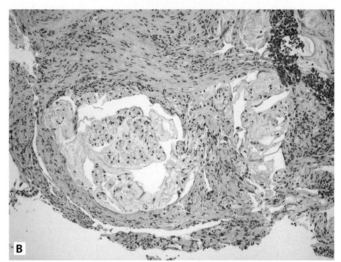

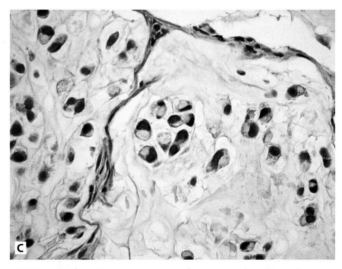

FIGURE 16-19. Mucinous carcinoma. **A.** Low-grade, well-differentiated adenocarcinoma. Low-grade mucinous columnar cells (goblet cells) form strips at the periphery of large mucin pools or form small glands. **B.** Poorly differentiated mucinous adenocarcinoma. **C.** High-grade, poorly differentiated carcinoma. Large mucin pools contain highly atypical cells, some with signet-ring morphology.

risk for diffuse gastric cancer, thousands of biopsies would be required,[24] which is not practical. In actual clinical practice, biopsies are performed to rule out malignancy only in symptomatic patients with endoscopic abnormalities. Nonetheless, to ensure appropriate diagnostic yield, clinicians should be encouraged to take multiple biopsies in a patient suspected of having cancer. The second cause of sampling error relates to the fact that some diffuse-type gastric carcinomas are deeply invasive but with no or limited involvement of the upper mucosal layer. Nonneoplastic mucosa overlying a malignant tumor often undergoes hyperplastic changes, further increasing the thickness of the "negative" zone of mucosa. Thus it is not uncommon that, even in some patients with evident pyloric obstruction, a mucosal biopsy may yield a negative result. Reexamination with deeper biopsy guided by endoscopic ultrasound (EUS) may eventually give rise to a positive result (Figure 16-27).

Another scenario is related to severe narrowing of the pylorus, which prevents the endoscope from proceeding properly and targeting the lesion to obtain a productive biopsy.

In these scenarios, the false-negative result is due to sampling error prior to the pathologist's interpretation, thus representing true negativity from the pathologist's point of view. Nevertheless, it is important to alert the clinician regarding possible insufficient or improper sampling, especially when the biopsy tissue is superficial and minute.

Interpretation Error

As discussed, diffuse signet-ring cell carcinomas may be small in size and patchy in distribution (Figure 16-28). Even when present in the biopsy, it is not rare for pathologists who see many biopsies daily, most of which are inflammatory in nature, to miss the tumor spot on the slides or fail to obtain deeper sections to avoid a histological sampling error. Another unique feature of diffuse or signet-ring cell carcinoma is the lack of dysplastic changes in the background mucosa (Figure 16-17),

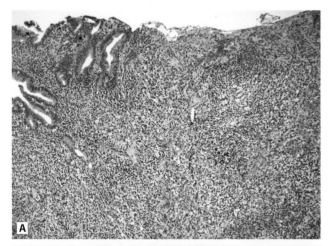

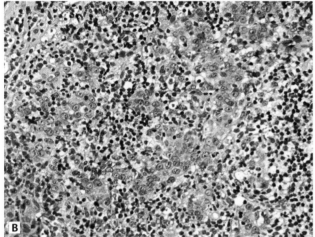

FIGURE 16-20. Medullary carcinoma. **A.** The tumor consists of sheets of poorly differentiated epithelial cells infiltrating the cardia mucosa, with ulceration, and abundant lymphoid tissue, including a lymphoid follicle. **B.** Higher magnification demonstrates the large tumor cells with vesicular nuclei with prominent nucleolus and significant intratumoral infiltration by small lymphocytes.

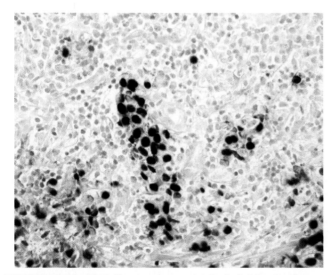

FIGURE 16-21. Medullary carcinoma. In situ hybridization for Epstein-Barr virus (EBV)–encoded small RNA (EBER) revealed positive staining in tumor cells.

and the small clusters of infiltrative tumor cells may be inconspicuous (Figure 16-28). In fact, in many cases, the few tumor cells sit among microscopically unremarkable glands. To avoid this type of mistake, the only approach is to be highly alert when evaluating gastric biopsies. Scrutiny at both scanning and high magnification of the entire biopsy or EMR specimen is always required. This will allow the pathologist to recognize a suspicious focus, even though a firm diagnosis cannot always be made solely on slides stained with hematoxylin and eosin (H&E). A simple workup with immunostain for cytokeratin (CAM5.2) may help confirm the epithelial nature of the infiltrative tumor cells. Some pathologists may also perform immunostaining for CD68 to rule out macrophages.

Missing the malignant diagnosis in this manner (interpretation error) is a false-negative result on the pathologist's part, which can be avoided in most cases if great caution is taken and high vigilance maintained.

Pseudoadenocarcinoma

There have been reports of some cases of fundic gland or chief cell–type adenocarcinoma, with prominent fundic glands (many with hypertrophy and dilation) focally "extending" into the muscularis mucosa. However, patchy superficial extension of benign gastric glands into the muscularis mucosae is not uncommon and should not be interpreted as invasion in nondysplastic background. All the patients in these reports had an excellent prognosis. Other studies found that these represent overdiagnosis.[25]

Gastric Involvement by Cancers from Other Primary Sites

It should be kept in mind that tumors from several other sites can be initially discovered in biopsies of the stomach mucosa due to upper gastrointestinal symptoms and relative ease in obtaining biopsies. These other tumors may secondarily involve the stomach as either a metastasis or direct invasion. In patients with the clinical history of a known primary, it is easy to perform additional special or immunohistochemical stains to confirm or rule out a metastasis. However, often there is a lack of such history. For example, invasive lobular carcinoma may involve the gastric mucosa in the form of diffuse or signet-ring cell carcinoma (Figure 16-29). When this possibility is suspected, immunostains for estrogen receptor (ER) and progesterone receptor (PR) often will help reach the correct diagnosis. Theoretically, the possibility of a metastatic carcinoma should be considered in every case of poorly differentiated or signet-ring cell carcinoma discovered in biopsy. However, it is neither ethical nor practical to perform a battery of immunostains on every tumor-positive gastric biopsy. Careful scrutiny at high power sometimes can identify unusual features that should prompt further investigation. For example, prominent intracytoplasmic secretions are not a feature of signet-ring cells. These cells are sometimes referred to as "targetoid" cells (Figure 16-29), which are quite distinct and should prompt further immunostains.

In addition, pancreatic ductal carcinoma sometimes invades the wall of stomach. Rarely, adenocarcinoma may

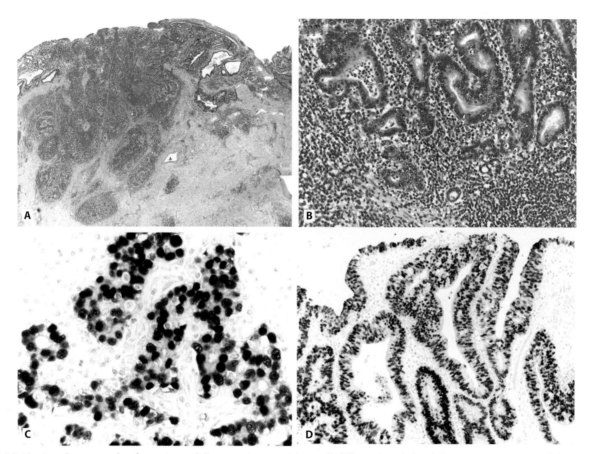

FIGURE 16-22. Another example of gastric medullary carcinoma with a well-differentiated glandular component toward the mucosal surface (**A**). The glandular component also exhibits increased intraepithelial lymphocytes (**B**). In situ hybridization demonstrated EBER (Epstein-Barr virus–encoded small RNA) in both carcinoma (**C**) and surface dysplastic glandular epithelium (**D**).

occur in a cystogastrostomy and present as a gastric mucosa mass at the pancreatogastric anastomosis.

Evaluation of Resected Specimens

Proper gross examination and strategic section-taking of resected specimen are essential for accurate microscopic examination and the final report with proper parameter recording. This principle also applies to EMR or ESD specimens. EMR and ESD specimens are preferably inked at the margins and well fixed by pinning on a wax block. Details on how to assess pathologic parameters for staging are discussed in other publications. Several issues that sometimes can cause ambiguity in practice are described here.

Staging as GEJ Cancer or Gastric Cancer

The common practice is that when the tumor midpoint is within 5 cm of the gastroesophageal junction (GEJ), it should be staged as esophageal cancer. However, it should be pointed out that this refers only to those tumors that involve the GEJ. Otherwise, the tumor should be staged as gastric cancer, even when it is close to the GEJ.

Margins

For the most part, evaluation of the proximal and distal margins is straightforward. Due to the tendency of diffuse-type gastric carcinoma to spread widely in the submucosa ("lateral spreading"), grossly negative end margins may be involved by tumor on microscopic evaluation. For this reason, it is preferable to ink the proximal and distal margins, which are to be processed for histology to include the entire circumference. If the tumor is grossly close (within 2 cm) to the margin, perpendicular sections should be taken to include the inked margin at one end of each section, with the entire circumference "blocked," to ensure accurate assessment. The radial margins are represented by the lesser and greater omentum (omental margin), which are almost always negative for tumor.

T4 Status

When tumor is grossly close to the serosa or there is gross abnormality of the serosa surface, the area should be inked and a well-oriented tissue section should be taken for accurate microscopic evaluation (Figure 16-30).

ANCILLARY TESTING

Ancillary tests, including immunohistochemistry (IHC), polymerase chain reaction (PCR), mutational analysis, and other modalities, are discussed in Chapter 7. For gastric adenocarcinomas, the following are either routinely applied or often requested in clinical trial settings:

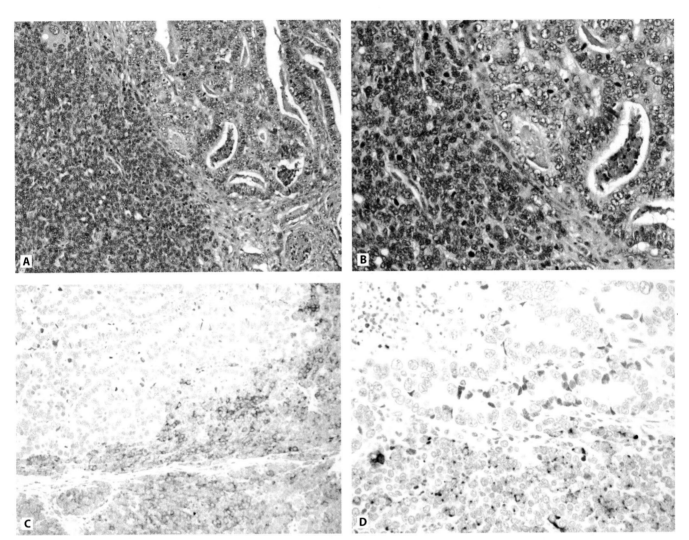

FIGURE 16-23. Mixed adenoendocrine carcinoma. This is a 3-cm tumor in the antrum of a patient who presented with gastrointestinal bleeding and anemia. **A.** Two distinctive components, the gland-forming, moderately differentiated adenocarcinoma and the endocrine tumor. **B.** The endocrine tumor has a high mitotic rate (33 per 10 high-power fields). **C.** Immunostaining for synaptophysin. **D.** Immunostaining for chromogranin. Both components were found in the lymph node metastasis.

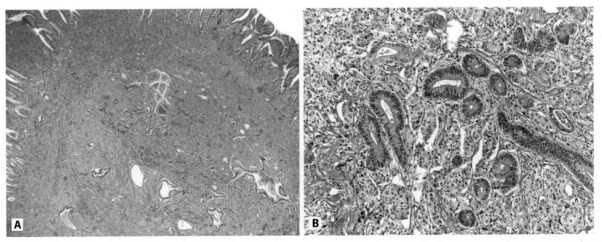

FIGURE 16-24. Gastric neuroendocrine tumor (NET; carcinoid tumor) with entrapped metaplastic glands. **A.** The tumor mostly occupies the submucosa, intermixed with small and dilated glands lined by metaplastic intestinal epithelium. **B.** Cytologic atypia is observed focally.

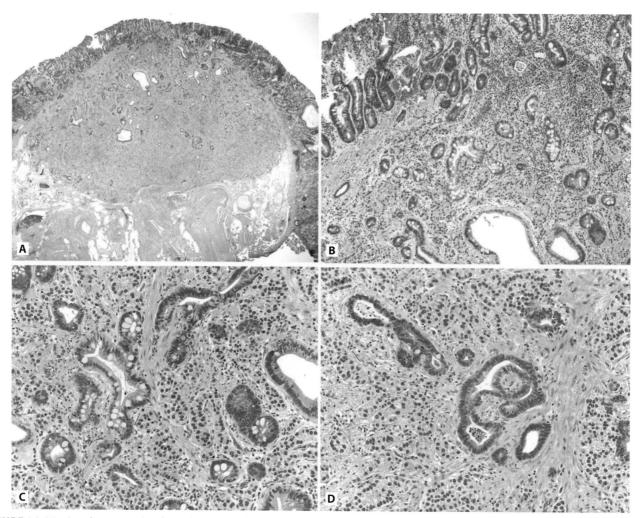

FIGURE 16-25. Another example of gastric neuroendocrine tumor (NET; carcinoid tumor) with entrapped glands. **A.** The lesion is well circumscribed and is connected directly at the top aspect with the intramucosal component. **B.** Higher magnification demonstrating the point of herniation of endocrine tumor along with benign glands where muscularis mucosa is interrupted. **C.** The deep glands retain the mixed-population epithelial cells. **D.** Focally, the glands may exhibit cytologic atypia, a reactive change to the surrounding endocrine tumor.

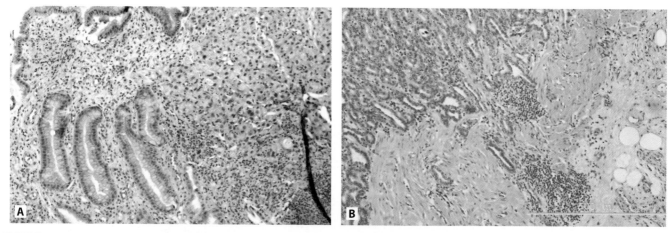

FIGURE 16-26. Superficial gastric adenocarcinomas. **A.** Intramucosal, poorly differentiated adenocarcinoma. **B.** Well-differentiated adenocarcinoma with superficial submucosal invasion.

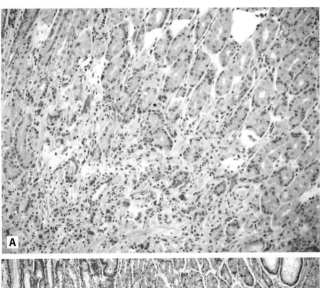

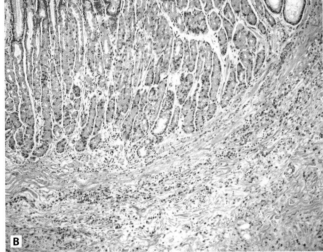

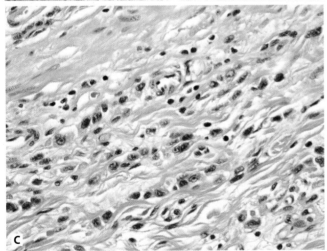

FIGURE 16-27. Poorly differentiated gastric carcinoma without superficial involvement. Despite symptoms and the endoscopic finding of linitis plastica, initial endoscopic biopsy was negative for cancer. Endoscopic ultrasound-guided needle biopsy obtained diagnostic materials. The overlying fundic mucosa was normal except for inconspicuous dysplastic glands at the base of fundic glands (**A**), which could be easily missed in superficial biopsy. The infiltrative carcinoma is mainly in the submucosa (**B**), focally with a single type of infiltration (mimicking breast lobular carcinoma) (**C**).

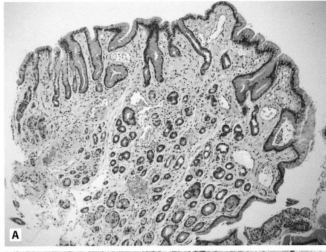

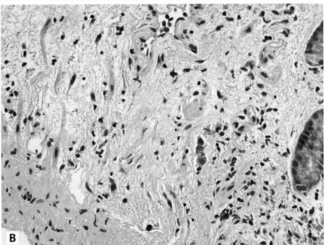

FIGURE 16-28. Invasive gastric adenocarcinoma in a biopsy. **A.** Most of the biopsy fragments exhibit marked foveolar hyperplasia. **B.** A single strip of malignant tumor cells in one biopsy fragment. Note the lack of dysplasia.

Immunostaining for p53. Nuclear p53 accumulation is reported to occur in about 60% of adenomas, as well as dysplastic foci in hyperplastic polyps.[26] This may be helpful when evaluating a focus in a biopsy that is suspicious for dysplasia in the background of atrophic gastritis with intestinal metaplasia. It must be noted that strong positive staining will help support the diagnosis of dysplasia in a suspected case. However, negative p53 staining does not necessarily exclude dysplasia.

Microsatellite instability (MSI): There are no consensus guidelines for testing patients for microsatellite instability high (MSI-H) or loss of mismatch repair (MMR) protein status. However, gastric adenocarcinomas in patients with Lynch syndrome are found to have deficient MMR proteins. Some patients may have somatic mutations, although rare. In our practice, for patients who otherwise meet the revised Bethesda guidelines for colorectal carcinoma, IHC for MMR protein will be performed to help identify potential Lynch syndrome.

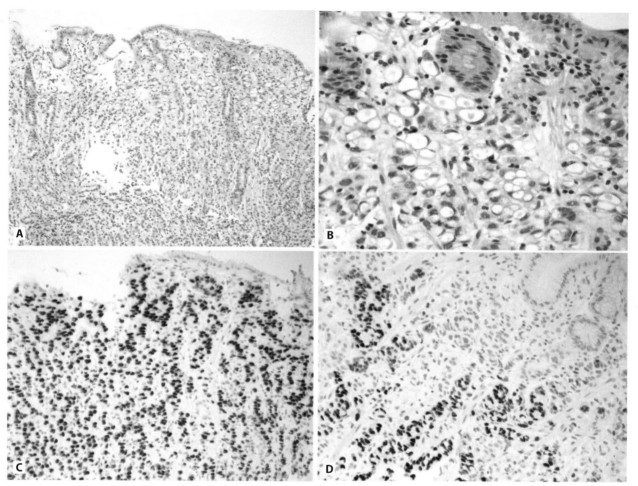

FIGURE 16-29. Metastatic lobular breast carcinoma to the stomach. **A.** Gastric biopsy from a woman with no prior history of malignancy revealed a diffuse-type, poorly differentiated adenocarcinoma with features suggestive of signet-ring cells. **B.** However, high-power view revealed cytoplasmic secretary material, an unusual feature for gastric signet-ring cell carcinomas. The tumor was positive for ER (**C**) and PR (**D**) immunohistochemically.

Epstein-Barr virus: As discussed previously, for a tumor with medullary morphology, in situ hybridization for EBER should be performed to rule out the EBV-related carcinoma (Figures 16-21 and 16-22).

Her2neu: It is believed that some gastric adenocarcinomas exhibit Her2 overexpression and may respond to anti-EGFR (anti–epidermal growth factor receptor) treatment. It is more prevalent in tumors of the intestinal type. Even though currently there has been no prognostic value identified in well-controlled analysis,[27] immunostaining for Her2 is performed in gastric carcinomas with metastatic disease. As discussed in Chapter 7, in situ hybridization for Her2 amplification status is recommended for tumors that exhibit 2+ staining, whether focal or diffuse (Figure 16-31).

MET: Overexpression of MET tyrosine kinase receptor is found in some gastric carcinomas[28] and is a potential treatment target for metastatic gastric carcinomas.[29] In the Western population, about 7%–20% of gastric cancers are found to have activated MET mutations. In clinical trial settings, immunostaining for MET is performed on gastric adenocarcinomas that have metastasized.

FIGURE 16-30. Tumor cell extending to the proximity of the serosa, indicating a T4a grade in the TNM system.

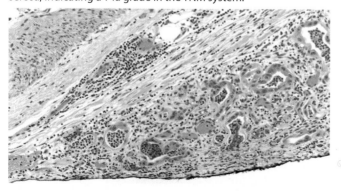

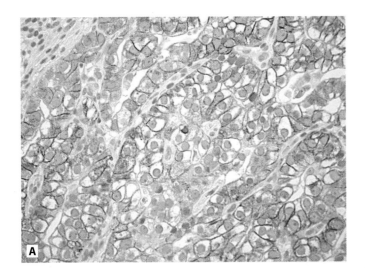

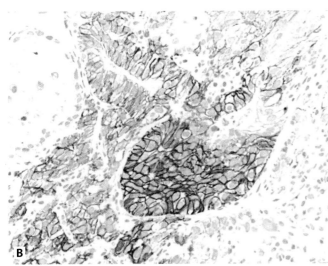

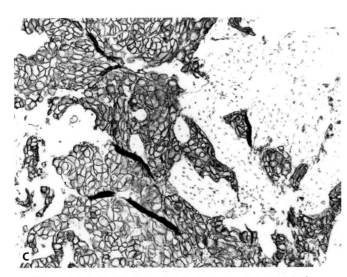

FIGURE 16-31. Her2 expression by immunostain. **A.** Moderately differentiated adenocarcinoma with 2+ staining. **B.** Focal 3+ immunostaining of the same tumor. **C.** Poorly differentiated gastroesophageal junctional (GEJ) adenocarcinoma with 3+ staining.

REFERENCES

1. Carneiro F, Huntsman DG, Smyrk TC, et al. Model of the early development of diffuse gastric cancer in E-cadherin mutation carriers and its implications for patient screening. *J Pathol.* 2004;203(2):681–687. PMID: 15141383.

2. Oliveira C, Moreira H, Seruca R, de Oliveira MC, Carneiro F. Role of pathology in the identification of hereditary diffuse gastric cancer: report of a Portuguese family. *Virchows Arch.* 2005;446(2):181–184. PMID: 15735979.

3. Barber ME, Save V, Carneiro F, et al. Histopathological and molecular analysis of gastrectomy specimens from hereditary diffuse gastric cancer patients has implications for endoscopic surveillance of individuals at risk. *J Pathol.* 2008;216(3):286–294. PMID: 18825658.

4. Vieth M, Kushima R, Borchard F, Stolte M. Pyloric gland adenoma: a clinico-pathological analysis of 90 cases. *Virchows Arch.* 2003;442(4): 317–321. PMID: 12715167.

5. Chen ZM, Scudiere JR, Abraham SC, Montgomery E. Pyloric gland adenoma: an entity distinct from gastric foveolar type adenoma. *Am J Surg Pathol.* 2009;33(2):186–193. PMID: 18830123.

6. Matsubara A, Sekine S, Kushima R, et al. Frequent GNAS and KRAS mutations in pyloric gland adenoma of the stomach and duodenum. *J Pathol.* 2013;229(4):579–587. PMID: 23208952.

7. Hassan A, Yerian LM, Kuan SF, Xiao SY, Hart J, Wang HL. Immunohistochemical evaluation of adenomatous polyposis coli, beta-catenin, c-Myc, cyclin D1, p53, and retinoblastoma protein expression in syndromic and sporadic fundic gland polyps. *Hum Pathol.* 2004;35(3): 328–334. PMID: 15017589.

8. Arnason T, Liang WY, Alfaro E, et al. Morphology and natural history of familial adenomatous polyposis-associated dysplastic fundic gland polyps. *Histopathology.* 2014;65(3):353–362. PMID: 24548295.

9. Garrean S, Hering J, Saied A, Jani J, Espat NJ. Gastric adenocarcinoma arising from fundic gland polyps in a patient with familial adenomatous polyposis syndrome. *Am Surg.* 2008;74(1):79–83. PMID: 18274437.

10. Sarre RG, Frost AG, Jagelman DG, Petras RE, Sivak MV, McGannon E. Gastric and duodenal polyps in familial adenomatous polyposis: a prospective study of the nature and prevalence of upper gastrointestinal polyps. *Gut.* 1987;28(3):306–314. PMID: 3032754. PMCID: 1432679.

11. Abraham SC, Nobukawa B, Giardiello FM, Hamilton SR, Wu TT. Fundic gland polyps in familial adenomatous polyposis: neoplasms with frequent somatic adenomatous polyposis coli gene alterations. *Am J Pathol.* 2000;157(3):747–754. PMID: 10980114. PMCID: 1885693.

12. Orlowska J, Jarosz D, Pachlewski J, Butruk E. Malignant transformation of benign epithelial gastric polyps. *Am J Gastroenterol.* 1995;90(12):2152–2159. PMID: 8540506.

13. Abraham SC, Singh VK, Yardley JH, Wu TT. Hyperplastic polyps of the stomach: associations with histologic patterns of gastritis and gastric atrophy. *Am J Surg Pathol.* 2001;25(4):500–507. PMID: 11257625.

14. Yao T, Kajiwara M, Kuroiwa S, et al. Malignant transformation of gastric hyperplastic polyps: alteration of phenotypes, proliferative activity, and p53 expression. *Hum Pathol.* 2002;33(10):1016–1022. PMID: 12395375.

15. Ahn JY, Son da H, Choi KD, et al. Neoplasms arising in large gastric hyperplastic polyps: endoscopic and pathologic features. *Gastrointest Endosc.* 2014;80(6):1005–1013 e2. PMID: 24929480.

16. Rugge M, Leandro G, Farinati F, et al. Gastric epithelial dysplasia. How clinicopathologic background relates to management. *Cancer.* 1995;76(3):376–382. PMID: 8625116.

17. Yamada H, Ikegami M, Shimoda T, Takagi N, Maruyama M. Long-term follow-up study of gastric adenoma/dysplasia. *Endoscopy.* 2004;36(5):390–396. PMID: 15100945.

18. Cho SJ, Choi IJ, Kim CG, et al. Risk of high-grade dysplasia or carcinoma in gastric biopsy-proven low-grade dysplasia: an analysis using the Vienna classification. *Endoscopy.* 2011;43(6):465–471. PMID: 21425043.

PART THREE

19. Fertitta AM, Comin U, Terruzzi V, et al. Clinical significance of gastric dysplasia: a multicenter follow-up study. Gastrointestinal Endoscopic Pathology Study Group. *Endoscopy.* 1993;25(4):265–268. PMID: 8330543.

20. Lauren P. The two histological main types of gastric carcinoma: diffuse and so-called intestinal-type carcinoma. An attempt at a histoclinical classification. *Acta Pathol Microbiol Scand.* 1965;64:31–49. PMID: 14320675.

21. Whitcomb E, Liu X, Xiao SY. Crohn enteritis-associated small bowel adenocarcinomas exhibit gastric differentiation. *Hum Pathol.* 2014;45(2):359–367. PMID: 24331840.

22. Sordal O, Qvigstad G, Nordrum IS, Sandvik AK, Gustafsson BI, Waldum H. The PAS positive material in gastric cancer cells of signet ring type is not mucin. *Exp Mol Pathol.* 2014;96(3):274–278. PMID: 24589859.

23. Uemura Y, Tokunaga M, Arikawa J, et al. A unique morphology of Epstein-Barr virus-related early gastric carcinoma. *Cancer Epidemiol Biomarkers Prev.* 1994;3(7):607–611. PMID: 7827592.

24. Fujita H, Lennerz JK, Chung DC, et al. Endoscopic surveillance of patients with hereditary diffuse gastric cancer: biopsy recommendations after topographic distribution of cancer foci in a series of 10 CDH1-mutated gastrectomies. *Am J Surg Pathol.* 2012;36(11):1709–1717. PMID: 23073328.

25. Singhi AD, Lazenby AJ, Montgomery EA. Gastric adenocarcinoma with chief cell differentiation: a proposal for reclassification as oxyntic gland polyp/adenoma. *Am J Surg Pathol.* 2012;36(7):1030–1035. PMID: 22472957.

26. Lauwers GY, Wahl SJ, Melamed J, Rojas-Corona RR. p53 expression in precancerous gastric lesions: an immunohistochemical study of PAb 1801 monoclonal antibody on adenomatous and hyperplastic gastric polyps [erratum appears in *Am J Gastroenterol.* 1994;89(2):300]. *Am J Gastroenterol.* 1993;88(11):1916–1919. PMID: 8237942.

27. Fisher SB, Fisher KE, Squires MH 3rd, et al. HER2 in resected gastric cancer: Is there prognostic value? *J Surg Oncol.* 2014;109(2):61–66. PMID: 24122802.

28. Janjigian YY, Tang LH, Coit DG, et al. MET expression and amplification in patients with localized gastric cancer. *Cancer Epidemiol Biomarkers Prev.* 2011;20(5):1021–1027. PMID: 21393565. PMCID: 3690490.

29. Catenacci DV, Henderson L, Xiao SY, et al. Durable complete response of metastatic gastric cancer with anti-Met therapy followed by resistance at recurrence. *Cancer Disc.* 2011;1(7):573–579. PMID: 22389872. PMCID: 3289149.

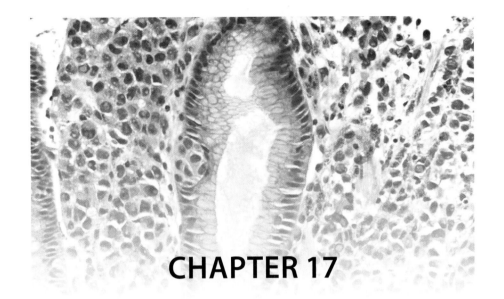

CHAPTER 17

Gastric Neuroendocrine Tumors and Other Rare Tumors

H. Aimee Kwak and Shu-Yuan Xiao

INTRODUCTION

Neuroendocrine tumors (NETs) of the stomach were discussed briefly as part of the general topics in Chapter 6. In this chapter, more details of these tumors are presented, particularly issues unique to the stomach. In addition, several other tumors that are rarely encountered in the stomach are discussed.

GASTRIC NEUROENDOCRINE TUMORS

There are multiple types of endocrine cells in the stomach (see also Chapter 6), three of which are well characterized in their roles of working together to regulate acid secretion from parietal cells. G cells are present in the antrum and secrete gastrin. D cells are located in the fundus and antrum and secrete somatostatin. Enterochromaffin-like (ECL) cells are seen in the fundus and body and secrete histamine 1. Of these, most NETs in the stomach arise from ECL cells.[2-4]

According to the World Health Organization (WHO) classification, gastric ECL cell NETs previously referred to as carcinoid tumors or well-differentiated neuroendocrine tumors are subtyped by clinicopathologic factors into well-differentiated types 1–3. In addition, other studies have proposed a type 4 gastric NET category to include neuroendocrine carcinoma (NEC), mixed endocrine-exocrine tumors, and some non-ECL cell tumors (Table 17-1).[5-7]

Types 1 and 2 are associated with secondary and primary hypergastrinemia, respectively. Type 1 tumor occurs as a result of decreased acid secretion seen in chronic atrophic gastritis (CAG).[8] In type 2 NETs there is ectopic secretions of gastrin from gastrinomas in Zollinger-Ellison syndrome (ZES) associated with multiple endocrine neoplasia type 1 (MEN 1).[8-10] Normal gastrin levels and sporadic occurrence characterize types 3 and 4.[11,12]

Epidemiology

The first reported cases of gastric NET were described in 1923 by Askanazy.[13] According to the SEER (Surveillance, Epidemiology, and End Results Program) database records from 1970 to 2008, gastric NETs comprise approximately 10% of gastrointestinal NETs. The incidence of gastric NETs has increased as demonstrated in a 5-decade analysis reporting a rise from 2.4 to 8.7% during 1969–1999, with 1–2 persons affected per 1 million people a year. This may be attributed partially to the increased use of endoscopy.[14] Multiple epidemiologic studies demonstrated an equal prevalence to slight predominance in females (1.4:1 to 2:1).[14-17]

Due to variable reporting and classification of the types of gastric NETs, the frequency of each type is not well established. Of the 3 conventional types, the largest case series on well-differentiated gastric NETs by Rindi et al demonstrated that the most common is type 1, followed by

TABLE 17-1. Neuroendocrine neoplasms of the stomach.[a]

Classification	Association	Frequency	Demographics	Location	Size	Outcome
Type 1	CAG	80%	F>M 40–50 years	Multicentric, body or fundus	Usually <1 cm	Usually benign
Type 2	ZES/MEN1	6%	M = F 50 years	Multicentric, body or fundus	Usually <1.5 cm	30% metastasize
Type 3	Sporadic	14%	M>F 55 years	Solitary, anywhere	33% of cases >2 cm	71% malignant
Type 4	Sporadic	Rare	M>F 63–70 years	Solitary, anywhere	Large	High-grade carcinoma, metastases common

Abbreviations: CAG, chronic atrophic gastritis; F, female; M, male; MEN1, multiple endocrine neoplasm type 1; ZES, Zollinger-Ellison syndrome.

[a]Data from Washington MK, Tang LH, Berlin J, et al. Protocol for the examination of specimens from patients with neuroendocrine tumors (carcinoid tumors) of the stomach. *Arch Pathol Lab Med.* 2010;134(2):187–191.[83]

types 3 and 2, respectively. These types were seen in 80%, 14%, and 6% of cases, respectively.[18] Multiple case reports have been published stating the rare frequency of type 4 tumors; however, when accounting for type 4 gastric NETs, the case series by Rindi et al and Borch et al showed a frequency of 7% and 14%, respectively.[5-7,11] Although type 1 is the most common gastric NET, it develops in only 0.7%–2.4% of patients with chronic atrophic gastritis.[19,20] In contrast, 20%–30% of patients with ZES associated with MEN 1 develop type 2 tumors.[21,22] There is a predominance of type 1 gastric NETs in females between 40 and 50 years of age, while type 3 occurs more frequently in males with a mean age of 55 years. Type 4 tumors are also increased in males with mean age of 63–70 years, while there is an equal prevalence of males and females in type 2 with a mean age of 50 years.[11,12,18,23] The overall 5-year rate of survival ranges from 63% to 82.7%.[14-17]

Clinical Presentation

Patients with type 1 gastric NETs can present with symptoms related to atrophic gastritis, often with anemia. Other patients are asymptomatic, presenting with an incidental nodule or polyp found on endoscopy. If present, symptoms are nonspecific and may include abdominal pain, anemia, nausea, upper gastrointestinal bleeding, and diarrhea.[11,24-26] On rare occasions, patients will develop carcinoid syndrome with paroxysmal flushing, diarrhea, and bronchospasm.[12,18]

Endoscopically, types 1 and 2 tumors demonstrate small (usually < 1–1.5 cm), multicentric, polypoid or submucosal lesions with occasional central erosion or ulceration; these are located in the gastric body or fundus. Types 3 and 4 NETs are larger, typically greater than 1 cm, and solitary, and can occur anywhere in the stomach.[18,27,28] When suspicious for a gastric NET, additional biopsies of the antrum, body, and fundus should be taken to help assess the NET type.[19,29] CAG (associated with type 1 tumors) is characterized by diffuse thinning or atrophy of the gastric mucosa but may also present as nodular mucosa paradoxically (see also Chapter 12). In contrast, ZES (associated with type 2 tumors) demonstrates diffuse gastric mucosa hypertrophy (see also Chapter 14),

with ulceration. The background mucosa is usually normal for type 3 NETs. Minimum biochemical tests in patients with type 1 and 2 lesions include serum gastrin and chromogranin A, while genetic testing should be performed if MEN 1 is suspected.[29] The size of the lesion and type of NET will guide further imaging studies and treatment.

Diagnosis and Histological Grading

The WHO classification designates neuroendocrine neoplasms of the stomach into well-differentiated NET and NEC.[30] Well-differentiated NETs are composed of nests or cords of uniform cells with finely granular, amphophilic-to-eosinophilic cytoplasm. The nuclei are round to oval and centrally placed; they have salt-and-pepper chromatin and no or inconspicuous nucleoli (Figure 17-1) (see also Chapter 6). Immunohistochemical features include positivity for chromogranin A and synaptophysin; evaluation for specific hormones should be performed when clinically indicated.[31] In NECs, the histology demonstrates diffuse sheets of small- to intermediate-size tumor cells with frequent necrosis, mitoses, angioinvasion, and deep-wall invasion (Figure 17-2). The tumor cells are weakly positive for or lack chromogranin A but retain strong positivity for synaptophysin or neuron-specific enolase.[28]

Histologically, type 1 NETs can be solitary but are often multiple. The surrounding background mucosa exhibits diffuse atrophic gastritis, with pyloric gland metaplasia or intestinal metaplasia (see also Chapter 12). In addition to NETs, there may be linear or nodular endocrine cell (ECL) hyperplasia (Figure 17-3).

Taken out of context, type 2 and type 1 NETs are indistinguishable from each other. Clinically, both are associated with hypergastrinemia. Therefore, evaluation of the background mucosa is critical, as type 2 tumors are associated with fundic gland hypertrophy and type 1 with atrophy accompanied by intestinal metaplasia (Figure 17-4).

In some cases, a gastrinoma may be identified, which can be in the duodenum or a periduodenal lymph node (Figure 17-5).

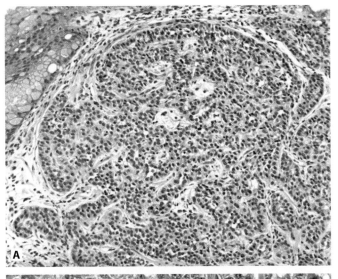

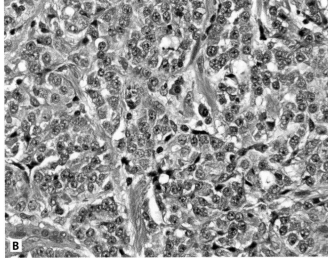

FIGURE 17-1. Well-differentiated neuroendocrine tumor. **A.** Monotonous uniform endocrine cells forming nest in the lamina propria. **B.** Tumor cells with moderate amount of cytoplasm and medium-size nuclei (slightly larger than the nuclei of intermixed plasma cells). The nuclei are characterized by fine or "open" chromatin and an inconspicuous nucleolus. There is no mitosis.

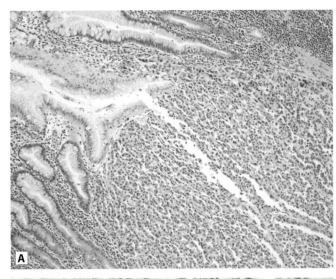

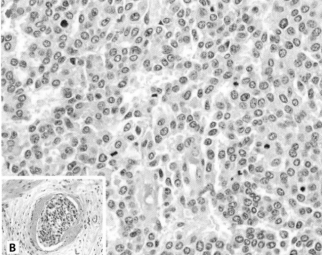

FIGURE 17-2. Poorly differentiated neuroendocrine carcinoma. **A.** The uniform tumor cells form a solid mass in the gastric mucosa. **B.** There is relatively abundant cytoplasm and round nuclei with cytologic features of a neuroendocrine tumor. Note the high mitotic count (Ki-67 index 40%; not shown). The insert demonstrates submucosal vascular invasion.

Type 3 NETs, as sporadic tumors, are not associated with increased serum gastrin levels. These usually present as solitary lesions, with the background body and antral mucosa being normal histologically (Figure 17-6).

Straightforward as it may seem, occasionally in mucosal biopsy specimens the morphologic features of an NET may not be obvious. For example, as shown in Figure 17-7, the tumor cells may exhibit a "plasmacytoid" appearance, with solid dark nuclei. The tumor cells are strongly positive for synaptophysin. Rarely, the tumor cells may assume a spindle cell morphology, mimicking a gastrointestinal stromal tumor (Figure 17-3C). The diagnosis can be elucidated by positive staining for neuroendocrine markers—most commonly, synaptophysin and chromogranin.

Histologic grading is based on a mitotic count of 50 high-power fields (HPFs) using a ×40 objective and Ki-67 index in the areas with highest labeling, counting at least 2000 nuclei in a resection specimen and less if it is a biopsy or cytology specimen.[30,32] Previous studies have demonstrated a correlation between increased immunoexpression of Ki-67 and worse prognosis in gastrointestinal NETs.[28,33–36] The grading scheme is made up of 3 tiers (G1–G3), with an increase in grade corresponding to an increase in the proliferation rate. Most well-differentiated NETs are categorized as G1, while G3 is reserved for PDNECs. Punctate necrosis can be seen in a G2 tumor, suggestive of an aggressive lesion.[37] Due to the mostly indolent clinical course and lack of data, detailed histologic grading is not necessary for type 1 and 2 gastric NETs, which are mostly G1 if graded (see the following discussion). However, sporadic (type 3) tumors are similar to their counterpart in other locations and thus are graded as described previously.

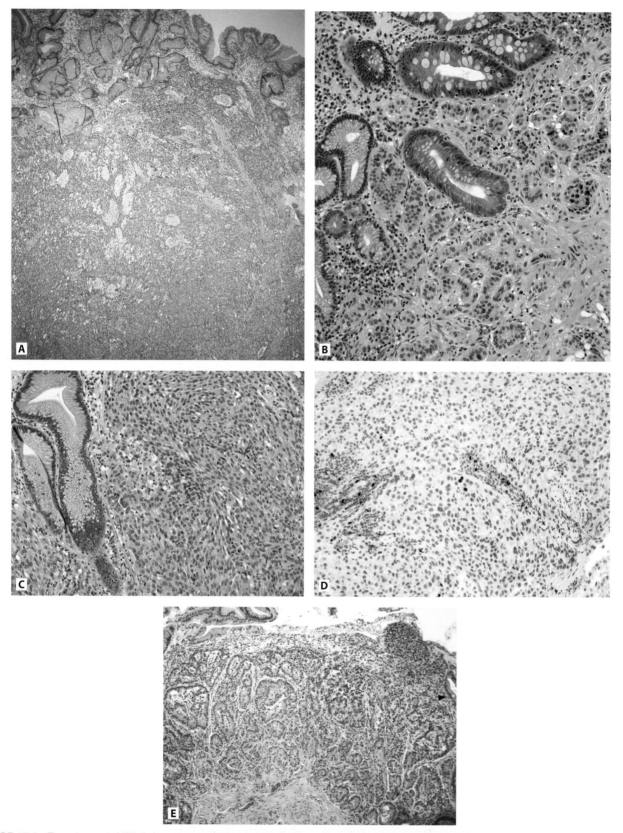

FIGURE 17-3. Type 1 gastric NET. **A.** Intramucosal tumor nests displaced gastric glands without clear demarcation from surrounding lamina propria. **B.** Small tumor cell clusters infiltrated the lamina propria and foveolar type as well as metaplastic intestinal glands. **C.** Occasionally and focally, the tumor cells may exhibit a spindle cell appearance, a potential pitfall that may exclude initial immunohistochemistry workup for endocrine markers if seen in small biopsy specimens. **D.** Immunostain demonstrating very low Ki-67 index. **E.** In this example, the tumor is characterized by trabecular as well as pseudoacinar patterns. Note intestinal metaplasia (arrowhead).

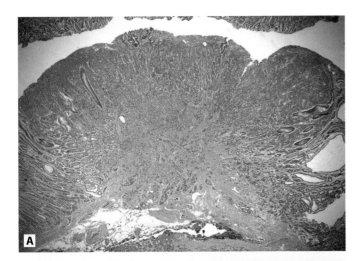

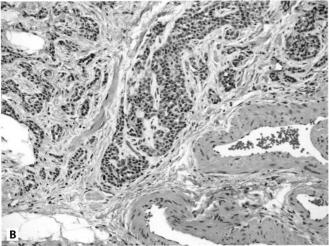

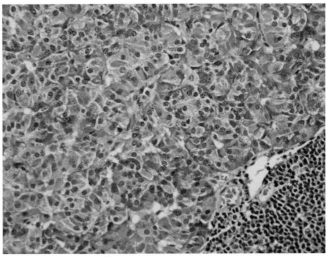

FIGURE 17-5. A gastrinoma involving a portal lymph node. The tumor cells show abundant bright eosinophilic fine granular cytoplasm; nuclei are eccentrically located and exhibit a typical "salt-and-pepper" texture. The patient had no other sites of gastrinoma identified.

FIGURE 17-4. Type 2 gastric NET. **A.** A well-circumscribed tumor nodule consisting of typical neuroendocrine cells. The surrounding mucosa (lateral edges) exhibits marked fundic gland hypertrophy with dilation. **B.** Endocrine tumor nests and clusters extend to the submucosa. Note the lack of mitotic figures or nuclear atypia.

Prognosis and Treatment

The prognosis and treatment of a gastric NET depends on the tumor type and size, and extent of the disease.

Type 1

Type 1 gastric NETs mostly are G1 (82.7%–100%), are limited to the mucosa and submucosa (82%), and have no associated mortality with prolonged follow-up.[11,26,36] Although usually benign, these tumors have a recurrence rate of 40%–64%, with a median time of 8–24 months. In addition, 3% of type 1 gastric NETs develop into poorly differentiated neuroendocrine carcinomas, and 5% will metastasize.[20,36,38,39] For localized type 1 gastric NETs smaller than 1 cm, endoscopic annual surveillance with or without resection is recommended, while lesions greater than 1 cm warrant an endoscopic ultrasound (EUS) to look for invasion beyond the submucosa, tumor extension into the muscularis propria, or local lymph node metastasis. Lesions greater than 1 cm and not involving the

muscularis propria can be removed by endoscopic mucosal resection (EMR). Surgical resection should be performed if a single lesion is greater than 2 cm, there are more than 6 lesions with 3–4 lesions greater than 1 cm, or there is local or distant disease spread.[29] Studies have shown that the use of somatostatin analogues (SSAs) in the presence of multiple lesions can reduce the number and size of the lesions, although long-term outcomes have not been determined.[40,41]

Type 2

Similar to type 1, type 2 gastric NETs are typically graded as G1; however, there is a slight increase in type 2 lesions invading beyond the submucosa (9%) or with metastatic disease (15%).[18,36] For lesions greater than 1–2 cm, EUS is performed to determine the extent of invasion. With the higher risk of local or distant metastasis, additional imaging (ie, computed tomography [CT], magnetic resonance imaging [MRI], and scintigraphy) is useful, and all lesions should be resected. Endoscopic resection is used if the extent is not beyond the submucosa, whereas if local lymph nodal invasion is present, surgical resection is performed. Annual endoscopic surveillance is recommended, and acid secretion is controlled with proton pump inhibitor therapy or SSAs.[42]

Type 3

The histologic grade for type 3 tumors can be G1 or G2 and is more commonly accompanied by invasion beyond the submucosa (about 70% of cases). The mortality rate ranges from 22% to 38%.[28,36,43] CT imaging is used to determine the extent of spread of the disease, and treatment is the same as for gastric adenocarcinomas, including surgical resection, chemotherapy, and peptide receptor radionuclide therapy.[44]

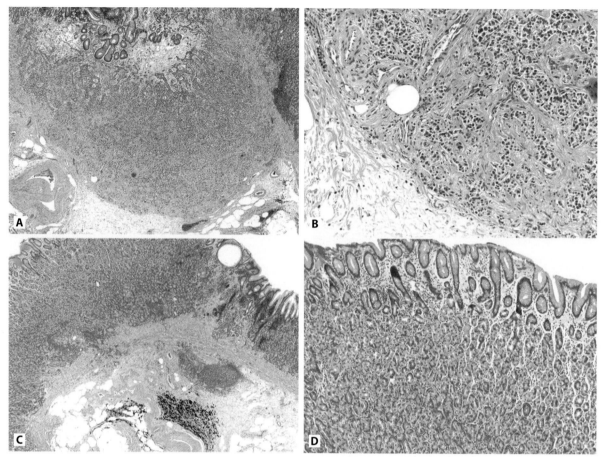

FIGURE 17-6. Type 3 gastric NET. **A.** The solitary tumor nodule involves the mucosa and submucosa. **B.** High-power view demonstrating endocrine tumor cell clusters in a fibrotic stromal background. **C.** The background gastric body mucosa is normal. **D.** Higher-power view demonstrating normal body mucosa without inflammation or intestinal metaplasia.

Type 4

By definition, NECs are a histologic grade 3. These tumors deeply invade the gastric wall and most commonly are metastatic. Treatment is similar to that for type 3 tumors.

Summary

Neuroendocrine tumors of the stomach are divided into 4 types by clinicopathologic features: Type 1 is associated with CAG; type 2 is associated with ZES/MEN 1; type 3 is sporadic; depending on the source, type 4 may include NEC, mixed endocrine and exocrine tumors, and non-ECL tumors. The clinical presentation is nonspecific, and the tumors are often incidental findings on endoscopic examination. Histology is important in making a diagnosis and guiding treatment. Noninvasive type 1 and lesions smaller than 1 cm can be endoscopically resected with annual endoscopic surveillance. Patients with lesions larger than 1 cm should have EUS to look for extent of the disease. Systemic therapy and surgical resection are used for type 3 tumors or extensive type 1 or 2 tumors.

MELANOMA

Melanoma of the stomach is mostly metastatic in origin. Primary gastric melanoma is rare, as evidenced by few published case reports, and comprises 2.7% of primary gastrointestinal melanomas.[45]

Clinical symptoms for gastric melanoma are nonspecific and include weight loss, epigastric pain, melena, anemia, nausea, emesis, and fatigue. In one case report of primary gastric melanoma, the patient's initial presenting system was left axillary swelling.[46] Endoscopically, these tumors manifest as an ulcerated, amelanotic, or pigmented mass. Histology of the tumor demonstrates spindled, pleomorphic, or discohesive cells. In the absence of melanin, immunohistochemical studies aid in the diagnosis and demonstrate immunoreactivity of the tumor cells with S100, melan A, and HMB45.[47–52]

The diagnosis of gastric primary origin may be difficult due to the absence of native melanocytes in the stomach. Rare cases of isolated melanosis in the gastric antrum have been reported, which may have been associated with an esophageal melanoma.[53,54] In some cases in which no other primary sites can be identified, some investigators believe that it may be due

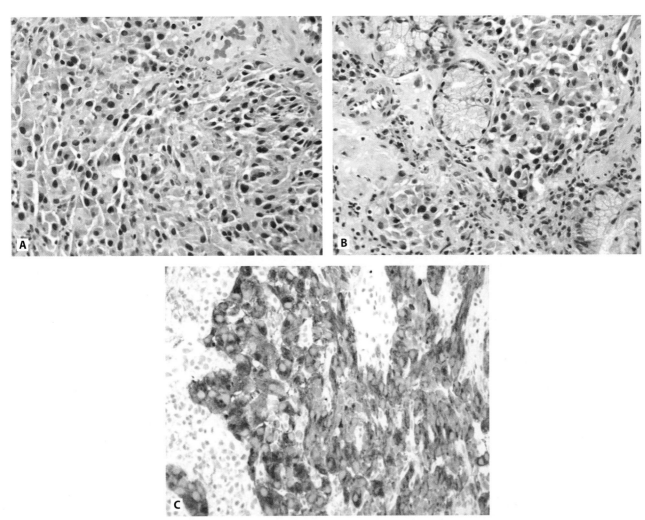

FIGURE 17-7. A type 1 gastric NET identified in mucosa biopsy. **A.** The tumor cells contain a solid dark nucleus, with abundant eosinophilic cytoplasm. **B.** The tumor cells are otherwise without high-grade features or mitosis. **C.** Immunohistochemically, the cells are strongly positive for synaptophysin. Despite the atypical morphology, this is a low-grade, well-differentiated NET.

to spontaneous regression of the primary lesion[55-57] rather than true primary gastric melanoma. Nevertheless, proposed diagnostic criteria for primary gastric melanomas include the lack of prior or concurrent melanoma of the skin or other sites, adjacent gastrointestinal epithelium demonstrating an in situ component, and pagetoid spread of melanotic cells into the superficial epithelium (Figure 17-8).

The current mainstay of therapy for primary gastric melanoma is surgical resection, whereas metastatic gastric melanoma with a known extraprimary location is often treated with chemoradiation therapy.[8] In advanced stages of primary gastric melanoma, chemotherapy in combination with immunotherapy is recommended.[46] Overall, the prognosis of primary gastric or metastatic melanoma is poor, with one study demonstrating a median survival of 5 months in patients diagnosed with primary gastric melanoma.[45] A review of cases has shown a 50% mortality rate in patients following their diagnosis of metastatic melanoma of the skin or melanoma involving visceral organs with an unknown primary.[58]

KAPOSI SARCOMA

Kaposi sarcoma was first described in five patients by Dr. Moritz Kaposi in 1872. Four variants were characterized based on the varying clinical and epidemiological presentations and are summarized in Table 17-2. All forms demonstrate the presence of human herpesvirus 8 (HHV-8) DNA sequence, and HHV-8 is thought to play a significant role in the pathogenesis.[59]

The most relevant variants of Kaposi sarcoma in the United States include the immunosuppression or iatrogenic and AIDS-related forms.[64,68] The third form primarily occurs in transplant patients, but also includes patients with collagen, vascular, or skin disorders, all of whom are receiving immunosuppressive therapy. Skin, viscera, and lymph nodes are affected.[64] In the United States, Kaposi sarcoma is the most common AIDS-associated tumor, also known as the "epidemic" or AIDS-related form. Similar to the immunosuppression-associated or iatrogenic form, AIDS-associated Kaposi sarcoma has a diffuse distribution in the body, but with earlier involvement of the lymph nodes and gastrointestinal tract.[67,68]

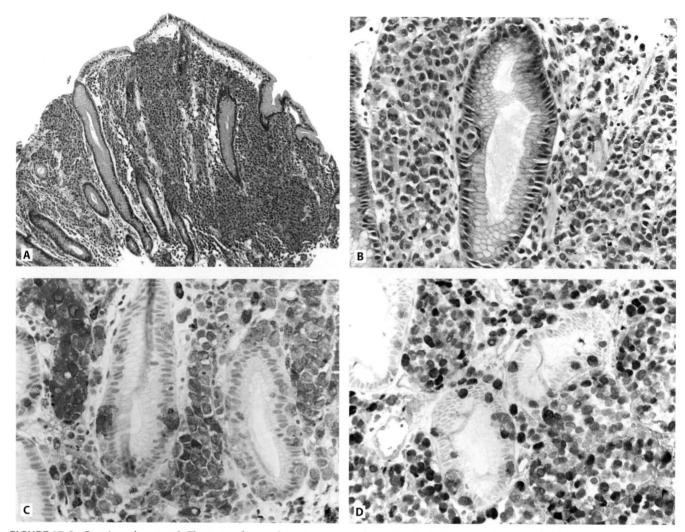

FIGURE 17-8. Gastric melanoma. **A.** The tumor forms a large intramucosal nodule, displacing normal gastric glands. **B.** Despite the seemingly uniform morphology, at higher-power view, the tumor cells are highly atypical, with large nuclei, some vesicular, with a prominent nucleolus. Some of the tumor cells contain cytoplasmic melanin granules. An intraepithelial tumor nest is evident. **C.** Immunostain for HMB-45 demonstrating scattered intramucosal melanocytes that otherwise are not evident on H&E staining. Some of the brown granules are negative for the stain and likely represent hemosiderin. **D.** Immunostain for S-100. Some of the positive cells in the epithelium are melanoma cells, but others likely represent in situ melanocytes due to lack of tumor cell morphology.

TABLE 17-2. Variants of Kaposi sarcoma.			
Variant	*Epidemiology*	*Affected sites*	*Other*
1. Classic	Elderly Mediterranean and Eastern European men[60]	Skin of lower extremities	Increased risk of developing a secondary malignancy, especially non-Hodgkin lymphoma[61]
2. Endemic or African	Sub-Saharan African adults and children[62,63]	Skin, lymph nodes	
3. Immunosuppression or iatrogenic	Patients on immunosuppressive therapy	Diffuse[64]	
4. Epidemic or AIDS related	Homosexual males, bisexual males, heterosexual females	Diffuse with early involvement of lymph nodes and gastrointestinal tract[68]	Decreased incidence since initiation of antiretroviral therapy[65,66]

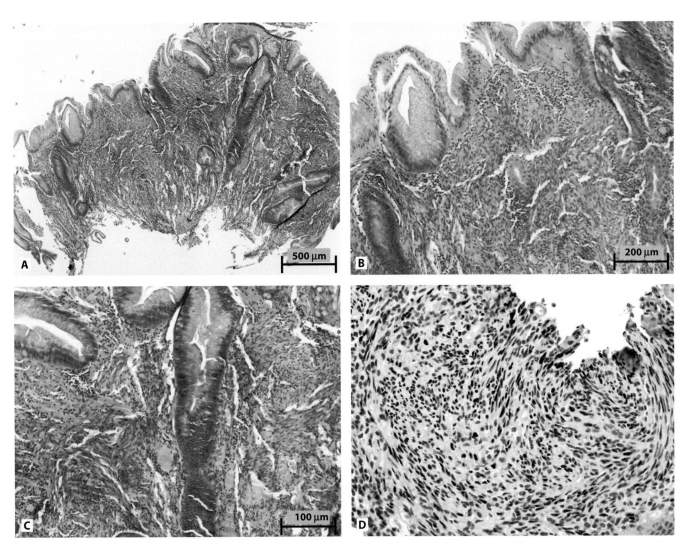

FIGURE 17-9. Kaposi sarcoma of the stomach from a patient with AIDS. **A.** There is marked expansion of the lamina propria by irregular spindle cell and vascular proliferation among foveolar glands. **B.** Higher-power view shows solid areas of atypical spindle cells. **C.** Both narrow, slit-like vascular spaces and dilated vascular spaces are evident. There is also mixed inflammatory cellular infiltration. **D.** Immuno-histochemically, the nuclei of the spindle cells are strongly positive for HHV-8 latency-associated nuclear antigen (LANA), confirming the diagnosis.

The most common clinical manifestations are multiple bluish-red patches on the skin, which can progress to form plaques, then nodules. Not only were they found classically on the face, limbs, and trunk, but also post-mortem findings demonstrated involvement by the gastrointestinal tract.[69] Although most patients with gastrointestinal manifestations of the disease are asymptomatic, there have been reports of patients presenting with anemia, obstruction, and perforation.[70–73] On endoscopic examination, Kaposi sarcoma is bluish red and forms polypoid lesions or plaques, which may have ulceration.[72–76] Histology usually shows a submucosal spindle cell proliferation forming slit-like spaces which is associated with extravasated red cells, plasma cells, hemosiderin, and eosinophilic hyaline globules (Figure 17-9). The cell

of origin is thought to be a lymphatic endothelial cell, given the immunohistochemical reactivity of the tumor cells for Fli-1, VEGFR-3 (vascular endothelial growth factor receptor 3), D2-40, CD34, CD31, and HHV-8[77–81] (Figure 17-9D).

Kaposi sarcoma is typically an indolent disease, and treatment depends on the variant, extent of the disease, and patient's symptoms. The initial step in treating immunosuppression and AIDS-associated forms is to restore immunity by changing immunosuppressive therapy or initiating antiretroviral therapy, respectively. Treatment can be divided into local or systemic and be used for reasons or to alleviate symptoms. These include compression stockings, topical therapy, surgery, cryotherapy, chemotherapy, radiotherapy, cytostatic agents, and immunomodulators.[82]

REFERENCES

1. Sachs G, Zeng N, Prinz C. Physiology of isolated gastric endocrine cells. *Annu Rev Physiol.* 1997; 59:243–256. PMID: 9074763.

2. Modlin IM, Zucker KA, Zdon MJ, Sussman J, Adrian TE. Characteristics of the spontaneous gastric endocrine tumor of mastomys. *J Surg Res.* 1988;44(3):205–215. PMID: 3343820.

3. Hakanson R, Larsson LI, Owman C, Snell KC, Sundler F. Fluorescence and electron microscopic histochemistry of endocrine-like cells in gastric mucosa and argyrophil tumor of *Praomys* (*Mastomys*) *natalensis.* Analysis of 5-hydroxytryptamine, histamine, histidine decarboxylase, and aromatic amino acid decarboxylase. *Histochimie.* 1973;37(1):23–38. PMID: 4770333.

4. Solcia E, Bordi C, Creutzfeldt W, et al. Histopathological classification of nonantral gastric endocrine growths in man. *Digestion.* 1988;41(4):185–200. PMID: 3072229.

5. Waisberg J, de Matos LL, do Amaral Antonio Mader AM, et al. Neuroendocrine gastric carcinoma expressing somatostatin: a highly malignant, rare tumor. *World J Gastroenterol.* 2006;12(24):3944–3947. PMID: 16804989. PMCID: 4087952.

6. Ronellenfitsch U, Strobel P, Schwarzbach MH, Staiger WI, Gragert D, Kahler G. A composite adenoendocrine carcinoma of the stomach arising from a neuroendocrine tumor. *J Gastrointest Surg.* 2007;11(11):1573–1575. PMID: 17436049.

7. Latta E, Rotondo F, Leiter LA, Horvath E, Kovacs K. Ghrelin- and serotonin-producing gastric carcinoid. *J Gastrointest Cancer.* 2012;43(2):319–323. PMID: 21424696.

8. Borch K, Renvall H, Liedberg G. Gastric endocrine cell hyperplasia and carcinoid tumors in pernicious anemia. *Gastroenterology.* 1985;88(3):638–648. PMID: 2578420.

9. Solcia E, Capella C, Fiocca R, Rindi G, Rosai J. Gastric argyrophil carcinoidosis in patients with Zollinger-Ellison syndrome due to type 1 multiple endocrine neoplasia. A newly recognized association. *Am J Surg Pathol.* 1990;14(6):503–513. PMID: 1970928.

10. Borch K, Renvall H, Liedberg G, Andersen BN. Relations between circulating gastrin and endocrine cell proliferation in the atrophic gastric fundic mucosa. *Scand J Gastroenterol.* 1986;21(3):357–363. PMID: 3715400.

11. Borch K, Ahren B, Ahlman H, Falkmer S, Granerus G, Grimelius L. Gastric carcinoids: biologic behavior and prognosis after differentiated treatment in relation to type. *Ann Surg.* 2005;242(1):64–73. PMID: 15973103. PMCID: 1357706.

12. Rindi G, Luinetti O, Cornaggia M, Capella C, Solcia E. Three subtypes of gastric argyrophil carcinoid and the gastric neuroendocrine carcinoma: a clinicopathologic study. *Gastroenterology.* 1993;104(4):994–1006. PMID: 7681798.

13. Zur M. VA. Pathogenese der Magenkarzinoide und ober ihren gelgentlichen Ursprung aus angeborenen epitheliaen Keimen in der Magenwand. *Dtsch Med Wochenschr.* 1923;49:49–51.

14. Modlin IM, Lye KD, Kidd M. A 5-decade analysis of 13,715 carcinoid tumors. *Cancer.* 2003;97(4):934–959. PMID: 12569593.

15. Yao JC, Hassan M, Phan A, et al. One hundred years after "carcinoid": epidemiology of and prognostic factors for neuroendocrine tumors in 35,825 cases in the United States. *J Clin Oncol.* 2008;26(18):3063–3072. PMID: 18565894.

16. Lawrence B, Gustafsson BI, Chan A, Svejda B, Kidd M, Modlin IM. The epidemiology of gastroenteropancreatic neuroendocrine tumors. *Endocrinol Metab Clin North Am.* 2011;40(1):1–18, vii. PMID: 21349409.

17. Tsikitis VL, Wertheim BC, Guerrero MA. Trends of incidence and survival of gastrointestinal neuroendocrine tumors in the United States: a seer analysis. *J Cancer.* 2012;3:292–302. PMID: 22773933. PMCID: 3390599.

18. Rindi G, Bordi C, Rappel S, La Rosa S, Stolte M, Solcia E. Gastric carcinoids and neuroendocrine carcinomas: pathogenesis, pathology, and behavior. *World J Surg.* 1996;20(2):168–172. PMID: 8661813.

19. Annibale B, Azzoni C, Corleto VD, et al. Atrophic body gastritis patients with enterochromaffin-like cell dysplasia are at increased risk for the development of type I gastric carcinoid. *Eur J Gastroenterol Hepatol.* 2001;13(12):1449–1456. PMID: 11742193.

20. Vannella L, Sbrozzi-Vanni A, Lahner E, et al. Development of type I gastric carcinoid in patients with chronic atrophic gastritis. *Aliment Pharmacol Ther.* 2011;33(12):1361–1369. PMID: 21492197.

21. Gibril F, Schumann M, Pace A, Jensen RT. Multiple endocrine neoplasia type 1 and Zollinger-Ellison syndrome: a prospective study of 107 cases and comparison with 1009 cases from the literature. *Medicine.* 2004;83(1):43–83. PMID: 14747767.

22. Lehy T, Cadiot G, Mignon M, Ruszniewski P, Bonfils S. Influence of multiple endocrine neoplasia type 1 on gastric endocrine cells in patients with the Zollinger-Ellison syndrome. *Gut.* 1992;33(9):1275–1279. PMID: 1358767. PMCID: 1379501.

23. Matsui K, Jin XM, Kitagawa M, Miwa A. Clinicopathologic features of neuroendocrine carcinomas of the stomach: appraisal of small cell and large cell variants. *Arch Pathol Lab Med.* 1998;122(11):1010–1017. PMID: 9822131.

24. Soga J. Early-stage carcinoids of the gastrointestinal tract: an analysis of 1914 reported cases. *Cancer.* 2005;103(8):1587–1595. PMID: 15742328.

25. Gough DB, Thompson GB, Crotty TB, et al. Diverse clinical and pathologic features of gastric carcinoid and the relevance of hypergastrinemia. *World J Surg.* 1994;18(4):473–479; discussion 479–480. PMID: 7725731.

26. Thomas D, Tsolakis AV, Grozinsky-Glasberg S, et al. Long-term follow-up of a large series of patients with type 1 gastric carcinoid tumors: data from a multicenter study. *Eur J Endocrinol.* 2013;168(2):185–193. PMID: 23132699.

27. Bordi C, Yu JY, Baggi MT, et al. Gastric carcinoids and their precursor lesions. A histologic and immunohistochemical study of 23 cases. *Cancer.* 1991;67(3):663–672. PMID: 1702355.

28. Rindi G, Azzoni C, La Rosa S, et al. ECL cell tumor and poorly differentiated endocrine carcinoma of the stomach: prognostic evaluation by pathological analysis. *Gastroenterology.* 1999;116(3):532–542. PMID: 10029611.

29. Delle Fave G, Kwekkeboom D, Van Cutsem E, et al. ENETS consensus guidelines for the management of patients with gastroduodenal neoplasms. *Neuroendocrinology.* 2012;95:74–87.

30. Rindi G AR, Bosman FT, et al. Nomenclature and classification of neuroendocrine neoplasms of the digestive system. In: Bosman TF, Carniero F, Hruban RH, Theise ND, eds. *WHO Classification of Tumours of the Digestive System.* 4th ed. Lyon, France: International Agency for Research on Cancer (IARC); 2010:13.

31. Capelli P, Fassan M, Scarpa A. Pathology—grading and staging of GEP-NETs. Best practice and research. *Clin Gastroenterol.* 2012;26(6):705–717. PMID: 23582914.

32. Kloppel G, Couvelard A, Perren A, et al. ENETS consensus guidelines for the standards of care in neuroendocrine tumors: towards a standardized approach to the diagnosis of gastroenteropancreatic neuroendocrine tumors and their prognostic stratification. *Neuroendocrinology.* 2009;90(2):162–166. PMID: 19060454.

33. Boo YJ, Park SS, Kim JH, Mok YJ, Kim SJ, Kim CS. Gastric neuroendocrine carcinoma: clinicopathologic review and immunohistochemical study of E-cadherin and Ki-67 as prognostic markers. *J Surg Oncol.* 2007;95(2):110–117. PMID: 17066436.

34. Safatle-Ribeiro AV, Ribeiro U Jr, Corbett CE, et al. Prognostic value of immunohistochemistry in gastric neuroendocrine (carcinoid) tumors. *Eur J Gastroenterol Hepatol.* 2007;19(1):21–28. PMID: 17206073.

35. Pelosi G, Bresaola E, Bogina G, et al. Endocrine tumors of the pancreas: Ki-67 immunoreactivity on paraffin sections is an independent predictor for malignancy: a comparative study with proliferating-cell nuclear antigen and progesterone receptor protein immunostaining, mitotic index, and other clinicopathologic variables. *Hum Pathol.* 1996;27(11):1124–1134. PMID: 8912819.

36. La Rosa S, Klersy C, Uccella S, et al. Improved histologic and clinico-pathologic criteria for prognostic evaluation of pancreatic endocrine tumors. *Hum Pathol.* 2009;40(1):30–40. PMID: 18715612.

37. Rindi G, Kloppel G, Alhman H, et al. TNM staging of foregut (neuro) endocrine tumors: a consensus proposal including a grading system. *Virchows Arch.* 2006;449(4):395–401. PMID: 16967267. PMCID: 1888719.

38. Bordi C. Gastric carcinoids. *Ital J Gastroenterol Hepatol.* 1999;31(Suppl 2):S94–S97. PMID: 10604110.

39. Merola E, Sbrozzi-Vanni A, Panzuto F, et al. Type I gastric carcinoids: a prospective study on endoscopic management and recurrence rate. *Neuroendocrinology.* 2012;95(3):207–213. PMID: 21811050.

40. Fossmark R, Sordal O, Jianu CS, et al. Treatment of gastric carcinoids type 1 with the gastrin receptor antagonist netazepide (YF476) results in regression of tumours and normalisation of serum chromogranin A. *Aliment Pharmacol Ther.* 2012;36(11–12):1067–1075. PMID: 23072686.

41. Moore AR, Boyce M, Steele IA, Campbell F, Varro A, Pritchard DM. Netazepide, a gastrin receptor antagonist, normalises tumour biomarkers and causes regression of type 1 gastric neuroendocrine tumours in a nonrandomised trial of patients with chronic atrophic gastritis. *PLoS One.* 2013;8(10):e76462. PMID: 24098507. PMCID: 3788129.

42. Jensen RT, Cadiot G, Brandi ML, et al. ENETS consensus guidelines for the management of patients with digestive neuroendocrine neoplasms: functional pancreatic endocrine tumor syndromes. *Neuroendocrinology.* 2012;95:98–119.

43. Rappel S, Altendorf-Hofmann A, Stolte M. Prognosis of gastric carcinoid tumours. *Digestion.* 1995;56(6):455–462. PMID: 8536814.

44. Pavel M, Baudin E, Couvelard A, et al. ENETS consensus guidelines for the management of patients with liver and other distant metastases from neuroendocrine neoplasms of foregut, midgut, hindgut, and unknown primary. *Neuroendocrinology.* 2012;95:157–176.

45. Cheung MC, Perez EA, Molina MA, et al. Defining the role of surgery for primary gastrointestinal tract melanoma. *J Gastrointest Surg.* 2008;12(4):731–738. PMID: 18058185.

46. Khaliq A, Siddappa PK, Thandassery RB, et al. Melanoma of stomach. *J Gastrointest Cancer.* 2012;43(4):630–633. PMID: 22125087.

47. Castro C, Khan Y, Awasum M, et al. Case report: primary gastric melanoma in a patient with dermatomyositis. *Am J Med Sci.* 2008;336(3):282–284. PMID: 18794626.

48. Lagoudianakis EE, Genetzakis M, Tsekouras DK, et al. Primary gastric melanoma: a case report. *World J Gastroenterol.* 2006;12(27):4425–4427. PMID: 16865791.

49. Yamamura K, Kondo K, Moritani S. Primary malignant melanoma of the stomach: report of a case. *Surg Today.* 2012;42(2):195–199. PMID: 22167480. PMCID: 3264870.

50. Ravi A. Primary gastric melanoma: a rare cause of upper gastrointestinal bleeding. *Gastroenterol Hepatol.* 2008;4(11):795–797. PMID: 21960901. PMCID: 3104388.

51. Alazmi WM, Nehme OS, Regalado JJ, Rogers AI. Primary gastric melanoma presenting as a nonhealing ulcer. *Gastrointest Endosc.* 2003;57(3):431–433. PMID: 12612539.

52. Slater JM, Ling TC, Slater JD, Yang GY. Palliative radiation therapy for primary gastric melanoma. *J Gastrointest Oncol.* 2014;5(1):E22–E26. PMID: 24490048. PMCID: 3904019.

53. Vuppalanchi R, Vakili ST, Kahi CJ. Isolated melanosis of the gastric antrum: an unusual endoscopic finding. *Clin Gastroenterol Hepatol.* 2007;5(1):e2. PMID: 17142108.

54. Alberti JE, Bodor J, Torres AD, Pini N. Melanoma maligno primitivo del esofago asociado a melanosis del esofago y del estomago [Primary malignant melanoma of the esophagus associated with melanosis of the esophagus and stomach]. *Acta Gastroenterol Latinoam.* 1984;14(2):139–148. PMID: 6535357.

55. Smith JL Jr, Stehlin JS Jr. Spontaneous regression of primary malignant melanomas with regional metastases. *Cancer.* 1965;18(11):1399–1415. PMID: 5844157.

56. High WA, Stewart D, Wilbers CR, Cockerell CJ, Hoang MP, Fitzpatrick JE. Completely regressed primary cutaneous malignant melanoma with nodal and/or visceral metastases: a report of 5 cases and assessment of the literature and diagnostic criteria. *J Am Acad Dermatol.* 2005;53(1):89–100. PMID: 15965428.

57. Panagopoulos E, Murray D. Metastatic malignant melanoma of unknown primary origin: a study of 30 cases. *J Surg Oncol.* 1983;23(1):8–10. PMID: 6843134.

58. Chang AE, Karnell LH, Menck HR. The National Cancer Data Base report on cutaneous and noncutaneous melanoma: a summary of 84,836 cases from the past decade. The American College of Surgeons Commission on Cancer and the American Cancer Society. *Cancer.* 1998;83(8):1664–1678. PMID: 9781962.

59. Chang Y, Cesarman E, Pessin MS, et al. Identification of herpesvirus-like DNA sequences in AIDS-associated Kaposi's sarcoma. *Science.* 1994;266:1865–1869.

60. Geddes M, Franceschi S, Barchielli A, et al. Kaposi's sarcoma in Italy before and after the AIDS epidemic. *Br J Cancer.* 1994;69(2):333–336. PMID: 8297730. PMCID: 1968687.

61. Safai B, Mike V, Giraldo G, Beth E, Good RA. Association of Kaposi's sarcoma with second primary malignancies: possible etiopathogenic implications. *Cancer.* 1980;45(6):1472–1479. PMID: 6244084.

62. Ziegler JL. Endemic Kaposi's sarcoma in Africa and local volcanic soils. *Lancet.* 1993;342(8883):1348–1351. PMID: 7901641.

63. Taylor JF, Templeton AC, Vogel CL, Ziegler JL, Kyalwazi SK. Kaposi's sarcoma in Uganda: a clinico-pathological study. *Int J Cancer.* 1971;8(1):122–135. PMID: 5118203.

64. Sampaio MS, Cho YW, Qazi Y, Bunnapradist S, Hutchinson IV, Shah T. Posttransplant malignancies in solid organ adult recipients: an analysis of the US National Transplant Database. *Transplantation.* 2012;94(10):990–998. PMID: 23085553.

65. Engels EA, Biggar RJ, Hall HI, et al. Cancer risk in people infected with human immunodeficiency virus in the United States. *Int J Cancer.* 2008;123(1):187–194. PMID: 18435450.

66. Robbins HA, Shiels MS, Pfeiffer RM, Engels EA. Epidemiologic contributions to recent cancer trends among HIV-infected people in the United States. *AIDS.* 2014;28(6):881–890. PMID: 24300545.

67. Mwakigonja AR, Pyakurel P, Kokhaei P, et al. Human herpesvirus-8 (HHV-8) sero-detection and HIV association in Kaposi's sarcoma (KS), non-KS tumors and non-neoplastic conditions. *Infect Agents Cancer.* 2008;3:10. PMID: 18590556. PMCID: 2499990.

68. Beral V, Peterman TA, Berkelman RL, Jaffe HW. Kaposi's sarcoma among persons with AIDS: a sexually transmitted infection? *Lancet.* 1990;335(8682):123–128. PMID: 1967430.

69. Breimer L. Original description of Kaposi's sarcoma. *BMJ.* 1994;308(6939):1303–1304. PMID: 8205038. PMCID: 2540175.

70. Yoshida EM, Chan NH, Chan-Yan C, Baird RM. Perforation of the jejunum secondary to AIDS-related gastrointestinal Kaposi's sarcoma. *Can J Gastroenterol.* 1997;11(1):38–40. PMID: 9113797.

71. Carratala J, Lacasa JM, Mascaro J, Torras JT. AIDS presenting as duodenal perforation due to Kaposi's sarcoma. *AIDS.* 1992;6(2):241–242. PMID: 1558729.

72. Kahl P, Buettner R, Friedrichs N, Merkelbach-Bruse S, Wenzel J, Carl Heukamp L. Kaposi's sarcoma of the gastrointestinal tract: report of two cases and review of the literature. *Pathol Res Pract.* 2007;203(4):227–231. PMID: 17379429.

73. Kibria R, Siraj U, Barde C. Kaposi's sarcoma of the stomach and duodenum in human immunodeficiency virus infection. *Dig Endosc.* 2010;22(3):241–242. PMID: 20642618.

74. Barrison IG, Foster S, Harris JW, Pinching AJ, Walker JG. Upper gastrointestinal Kaposi's sarcoma in patients positive for HIV antibody without cutaneous disease. *BMJournal.* 1988;296(6615):92–93. PMID: 3122968. PMCID: 2544701.

75. Mansfield SA, Stawicki SP, Forbes RC, Papadimos TJ, Lindsey DE. Acute upper gastrointestinal bleeding secondary to Kaposi sarcoma as initial presentation of HIV infection. *J Gastrointest Liver Dis.* 2013;22(4):441–445. PMID: 24369327. PMCID: 4097021.

76. Arora M, Goldberg EM. Kaposi sarcoma involving the gastrointestinal tract. *Gastroenterol Hepatol.* 2010;6(7):459–462. PMID: 20827371. PMCID: 2933764.

77. Folpe AL, Veikkola T, Valtola R, Weiss SW. Vascular endothelial growth factor receptor-3 (VEGFR-3): a marker of vascular tumors with presumed lymphatic differentiation, including Kaposi's sarcoma, kaposiform and Dabska-type hemangioendotheliomas, and a subset of angiosarcomas. *Mod Pathol.* 2000;13(2):180–185. PMID: 10697276.

78. Folpe AL, Chand EM, Goldblum JR, Weiss SW. Expression of Fli-1, a nuclear transcription factor, distinguishes vascular neoplasms from potential mimics. *Am J Surg Pathol.* 2001;25(8):1061–1066. PMID: 11474291.

79. Fukunaga M. Expression of D2-40 in lymphatic endothelium of normal tissues and in vascular tumours. *Histopathology.* 2005;46(4): 396–402. PMID: 15810951.

80. Russell Jones R, Orchard G, Zelger B, Wilson Jones E. Immunostaining for CD31 and CD34 in Kaposi sarcoma. *J Clin Pathol.* 1995;48(11):1011–1016. PMID: 8543622. PMCID: 503005.

81. Hammock L, Reisenauer A, Wang W, Cohen C, Birdsong G, Folpe AL. Latency-associated nuclear antigen expression and human herpes virus-8 polymerase chain reaction in the evaluation of Kaposi sarcoma and other vascular tumors in HIV-positive patients. *Mod Pathol.* 2005;18(4):463–468. PMID: 15578080.

82. Ruocco E, Ruocco V, Tornesello ML, Gambardella A, Wolf R, Buonaguro FM. Kaposi's sarcoma: etiology and pathogenesis, inducing factors, causal associations, and treatments: facts and controversies. *Clin Dermatol.* 2013;31(4):413–422. PMID: 23806158.

83. Washington MK, Tang LH, Berlin J, et al. Protocol for the examination of specimens from patients with neuroendocrine tumors (carcinoid tumors) of the stomach. *Arch Pathol Lab Med.* 2010;134(2):187–191. PMID: 20121605.

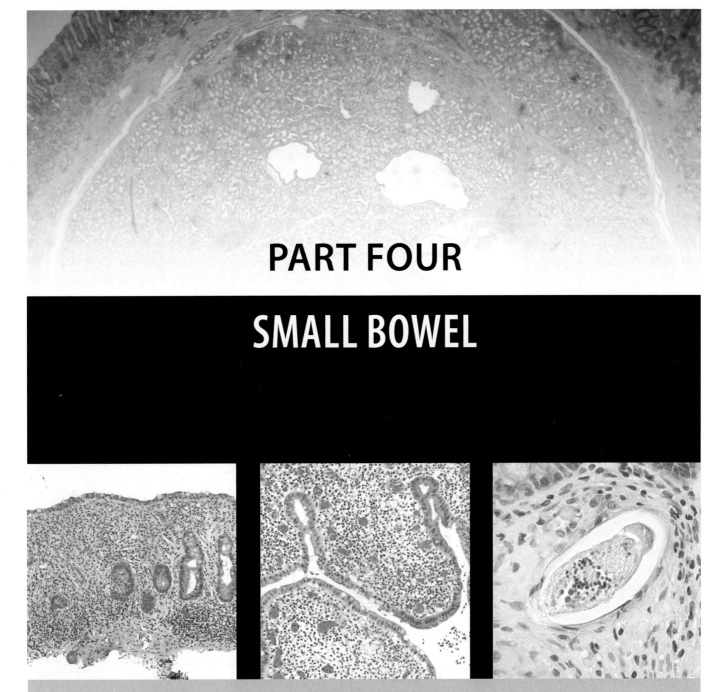

PART FOUR

SMALL BOWEL

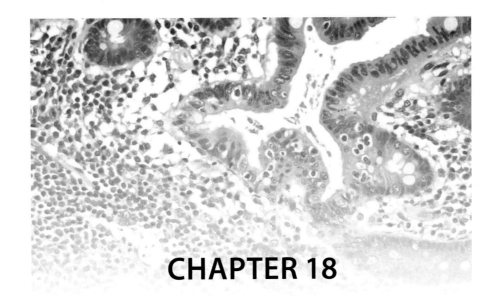

CHAPTER 18

Celiac Disease and Related Conditions

INTRODUCTION

Biopsies of the small bowel, most commonly the duodenum, are performed as part of the diagnostic workup for celiac disease or gluten-sensitive enteropathy (GSE). Several questions should be considered and addressed during microscopic evaluation of these biopsies (Table 18-1). Answers to these questions partially depend on the clinical setting and in turn greatly help clinical decision making.

In this chapter, the typical histologic features of celiac disease in small-bowel mucosa biopsies are described, followed by a discussion of the diagnostic criteria as well as pitfalls. Refractory and collagenous sprue and enteropathy-associated T-cell lymphoma (EATL) are also discussed. Celiac disease–associated small-bowel adenocarcinoma is covered in Chapter 22.

CLINICAL BACKGROUND

Celiac disease is a disorder mainly of a genetic predisposition. It usually develops and is diagnosed during childhood and adolescence. However, with increasing awareness and variable expression (penetrance) of the disease, an increasing number of cases are diagnosed in adults as well, including elderly persons. In general, patients with celiac disease present with gastrointestinal symptoms such as abdominal pain and malabsorption. In children, additional problems can present as consequences of impaired growth and development, such as dental enamel defects, osteoporosis, short stature, delayed puberty, and persistent iron deficiency anemia. It is not uncommon for these patients to have dermatitis herpetiformis (DH). Other disorders that likely accompany celiac disease include type 1 diabetes, Down syndrome, and selective immunoglobulin (Ig) A deficiency. It should be noted that gastrointestinal symptoms and malabsorption may be lacking in some adult patients.

Susceptibility to Celiac Disease

Most patients with celiac disease carry one of two major histocompatibility complex (MHC) class II alleles: the HLA DQA1 *0501-DQB1*02 (**DQ2**) and HLA-DQA1*0301-DQB1* 0302 (**DQ8**). About 30% of the general population in North America is DQ2 positive. Most celiac patients (86%–100%) have the DQ2 background, and homozygosity for DQ2 alleles may be associated with early onset of the disease. Nearly all celiac patients without HLA-DQ2 have the HLA-DQ8 antigen (encoded by DQB1*0302 and DQA1*0301). In other words, absence of DQ2 and DQ8 essentially excludes the diagnosis of celiac disease.

Other Disease Associations

Some patients with celiac disease have concurrent eosinophilic esophagitis.[1-3] Patients may also exhibit histologic changes of lymphocytic gastritis if the stomach is biopsied (see Chapter 12). In addition, patients with celiac or collagenous sprue may show histologic features of microscopic colitis when colonoscopic biopsies are obtained, or have bona fide concurrent microscopic colitis.[4-8]

TABLE 18-1. Questions to address when evaluating biopsies for celiac disease.

1. Are histologic changes characteristic of celiac disease present?

2. If not, what might be the likely underlying disease that can explain the symptoms?

3. How did the patient with an established diagnosis of celiac disease respond to a gluten-free diet (GFD)?

4. If the patient did not respond to a strict GFD, can a diagnosis of refractory sprue be made, and what is the subtype?

5. Are mimics of celiac disease ruled out?

6. For a patient with refractory sprue, is there evidence of enteropathy-associated T-cell lymphoma?

Laboratory Tests

Several serologic tests and HLA typing are available that are a necessary part of the diagnostic workup. These may be performed in patients with a clinical suspicion of the disease or after biopsies reveal histologic changes that are suggestive of the diagnosis. Currently, serum IgA anti–tissue transglutaminase (tTG), IgA anti–endomysium antibody (EMA), and anti–deamidated glidian peptide (DGP) are considered to have the best diagnostic value in terms of sensitivity and specificity. However, 0.1%–0.6% of healthy blood donors in Europe, the United States, and Brazil have selective IgA deficiency (a serum IgA level below 5 mg/dL); while celiac disease occurs with increased frequencies in these populations, these patients will not be diagnosed if the serologic IgA markers are used. Therefore, clinical symptoms and other tests play more important roles in these patients. For genetic testing, probes for HLA-DQ2 and HLA-DQ8 both have high sensitivity but poor specificity, yielding a low positive predictive value but a high negative predictive value for celiac disease. Therefore, diagnosis of celiac disease should be based on multiple parameters, as discussed next (Table 18-2).

TABLE 18-2. Diagnostic markers for celiac disease.

Clinical history	Most important! (patient age, drug history, etc)
HLA alleles[a]	DQ2
	DQ8
Antibodies[b]	IgA anti–tissue transglutaminase (tTG)
	IgA anti–endomysium antibody (EMA)
	Anti–deamidated gliadin peptide (DGP)
Biopsy	Villous blunting, increased IELs, crypt hyperplasia
Clinical outcome	Response to GFD

Abbreviations: GFD, gluten-free diet; IEL, intraepithelial lymphocyte; IgA, immunoglobulin A.

[a] High sensitivity, low specificity.

[b] Excellent sensitivity and specificity, but false negativity in patients with IgA deficiency.

Diagnosis

For patients with symptoms of celiac disease or at increased risk for celiac disease, the diagnostic workup should be a combination of clinical history, HLA antigen typing, positive celiac serological tests, and biopsy findings (see the next section) (Table 18-2). Due to variation of mucosal architecture in different regions of the intestine, optimal biopsies should be obtained from the distal duodenum. Not uncommonly, duodenal biopsies obtained for indications other than suspicion for celiac disease show microscopic features of celiac disease, prompting further serological testing and leading to the diagnosis of celiac disease. The diagnosis is considered definitive when there is complete symptom resolution after treatment with a strict gluten-free diet (GFD) in a previously symptomatic individual with characteristic histologic changes on biopsy.

■ HISTOPATHOLOGY OF CELIAC DISEASE AND EVALUATION OF BIOPSIES

The classic histologic changes of celiac disease in small-bowel biopsies are marked villous blunting, crypt hyperplasia, and marked intraepithelial lymphocytosis (IELs) (Figure 18-1). Although pathognomic in the proper clinical context, this celiac histologic "triad" is not entirely specific. On the other hand, this triad may not always be present in a given biopsy and can vary depending on the phase or stage of disease, treatment history, location of the biopsy, and changes introduced during sample collection and processing.

Sometimes, biopsies from the stomach of celiac patients reveal significant lymphoplasmacytic infiltration in the lamina propria with increased IELs, which render the histologic diagnosis of "lymphocytic gastritis." When lacking active neutrophilic infiltration and *Helicobacter pylori* infection, the most common association of this histologic finding is underlying celiac disease. Therefore, the duodenal mucosa should be carefully evaluated and biopsied to rule out this possibility.

FIGURE 18-1. Typical histology of celiac disease. There is complete loss of villi, replaced by crypt hyperplasia, and intraepithelial lymphocytosis.

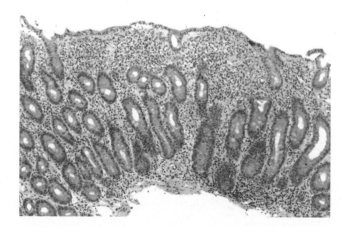

VILLOUS ARCHITECTURAL ABNORMALITY

For assessment of villous architectural abnormality, several pitfalls should be recognized: (1) The presence of Brunner's glands in the bulb and the second portion of the duodenum may cause at least focal villous shortening or even flattening (Figure 18-2A). (2) Peptic injury may make the villi appear irregular or shorter (Figure 18-2B). (3) Random orientation of the biopsy fragments during the embedding process results in unavoidable tangential sectioning (Figure 18-2C). (4) Certain diets increase the frequency of focal or patchy villous fusion (Figure 18-2D), giving rise to the impression of flattening.

In untreated celiac disease, villous blunting is usually extensive. Therefore, one should be cautious when only one or two foci of villous "atrophy" or "blunting" is seen on a biopsy to avoid overcalling celiac disease (except for treated cases). Likewise, one should not rely on biopsies of the bulb alone when evaluating villous architecture unless the flattening is diffuse and overwhelming. Also, mucosal changes may be patchy in distribution and vary in severity in treated celiac disease or in patients who are early in the development of the disease because an increasing number of patients are now being evaluated earlier due to family history, partial symptoms, and increased awareness among the general population. Therefore, the pathologist needs to be vigilant not to miss subtle early lesions.

Intraepithelial Lymphocytes and Lymphocytosis

Lymphocytes, mostly cytotoxic T cells ($CD3^+$/$CD8^+$) with a minor component of T helper cells ($CD3^+$/$CD4^+$), are a normal component of the small-bowel epithelium. These IELs are more concentrated at foci overlying lymphoid follicles, lined by the specialized epithelial cells termed *microfold* or *M cells* (Figure 18-3). Normally, the distribution of IELs is denser in the jejunum compared to the duodenum. There is much debate regarding the "normal" density of IELs in the duodenum. From a practical point of view, a count of 20 to 25 per 100 villous epithelial cells on sections stained with

FIGURE 18-2. Pitfalls in assessing villous abnormalities. **A.** Flattening of villi over Brunner's gland. **B.** Complete villous replacement by crypts from healed ulcer from peptic injury (nonsteroidal anti-inflammatory drugs). **C.** Tangential sectioning caused by poor orientation of specimen. **D.** Focal fusing of villi as a nonspecific change or variant.

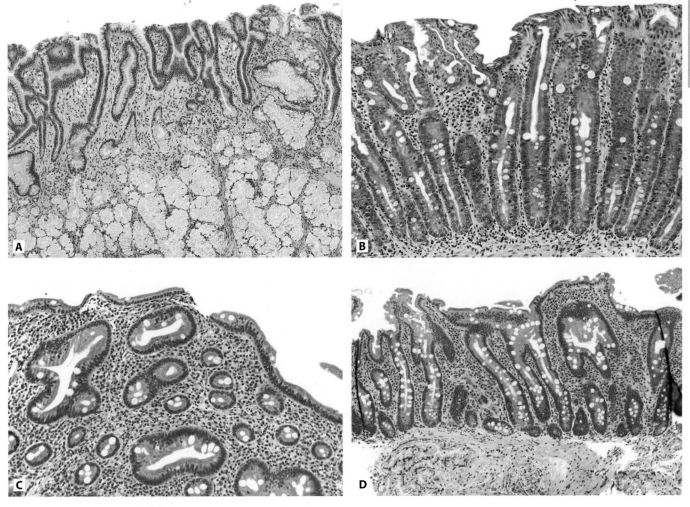

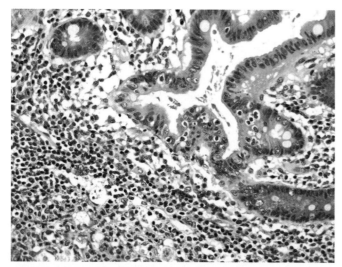

FIGURE 18-3. M cells. The epithelial cells immediately overlying a lymphoid follicle are specialized with intraepithelial lymphocytes.

hematoxylin and eosin (H&E) is considered the upper limit of normal by most pathologists.[9] In most bona fide cases of celiac disease, however, an increase in IELs is marked and readily recognizable without performing an actual count (Figure 18-4). When subtle, the counting should be done in a meticulous and consistent way to avoid errors due to suboptimal processing, thicker sectioning, or areas overlying lymphoid follicles, which usually lead to a higher count.

Some pathologists use immunostain for CD3 to highlight IELs for counting. It has been suggested that immunostaining only makes the IELs easier to recognize and should yield the same count as H&E stain. Nonetheless, in our experience this consistently leads to a much greater number of IELs than using H&E stain (Figure 18-5). It should be recognized that the so-called normal range is technique dependent. H&E stain is always less sensitive than immunostain in identifying

FIGURE 18-4. Flattened duodenal mucosa with marked intraepithelial lymphocytosis.

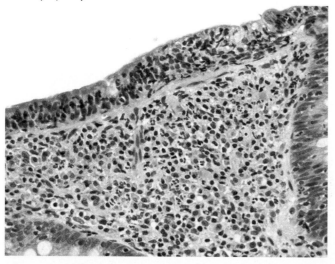

cells with a certain immunophenotype. Knowledge regarding the clinicopathologic correlation of celiac disease was mostly based on excellent studies without the use of the CD3 marker. For example, in the work of Marsh,[10] which described the diagnostic criteria of celiac disease in a more systemic manner, no immunostain was used for IEL counting. Thus, only H&E sections of the biopsy are used for evaluation of number of IELs in our practice for the purpose of initial diagnosis. Nevertheless, for cases of refractory sprue (RS), these immunomarkers are used as a part of the diagnostic workup (see below).

Increase in IELs in the Background of Normal Villous Architecture

As mentioned, with increasing awareness of celiac disease, patients who are at increased risk due to a celiac family history may seek medical attention earlier than in the past, usually with minimal or no symptoms. Biopsies from these patients often yield a normal or mildly abnormal histology. That is, before the disease is fully expressed clinically, the biopsies may show normal villi but with a variable degree of increase in IELs (Figure 18-6). Early studies of relatives of patients with celiac disease or asymptomatic patients commonly showed this histology. Studies based on small series have shown a significant proportion of patients with this histologic pattern either developed full-blown celiac disease or were found to be positive for celiac serology at follow-up. However, other studies with larger numbers of subjects failed to confirm this finding. For example, in the study by Lahdeaho et al, 236 patients were followed up for 8 to 25 years and only 2% developed celiac disease.[11]

Increased IELs with normal villous architecture can occur in many other conditions, including *H. pylori* gastritis, injury induced by nonsteroidal anti-inflammatory drugs (NSAIDs), cow's milk protein intolerance, and other autoimmune disorders, to name a few. This is also seen in treated celiac disease. Hence, specificity of this microscopic pattern is low for celiac disease, leading to a poor predictive value for this diagnosis in an unselected patient population. Another potential reason for the low predictive value of increased IELs may be associated with the low threshold for increased density of IELs used. In some early publications, such as the one by Marsh,[10] when describing this lesion, the photomicrograph showed IELs in a density that can be readily recognized as increased without counting (similar to the lesion illustrated in Figure 18-4). In contrast, in current practice, not only are we taught to count IELs per 100 epithelial cells, but also many pathologists use immunostain for CD3 to increase the sensitivity for counting IELs, as discussed previously. This makes the pool of biopsies with "abnormal" IELs much larger and thus much lower in specificity for celiac disease.

Another issue concerning the evaluation of IELs in normal villi is the difference in the number of IELs between the tip and the base of villi. Normally, there is a higher number of IELs toward the crypts. Therefore, this region should be avoided when assessing the density of IELs, and evaluation should be focused on the tip of the villi (Figure 18-6B).

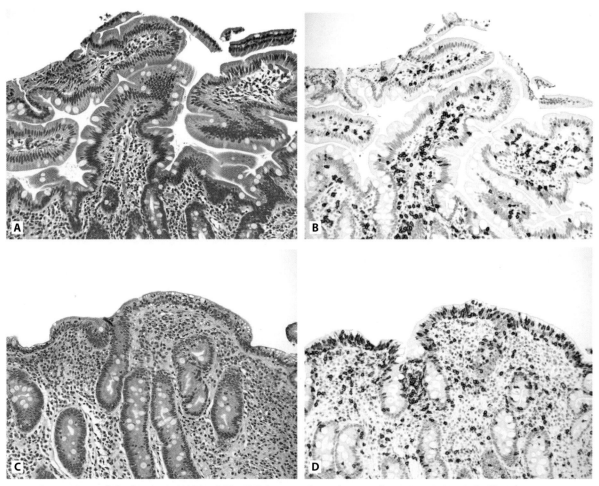

FIGURE 18-5. Comparison of IEL density in H&E and CD3 IHC (immunohistochemistry) staining. **A.** Normal villi with no increase in IELs. **B.** The same field showing "increased" IELs at tip of the villi when immunostain for CD3 is applied. **C.** Celiac disease with villous blunting and increased IELs. **D.** The same field stained for CD3 revealing a much greater density of IELs.

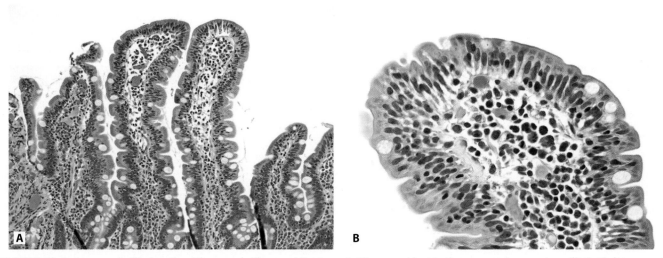

FIGURE 18-6. Increase in IEL density with normal villous architecture. **A.** IELs are evident in these normal-appearing villi. **B.** Higher magnification shows IELs at the tip of a villus.

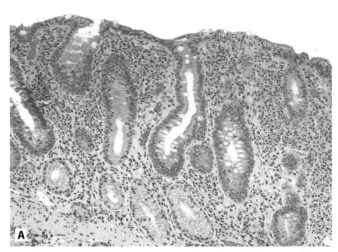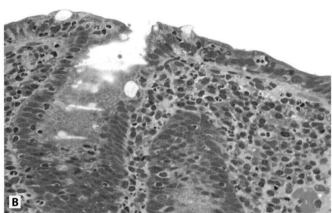

FIGURE 18-7. Neutrophilic infiltration in celiac disease. **A.** Duodenal mucosa with complete villous blunting and intraepithelial lymphocytes (IELs). In addition, there are neutrophils infiltrating. **B.** Higher magnification showing neutrophils in crypt and surface epithelium.

In general, increased IELs should be identified in at least 4 villi to be considered significant.

Neutrophils in Celiac Disease

Many authors emphasized that neutrophilic infiltration is inconsistent with the diagnosis of celiac disease. In reality, it is not uncommon to find neutrophilic infiltration in the lamina propria as well as epithelium in duodenal biopsies from patients with celiac disease (Figure 18-7), in up to 28% of adult and 56% of pediatric patients.[12] The significance of this is unknown but may be related to local bacterial overgrowth due to reduced mucosal immunity, which in turn causes secondary neutrophilic reaction. Regardless, the presence of neutrophilic infiltration in a duodenal biopsy that otherwise exhibits typical features of celiac disease should not persuade the pathologist to exclude the diagnosis (Figure 18-7).

Histologic Grading of Severity of Celiac Disease (Marsh Types)

To compare histologic abnormalities in different clinical settings, Marsh introduced a scheme to categorize the small-bowel mucosal changes[10] based on severity of individual morphologic changes, including villous atrophy, crypt hyperplasia, and degree of intraepithelial lymphocytosis. Notably, the normal number of IELs was not defined in the description. An updated classification was later proposed that included 40 IELs/100 enterocytes as the normal upper limit.[13] This updated Marsh-Oberhuber classification (Table 18-3) describes 5 histologic types (Figure 18-8): preinfiltrative (type 0), infiltrative (type 1), infiltrative-hypertrophic (type 2), flat-destructive (type 3), and atrophic-hypoplastic (type 4). The preinfiltrative lesion (type 0) refers to normal mucosa seen predominantly in patients with DH, but without evidence of malabsorption.

TABLE 18-3. Marsh classification of celiac disease.[a]

Type	IELs	Villi	Crypts
Preinfiltrative (type 0)	Normal	Normal	Normal
Infiltrative (type 1)	Increased	Normal	Normal
Infiltrative-hyperplastic (type 2)	Increased	Normal	Hyperplastic
Destructive type 3a	Increased	Mild blunting	Hyperplastic
Destructive type 3b	Increased	Moderate blunting	Hyperplastic
Destructive type 3c	Increased	Severe blunting (flat)	Hyperplastic
Hypoplastic type 4	Increased	Severe blunting (flat)	Atrophic

Abbreviation: IEL, intraepithelial lymphocyte.

Note: Type 1 is most frequently seen in patients with dermatitis herpetiformis, asymptomatic patients, and first-degree relatives of patients with celiac disease. Type 2 is rarely encountered in pathology practice. Types 3a, 3b, and 3c are mostly seen in classically symptomatic patients with celiac. Type 4 is rare and may be seen in patients with refractory sprue.

[a]Data from Marsh MN. Gluten, major histocompatibility complex, and the small intestine. A molecular and immunobiologic approach to the spectrum of gluten sensitivity ('celiac sprue'). *Gastroenterology.* 1992;102(1):330–354; Oberhuber G, Granditsch G, Vogelsang H. The histopathology of coeliac disease: time for a standardized report scheme for pathologists. *Eur J Gastroenterol Hepatol.* 1999;11(10):1185–1194.[10,13]

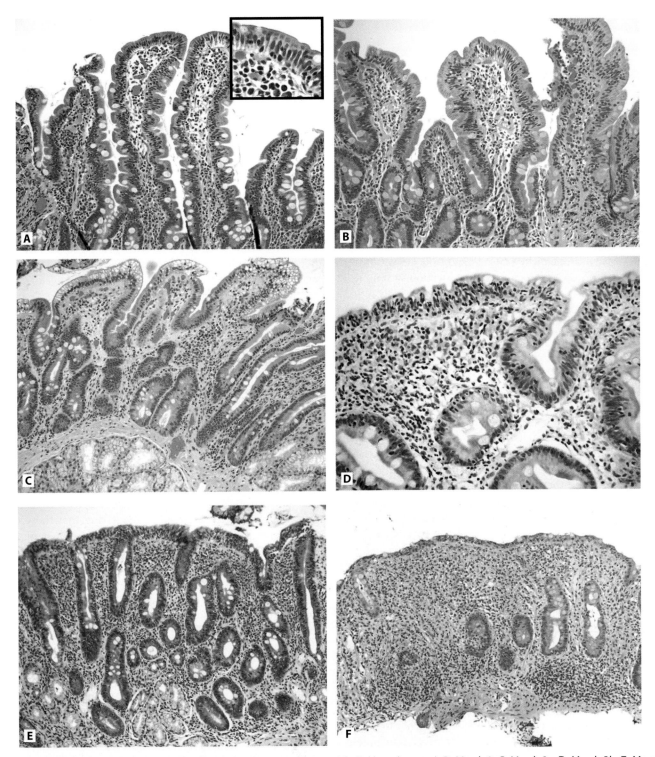

FIGURE 18-8. Marsh lesion types: **A.** Marsh 1 (insert: increased intraepithelial lymphocytes); **B.** Marsh 2; **C.** Marsh 3a; **D.** Marsh 3b; **E.** Marsh 3c; **F.** Marsh 4.

Although the "Marsh" types are sometimes referred to as "lesions," these should not be used as diagnostic terms. For example, one cannot list as a final diagnosis "March type 0 celiac disease" in the pathology report because it represents normal mucosa. Similarly, one cannot objectively assign a type 1 lesion as diagnostic of celiac disease because an increase in IELs with normal villous architecture can be seen in many other conditions, with celiac cases only representing a small subset of unselected patients with this finding. It must be emphasized that the Marsh type should be considered a grading tool for research purposes when all the specimens studied are processed consistently under

TABLE 18-4. Immunophenotype of type 1 and type 2 refractory celiac disease.

	IELs	LP lymphocytes	Flow cytometry
Type 1	CD3⁺/CD8⁺ TCR-β	CD3⁺/CD4⁺	Normal T-cell phenotype
Type 2	CD3⁺/CD8⁻ or CD3⁻/CD8⁻ TCR-γ, -δ	CD3⁺/CD4⁺ May be TIA⁺ (cytoplasmic)	Intracytoplasmic CD3ε, surface CD103, lack of CD8

Abbreviations: IEL, intraepithelial lymphocyte; LP, lamina propria; TCR, T-cell receptor.

similar conditions or as a "measurable" parameter for monitoring disease progress or histologic treatment response. For example, after treatment, a change from a Marsh type 3b to type 2 does provide a rough "quantification" of improvement in a patient with established celiac diagnosis. However, in a diagnostic workup, due to variation in location of sampling and specimen orientation, grading may not accurately reflect overall clinical disease severity. We believe that a Marsh score should be provided only if the clinician understands the true meaning as well as the limitations, therefore avoiding erroneous conclusions regarding the nature and severity of disease.

Follow-up biopsies are performed for various indications in patients with celiac disease after treatment with a GFD, such as poor clinical response, unresolving celiac serology, or inconclusive initial diagnosis. Rebiopsy is controversial for patients who have exhibited good clinical response and is thus not performed routinely in these patients. Studies have shown that while there may be some degree of histologic response in many patients, complete histologic resolution is expected only in a small subset of adult patients (about 20%–30%) who undergo rebiopsy[14,15] as compared to a much higher proportion in pediatric patients.

Refractory Celiac Disease

Refractory celiac disease (RCD) is defined as persistent or recurrent malabsorptive symptoms and villous atrophy despite strict adherence to a GFD for at least 6 months in the absence of other causes of nonresponsive treated celiac disease or overt malignancy. Thus, the diagnosis of RCD or RS should be made with careful clinical review of treatment history, confirmation of the initial diagnosis, and exclusion of other disorders that may have similar clinical symptoms or complications of celiac disease. Strict adherence to a GFD for 6 months or longer is the basic requirement. Any potential contamination that may have adversely led to ingestion of gluten should be excluded before the patient is deemed refractory to dietary treatment and subjected to steroid therapy. Usually, when RCD is clinically suspected, a repeat endoscopic evaluation with biopsy is performed to confirm the lack of histologic response as well as for the potential phenotypic study of the lesional lymphocytic populations.

To stratify patients for treatment and prognosis, RCD is further classified into two types.[16–18] Type 1 disease is expected to respond with a higher frequency to steroids, as opposed to most type 2 cases. As a part of the histology workup for RCD, a panel of immunostains is recommended to evaluate the phenotype of IELs (Table 18-4). Even if a patient responds to steroids, the clinicians may still request an immunohistochemical "T-cell panel" to be performed to ensure that they are not dealing with type 2 RCD; responding to steroids does not exclude the that diagnosis.

The histologic manifestations on H&E-stained sections of the two types of RCD are nearly identical. Immunohistochemically, type 1 RCD is characterized by IELs with normal cytotoxic T-cell phenotype, with coexpression of CD3, CD8, and T-cell receptor β (TCR-β) (Figure 18-9). In contrast, in type 2 RCD, most of the IELs exhibit loss of CD8 (Figure 18-10) and, rarely, cell surface CD3. This being said, immunohistochemically, loss of cell surface CD3 with preservation of cytoplasmic CD3 is difficult to recognize in practice. This is why flow cytometry using fresh tissue to access the IEL phenotype is also used for this purpose.

Some cases of type 2 RCD may demonstrate clonal TCR gene rearrangement as well,[19,20] suggesting that these cases may represent an evolving EATL (see below).[17] It must be noted that "clonality" of T cells by gene arrangement study may also be caused by the limited number of lymphocytes analyzed in biopsies. When only a small number of lymphocytes are analyzed by polymerase chain reaction (PCR), the predominant cluster of T-cell genes may be amplified during the procedure, giving rise to the identification of monoclonality. Therefore, for biopsies that otherwise exhibit the "usual" microscopic changes of celiac sprue, the value of clonality studies is not clear because they may add more uncertainties to the clinical decision making, not to mention the added costs.

Collagenous Sprue

Some patients initially respond to a GFD as in typical celiac disease but later may relapse or develop resistance to treatment. A subset of these patients exhibits biopsy findings of thickened subepithelial collagen layer focally or diffusely in addition to increased IELs and villous abnormality (Figure 18-11). The term *collagenous sprue* was coined for this condition.[21] Rarely, patients present initially with histologic features of collagenous sprue without a prior history of conventional celiac disease.[22,23]

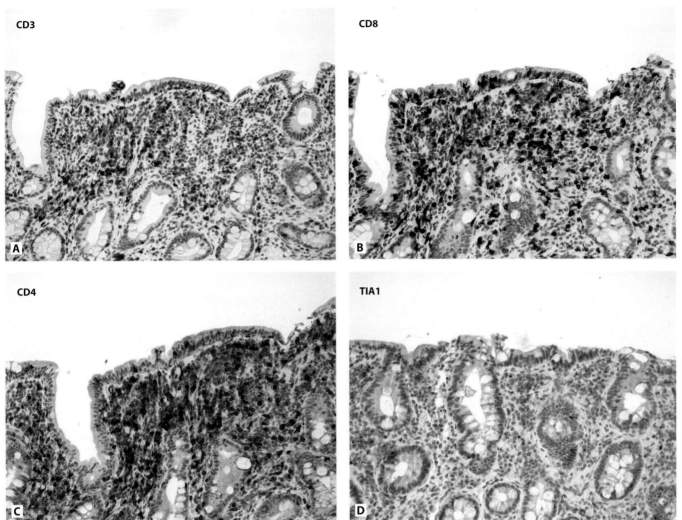

FIGURE 18-9. Type 1 refractory celiac disease: immunohistochemistry (IHC) pattern. Immunostain for CD3 highlighted the IEL population as well as CD8. CD4 mostly highlights a lamina propria population. Rare TIA1 cells in the lamina propria are also appreciated.

The natural history of collagenous sprue is unknown. The disease is characterized clinically by chronic or persistent diarrhea, refractory malabsorption, progressive weight loss, and multiple nutrient deficiencies. It is not clear if collagenous sprue represents disease progression from celiac disease or a unique disease entity with features that overlap with celiac disease. Some patients with this clinically complex disorder may have metachromatic or synchronic colonic disease, including lymphocytic or collagenous colitis.[22,23]

Immunophenotypically, the IELs in collagenous sprue are CD3+ and CD8+ in most patients, but some patients with collagenous sprue have IELs that are CD3+ but CD8−.

■ DIFFERENTIAL CONSIDERATIONS

As described, the microscopic changes of celiac disease range from minimum to severe, with increasing specificity for the diagnosis (Table 18-3). Each of these histologic patterns or

Marsh types can be seen in some other disorders, which should be considered in the differential diagnosis. These are listed in Table 18-5 as a quick reference.

Of the celiac mimics, tropical sprue most resembles celiac disease clinically and histologically and is underrecognized. This disorder affects both people who reside in the tropical areas and those who travel there. It is the latter group that may cause differential difficulties.[24–27] Aside from travel history, additional clues that suggest tropical sprue include prominent infiltration by eosinophils.[27] In addition, tropical sprue rarely causes complete villous blunting (Marsh 3c lesion).

Another increasingly recognized mimic of celiac disease is enteropathy caused by olmesartan, an angiotensin II receptor antagonist, and related drugs.[28–31] Most of these patients present with abdominal pain, diarrhea, and weight loss. Small-bowel biopsies reveal features characteristic of celiac disease (many with Marsh type 3a or 3b). Most recently, we encountered a case of villous blunting enteropathy related to

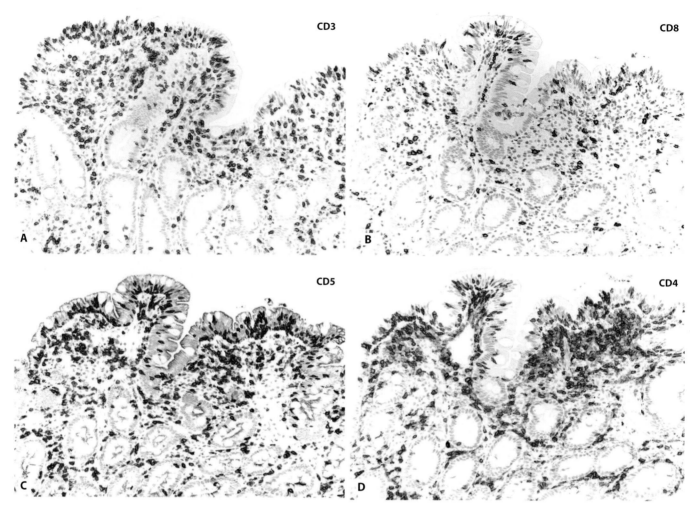

FIGURE 18-10. Type 2 refractory celiac disease: IHC pattern. Immunostain for CD3 highlighted most of the IEL population as compared to immunostain for CD5; loss of cell surface CD3 is difficult to appreciate on immunostain as the cytoplasmic CD3 is preserved. However, there is marked loss of the CD8 population. CD4 mostly highlights a lamina propria population.

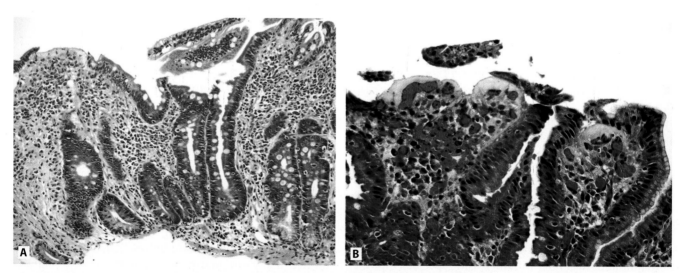

FIGURE 18-11. Collagenous sprue. **A.** Prominent subepithelial collagen layer causing partial sloughing of epithelium in a background of marked villous blunting and increase in IELs. **B.** A trichrome stain highlights the thickened collagen layer.

TABLE 18-5. Various microscopic patterns and their significance.

Normal histology

  Normal

  Latent celiac disease if positive celiac serology

Increased IELs and normal villous architecture

  Latent, evolving, or early (Marsh type 1) celiac disease if positive celiac serology

  Treated celiac disease

  Drug-induced changes (such as NSAIDs)

  Changes associated with *Helicobacter pylori* gastritis

  Cow's milk protein intolerance

  Acute viral gastroenteritis

  Other immune disorders

Increased IELs and villous blunting

  Celiac disease (including refractory sprue)

  Drug-induced changes (eg, olmesartan, simvastatin)

  Tropical sprue

  Common variable immune deficiency

  Autoimmune enteropathy

Increased IELs and villous blunting and thickened subepithelial collagen layer

  Collagenous sprue

  Autoimmune enterocolitis

Abbreviation: IEL, intraepithelial lymphocyte; NSAID, nonsteroidal anti-inflammatory drug.

simvastatin therapy (Figure 18-12), which had been reported only once in the literature.[32]

Some patients with a diagnosis of celiac disease will initially respond to a GFD but subsequently relapse. These patients are considered to have RS. Interestingly, most of these patients will have negative celiac serology. Because patients with so-called RS are usually elderly (median age 69 years) and thus often on medications, the possibility of drug-related enteropathy, such as olmesartan enteropathy, should be considered.[30]

CHRONIC ULCERATIVE JEJUNOILEITIS

The term *chronic ulcerative jejunoileitis* is mainly a clinical designation to conditions that are characterized by multiple chronic ulcers, which may be complicated by, or progress to, strictures. Most cases involve the proximal jejunum and, less frequently, other regions of the small bowel. The stomach or colon may also be affected rarely. The median age of patient presentation is 60 years. Clinical manifestations include abdominal pain, weight loss, malabsorption, and protein-losing enteropathy. Some patients may present with deceptively bland bowel perforation.

Pathologically, the underlying disease process of chronic ulcerative jejunoileitis may be just benign inflammation; however, it can be a manifestation of EATL.[33]

ENTEROPATHY-ASSOCIATED T-CELL LYMPHOMA

Arising in the intestine, EATL is a rare form of primary extranodal T-cell lymphoma. It may develop as a complication of long-term RCD, mostly type 2, and is associated with poor prognosis, with a median overall survival of about 10 months.

The most common sites of involvement by EATL are the proximal jejunum and ileum, with the duodenum and other sites involved less frequently. It usually manifests as multiple ulcers or ulcerated mucosal masses but can present with small-bowel perforation. Histologic findings include flattened mucosa with total villous atrophy, crypt hyperplasia, and markedly increased density of lymphocytic infiltration in the lamina propria and submucosa as well as in the crypt and surface epithelium. The lymphocytic infiltration is usually so severe that it obscures the epithelium of the mucosa (Figure 18-13).

Enteropathy-associated T-cell lymphoma is divided into 2 types (WHO Classification of Lymphoid Neoplasm 2008). Type I EATL is characterized by the presence of pleomorphic-to-anaplastic tumor cells (80% of cases) and a high rate of association with celiac disease (up to 70% of cases), with mucosal changes of celiac disease in adjacent mucosa. Type II EATL is characterized by monomorphic and small- to medium-size tumor cells and is rarely preceded by celiac disease. The background small-bowel mucosa shows enteropathy changes in less than 50% of cases of type II EATL. However, the typing is mainly determined based on immunophenotype of the lesional lymphocytes, as discussed next.

EATL Type I

Type I EATL is more common in Europe, and more than half of the patients have a history of celiac disease.[34] Confirmation of diagnosis requires a combination of histologic and immunohistochemical findings and demonstration of clonal rearrangement of TCR-β or -γ genes. The tumor cells are CD3+ and TIA1+ (cytotoxic granule-associated proteins) and negative for CD56 (Figure 18-13). Other immunomarkers include CD5−, CD8−/+, CD4−, and CD103+. IELs in the adjacent mucosa may show clonal TCR gene rearrangement or an aberrant immunophenotype (CD3+, CD5−, CD8−, and CD4−), indicating that it occurs in a background of RCD.

EATL Type II

Type II EATL is more common in Asia and has a much lower frequency of occurring in a background of celiac disease. Histologically, it is characterized by monotonous small- to medium-size cells.[34,35] In a small series, mild villous atrophy

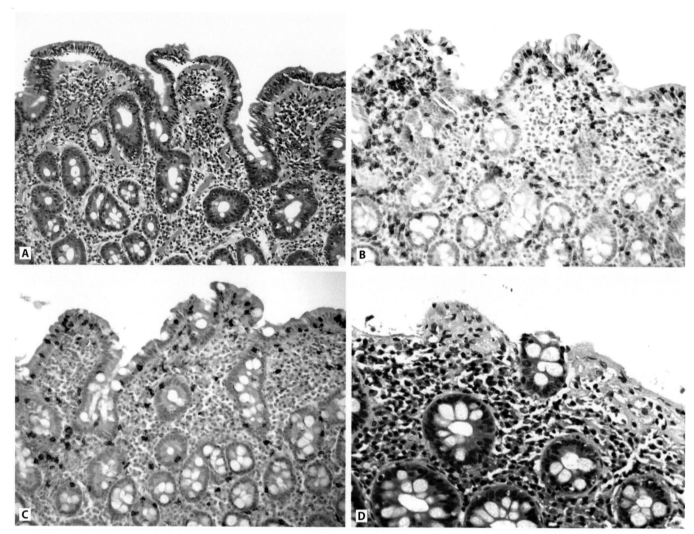

FIGURE 18-12. Simvastatin-induced enteropathy. A 79-year-old woman presented with abdominal pain and diarrhea. Endoscopic biopsies revealed villous blunting enteropathy as well as changes of collagenous colitis. The patient initially responded to a gluten-free diet (GFD) but symptoms rebounded. Celiac workup, including HLA DQ2/8 and serology, was negative. The patient was taking oral simvastatin. Her symptoms improved after cessation of the drug. Duodenal biopsy showed the (**A**) moderate-to-severe villous atrophy, with increase in IELs. **B.** CD3 immunostain. **C.** CD8 immunostain. **D.** Colon biopsy showing collagenous colitis.

was noted in 2 of 18 cases, with no crypt hyperplasia.[35] The IELs are immunohistochemically characterized by expression of CD56 (>90%) and CD8 (80%).[36] The IELs express γδ TCR in 65% of cases.[35] The immunohistochemical markers are listed in Table 18-6.

Based on the lack of association with celiac disease, Chan et al proposed that type II EATL be separated from the EATL category as a distinct form of lymphoma, namely, "monomorphic intestinal T-cell lymphoma."[35]

For differential consideration, other types of lymphoma that arise in or secondarily involve the small-bowel mucosa should be excluded based on clinical, histologic, and immunophenotype features. For example, Mediterranean lymphoma, also known as immunoproliferative small-intestinal

disease (IPSID), is a B-cell lymphoma arising from a background of diffuse plasmacytosis[37] that occurs mainly in the Middle East and North Africa. Biopsies reveal dense lamina propria infiltration consisting primarily of plasma cells and some large undifferentiated cells. While mild alteration of the villous and crypt architecture may be present due to expansion of the lamina propria by tumor infiltrate, there is no association with celiac disease. Despite many histologic similarities in small-bowel biopsy, in contrast to EATL, Mediterranean lymphoma has no significant intraepithelial lymphocytosis. The B-cell phenotype can be readily demonstrated immunohistochemically.

Follicular lymphoma, mucosa-associated lymphoid tissue (MALT) lymphoma, and mantle cell lymphoma can all

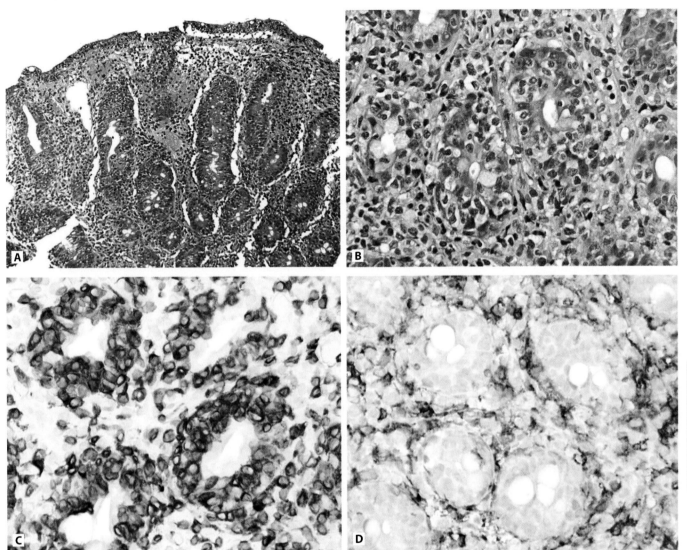

FIGURE 18-13. Type I EATL. The 54-year-old female patient had a history of refractory sprue and presented with abdominal pain and weight loss on a GFD. Biopsies from the duodenum and jejunum showed marked lymphocytic proliferation. **A.** Both surface and crypt epithelium were involved. **B.** Small- and medium-size lymphocytes with pleomorphic features infiltrated the epithelium. **C.** The intraepithelial lympho-cytes were positive for CD3 and 20% positive for CD8 (not shown). **D.** Staining for CD4 only highlighted the lamina propria lymphocytes. The tumor cells were negative for CD56 (not shown) and 100% Ki-67 index (not shown).

be seen in the small-bowel mucosa. Endoscopically, these tumors also present as ulcer, mass, or polypoid protrusions.

TABLE 18-6. Comparison of types 1 and 2 enteropathy-associated T-cell lymphoma.

	Type I (about 80%)	Type II (about 20%)
Preceded by celiac disease	Yes	Less frequently
	Yes	Infrequent
Adjacent mucosa with enteropathic changes	Pleomorphic to ana-plastic tumor cells	Monomorphic, small-to medium-size cells
Morphology	CD3+, TIA1+, often CD8-	CD56+, CD8+
Tumor cell phenotype	CD56-	

Similar to Mediterranean lymphoma, these lymphomas also lack significant intraepithelial lymphocytosis, and immuno-phenotype studies will confirm the B-cell nature.

■ SUMMARY

The discussions in this chapter centered on the diagnosis of celiac disease and expanded to disorders that may complicate or share clinical and pathologic features with celiac disease. The latter should be included in differential considerations when examining small-bowel biopsies for the general clini-cal symptoms of malabsorption. Key points to be kept in mind include the following: (1) Assessment of IELs should be based on H&E section; (2) neutrophils may be a part of celiac disease pathology; (3) histologic findings usually seen in celiac disease are nonspecific, so clinical, endoscopic, and serologic findings are critical; (4) even for "typical" Marsh 3 histology, other disorders should be excluded, such as tropical sprue or drug-induced sprue-like enteropathy; (5) RS should be diagnosed only after adherence to a GFD; (6) distinction between type 1 and type 2 RS is partly based on the immunophenotype of IELs with or without molecular testing for T-cell clonality.

REFERENCES

1. Soon IS, Butzner JD, Kaplan GG, deBruyn JC. Incidence and prevalence of eosinophilic esophagitis in children. *J Pediatr Gastroenterol Nutr.* 2013;57(1):72–80. PMID: 23539047.

2. Stewart MJ, Shaffer E, Urbanski SJ, Beck PL, Storr MA. The association between celiac disease and eosinophilic esophagitis in children and adults. *BMC Gastroenterol.* 2013;13:96. PMID: 23721294. PMCID: PMC3682941.

3. Thompson JS, Lebwohl B, Reilly NR, Talley NJ, Bhagat G, Green PH. Increased incidence of eosinophilic esophagitis in children and adults with celiac disease. *J Clin Gastroenterol.* 2012;46(1):e6–e11. PMID: 21778897.

4. Fine KD, Lee EL, Meyer RL. Colonic histopathology in untreated celiac sprue or refractory sprue: is it lymphocytic colitis or colonic lymphocytosis? *Hum Pathol.* 1998;29(12):1433–1440. PMID: 9865829.

5. Gillett HR, Freeman HJ. Prevalence of celiac disease in collagenous and lymphocytic colitis. *Can J Gastroenterol.* 2000;14(11):919–921. PMID: 11125181.

6. Matteoni CA, Goldblum JR, Wang N, Brzezinski A, Achkar E, Soffer EE. Celiac disease is highly prevalent in lymphocytic colitis. *J Clin Gastroenterol.* 2001;32(3):225–227. PMID: 11246349.

7. Padmanabhan V, Callas PW, Li SC, Trainer TD. Histopathological features of the terminal ileum in lymphocytic and collagenous colitis: a study of 32 cases and review of literature. *Mod Pathol.* 2003;16(2):115–119. PMID: 12591963.

8. Verkarre V, Asnafi V, Lecomte T, et al. Refractory coeliac sprue is a diffuse gastrointestinal disease. *Gut.* 2003;52(2):205–211. PMID: 12524401.

9. Hayat M, Cairns A, Dixon MF, O'Mahony S. Quantitation of intraepithelial lymphocytes in human duodenum: what is normal? *J Clin Pathol.* 2002;55(5):393–394. PMID: 11986350. PMCID: 1769642.

10. Marsh MN. Gluten, major histocompatibility complex, and the small intestine. A molecular and immunobiologic approach to the spectrum of gluten sensitivity ("celiac sprue"). *Gastroenterology.* 1992;102(1):330–354. PMID: 1727768.

11. Lahdeaho ML, Kaukinen K, Collin P, et al. Celiac disease: from inflammation to atrophy: a long-term follow-up study. *J Pediatr Gastroenterol Nutr.* 2005;41(1):44–48. PMID: 15990629.

12. Moran CJ, Kolman OK, Russell GJ, Brown IS, Mino-Kenudson M. Neutrophilic infiltration in gluten-sensitive enteropathy is neither uncommon nor insignificant: assessment of duodenal biopsies from 267 pediatric and adult patients. *Am J Surg Pathol.* 2012;36(9):1339–1345. PMID: 22531172.

13. Oberhuber G, Granditsch G, Vogelsang H. The histopathology of coeliac disease: time for a standardized report scheme for pathologists. *Eur J Gastroenterol Hepatol.* 1999;11(10):1185–1194. PMID: 10524652.

14. Bardella MT, Velio P, Cesana BM, et al. Coeliac disease: a histological follow-up study. *Histopathology.* 2007;50(4):465–471. PMID: 17448022.

15. Hutchinson JM, West NP, Robins GG, Howdle PD. Long-term histological follow-up of people with coeliac disease in a UK teaching hospital. *QJM.* 2010;103(7):511–517. PMID: 20519276.

16. Arguelles-Grande C, Brar P, Green PH, Bhagat G. Immunohistochemical and T-cell receptor gene rearrangement analyses as predictors of morbidity and mortality in refractory celiac disease. *J Clin Gastroenterol.* 2013;47(7):593–601. PMID: 23470642.

17. Daum S, Hummel M, Weiss D, et al. Refractory sprue syndrome with clonal intraepithelial lymphocytes evolving into overt enteropathy-type intestinal T-cell lymphoma. *Digestion.* 2000;62(1):60–65. PMID: 10899727.

18. Rubio-Tapia A, Murray JA. Classification and management of refractory coeliac disease. *Gut.* 2010;59(4):547–557. PMID: 20332526. PMCID: 2861306.

19. Daum S, Ipczynski R, Schumann M, Wahnschaffe U, Zeitz M, Ullrich R. High rates of complications and substantial mortality in both types of refractory sprue. *Eur J Gastroenterol Hepatol.* 2009;21(1):66–70. PMID: 19011576.

20. Verbeek WH, von Blomberg BM, Coupe VM, Daum S, Mulder CJ, Schreurs MW. Aberrant T-lymphocytes in refractory coeliac disease are not strictly confined to a small intestinal intraepithelial localization. *Cytometry B Clin Cytom.* 2009;76(6):367–374. PMID: 19444812.

21. Weinstein WM, Brow JR, Parker F, Rubin CE. The small intestinal mucosa in dermatitis herpetiformis. II. Relationship of the small intestinal lesion to gluten. *Gastroenterology.* 1971;60(3):362–369. PMID: 5554078.

22. Maguire AA, Greenson JK, Lauwers GY, et al. Collagenous sprue: a clinicopathologic study of 12 cases. *Am J Surg Pathol.* 2009;33(10):1440–1449. PMID: 19641452.

23. Vakiani E, Arguelles-Grande C, Mansukhani MM, et al. Collagenous sprue is not always associated with dismal outcomes: a clinicopathological study of 19 patients. *Mod Pathol.* 2010;23(1):12–26. PMID: 19855376.

24. Ghoshal UC, Ghoshal U, Ayyagari A, et al. Tropical sprue is associated with contamination of small bowel with aerobic bacteria and reversible prolongation of orocecal transit time. *J Gastroenterol Hepatol.* 2003;18(5):540–547. PMID: 12702046.

25. Kakar S, Nehra V, Murray JA, Dayharsh GA, Burgart LJ. Significance of intraepithelial lymphocytosis in small bowel biopsy samples with normal mucosal architecture. *Am J Gastroenterol.* 2003;98(9):2027–2033. PMID: 14499783.

26. Owens SR, Greenson JK. The pathology of malabsorption: current concepts. *Histopathology.* 2007;50(1):64–82. PMID: 17204022.

27. Brown IS, Bettington A, Bettington M, Rosty C. Tropical sprue: revisiting an underrecognized disease. *Am J Surg Pathol.* 2014;38(5):666–672. PMID: 24441659.

28. DeGaetani M, Tennyson CA, Lebwohl B, et al. Villous atrophy and negative celiac serology: a diagnostic and therapeutic dilemma. *Am J Gastroenterol.* 2013;108(5):647–653. PMID: 23644957.

29. Greywoode R, Braunstein ED, Arguelles-Grande C, Green PH, Lebwohl B. Olmesartan, other antihypertensives, and chronic diarrhea among patients undergoing endoscopic procedures: a case-control study. *Mayo Clin Proc.* 2014. PMID: 25023670.

30. Rubio-Tapia A, Herman ML, Ludvigsson JF, et al. Severe sprue-like enteropathy associated with olmesartan. *Mayo Clin Proc.* 2012;87(8):732–738. PMID: 22728033. PMCID: 3538487.

31. Stanich PP, Yearsley M, Meyer MM. Olmesartan-associated sprue-like enteropathy. *J Clin Gastroenterol.* 2013;47(10):894–895. PMID: 23751857.

32. Chagnon JP, Cerf M. Simvastatin-induced protein-losing enteropathy. *Am J Gastroenterol.* 1992;87(2):257. PMID: 1734709.

33. Daum S, Weiss D, Hummel M, et al. Frequency of clonal intraepithelial T lymphocyte proliferations in enteropathy-type intestinal T cell lymphoma, coeliac disease, and refractory sprue. *Gut.* 2001;49(6):804–812. PMID: 11709515. PMCID: 1728529.

34. Delabie J, Holte H, Vose JM, et al. Enteropathy-associated T-cell lymphoma: clinical and histological findings from the international peripheral T-cell lymphoma project. *Blood.* 2011;118(1):148–155. PMID: 21566094.

35. Chan JK, Chan AC, Cheuk W, et al. Type II enteropathy-associated T-cell lymphoma: a distinct aggressive lymphoma with frequent gammadelta T-cell receptor expression. *Am J Surg Pathol.* 2011;35(10):1557–1569. PMID: 21921780.

36. Zettl A, deLeeuw R, Haralambieva E, Mueller-Hermelink HK. Enteropathy-type T-cell lymphoma. *Am J Clin Pathol.* 2007;127(5): 701–706. PMID: 17511112.

37. Fine KD, Stone MJ. Alpha-heavy chain disease, Mediterranean lymphoma, and immunoproliferative small intestinal disease: a review of clinicopathological features, pathogenesis, and differential diagnosis. *Am J Gastroenterol.* 1999;94(5):1139–1152. PMID: 10235185.

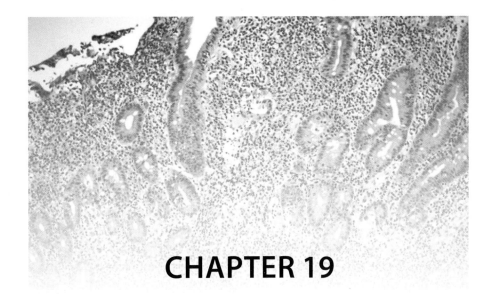

CHAPTER 19

Small-Bowel Involvement in Ulcerative Colitis

■ INTRODUCTION

In the broad sense, the small bowel can be affected by inflammatory bowel disease (IBD) in several different manners (Table 19-1). As well-accepted dogma, Crohn disease can affect any segment of the gastrointestinal (GI) tract, including the small bowel, with chronic gland or crypt-destroying inflammation, deforming the mucosal architecture (see Chapter 4); in contrast, classic ulcerative colitis (UC) only affects the colon. However, it is also well known that limited small-bowel inflammation can be seen in the form of backwash ileitis associated with pancolitis or pouchitis following ileal pouch–anal anastomosis (IPAA) after total proctocolectomy (see Chapter 26). Other than these scenarios, if significant active inflammation is seen involving the small bowel or the upper GI tract in a patient considered to have UC, questions will be raised regarding the appropriateness of the diagnosis of UC.

The past two decades brought the recognition that significant inflammatory diseases (ie, gastroduodenitis or ulcerative duodenitis) can occur in patients with bona fide UC; this is relatively more common in pediatric patients.[1-5] Lack of familiarity with these exceptions to the conventional "rule" of IBD may lead to difficulty or error in diagnosis and clinical management. Therefore, different types of small-bowel involvement in UC are the focus of discussion in this Chapter; small-bowel involvement by Crohn disease is discussed in Chapter 4.

■ BACKWASH ILEITIS

As discussed in Chapter 26, the distal 10–15 cm of terminal ileum can have both endoscopic and histologic evidence of active inflammation in some patients with severely active ulcerative pancolitis. In most cases, the histologic changes are mild (Figure 19-1). The villi may appear slightly shortened (Figure 19-1A), but with preserved overall architecture and scattered neutrophilic infiltration of the villous and crypt epithelium (Figure 19-1B). In general, the histologic changes in backwash ileitis lack significant villous or crypt architectural distortion, pyloric gland metaplasia, or granulomas (Figure 19-2). If the last abnormalities are noted, a diagnosis of Crohn enteritis should be considered and discussed with the treating physician. It may be ruled out through careful review of clinical history (including drug history), serology, and radiologic, endoscopic, and overall pathologic findings.

■ DUODENITIS OR GASTRODUODENITIS IN PATIENTS WITH ULCERATIVE COLITIS

Individual case reports and designed case reviews in the 1990s described upper GI inflammation in patients with UC.[1-3] The earliest report dated to 1960 and described 2 patients with "ulcerative duodenitis" and UC, but with no histology provided.[6] In a prospective study of pretreated pediatric patients with IBD, Ruuska et al[1] reported that 75% of 47 patients with UC had some degree of inflammation involving the

TABLE 19-1. Small-bowel involvement in irritable bowel disease.

Crohn enteritis (see Chapter 4)

    Terminal ileum: often biopsied or seen in resected specimens; most commonly affected by Crohn disease

    Duodenitis: often biopsied, particularly in pediatric patients

    Jejunum: rarely biopsied

Backwash ileitis

    Associated with active ulcerative pancolitis

Pouchitis

    Acute and chronic inflammation of mucosa of ileal pouch–anal anastomosis

Prepouch enteritis

De novo Crohn disease of pouch

Gastroduodenitis in patients with ulcerative colitis

    Common if mild nonspecific inflammation

    Rare if unequivocal chronic active duodenitis is considered

Diffuse ulcerative duodenitis after colectomy for ulcerative colitis

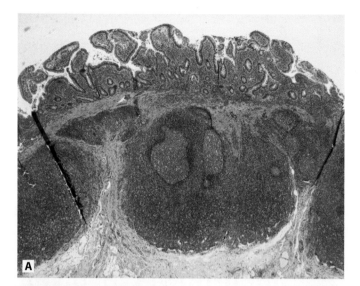

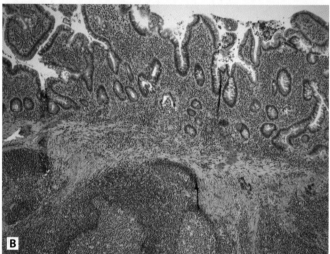

FIGURE 19-1. Backwash ileitis in terminal ileum as part of the total proctocolectomy for severely active ulcerative pancolitis. **A.** Terminal ileum with slightly shortened villi and prominent submucosal lymphoid follicles. **B.** Mild inflammatory cellular infiltration with neutrophilic infiltration of the villous and crypt epithelium.

esophageal, gastric, or duodenal mucosa, either endoscopically or radiologically. Duodenal ulcer was seen endoscopically in 2 of 47 patients with UC. However, histologic examination only found "nonspecific inflammation" in 3 of 34 patients with UC.[1]

Kaufman et al reported gastroduodenitis in 4 of 5 pediatric patients thought to have Crohn disease with pancolitis, but subsequently these cases were diagnosed as UC on examination of subtotal proctocolectomy.[2] Other case reports[3,5] described similar findings, including one patient with left-side colitis and ulcerative duodenitis.[3] Interestingly, none of the patients had granulomas in the duodenal biopsy or resection.[3,5] In a well-controlled study in which "blinded" histologic review of cases of both UC and Crohn disease were performed,[7] a significant proportion of patients with UC (2 of 13) were found to have "moderate-to-severe duodenitis." However, none of the UC patients had duodenal cryptitis (as compared to 26% of those with Crohn disease) or granulomas; none of the duodenal biopsies was reported to have "chronic inflammation,"[7] indicating nonspecific changes.

In a more recent study in which upper GI endoscopy was performed in 250 patients with UC, it was found that 19/250 (7.6%) of these patients had gastroduodenitis, defined endoscopically as friable mucosa, granular mucosa, or conditionally, multiple aphthae.[8] These findings appeared to be associated with pancolitis and a lower dose of prednisolone.[8] However, more than half of the patients in this cohort were postcolectomy patients (see next section), and histologic review was limited. Therefore, it is difficult to evaluate the significance of the conclusion from this study. In contrast, Sonnenberg et al, after analyzing 5493 cases with both colonoscopy and upper GI endoscopy, including 280 cases with UC, found 3% of patients with UC had features of active duodenitis (neutrophilic infiltration of epithelium) without villous architectural change.[9]

Based on careful review of published data, personal communications, and experience, it is safe to say that if strict histologic criteria are applied, such as unequivocal villous and crypt architectural distortion or granulomas, bona fide active chronic duodenitis is rare in patients with UC.[9–11] The presence of these lesions should still be considered diagnostically specific for Crohn disease unless the patient had a recent colectomy.

DIFFUSE GASTROENTERITIS AFTER TOTAL COLECTOMY FOR UC

Among patients who underwent total colectomy for uncontrollable UC, some develop postoperative severe upper GI symptoms and are found to have severe gastroduodenitis.[4,8,12–17]

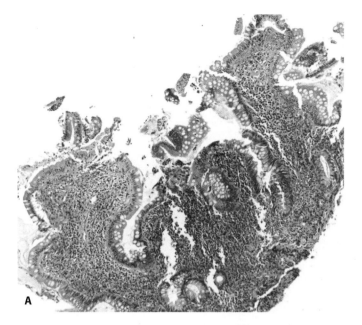

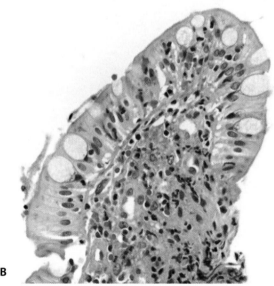

FIGURE 19-2. Biopsy of the terminal ileum showing mild villous abnormality (**A**) but without evident chronicity, such as pyloric gland metaplasia or granulomas. Focal neutrophilic infiltration is evident (**B**).

Valdez et al described 4 patients with UC who developed diffuse duodenitis after colectomy[4]; of these, 3 were younger than 18 years of age. All the patients had severe ulcerative pancolitis. Retrospective review found that 1 patient had focal mucosal distortion in duodenal biopsy. Follow-up did not find features of Crohn disease in 12–54 months. In another paper from the same group, diffuse duodenitis was found in 40% (4 of 10) of the patients with UC who had colectomy.[14]

Several other groups reported similar occurrences of diffuse ulcerative duodenitis after total colectomy for severe UC.[8,12,13] The reported prevalence of gastritis/duodenitis following proctocolectomy for UC ranged from 7.4% to 11%.[12,13]

and the occurrence seemed to be associated with pancolitis and development of pouchitis.[12]

Based on these reports, development of diffuse duodenitis after colectomy is not rare. Therefore, it should not necessarily lead to a change of the diagnosis to Crohn disease in patients who otherwise meet the clinical and pathologic features of UC.[4,8,11]

In post-colectomy UC-associated gastroduodenitis, the histologic findings in the duodenal mucosa are characterized by diffuse, villous-destroying active inflammation, accompanied by dense lymphoplasmacytic infiltration in lamina propria (Figure 19-3). Reexamination of clinical and endoscopic findings, as well as the colectomy specimen, confirmed the diagnosis of UC in these patients. It is important to reaffirm the diagnosis of UC for these patients because this unusual finding will not adversely affect the outcome of ileal pouch–anal anastomosis (IPAA). Also, the upper GI inflammation often responds well with anti-IBD treatment.

■ INFLAMMATORY DISEASES OF THE J POUCH

The curative surgery for severe or refractory UC is total proctocolectomy followed by the construction of an IPAA (or J pouch). Mild-to-severe inflammatory diseases of the pouch may develop in a subset of patients, leading to pouch dysfunction. The full spectrum of these disorders is discussed in Chapter 26 on UC. In this chapter, the discussion emphasizes the distinction between chronic pouchitis and Crohn disease of the pouch.

As described in Chapter 26, active pouchitis without significant mucosal architectural distortion ranges from mild (Figure 19-4) to more severe with erosion or ulcer (Figure 19-5). In many instances, acute pouchitis is diagnosed based on clinical symptoms and endoscopic findings and is not biopsied for histologic confirmation.[18] It should be noted that in an asymptomatic patient with normal endoscopic findings, a few intraepithelial neutrophils should not be considered diagnostic of acute pouchitis.

Depending on time since the pouch was established, the normal small-bowel mucosa that constitutes the pouch undergoes various degrees of adaptive change. Therefore, mild or partial blunting of the villi is considered normal and not a sign of chronic pouchitis. However, unequivocal loss of villi, branching of hyperplastic crypts (Figure 19-6A), and pyloric gland metaplasia (Figure 19-6B) are considered features of chronic pouchitis.

Crohn disease can develop in the J pouch of some patients whose original diagnosis of UC may have been incorrect. However, it can also occur, in a rate as high as 12%, as de novo Crohn disease (Figures 19-7 and 19-8) in patients with well-documented UC[19] Such disease can lead to over 40% loss of the pouch.[20] Diagnosis of pouch Crohn diseases to a large extent relies on clinical findings of fistula or other perianal diseases that developed more than 3 months after ileostomy closure.[18,19] Multiple mucosal ulcers (5 or more) involving the mucosa proximal to the pouch are also considered diagnostic features for Crohn disease.

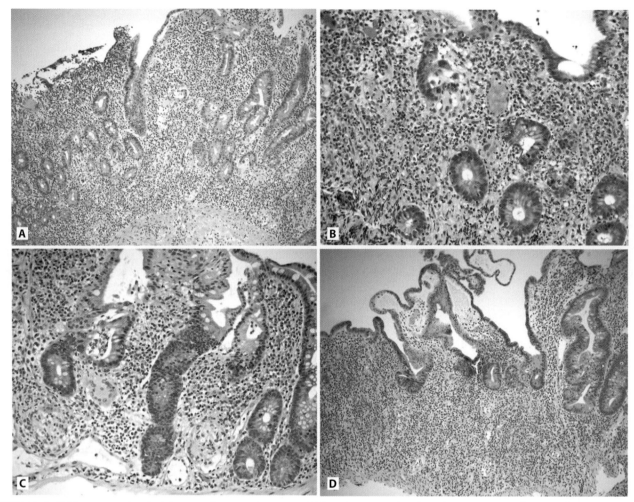

FIGURE 19-3. Diffuse gastroduodenitis postcolectomy. A 24-year-old female patient developed watery output from an ileostomy. **A** and **B.** Severe chronic active duodenitis. **C.** Pouch. **D.** Rectum.

FIGURE 19-4. Mild acute or active pouchitis. Biopsy of the pouch mucosa shows focal neutrophilic infiltration in cluster in the crypt (cryptitis) but no evident architectural distortion.

FIGURE 19-5. Focal superficial ulcer in a case of active pouchitis.

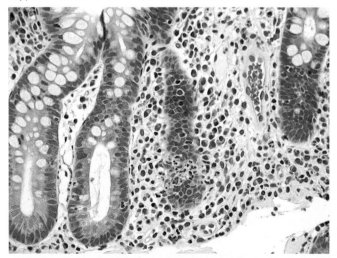

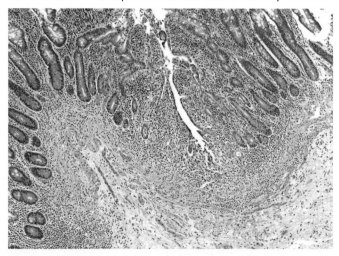

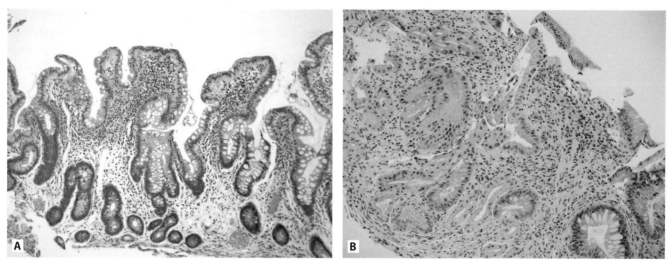

FIGURE 19-6. Chronic pouchitis. Normal villous and crypt architecture is deformed (**A**); many crypts are replaced by pyloric gland metaplasia (**B**).

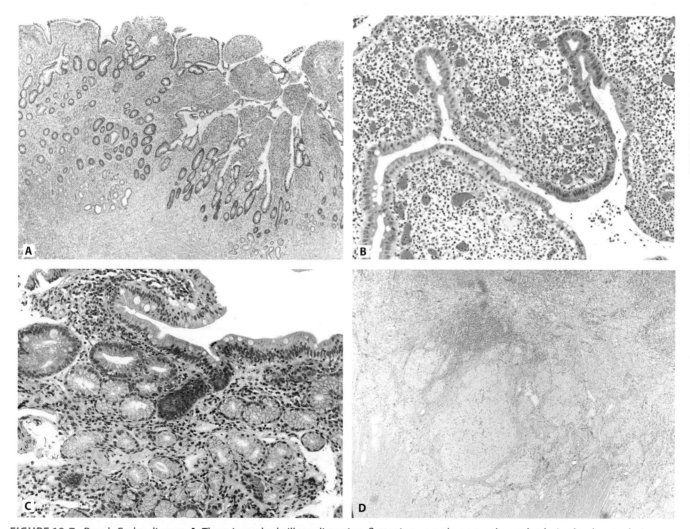

FIGURE 19-7. Pouch Crohn disease. **A.** There is marked villous distortion, flattening, crypt hypertrophy, and pyloric gland metaplasia. **B.** In addition to mixed inflammatory cellular infiltration in lamina propria, there is prominent neutrophilic infiltration of the epithelium in active disease. **C.** Although pyloric gland metaplasia is prominent and involves the superficial mucosa, it is not specific or diagnostic of Crohn disease, as it can be seen in chronic pouchitis as well. **D.** In resected specimens prominent nerve hypertrophy may also be present.

PART FOUR

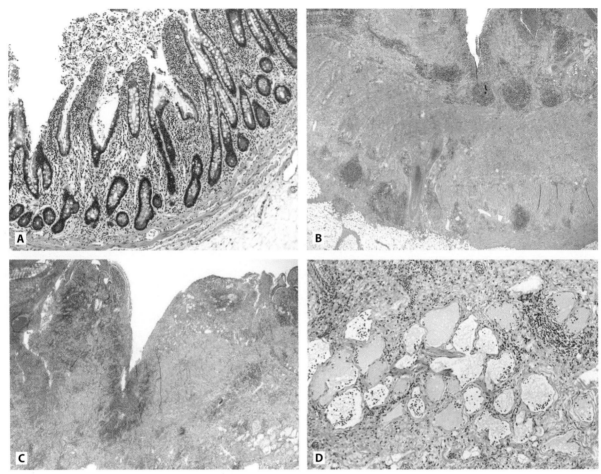

FIGURE 19-8. J-pouch resection due to de novo Crohn disease in a patient with well-documented ulcerative colitis. **A.** Mildly involved area exhibiting only minimal villous change. **B.** Transmural chronic inflammation evidenced by submucosal as well as intramuscular lymphoid "beading." **C.** Knifelike fissuring ulcer. **D.** Prominent submucosal lymphangiectasia.

Histologically, the pouch exhibits features otherwise typical of small-bowel Crohn disease, with villous deformity (Figure 19-7), active neutrophilic infiltration (Figure 19-7B), pyloric gland metaplasia (Figure 19-7C), or epithelioid granulomas. Ulcers (Figure 19-8) and inflammatory polyps can be seen in severe cases. In resected specimens, transmural inflammation, deep fissuring ulcers, or intramural abscess may also be identified (Figure 19-8).

SUMMARY

Although mild nonspecific inflammation of gastric or duodenal mucosa can occur in patients with UC, particularly in pediatric patients, bona fide chronic active duodenitis is rare. In precolectomy patients, the presence of crypt- or villi-destroying duodenitis or epithelioid granuloma supports the diagnosis of Crohn disease. However, diffuse ulcerative duodenitis in patients with post-colectomy UC should not be considered as evidence for Crohn disease on its own. Similarly, active inflammation of the distal terminal ileum in patients with active ulcerative pancolitis without unequivocal chronicity (pyloric gland metaplasia, epithelioid

granuloma, marked villous deformity) represents backwash ileitis, not Crohn disease. Various histologic changes in pouchitis (granulomas, pyloric gland metaplasia) are not predictive of Crohn disease; this diagnosis should rely more on clinical and endoscopic findings.

REFERENCES

1. Ruuska T, Vaajalahti P, Arajarvi P, Maki M. Prospective evaluation of upper gastrointestinal mucosal lesions in children with ulcerative colitis and Crohn's disease. *J Pediatr Gastroenterol Nutr*. 1994;19(2): 181–186. PMID: 7815240.
2. Kaufman SS, Vanderhoof JA, Young R, Perry D, Raynor SC, Mack DR. Gastroenteric inflammation in children with ulcerative colitis. *Am J Gastroenterol*. 1997;92(7):1209–1212. PMID: 9219802.
3. Mitomi H, Atari E, Uesugi H, et al. Distinctive diffuse duodenitis associated with ulcerative colitis. *Dig dis Sci*. 1997;42(3):684–693. PMID: 9073157.
4. Valdez R, Appelman HD, Bronner MP, Greenson JK. Diffuse duodenitis associated with ulcerative colitis. *Am J Surg Pathol*. 2000; 24(10):1407–1413. PMID: 11023103.
5. Terashima S, Hoshino Y, Kanzaki N, Kogure M, Gotoh M. Ulcerative duodenitis accompanying ulcerative colitis. *J Clin Gastroenterol*. 2001;32(2):172–175. PMID: 11205658.

6. Thompson JW 3rd, Bargen JA. Ulcerative duodenitis and chronic ulcerative colitis: report of two cases. *Gastroenterology*. 1960;38:452–455. PMID: 13838088.

7. Tobin JM, Sinha B, Ramani P, Saleh AR, Murphy MS. Upper gastrointestinal mucosal disease in pediatric Crohn disease and ulcerative colitis: a blinded, controlled study. *J Pediatr Gastroenterol Nutr*. 2001;32(4):443–448. PMID: 11396811.

8. Hori K, Ikeuchi H, Nakano H, et al. Gastroduodenitis associated with ulcerative colitis. *J Gastroenterol*. 2008;43(3):193–201. PMID: 18373161.

9. Sonnenberg A, Melton SD, Genta RM. Frequent occurrence of gastritis and duodenitis in patients with inflammatory bowel disease. *Inflamm Bowel Dis*. 2011;17(1):39–44. PMID: 20848539.

10. Genta RM, Sonnenberg A. Non-*Helicobacter pylori* gastritis is common among paediatric patients with inflammatory bowel disease. *Aliment Pharmacol Ther*. 2012;35(11):1310–1316. PMID: 22486730.

11. Uchino M, Matsuoka H, Bando T, et al. Clinical features and treatment of ulcerative colitis-related severe gastroduodenitis and enteritis with massive bleeding after colectomy. *Int J Colorectal Dis*. 2014;29(2):239–245. PMID: 24105365.

12. Shen B, Wu H, Remzi F, Lopez R, Shen L, Fazio V. Diagnostic value of esophagogastroduodenoscopy in patients with ileal pouch-anal anastomosis. *Inflamm Bowel Dis*. 2009;15(3):395–401. PMID: 18972552.

13. Hisabe T, Matsui T, Miyaoka M, et al. Diagnosis and clinical course of ulcerative gastroduodenal lesion associated with ulcerative colitis: possible relationship with pouchitis. *Dig Endosc*. 2010;22(4):268–274. PMID: 21175478.

14. Lin J, McKenna BJ, Appelman HD. Morphologic findings in upper gastrointestinal biopsies of patients with ulcerative colitis: a controlled study. *Am J Surg Pathol*. 2010;34(11):1672–1677. PMID: 20962621.

15. Endo K, Kuroha M, Shiga H, et al. Two cases of diffuse duodenitis associated with ulcerative colitis. *Case Rep Gastrointest Med*. 2012;2012:396521. PMID: 23119193. PMCID: PMC3483663.

16. Chiba M, Ono I, Wakamatsu H, Wada I, Suzuki K. Diffuse gastroduodenitis associated with ulcerative colitis: treatment by infliximab. *Dig Endosc*. 2013;25(6):622–625. PMID: 24164601.

17. Uchino M, Ikeuchi H, Bando T, et al. Diffuse gastroduodenitis and enteritis associated with ulcerative colitis and concomitant cytomegalovirus reactivation after total colectomy: report of a case. *Surg Today*. 2013;43(3):321–324. PMID: 22965486.

18. Murrell ZA, Melmed GY, Ippoliti A, et al. A prospective evaluation of the long-term outcome of ileal pouch-anal anastomosis in patients with inflammatory bowel disease-unclassified and indeterminate colitis. *Dis Colon Rectum*. 2009;52(5):872–878. PMID: 19502850.

19. Shen B. Diagnosis and management of postoperative ileal pouch disorders. *Clin Colon Rectal Surg*. 2010;23(4):259–268. PMID: 22131896. PMCID: PMC3134805.

20. Gu J, Stocchi L, Kiran RP, Shen B, Remzi FH. Do clinical characteristics of de novo pouch Crohn's disease after restorative proctocolectomy affect ileal pouch retention? *Dis Colon Rectum*. 2014;57(1):76–82. PMID: 24316949.

PART FOUR

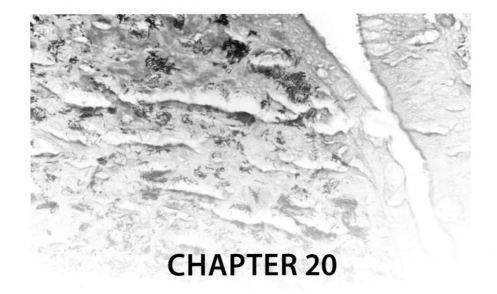

CHAPTER 20

Small-Bowel Infections

Katherine Sun and Shu-Yuan Xiao

INTRODUCTION

Most small-bowel infections that come to the surgical pathologist's attention are from immune-suppressed or immunocompromised patients, often as part of a systemic opportunistic infection. Isolated small-bowel infections in healthy individuals are less common and usually are not biopsied. For example, acute and self-limited virus-induced enteritis is usually diagnosed by serology or stool examinations and rarely requires histologic diagnosis. However, certain parasitic, fungal, or bacterial organisms lead to significant histologic abnormalities and can be encountered in small-bowel specimens. Familiarity with these microscopic features and the ability to identify the underlying etiologic agent are critical for correct diagnosis. Selected infectious disorders are discussed in this chapter.

PARASITES

Protozoal diseases, such as giardiasis, toxoplasmosis, leishmaniasis, and that caused by *Trypanosome cruzi* can cause insidious infections in pet animals and be transmitted to humans.[1,2] Fortunately, infestations in healthy individuals usually pose no immediate risk of symptomatic illness. However, in immunocompromised individuals, infection with these organisms can lead to clinically significant or devastating disorders. Several helminthes, such as *Schistosoma*, are occasionally encountered in small-bowel tissue. Recognition of these infections relies heavily on increased alertness by the

pathologist and knowledge of the morphologic features associated with these organisms.

Giardia lamblia

Giardia lamblia can infect both immunocompetent and immunocompromised patients. The most common place to come across this parasite is the duodenum, but they can be found in other segments of the gastrointestinal tract as well, including the stomach.[3] Of note, patients with celiac disease are more prone to infection. Coinfection of *Giardia* and Whipple disease may occur as well.[4,5]

Histologically, most cases of giardiasis do not show significant abnormality of the mucosa. Some cases can exhibit changes similar to that of an underlying disease, such as celiac disease. Usually, there is no or only minimal inflammatory infiltration. Rarely, nonceliac cases may show mild villous shortening with active inflammation (neutrophilic infiltration). The *Giardia* trophozoites can be found on the luminal surface of the mucosa, ranging from scarce to numerous (usually in immunocompromised hosts). The parasites appear as sickle, new moon, or pear shape, depending on the orientation during sectioning of the specimen (Figure 20-1). In the pear-shaped trophozoites, sometimes two nuclei can be seen, making the organisms look like a stingray (Figure 20-2).

In immunocompromised patients, the clinical background and GI symptoms often lead to a search for an infectious etiology, including stool examination for parasites, and the pathologist may have already been alerted to look

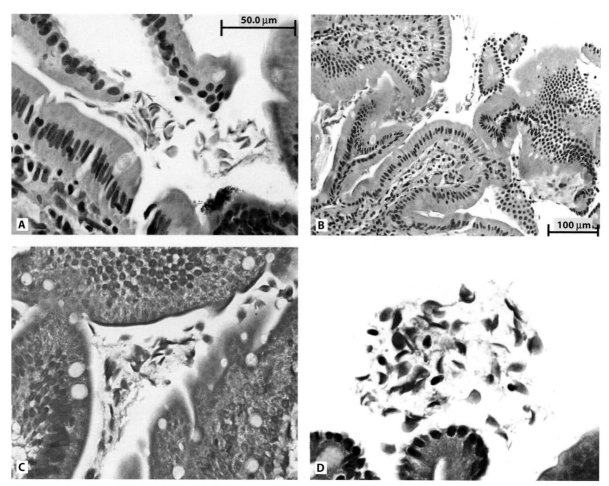

FIGURE 20-1. Duodenal giardiasis in a patient with AIDS and long-standing diarrhea and weight loss. **A** and **B.** Numerous trophozoites are present in the duodenal biopsy H&E stain). **C.** Trophozoites highlighted by PAS stain. **D.** Trophozoites highlighted by trichrome stain.

FIGURE 20-2. Duodenal giardiasis. A partially sectioned pear-shaped trophozoite with two nuclei resembling stingray eyes.

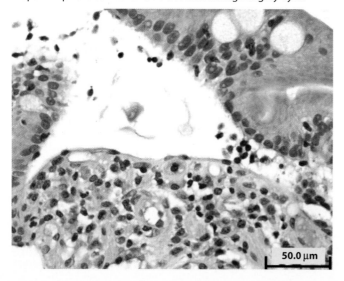

for parasites in the biopsy. Therefore, reaching the correct diagnosis may not pose much of a challenge because the parasites may have already been detected and be numerous and easy to recognize (Figures 20-1 and 20-3). Other tools that can help the pathologist recognize the parasite are several types of special stains. The trophozoites can be made more prominent to visualize by Giemsa or trichrome stain (Figure 20-1D). They also stain positive for CD117 (Figure 20-3B). However, these special studies are seldom necessary in most cases, as discussed previously. On the other hand, in immunocompetent patients the trophozoites can be scarce. Special stains or immunohistochemical stains can be used when there is a high clinical suspicion for *Giardia* and the parasites cannot be identified on routine H&E stained sections. In addition, when the biopsy reveals features that are suggestive of celiac disease in a patient with negative laboratory tests (HLA haplotype, celiac serology, etc.), *Giardia* should always be a part of the differential diagnosis.[6]

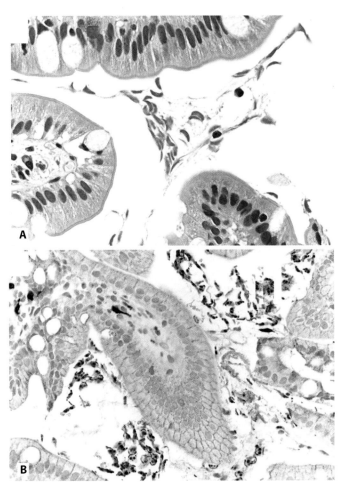

FIGURE 20-3. Another case of duodenal giardiasis, with parasites visible on H&E stain (**A**) and CD117 immunostain (**B**).

Leishmania

A major clinical manifestation of intestinal leishmaniasis is malabsorption. Histologically, the findings include infiltration by parasite-containing macrophages into villi,[7,8] sometimes with mild villous atrophy and mild lymphoplasmacytic infiltration.[7] Granuloma formation may be seen as well. In patients with AIDS, there have been rare coinfections of *Leishmania* and *Mycobacteria avium-intracellulare* (MAI) reported in the same duodenal biopsy.[8,9]

Cryptosporidium

Cryptosporidium parvum is the most common of the cryptosporidia to infect humans. In immunocompetent patients, it causes mild diarrhea, but in patients with AIDS, it causes severe enteritis. Histologic diagnosis in small-bowel biopsies requires the pathologist to carefully search at high magnification. The organisms (sporozoites) can be recognized by the clusters they form at the apical surface of the intestinal epithelium (Figure 20-4). These clusters are occasionally encompassed by a membrane made of the cytoplasm of the epithelial cells in the form of surface "vacuoles." The sporozoites appear small, round, or oval shaped and are basophilic (Figure 20-4B).

In most cases, the background small-bowel mucosa exhibits normal histology. However, rare cases may show mild villous atrophy or active duodenitis (Figure 20-4A).

Cyclospora cayetanensis

Cyclospora cayetanensis most commonly infects the small bowel and causes self-limited watery diarrhea in immunocompetent individuals or prolonged diarrhea in immunocompromised patients that may simulate tropical sprue and may be associated with biliary disease. The sporozoites are ingested with contaminated food or water, and the sporozoites enter the epithelial cells of the small intestine. Endoscopy findings include marked erythema of the small intestinal mucosa. Biopsies of the duodenum and the jejunum reveal villous blunting and atrophy, as well as crypt hyperplasia of varying degrees. On tissue sections, merozoites are 8 to 10 μm in diameter and are normally located within the supranuclear cytoplasm of the enterocytes but can also be seen on the epithelial cell surface (Figures 20-4C and 20-4D). The parasites are round, ovoid, or crescent and are sometimes located in a parasitophorous vacuole. They are acid fast with modified kinyoun and are positive with auramine, but they do not stain with GMS or PAS stain. The round or ovoid form of *Cyclospora* may be confused with *Cryptosporidium*, but *Cyclospora* is much larger (8 to 10 μm vs *Cryptosporidium* at 2 to 5 μm). The crescent-shaped *Cyclospora* is similar in appearance with *Isospora belli*, but *Isospora* is generally larger and stains positive for GMS, PAS, and Giemsa stains.

Strongyloides

Strongyloides stercoralis can infest both immunocompetent and immunocompromised patients. This infection occurs by the larvae of the nematode in the soil entering a human host through the skin. Later, the larvae travel to the lungs through the circulatory system, are coughed up, and then are swallowed. The larvae can invade the mucosa of the jejunum and the duodenum, where they mature into adults. In immunocompetent patients, the infestation may be asymptomatic even though the parasites can be identified in the upper small bowel. However, in immunocompromised patients, a systemic infection may occur, leading to a hyperinfective syndrome with the parasites identified in multiple sites.[10] Infestation of the colon may manifest as eosinophilic granulomatous enterocolitis.[11] Although the diagnosis is usually made by stool examination, the parasite may first be visualized in small-bowel tissue (Figure 20-5). Some prominent features of the parasite larvae are that they contain a tiny buccal capsule and cylindrical esophagus without a posterior bulb, but these features may not be seen in tissue sections.

Schistosomiasis

Worldwide, it is estimated that more than 200 million people are infected with schistosomiasis.[12] Even though this infection is second only to malaria as the most important parasitic

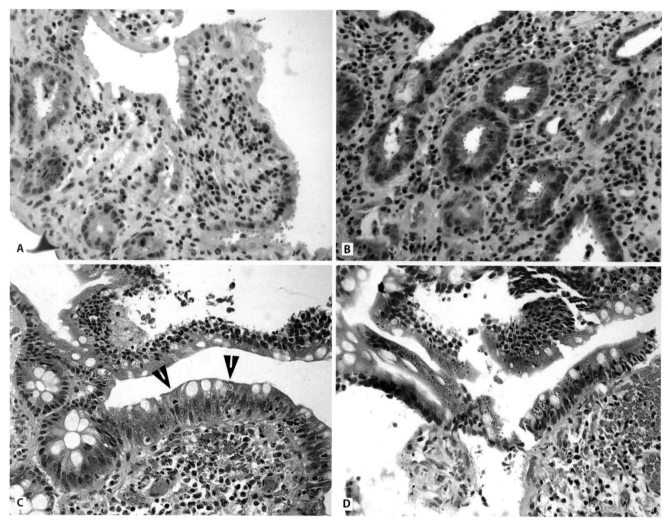

FIGURE 20-4. **A** and **B.** Duodenal cryptosporidiosis. **A.** The duodenal mucosa exhibits focal active inflammation. Numerous sporozoites are attached to the surface of epithelium. **B.** Organisms on the crypt epithelium. **C** and **D.** Duodenal cyclosporiasis. **C.** The parasites in the supranuclear cytoplasm of absorptive cells in a double "banana" shape (arrowheads). **D.** Numerous parasites in the cytoplasm as well as the cell surface.

disease, it is underrecognized, particularly in areas where the parasite is not endemic. The infection occurs by direct contact of skin with contaminated freshwater. There are currently three species that infect humans: *Schistosoma mansoni*, *S. japonicum*, or *S. haematobium*.

Diagnosis is usually made by stool examination for parasite eggs (urine for *S. haematobium*). For the pathologist, histologic changes suggestive of schistosomiasis may be seen with or without parasite eggs in tissue specimens (Figure 20-6). After infestation and maturation in blood vessels, the parasites produce eggs, some of which can be contained in the bowel (Figure 20-6) or bladder wall. Therefore, parasite eggs may be identified in the bowel wall, usually associated with granulomas (Figure 20-6). The presence of eggs combined with an inflammatory response may lead to ulceration or focal polyps. However, it is often the case that the overlying mucosa is normal (Figure 20-6A).

FUNGAL INFECTIONS

Most fungal infections of the small bowel are part of a systemic infection, such as with *Candida*, *Histoplasma*, *Aspergillus*, or *Mucor*. They often occur in the immunocompromised or chronically debilitated patients, particularly *Aspergillus* and *Mucor*. Small-bowel involvement by *Candida* occurs in about 20% of patients with systemic infection, and *Aspergillus* most often occurs in hospitalized patients.

Histoplasmosis

Histoplasma capsulatum usually infects the small bowel, colon, and liver simultaneously, mostly in the immunocompromised. However, in endemic areas, there can be heavy inhalation of spores, and disease can occur in normal individuals as well. This organism induces a mucosal and submucosal granulomatous inflammation that may

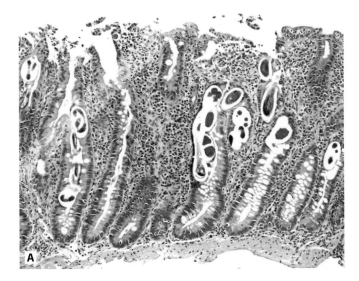

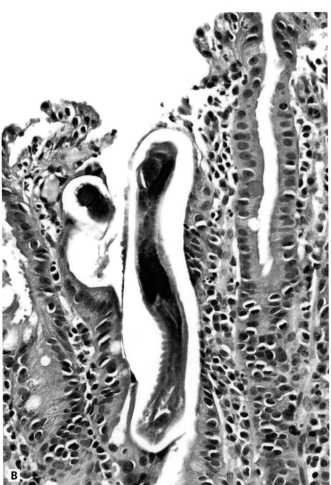

FIGURE 20-5. *Strongyloides* infestation of the small bowel. **A.** Small-bowel mucosa exhibiting total loss of villi and crypt hypertrophy, with many larvae invading the crypts. **B.** Complete longitudinal section of a larva with tiny buccal capsule and cylindrical esophagus.

lead to ulcers, pseudopolyps, or perforation. Milder cases may exhibit accumulation of clusters of macrophages in the lamina propria with a foamy appearance (Figure 20-7) and mild villous shortening, which somewhat resembles the changes seen in Whipple disease (discussed in a separate section that follows). However, cases that are more severe demonstrate well-formed granulomas that may have necrosis and involve both the mucosa and the submucosa. Also, severe cases may be associated with ulceration. The organisms are strongly positive for GMS (Figure 20-7), and they have easily recognizable yeast morphology. The capsule of the organism stains positive for PAS.

Mucormycosis

Mucor infection of the GI tract is rare, with the small bowel the least-frequent site after the stomach and colon. Most infections occur in patients with hematologic malignancies, chemotherapy-induced neutropenia, and steroid use. *Mucor* is characterized by ribbon-like, broad hyphae with irregular, right-angled branching. Small-bowel mucormycosis is rarely associated with perforation.

Other fungal infections, such as aspergillosis and candidiasis, rarely involve the small bowel as part of a systemic opportunistic infection and are not further discussed in this chapter. It suffices to mention that, occasionally, these patients may initially present with small-bowel infarction or perforation. These cases require high alertness by the pathologist to recognize the underlying etiology.

■ BACTERIAL INFECTIONS

Whipple Disease

The rare Whipple disease, although it frequently involves the small bowel, is a systemic infection involving not only other segments of the GI tract and liver but also other systems. These include culture-negative endocarditis, central nervous system infection, joint infection, and so on.[13] Lymphadenopathy occurs in 50% of cases. The disease was first described in 1907 by George Whipple[14] in a fatal case thought to be of an enteropathy related to fat or fatty acid disorders, referred to as "intestinal lipodystrophy." The infectious nature of the disease was recognized in the 1960s when bacterial forms were identified by electron microscopy[15,16] that stained positive by diastase-resistant periodic acid–Schiff staining (dPAS). Study of the r16 RNA species confirmed the organism is a new bacterial species related to the actinomycete branch (gram-positive bacilli)[17,18] and is termed *Tropheryma whipplei*. Culture of the bacteria has only recently become successful. The infection is only seen in humans, but a specific host risk factor for infection has not yet been identified.[19] The most important job for the pathologist is to recognize the disease because treatment with antibiotics is effective, but without them the clinical course is often fatal.

Symptoms associated with GI infection include abdominal pain, malabsorption syndrome with diarrhea,

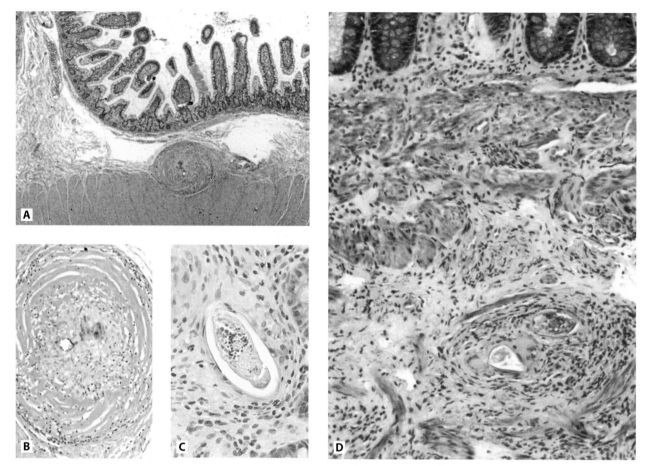

FIGURE 20-6. Schistosomiasis. **A.** "Egg granuloma" in the submucosa, with the overlying normal small-bowel mucosa. **B.** Granuloma surrounding an egg with lateral spine, characteristic of *Schistosoma mansoni*. **C.** An egg in the lamina propria. **D.** Eggs in tissue sections highlighted by Mason trichrome stain.

and weight loss. The changes associated with the disease are mostly seen in the jejunum and ileum and less frequently in the duodenum. Endoscopically, the affected mucosa exhibits coarse granularity, often with yellow-white discolorization or plaques. Histologically, the small-bowel biopsy is characterized by lamina propria infiltration with densely arranged clusters of foamy cells (Figure 20-8). Depending on the amount of bacterial infiltration, there may be varying degrees of villous blunting (Figure 20-9). There is usually no significant inflammatory cellular infiltration, and with effective treatment, the villous architecture returns to normal with marked reduction in the amount of organisms present (Figure 20-9D).

The main differential diagnosis with infiltration by foamy macrophages is MAI. Both organisms stain positive with dPAS stain; however, the latter is also positive for the acid-fast stain (Figure 20-10). An immunostain for *T. whipplei* antigen is also available and has been found to be specific[20,21] (interestingly, this allowed the confirmation of the first case described by Dr. Whipple[21]). Although the organism can be cultured, it can only be done in a few research laboratories and takes several weeks to yield a result; therefore, culture is not considered to be diagnostically appropriate.

Mycobacteria avium-intracellulare

Mycobacteria avium-intracellulare causes disease almost exclusively in patients with AIDS. Fortunately, because of the progress in treatment of HIV infection, MAI infection has become much less common. Histologically, small-bowel lesions closely resemble those of Whipple disease (discussed previously) with organism-filled foamy macrophages expanding the lamina propria of the mucosa and villi. However, as mentioned, MAI demonstrates diffuse and strong positivity with acid-fast staining (Figure 20-10), whereas Whipple bacilli are negative. Another histologic feature that can differentiate the two organisms is that scattered fat droplets may be mixed with foamy macrophages in Whipple disease but is never seen in MAI.

Tuberculosis

There has been a noticeable increase in tuberculosis (TB) prevalence worldwide in the last 2 decades, including the emergence

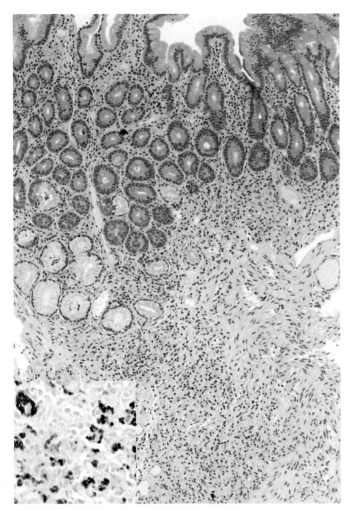

FIGURE 20-7. Histoplasmosis. Small-bowel mucosa and submucosa are infiltrated by clusters of foamy histiocytes. Grocott methenamine silver (GMS) stain highlights numerous yeast forms of the fungus (insert).

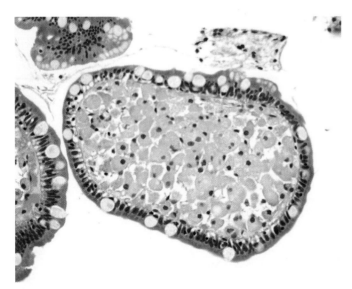

FIGURE 20-8. Whipple disease. Villi filled with large foamy macrophages in lamina propria.

of multidrug-resistant strains. In contrast to MAI, TB can cause severe enterocolitis with various complications and pose a great challenge to treatment. Like Crohn disease, the ileocecal region is most frequently affected, with chronic inflammation and tissue response forming tubercles, which often lead to ulceration. Histologically, the lesions are characterized by mucosal and submucosal epithelioid and giant cell granulomas, which often have caseating necrosis (Figure 20-11). There may be mucosal ulceration, perforation, obstruction, or fistula formation, similar to Crohn disease. In a series looking at nontraumatic small-bowel perforations, about 30% of cases were found to be due to TB.[22] The differential diagnoses include Crohn disease (discussed in Chapter 4), Behçet disease (BD), fungal enteritis (discussed previously), *Yersinia* infection, and other infections. The key to reaching the correct diagnosis relies on a high level of suspicion for the disease and a battery of ancillary tests, such as an acid-fast stain, culture, or a polymerase chain reaction for the detection of the organism.

There are other histologic features that may be of help with differential diagnoses. In TB, the epithelioid granulomas tend to be multiple and larger, frequently have caseating necrosis, and are often associated with mucosal ulceration. The background mucosa usually lacks chronic changes, such as villous or crypt architectural distortion, and the background inflammation is usually minimal or mild. In contrast, in Crohn disease, granulomas are small or inconspicuous (clusters of epithelioid histiocytes) and non-necrotizing, and there is multifocal mucosal inflammation.[23]

Bacterial Overgrowth

Bacterial overgrowth in the small bowel may be related to slowed "clearing" of organisms. This can be caused by achlorhydria, a blind loop or adhesions related to prior surgery, or other types of bowel obstruction. In addition, immunodeficiency, motility disorders (amyloidosis), ischemia, and small-bowel bypass can contribute to increased bacterial infection.[24] Understandably, a damaged mucosal barrier makes it more "vulnerable" to bacterial colonization (in drug-, toxin-, or radiation-induced injury, eg). Bacterial overgrowth may be a cause for malabsorption.[25]

Histologic findings in most mild cases consist of normal villous architecture without significant inflammation. Some cases may exhibit mild villous atrophy with increased lymphocytic infiltration and epithelial reactive changes. Patchy crypt hyperplasia may also be seen. Occasionally, bacterial colonies can be visualized with careful scrutiny at higher magnification.

■ VIRAL INFECTIONS

Many types of viral infections cause acute gastroenteritis. Most can be diagnosed by serology, stool antigen examination using enzyme-linked immunosorbent assay (ELISA or enzyme immunoassay [EIA]), or electron microscopy and seldom require a biopsy for histologic examination.

PART FOUR

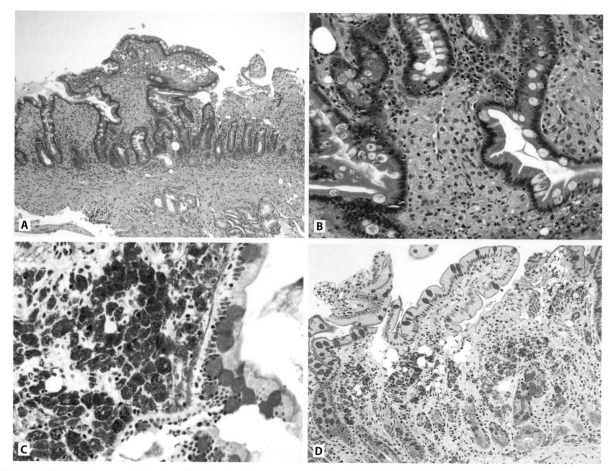

FIGURE 20-9. Whipple disease. **A.** Duodenal biopsy with partial villous blunting and lamina propria expansion by macrophage with pale "foamy" cytoplasm. There is no significant inflammatory infiltration. **B.** The macrophages are tightly "packed." **C.** Diastase-resistant periodic acid–Schiff (dPAS) stain, highlighting densely arranged organisms. **D.** dPAS stain of rebiopsy after antibiotic treatment showing recovery of normal villous architecture. Residual macrophages contain a reduced number of PAS-positive organisms.

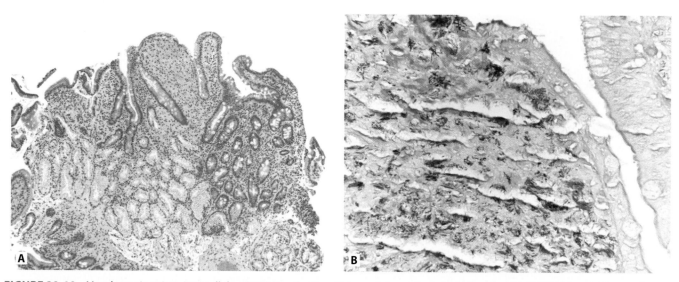

FIGURE 20-10. *Mycobacteria avium-intracellulare* (MAI) in a duodenal biopsy from a 28-year-old female with HIV/AIDS and CD4 T-cell count of 17. Endoscopically, there was diffuse mottling in the duodenum. **A.** Foci of foamy macrophage infiltration is evident. **B.** Acid-fast stain highlights the bacilli of MAI.

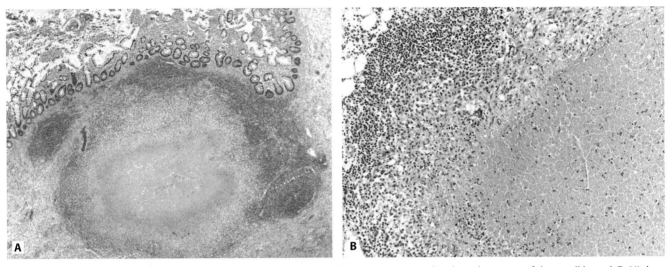

FIGURE 20-11. Small-bowel tuberculosis. **A.** Multiple caseating granulomas are scattered in the submucosa of the small bowel. **B.** Higher-power view showing extensive central necrosis surrounded by a rim of epithelioid histiocytes.

However, with increased use of therapies that reduce host immunity, cases of small-bowel injury due to viruses may be encountered in the biopsy and, rarely, resected specimens.

Adenovirus

Adenoviral gastroenteritis mostly occurs in children (enteric adenovirus) and seldom comes to the pathologist's attention unless prominent lymphoid hyperplasia of the ileum leads to an intussusception. The virus also causes problems in patients with immunosuppression, such as those with stem cell transplantation or solid-organ transplantation (discussed in Chapter 2). The histologic changes may include a nonspecific inflammatory infiltration, sometimes with epithelial injury. Careful examination may reveal cytopathic changes in the form of dark-purple smudged nuclei (Figure 20-12) or intranuclear inclusion bodies with an inconspicuous clear halo. Immunostain is fairly sensitive and specific (Figure 20-12D), but in situ hybridization is also used in some laboratories.

Cytomegalovirus

For small-bowel cytomegalovirus (CMV) infection, the clinical setting is usually immunosuppression, such as in HIV infection or in transplant recipients. Histologically, the infection can be associated with minimal mucosal changes or marked acute inflammation, erosion, or ulceration (Figure 20-13) with various forms of viral cytopathic changes (inclusions). An immunohistochemical stain can be used to help identify the viral inclusions or for confirmation of the presence of the virus (Figure 20-14).

■ SUMMARY

Most of the disorders discussed in this chapter represent small-bowel involvement as part of a systemic infection. With appropriate clinical and laboratory information, the diagnosis is usually that of confirmation and may be straightforward in many patients. Occasionally, clinical laboratory information may not be readily available and the disorder not clinically suspected. In such instances, discovering an infectious etiology from a small-bowel biopsy offers critical guidance to clinical management. Familiarity with the different histologic patterns and the selected use of special and immunohistochemical stains is essential for the recognition of these infectious agents.

■ REFERENCES

1. Himsworth CG, Skinner S, Chaban B, et al. Multiple zoonotic pathogens identified in canine feces collected from a remote Canadian indigenous community. *Am J Trop Med Hyg.* 2010;83(2):338–341. PMID: 20682878. PMCID: 2911181.

2. Esch KJ, Petersen CA. Transmission and epidemiology of zoonotic protozoal diseases of companion animals. *Clin Microbiol Rev.* 2013;26(1):58–85. PMID: 23297259. PMCID: 3553666.

3. Doglioni C, De Boni M, Cielo R, et al. Gastric giardiasis. *J Clin Pathol.* 1992;45(11):964–967. PMID: 1452790. PMCID: 495025.

4. Bassotti G, Pelli MA, Ribacchi R, et al. *Giardia lamblia* infestation reveals underlying Whipple's disease in a patient with longstanding constipation. *Am J Gastroenterol.* 1991;86(3):371–374. PMID: 1705390.

5. Fenollar F, Lepidi H, Gerolami R, Drancourt M, Raoult D. Whipple disease associated with giardiasis. *J Infect Dis.* 2003;188(6):828–834. PMID: 12964113.

6. DeGaetani M, Tennyson CA, Lebwohl B, et al. Villous atrophy and negative celiac serology: a diagnostic and therapeutic dilemma. *Am J Gastroenterol.* 2013;108(5):647–653. PMID: 23644957.

7. Muigai R, Gatei DG, Shaunak S, Wozniak A, Bryceson AD. Jejunal function and pathology in visceral leishmaniasis. *Lancet.* 1983;2(8348):476–479. PMID: 6136644.

8. Wang J, Vanley C, Miyamoto E, Turner JA, Peng SK. Coinfection of visceral leishmaniasis and *Mycobacterium* in a patient with acquired immunodeficiency syndrome. *Arch Pathol Lab Med.* 1999;123(9):835–837. PMID: 10458835.

9. Velasco M, Flores L, Guijarro-Rojas M, Roca V. Simultaneous intestinal leishmaniasis and mycobacterial involvement in a patient with acquired immune deficiency syndrome. *J Clin Gastroenterol.* 1998;27(3):271–273. PMID: 9802464.

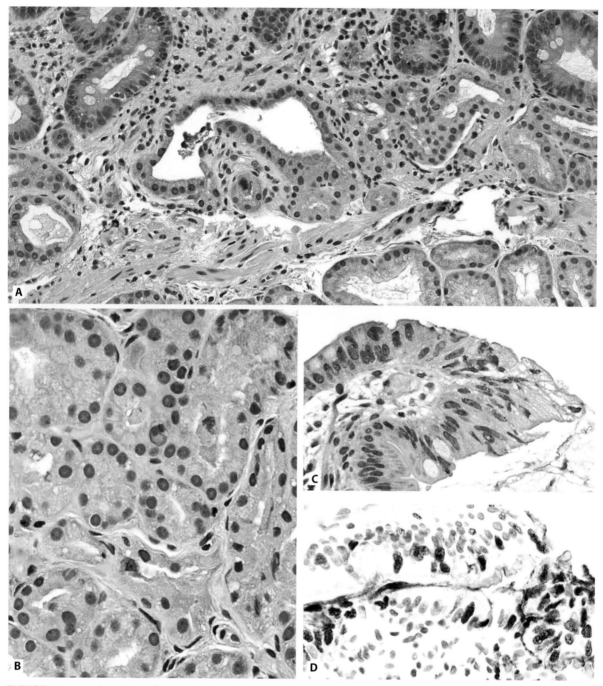

FIGURE 20-12. Adenovirus infection in the duodenum of a patient with a stem cell transplant. There is mild duodenitis. Irregular "smudged" nuclei are found in epithelial cells (**A**), Brunner glands (**B**), and villi (**C**). Immunostaining for adenovirus confirmed the findings (**D**).

10. Haque AK, Schnadig V, Rubin SA, Smith JH. Pathogenesis of human strongyloidiasis: autopsy and quantitative parasitological analysis. *Mod Pathol.* 1994;7(3):276–288. PMID: 8058699.

11. Gutierrez Y, Bhatia P, Garbadawala ST, Dobson JR, Wallace TM, Carey TE. *Strongyloides stercoralis* eosinophilic granulomatous enterocolitis. *Am J Surg Pathol.* 1996;20(5):603–612. PMID: 8619425.

12. Centers for Disease Control and Prevention (CDC). Parasites—schistosomiasis. http://www.cdc.gov/parasites/schistosomiasis/. Updated November 7, 2012.

13. Bayless TM, Knox DL. Whipple's disease: a multisystem infection. *N Engl J Med.* 1979;300(16):920–921. PMID: 85261.

14. Whipple GH. A hitherto undescribed disease characterized anatomically by deposits of fat and fatty acids in the intestinal and mesenteric lymphatic tissues. *Bull Johns Hopkins Hosp.* 1907;18:382–391.

15. Yardley J, Hendrix T. Combined electron and light microscopy in Whipple's disease. *Bull Johns Hopkins Hosp.* 1961;109:80–98.

16. Kent TH, Layton JM, Clifton JA, Schedl HP. Whipple's disease: light and electron microscopic studies combined with clinical studies suggesting an infective nature. *Lab Investig.* 1963;12:1163–1178. PMID: 14098348.

17. Wilson KH, Blitchington R, Frothingham R, Wilson JA. Phylogeny of the Whipple's-disease-associated bacterium. *Lancet.* 1991;338(8765):474–475. PMID: 1714530.

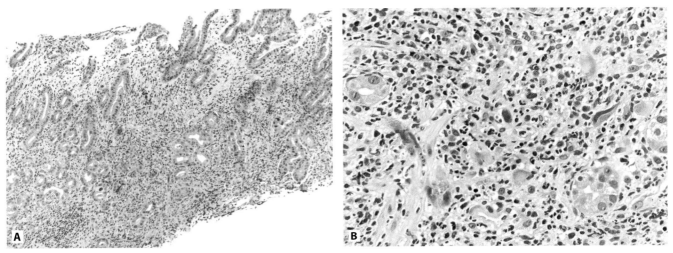

FIGURE 20-13. Cytomegalovirus (CMV) duodenitis in a patient with Hodgkin lymphoma. **A.** Diffuse peptic-type duodenitis with erosion. **B.** Many viral inclusion bodies are present in both epithelial and mesenchymal cells.

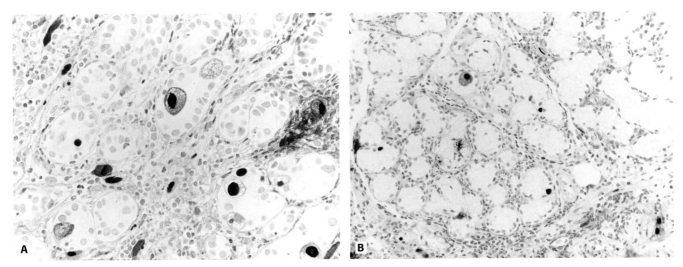

FIGURE 20-14. Immunostain for CMV in the case in Figure 20-13. **A.** Predominantly nuclear staining in epithelial and in mesenchymal cells, with slight cytoplasmic staining or "spillover." **B.** Positive staining in some Brunner gland epithelia that were not evident in section stained with hematoxylin and eosin (H&E).

PART FOUR

18. Relman DA, Schmidt TM, MacDermott RP, Falkow S. Identification of the uncultured bacillus of Whipple's disease. *N Engl J Med*. 1992;327(5):293–301. PMID: 1377787.

19. Keren DF. Whipple's disease: a review emphasizing immunology and microbiology. *Crit Rev Clin Lab Sci*. 1981;14(2):75–108. PMID: 6165517.

20. Lepidi H, Fenollar F, Gerolami R, et al. Whipple's disease: immunospecific and quantitative immunohistochemical study of intestinal biopsy specimens. *Hum Pathol*. 2003;34(6):589–596. PMID: 12827613.

21. Dumler JS, Baisden BL, Yardley JH, Raoult D. Immunodetection of *Tropheryma whipplei* in intestinal tissues from Dr. Whipple's 1907 patient. *N Engl J Med*. 2003;348(14):1411–1412. PMID: 12672878.

22. Nadkarni KM, Shetty SD, Kagzi RS, Pinto AC, Bhalerao RA. Small-bowel perforations. A study of 32 cases. *Arch Surg*. 1981;116(1):53–57. PMID: 7469733.

23. Pulimood AB, Ramakrishna BS, Kurian G, et al. Endoscopic mucosal biopsies are useful in distinguishing granulomatous colitis due to Crohn's disease from tuberculosis. *Gut*. 1999;45(4):537–541. PMID: 10486361. PMCID: 1727684.

24. Passaro E Jr, Drenick E, Wilson SE. Bypass enteritis. A new complication of jejunoileal bypass for obesity. *Am J Surg*. 1976;131(2):169–174. PMID: 1251958.

25. Owens SR, Greenson JK. The pathology of malabsorption: current concepts. *Histopathology*. 2007;50(1):64–82. PMID: 17204022.

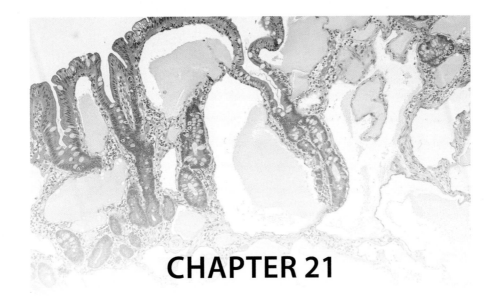

CHAPTER 21

Small-Bowel Polyps and Nodules

Deborah A. Giusto and Shu-Yuan Xiao

■ INTRODUCTION

Several categories of disorders, including neoplastic, hamartomatous, and inflammatory, manifest as polyps or nodules in the small bowel. Most of these polyps are encountered in the duodenum, although lesions located in other portions of the small bowel are increasingly biopsied or resected with advances in enteroscopic technology.

With improved endoscopic ultrasound (EUS) and other imaging techniques, the localization of a lesion to a specific layer of the bowel wall can be accurately achieved in most cases. Knowing which layer a lesion arises from (ie, intramucosal, submucosal, or intramural) is helpful in narrowing down the differential diagnosis (Table 21-1). For example, polyps and nodules that involve the surface epithelium usually include nodular peptic injury, small-bowel or duodenal adenomas, and other syndromic polyps. These clinically significant lesions often exhibit histologic features that are familiar to most pathologists and do not pose diagnostic difficulty. Less-common lesions, mostly arising in the submucosa, may only have subtle changes in superficial biopsies and thus are more difficult to recognize microscopically. Although many of these lesions are benign, a few of them may be misdiagnosed due to associated reactive changes in the surface epithelium. Therefore, it is important to be familiar with the seemingly "insignificant" or "miscellaneous" lesions of the small bowel to provide an accurate diagnosis without unnecessary repeated biopsies.

In this chapter, polyps caused by proliferations of the surface and glandular epithelium are discussed, as are benign mesenchymal lesions, which often present as polypoid lesions endoscopically. Neuroendocrine tumors are also often included in mucosal biopsies, but these lesions seldom cause difficulty diagnostically (they are discussed in Chapter 23).

■ GASTRIC FOVEOLAR METAPLASIA

Biopsies from the duodenal bulb that are described as a "raised" mucosal abnormality, nodule, or polyp may represent one of a variety of underlying pathologic processes. The most common of these is peptic injury. This process is characterized by surface gastric foveolar metaplasia with prominent Brunner glands (BGs) (Figure 21-1). There may be active inflammatory cellular infiltration (mostly consisting of neutrophils), causing peptic duodenitis (Figure 21-2), with or without erosions or ulcerations. The term *peptic injury* is generic and histologic features are nonspecific, with the underlying etiology ranging from infection to chemical (eg, nonsteroidal anti-inflammatory drugs [NSAIDs]). The mucosa overlying a mass often exhibits changes resembling peptic injury. Not infrequently, there may be marked reactive atypia in the epithelium, which should not be mistaken for adenomatous change (Figure 21-3).

TABLE 21-1. Small-bowel polyps or nodules.

Polyps or lesions with epithelial dysplasia

    Duodenal adenoma

    Ampullary adenoma

Other epithelial polyps

    Hyperplastic polyp

    Inflammatory polyp

    Sessile serrated polyp

    Hamartomatous polyp

Polyp or nodules with prominent Brunner glands

    Brunner gland hyperplasia

    Brunner gland adenoma

    Brunner gland hamartoma

    Brunner gland duct cyst

    Brunner gland duct adenoma

Other polyps or nodules with glandular component

    Gastric gland heterotopia

    Ectopic pancreas rest

    Endometriosis

    Neuroendocrine tumor (carcinoid tumor) (Chapter 23)

Polyps with lamina propria "empty spaces"

    Lymphangiectasia

    Lymphangioma

    Lymphangiomatosis

    Pseudolipomatosis

Submucosal mesenchymal nodule or mass

    Inflammatory fibroid polyp (Chapter 23)

    Lipoma

    Adenomyoma or groove pancreatitis

    Leiomyoma (Chapter 23)

    Gastrointestinal stromal tumor (Chapter 23)

    Neurofibroma (Chapter 23)

    Gangliocytic paraganglioma (Chapter 23)

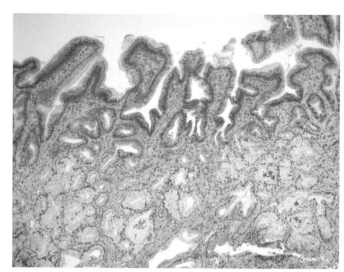

FIGURE 21-1. Peptic injury. Foveolar metaplasia with prominent Brunner glands.

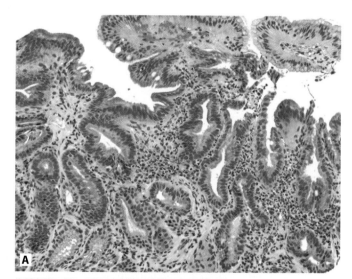

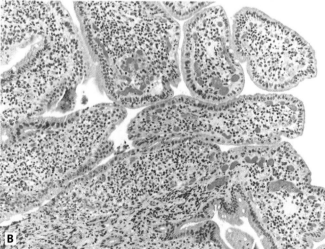

FIGURE 21-2. Peptic duodenitis. Foveolar metaplasia with neutrophilic infiltration, predominantly in the lamina propria (**A**) or in the epithelium (**B**).

GASTRIC GLAND HETEROTOPIA

A biopsy of a nodule or polyp may show seemingly normal gastric fundic glands, often covered by foveolar epithelium. This finding can sometimes raise the question of whether the specimen represents a mislabeled gastric biopsy. However, careful examination will always lead to the identification of scarce intestinal epithelium or goblet cells. In addition, the tightly packed glands often assume a lobular or nodular configuration rather than the straight tubular configuration of normal fundic glands (Figure 21-4). With proper endoscopic correlation, the diagnosis of gastric fundic gland heterotopia

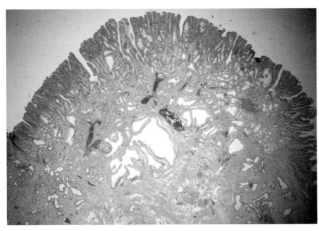

FIGURE 21-3. Mucosa overlying an adenomyoma exhibiting marked reactive atypia. The initial biopsy was overdiagnosed as a duodenal adenoma.

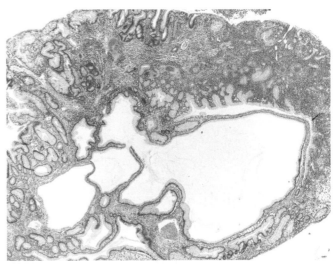

FIGURE 21-5. Duodenal pyloric gland adenoma from a large duodenal polyp from a 70-year-old female patient. The normal intestinal mucosa is replaced by gastric-type mucosa with mucous-type glands, with dilation, and inflammatory infiltration in lamina propria.

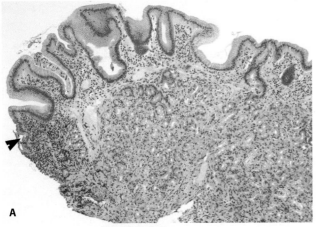

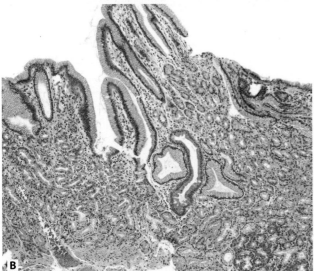

FIGURE 21-4. Gastric fundic gland heterotopia. **A.** Duodenal bulb nodule, with mostly lobular fundic-type glands. The surface is largely replaced by foveolar epithelium, with rare residual goblet cells (arrowhead). **B.** Another example of fundic gland heterotopia with a focus of pancreatic acinar metaplasia (lower right corner).

is usually not problematic. Rarely, the glandular component is more mucinous in nature, or there are other minor components, such as pancreatic acinar metaplasia (Figure 21-4B).

■ PYLORIC GLAND ADENOMA

Pyloric gland adenomas (PGAs) outside the stomach are most common in the gallbladder but can also be seen in many other locations, including the small bowel.[1] PGAs from all locations exhibit similar microscopic appearance, consisting of proliferating mucous glands of pylorus type (Figure 21-5).[1-4] Despite the name, most of these tumors have nothing to do with gastric mucosa, either native or metaplastic, other than the fact that this type of gland is most prominent in the normal antrum or pylorus. Rarely, PGAs may occur in gastric gland heterotopia (Figure 21-5). The pathogenesis of PGAs in extragastric sites is unknown. However, it is not uncommon to see pyloric gland metaplasia in these locations (gallbladder, small bowel, and colon) in response to chronic inflammatory injury.

■ HYPERPLASTIC AND INFLAMMATORY POLYPS

Hyperplastic polyps are rare in the small bowel. Contributing to this "rarity" is the reluctance of the pathologist to make such a diagnosis and the use of a descriptive diagnosis instead. For example, we do occasionally see small-bowel polyps exhibiting glandular hypertrophy with serrated configuration, similar to colonic hyperplastic polyps (Figure 21-6). Some of these polyps may contain thin strands of smooth muscle, resembling a Peutz-Jeghers polyp but in a patient unlikely to have the syndrome (older age, no previous history, isolated polyp).

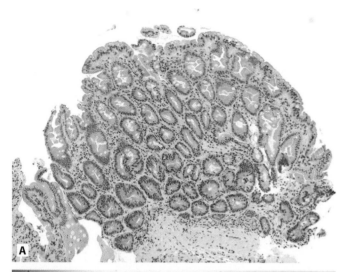

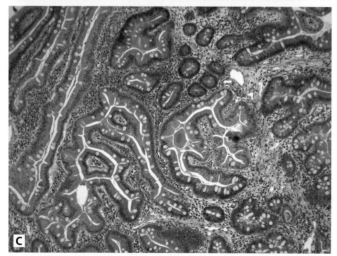

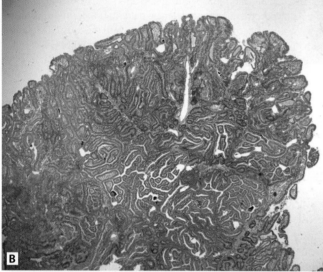

FIGURE 21-6. Small-bowel hyperplastic polyps. **A.** A polypoid lesion with focal serrated configuration toward the surface. **B.** Another polyp with rather complex hypertrophy of glands. **C.** There are focal serration and mild villous attenuation at the surface.

Some pathologists may choose the term *hamartomatous-like polyp* instead of calling it a hyperplastic polyp.

Hyperplastic polyps can occur in any portion of the small bowel. Microscopically, they are characterized by a proliferation of normal small-bowel crypts with or without attenuation of surface villous architecture (Figure 21-6B). The glands are different from normal small-bowel crypts, which are short and inconspicuous. Some pathologists also use the term *inflammatory polyp* to describe these polyps. However, true inflammatory polyps should not exhibit prominent glandular proliferation and instead are characterized by changes in the normal mucosal architecture accompanied by various degrees of inflammatory cellular infiltration. Occasionally, the surface erosion leads to a prominent stromal reaction, including capillary proliferation, which resembles a pyogenic granuloma (Figure 21-7A). In the small bowel, inflammatory polyps usually occur in the setting of Crohn disease (discussed in Chapter 4). Occasionally, they occur in a segment of ileum adjacent to an ileostomy stoma in patients without Crohn disease (Figure 21-7A).

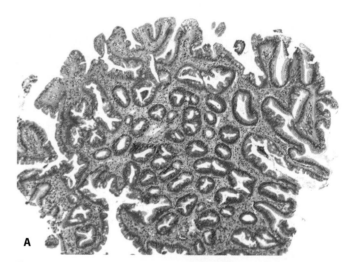

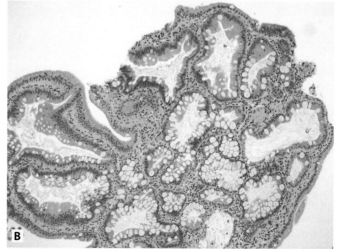

FIGURE 21-7. **A.** Inflammatory polyp occurring adjacent to an ileostomy stoma. **B.** Duodenal polyp with prominent serration.

Understandably, due to the rarity of small-bowel hyperplastic polyps, it is not clear if the term *serrated polyp*, due to the obvious serration of the glands, is a better fit for them (Figure 21-7B). Rare reports describe *K-ras* or *BRAF* mutations in some of these polyps.[5]

PEUTZ-JEGHERS POLYP

The hamartomatous polyps of Peutz-Jeghers syndrome occur most commonly in the jejunum and ileum, distinguishing them from components of other polyposis syndromes. Histologically, the small-intestinal polyps are distinctive in that they have relatively normal small-bowel epithelium and lamina propria overlying a complex, arborizing smooth muscle framework arising from the muscularis mucosa (Figure 21-8).

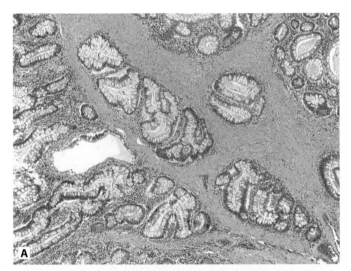

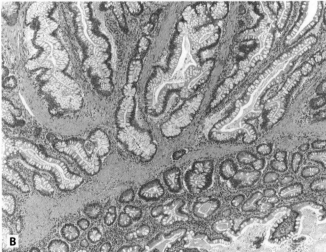

FIGURE 21-8. Small-bowel Peutz-Jeghers polyp. **A.** Toward the base of the polyp, it is evident that the mucosa, along with the thickened muscularis mucosa, proliferates and "branches" out. **B.** More delicate muscle strands are evident in the more superficial zone of the proliferating glands.

SMALL-BOWEL ADENOMAS

Small-bowel adenomas, the precursor to small-bowel adenocarcinomas, can be either polypoid (Figure 21-9A) or sessile (Figure 21-9B). The microscopic architecture can be described in the same way as colorectal adenomas: tubular, villous, or tubulovillous. However, owing to the native villous architecture of the small-bowel mucosa and the fact that a villous designation in small-bowel adenomas is not associated with a more aggressive outcome,[6] we prefer to simply refer to these lesions as adenomas without further architectural designation.

The cells lining the surface and glands in adenomatous lesions have varying degrees of dysplasia, which are designated as either low or high grade. In low-grade dysplasia, the lining cells are pseudostratified, columnar, and mucin depleted with elongated, hyperchromatic, so-called pencil-shaped nuclei (Figure 21-10). High-grade dysplasia is characterized by a pleomorphic population of cells with enlarged, round, irregular nuclei and more severe loss in polarity (Figure 21-11).

In addition to macroscopic polyps, microscopic adenomas of grossly unremarkable mucosa are common in familial adenomatous polyposis (FAP).[7] It is not uncommon for small-bowel adenomas to have endocrine cells or Paneth cells intermixed, particularly in patients with FAP (Figure 21-10B), which is possibly related to a defect in stem cell regulation.[7] Their presence near the surface may be useful in differentiating reactive changes from neoplasia. Interestingly, increased Paneth cells have also been described in a proportion of colonic adenomas.[8] There is insufficient data in the literature to determine if the degree of dysplasia in small-bowel adenomas carries any prognostic significance; however, a number of studies on colorectal adenomas have demonstrated that high-grade dysplasia is not independently associated with increased risk of future advanced adenomas or carcinoma.[9-11] For this reason, in our practice, the degree of dysplasia is not included in the diagnosis of colorectal or small-bowel adenomas.

In patients with FAP, adenomas can also occur in the ampulla, where they exhibit histologic features identical to those seen in the duodenum (Figure 21-12).

BRUNNER GLAND ADENOMA, HYPERPLASIA, AND HAMARTOMA

The Brunner gland (BG) adenoma, hyperplasia, and hamartoma lesions are usually small polyps incidentally identified in the duodenum, which are then biopsied or removed by endoscopic mucosal resection. Rarely, a very large lesion requires surgical resection.

Both BG adenoma (Figure 21-13) and hyperplasia (Figure 21-14) consist of prominent BGs. However, beyond this there are no widely agreed-on criteria regarding the distinction between these two entities. Some pathologists use these two terms interchangeably. Therefore, the biopsy

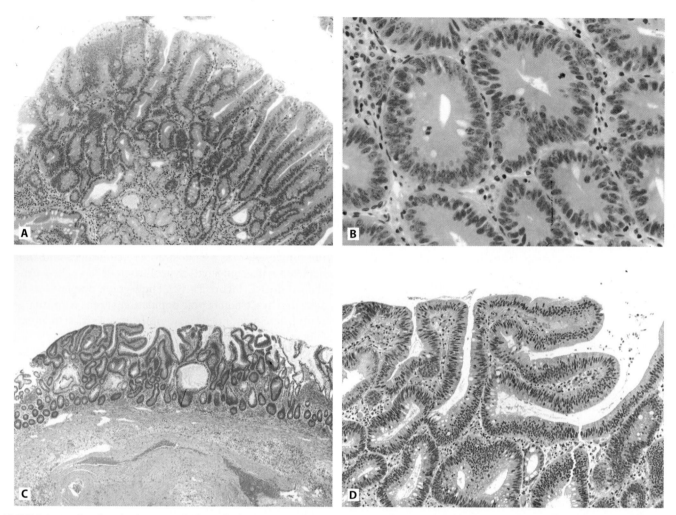

FIGURE 21-9. Duodenal adenomas. **A.** Typical adenomatous change involving the partially transformed villi and crypts. **B.** High-power view illustrating nuclear enlargement and hyperchromasia involving the basal aspect of the epithelium (low-grade dysplasia). **C.** A sessile (flat) adenoma arising in the terminal ileum in a field of previous radiation therapy. The mucosa is focally thickened due to proliferation of adenomatous glands and villi. **D.** The cells are characterized by overlapping, elongated nuclei.

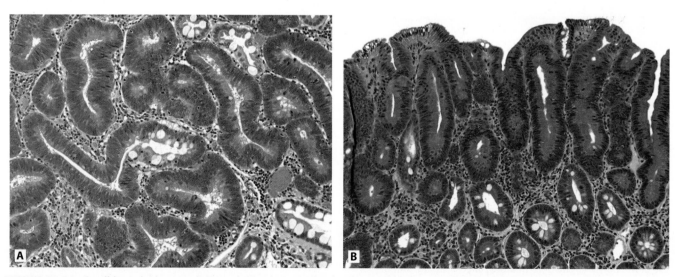

FIGURE 21-10. Small-bowel adenoma, low-grade dysplasia. **A.** The dysplastic epithelium shows pseudostratified, elongated nuclei and mucin depletion. **B.** Duodenal adenoma in familial adenomatous polyposis syndrome. There is low-grade dysplasia with increased inter-mixed Paneth cells.

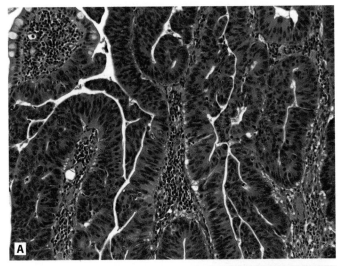

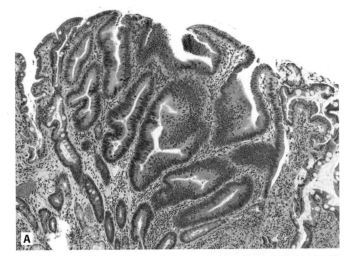

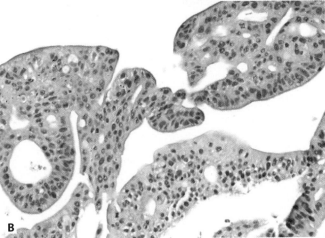

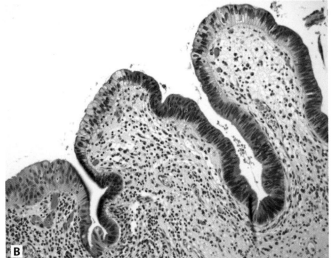

PART FOUR

FIGURE 21-11. Small-bowel adenoma, high-grade dysplasia.
A. Compared to low-grade dysplasia, an adenoma with high-grade dysplasia has more complex architecture with epithelial infolding and cribriform appearance. There is greater loss of polarity with near-complete mucin depletion. The nuclei have increased atypia.
B. High-grade dysplasia of the pancreatobiliary type is seen arising from the ampulla.

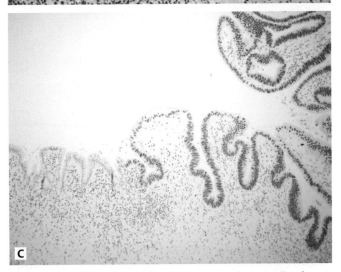

diagnosis is usually "duodenal mucosa with prominent Brunner glands" without further characterization.

Morphologically, in BG adenoma, the mass should assume an expanding or pushing growth pattern with a relatively clear demarcation from the surrounding normal tissue (Figure 21-13). In contrast, BG hyperplasia is characterized by haphazardly arranged gland lobules (Figure 21-14). With this understanding, only rare cases can be diagnosed as BG adenomas, and the diagnosis should only be rendered in polypectomy or surgical section specimens in which the border between the lesion and normal tissue can be fully evaluated.

The BG hamartoma (Figure 21-15) is characterized by a local mass lesion consisting of heterogeneous normal components of the BG and other submucosal tissue, such as fat and fibrovascular tissues. This lesion is usually not confused with a BG adenoma or hyperplasia.

FIGURE 21-12. Duodenal adenoma arising in the ampulla of Vater. **A.** Adenomatous change (low-grade dysplasia) is seen in a background of small-bowel–type epithelium. **B.** Another example showing an intestinal-type adenoma occurring in the background of pancreatobiliary epithelium of the ampulla. **C.** An immunostain for CDX2 confirmed the phenotypic difference.

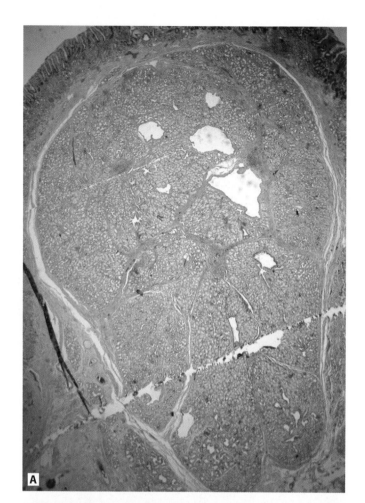

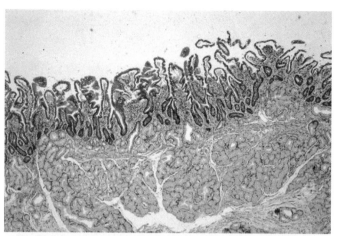

FIGURE 21-14. Brunner gland hyperplasia. This was a biopsy targeting a mucosal nodule, which showed prominent Brunner glands overlined by essentially normal mucosa.

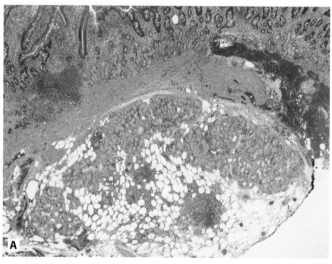

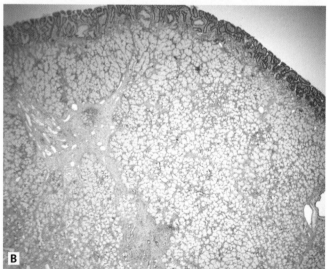

FIGURE 21-13. Brunner gland adenoma. **A.** A well-circumscribed nodule of normal-appearing Brunner glands is seen in solid lobular configuration. **B.** A larger mass resected surgically and examined in frozen section shows a solid arrangement of benign Brunner glands with the overlying mucosa stretched flat.

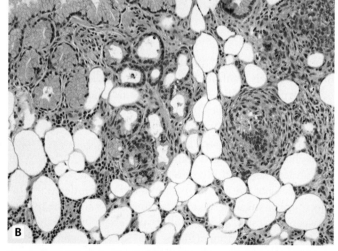

FIGURE 21-15. Brunner gland hamartoma. **A.** This submucosal lesion consists of a mixture of Brunner glands, blood vessels, and adipose tissue in a well-circumscribed pattern. **B.** There is also focal periductal inflammatory infiltration.

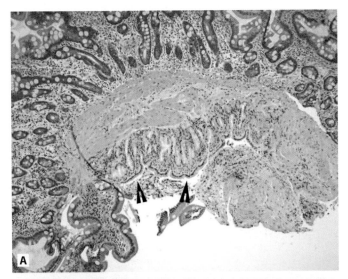

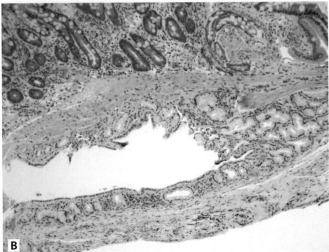

FIGURE 21-16. Brunner gland duct cyst in a biopsy of a raised lesion in the duodenum. **A.** In initial sections, the submucosal Brunner glands appeared unremarkable. However, there is continuous epithelial lining along the base of the cluster of glands (arrowheads). **B.** Deeper sections clearly demonstrate a cystically dilated duct.

BRUNNER GLAND DUCT CYST AND BRUNNER GLAND DUCT ADENOMA

Another polyploid lesion that may be encountered in biopsy or endoscopic mucosal resection consists of BGs with a cystically dilated duct (Figure 21-16). Occasionally, in larger lesions, intraductal papillary growth may be present, exhibiting a gastric epithelial morphology, which mimics the microscopic appearance of pancreatic branch duct intraductal papillary mucinous neoplasia (BD-IPMN).[12] We recently named this lesion Brunner gland duct adenoma (BGDA)[13] (Figure 21-17).

ADENOMYOMA (AND GROOVE PANCREATITIS)

Although adenomyomas are most common in the duodenum, they can be seen in any segment of the small intestine or gastrointestinal tract. Adenomyomas are small to large,

nodular or polyploid lesions consisting of a focal proliferation of benign glands intermixed with smooth muscle fibers (Figure 21-18). The glandular component may be intestinal or pancreatobiliary in phenotype. The surface epithelium often shows foveolar metaplasia. When these lesions are resected endoscopically, the diagnosis should be straightforward. However, in biopsies, the submucosal lesion may not be evident, with only the edge present in the material sampled, and the erosion with reactive atypia of the overlying mucosa may lead to an erroneous diagnosis of a duodenal adenoma (Figure 21-3).

The so-called groove pancreatitis represents a special form of the same disease. The common histologic picture is bland-appearing glands or ducts intermixed with smooth muscle bundles (Figure 21-19). The endoscopic and macroscopic description may seem alarming, raising the possibility of an invasive adenocarcinoma, but the lack of histologic evidence of cytologic atypia or desmoplasia confirms the benign nature of this lesion.

It is believed (quite reasonably) that most gastrointestinal tract adenomyomas result from remnants of ectopic pancreatic tissue. It is not uncommon to see ectopic pancreas in the duodenal wall, particularly in the ampullary region.

LYMPHANGIECTASIA AND LYMPHANGIOMA

Lymphangiectasias are solitary or multiple polyploid lesions that are microscopically characterized by dilation of either native or proliferating lymphatic vessels. These lesions can be encountered in either mucosal biopsies or resected specimens.

Endoscopically, individual lymphangiectasias appear as nondescript polyps or nodules, often with a white, shining external appearance. Microscopically, the lesions range from a single dilated lymphatic (lacteal) filling the core of a villus (Figure 21-20) to prominent, anastomosing, dilated lymphatic channels involving multiple villi (Figure 21-21). This lesion may indicate a downstream obstruction to lymph return but most likely is simply the result of poor bowel preparation.

In lymphangioma, the anastomosing dilated lymphatics form a discrete submucosal nodule, which may focally involve the mucosal lamina propria (Figure 21-22A). The submucosal portion of the lesion may not be evident in small endoscopic mucosal biopsies. The lesion may be multifocal, a process sometimes termed *lymphangiomatosis*. Along with lymph fluid, foamy macrophages may be evident in lymphangioma or lymphangiomatosis (Figure 21-22B)

ENDOMETRIOSIS

Endometriosis can occur in the small-bowel wall, where it sometimes presents as a mucosal polyp or intramural nodule or mass, which occasionally results in small-bowel obstruction[14,15] (Figure 21-23). The differential diagnosis, both radiographically and endoscopically as well as pathologically, may include an invasive adenocarcinoma. However, recognizing the typical morphological features of endometrial glands

MUC6 MUC5AC

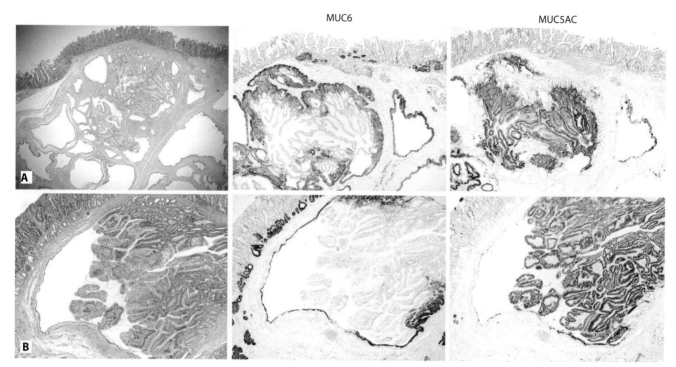

FIGURE 21-17. Brunner gland duct adenoma. Polypoid lesions that are away from the major and minor papilla may contain Brunner glands with a centrally dilated duct, with the latter exhibiting focal solid-to-papillary growth as well as the gastric foveolar type mucin, MUC5AC. **A.** An example with a configuration of multiple microcysts. **B.** An example with a single large cyst. Both exhibit positive MUC6 staining in lining epithelium (in contrast to the intracystic growth).

with associated stroma (Figure 21-23) should make the histologic diagnosis straightforward.

PSEUDOLIPOMATOSIS

Like similar lesions described in the colonic mucosa,[16,17] these gas-entrapping lamina propria lesions are also seen in small-bowel biopsies (Figure 21-24). The lack of lining of the spaces distinguishes this entity from lymphangiectasia.

LIPOMA

Lipomas are benign tumors composed of mature adipose tissue that makes up 1.6%–8% of small-intestinal tumors.[18–20] In a study examining only benign small-intestinal tumors, 26% were lipomas, which most commonly occurred in the ileum.[21] Patients can present with paroxysmal abdominal pain, obstruction, bleeding, and intussusception. A greater incidence of intussusception has been observed in tumors larger than 4 cm[22]

FIGURE 21-18. Adenomyoma. **A.** A submucosal dilated duct is intermixed with smooth muscle bundles. The overlying mucosa exhibits foveolar metaplasia. **B.** Another case of adenomyoma consisting of small submucosal glands, mainly of pancreatobiliary type with scattered goblet cells, intermixed with smooth muscle bundles.

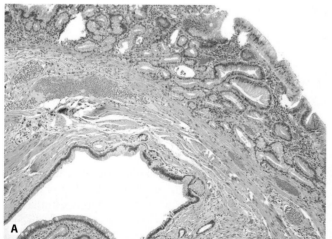
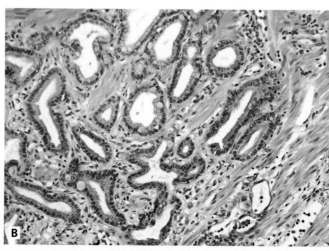

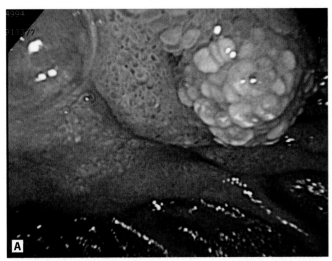

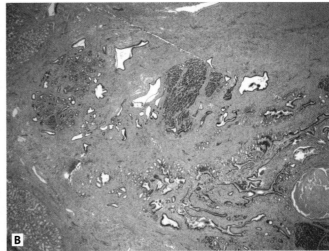

FIGURE 21-19. Groove pancreatitis presented as a duodenal polyp. **A.** Endoscopic image of what was considered a duodenal villous polyp with intramural "invasion into head of pancreas." Mucosal biopsy only revealed nonspecific peptic injury. **B.** Whipple procedure revealed a densely fibrotic area between the head of the pancreas and the duodenum, with residual atrophic pancreatic parenchyma and dilated ducts containing inspissated mucin.

(Figure 21-25). Endoscopically, lipomas have a characteristic "tent" or "cushion" sign.[23] In a case series of 14 patients, small-intestinal lipomas ranged from 2 to 6 cm in greatest dimension, were well circumscribed, and originated from the submucosal layer. Histology reveals mature adipose tissue, with 9 of 14 lipomas lined by necrotic and ulcerated mucosa.[22] Four of 14 lipomas also displayed inflammatory fibrous hyperplasia with septa extending into the adipose tissue.[22] Treatment is endoscopic or surgical resection, and the prognosis is excellent.

■ REFERENCES

1. Vieth M, Kushima R, Borchard F, Stolte M. Pyloric gland adenoma: a clinico-pathological analysis of 90 cases. *Virchows Arch*. 2003;442(4): 317–321. PMID: 12715167.

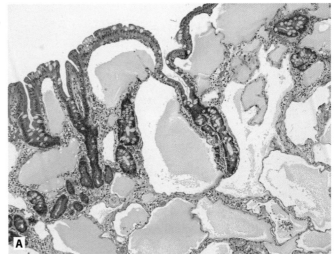

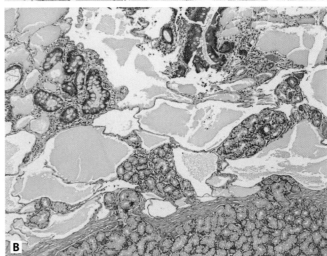

FIGURE 21-20. Mild lymphangiectasia. Dilation of individual lacteals of the small-bowel villi.

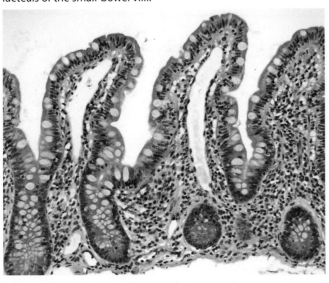

FIGURE 21-21. Lymphangiectasia. Dilation of more complex intramucosal lymphatics involving multiple adjacent villi (**A**) and separating small-bowel glands (**B**).

PART FOUR

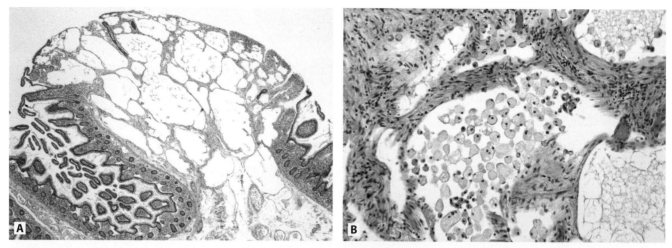

FIGURE 21-22. Lymphangioma. **A.** A solitary lesion consisting mainly of proliferating submucosal lymphatics with dilation, focally extending to the mucosa. **B.** Lymphangiomatosis, with many foamy macrophages in the dilated lymphatic channels.

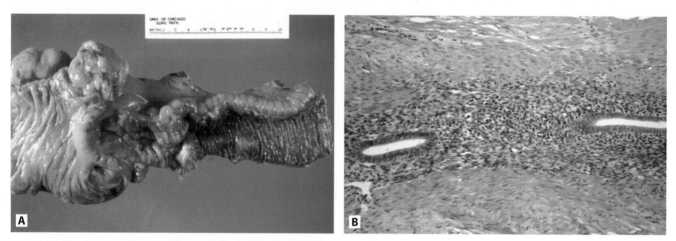

FIGURE 21-23. Endometriosis. **A.** A mass lesion in the terminal ileum caused obstruction. **B.** Simple glands lined by columnar epithelium with hyperchromatic nuclei may be mistaken for dysplasia, surrounded by endometrial stroma.

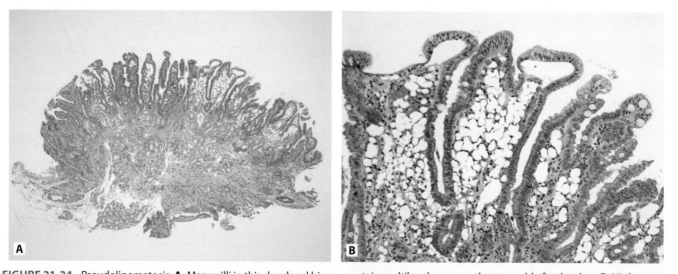

FIGURE 21-24. Pseudolipomatosis. **A.** Many villi in this duodenal biopsy contain multilocular spaces that resemble fat droplets. **B.** High-power view demonstrates mostly gas trapped in the lamina propria without an endothelial lining.

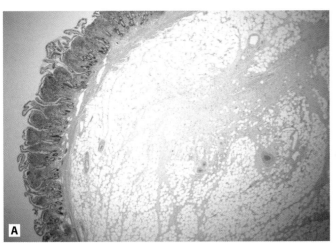
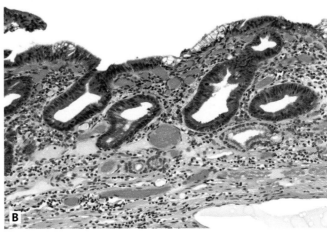

FIGURE 21-25. Duodenal lipoma. **A.** Well-circumscribed submucosal mass consisting of mature adipocytes. **B.** The overlying mucosa exhibits focal foveolar metaplasia with reactive changes.

2. Bakotic BW, Robinson MJ, Sturm PD, Hruban RH, Offerhaus GJ, Albores-Saavedra J. Pyloric gland adenoma of the main pancreatic duct. *Am J Surg Pathol*. 1999;23(2):227–231. PMID: 9989851.

3. Kato N, Akiyama S, Motoyama T. Pyloric gland-type tubular adenoma superimposed on intraductal papillary mucinous tumor of the pancreas. Pyloric gland adenoma of the pancreas. *Virchows Arch*. 2002;440(2):205–208. PMID: 11964052.

4. Albores-Saavedra J, Chable-Montero F, Gonzalez-Romo MA, Ramirez Jaramillo M, Henson DE. Adenomas of the gallbladder. Morphologic features, expression of gastric and intestinal mucins, and incidence of high-grade dysplasia/carcinoma in situ and invasive carcinoma. *Hum Pathol*. 2012;43(9):1506–1513. PMID: 22386521.

5. Rosty C, Buchanan DD, Walters RJ, et al. Hyperplastic polyp of the duodenum: a report of 9 cases with immunohistochemical and molecular findings. *Hum Pathol*. 2011;42(12):1953–1959. PMID: 21733555.

6. Perzin KH, Bridge MF. Adenomas of the small intestine: a clinico-pathologic review of 51 cases and a study of their relationship to carcinoma. *Cancer*. 1981;48(3):799–819. PMID: 7248908.

7. Domizio P, Talbot IC, Spigelman AD, Williams CB, Phillips RK. Upper gastrointestinal pathology in familial adenomatous polyposis: results from a prospective study of 102 patients. *J Clin Pathol*. 1990;43(9):738–743. PMID: 2170464. PMCID: PMC502752.

8. Pai RK, Rybicki LA, Goldblum JR, Shen B, Xiao SY, Liu X. Paneth cells in colonic adenomas: association with male sex and adenoma burden. *Am J Surg Pathol*. 2013;37(1):98–103. PMID: 23232853.

9. Martinez ME, Baron JA, Lieberman DA, et al. A pooled analysis of advanced colorectal neoplasia diagnoses after colonoscopic polypectomy. *Gastroenterology*. 2009;136(3):832–841. PMID: 19171141. PMCID: PMC3685417.

10. van Stolk RU, Beck GJ, Baron JA, Haile R, Summers R. Adenoma characteristics at first colonoscopy as predictors of adenoma recurrence and characteristics at follow-up. The Polyp Prevention Study Group. *Gastroenterology*. 1998;115(1):13–18. PMID: 9649453.

11. Bonithon-Kopp C, Piard F, Fenger C, et al. Colorectal adenoma characteristics as predictors of recurrence. *Dis Colon Rectum*. 2004;47(3):323–333. PMID: 14991494.

12. Xiao SY. Intraductal papillary mucinous neoplasm of the pancreas: an update. *Scientifica*. 2012;2012:893632. PMID: 24278753. PMCID: 3820567.

13. Alpert L, Whitcomb E, Westerhoff M, Hart J, Xiao S-Y. Brunner gland duct adenoma mimicking pancreatic intraductal papillary mucinous neoplasm. *Modern Pathology*. 2015;28(S2):145A.

14. Croom RD 3rd, Donovan ML, Schwesinger WH. Intestinal endometriosis. *Am J Surg*. 1984;148(5):660–667. PMID: 6496859.

15. Jiang W, Roma AA, Lai K, Carver P, Xiao SY, Liu X. Endometriosis involving the mucosa of the intestinal tract: a clinicopathologic study of 15 cases. *Mod Pathol*. 2013;26(9):1270–1278. PMID: 23579618.

16. Snover DC, Sandstad J, Hutton S. Mucosal pseudolipomatosis of the colon. *Am J Clin Pathol*. 1985;84(5):575–580. PMID: 4061380.

17. Waring JP, Manne RK, Wadas DD, Sanowski RA. Mucosal pseudolipomatosis: an air pressure-related colonoscopy complication. *Gastrointest Endosc*. 1989;35(2):93–94. PMID: 2714610.

18. Dudiak KM, Johnson CD, Stephens DH. Primary tumors of the small intestine: CT evaluation. *Am J Roentgenol*. 1989;152(5):995–998. PMID: 2705358.

19. Darling RC, Welch CE. Tumors of the small intestine. *N Engl J Med*. 1959;260(9):397–408. PMID: 13632900.

20. Raiford T. Tumors of the small intestine. *Arch Surg*. 1932;25(1):122–177.

21. Wilson JM, Melvin DB, Gray G, Thorbjarnarson B. Benign small bowel tumor. *Ann Surg*. 1975;181(2):247–250. PMID: 1078626. PMCID: 1343763.

22. Fang SH, Dong DJ, Chen FH, Jin M, Zhong BS. Small intestinal lipomas: diagnostic value of multi-slice CT enterography. *World J Gastroenterol*. 2010;16(21):2677–2681. PMID: 20518091. PMCID: 2880782.

23. De Beer RA, Shinya H. Colonic lipomas. An endoscopic analysis. *Gastrointest Endosc*. 1975;22(2):90–91. PMID: 1193347.

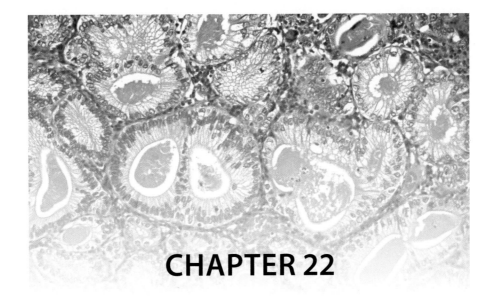

CHAPTER 22

Small-Bowel Adenocarcinoma

Emma Whitcomb and Shu-Yuan Xiao

BACKGROUND AND CLINICAL FEATURES

While the small bowel comprises 75% of the length of the gastrointestinal tract, adenocarcinoma of the small bowel is remarkably rare, representing less than 2% of all gastrointestinal malignancies.[1] A number of plausible explanations have been proposed for the relative rarity of small-bowel adenocarcinoma, including (1) rapid transit time and dilution of luminal contents, leading to reduced carcinogen exposure and decreased mechanical trauma; (2) low levels of colonizing bacteria, thus decreased bile salt conversion into carcinogenic substances; (3) increased concentration of detoxifying mucosal enzymes, such as benzpyrene hydroxylase; and (4) abundance of lymphoid tissue, resulting in a high degree of immunosurveillance.[1-3]

When small-bowel adenocarcinoma does arise, it usually presents in the sixth decade and is slightly more common in male patients.[4] In approximately 10%–20% of cases, an underlying hereditary or inflammatory condition is present.[5] The prognosis is dismal, with an overall 5-year survival of 26%.[4] Clinical detection of small-bowel adenocarcinoma is challenging due to vague presenting symptoms and the insensitivity of small-bowel imaging techniques. Thus, small-bowel adenocarcinoma is often diagnosed at a later stage, with synchronous metastases or lymph node involvement in 30%–40% of cases.[6,7] In recent years, newly developed imaging techniques such as capsule endoscopy and double-balloon enteroscopy have the potential to achieve earlier diagnosis; however, neither modality is currently widely used.

In general, sporadic small-bowel adenocarcinoma is thought to evolve through an adenoma-carcinoma sequence similar to colonic adenocarcinoma. Most tumors arise in the duodenum (~60%), followed by the jejunum (~30%) and ileum (~10%).[4] Ampullary adenomas and adenocarcinomas, which can arise from both duodenal and pancreatobiliary epithelium, are conventionally considered a distinct entity and are discussed in a separate section in this chapter.

PATHOLOGIC FEATURES

The majority of small-bowel adenocarcinomas microscopically resemble colorectal adenocarcinoma and are graded as well, moderately, and poorly differentiated. The determination of differentiation should be primarily based on the percentage of glandular architecture. Well-differentiated tumors have over 75% well-formed glands (Figure 22-1), moderately differentiated tumors have 25%–75% well-formed glands (Figure 22-2), and poorly differentiated tumors have less than 25% well-formed glands (Figure 22-3). Some tumors consist of solid sheets of cells with no apparent glandular differentiation and require immunohistochemical staining to confirm the epithelial origin; these are diagnosed as undifferentiated carcinoma (Figure 22-4). While histologic grading of these tumors is used in common practice, the prognostic significance has not been well established. In a recent study of 491 cases of small-bowel adenocarcinomas, tumor differentiation was not shown to be an independent predictor of survival.[4]

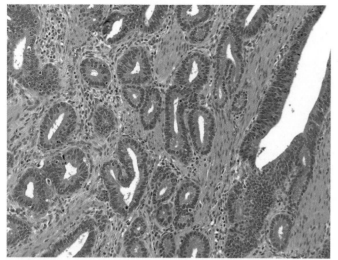

FIGURE 22-1. Well-differentiated small-bowel adenocarcinoma. The infiltrating tumor is composed entirely of well-formed glands of varying sizes and shapes and only occasional glandular crowding.

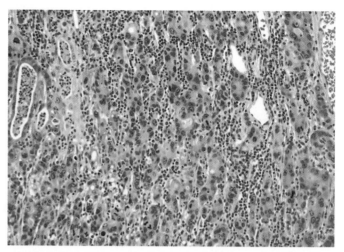

FIGURE 22-3. Poorly differentiated adenocarcinoma. The malignant cells infiltrate in cords and as single cells, with rare gland formation.

Occasionally, small-bowel adenocarcinomas have a mucinous component in which clusters and single tumor cells appear to float in pools of pale blue mucin by H&E stain (Figure 22-5). By definition, if the mucinous component comprises over 50% of the tumor, it is designated mucinous adenocarcinoma. The prognostic significance of this subtype in the small intestine is unknown, although in the colon it may carry a slightly worse prognosis.[8] Signet-ring carcinomas are also described in the small bowel, albeit in a minority of cases, and are also thought to have a worse prognosis than conventional adenocarcinoma (Figure 22-6).

In our experience, occasionally small-bowel adenocarcinomas exhibit morphologic resemblance to gastric tubular-type adenocarcinomas (Figure 22-7) rather than intestinal type, particularly in the setting of Crohn disease (see further discussion in this chapter). The invasive tumor consists

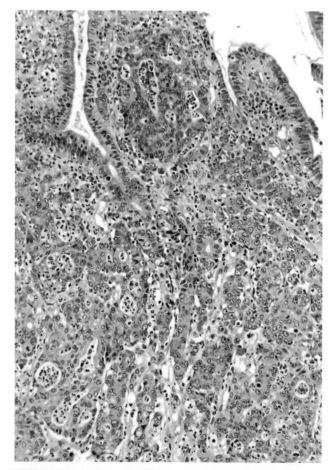

FIGURE 22-2. Moderately differentiated adenocarcinoma. The tumor consists of cords and sheets of malignant cells, with focal gland formation.

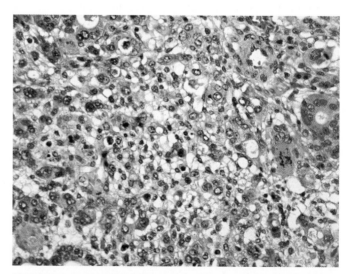

FIGURE 22-4. Undifferentiated type. This tumor is composed of sheets of highly atypical malignant cells. Immunohistochemical staining is required to confirm gastrointestinal origin.

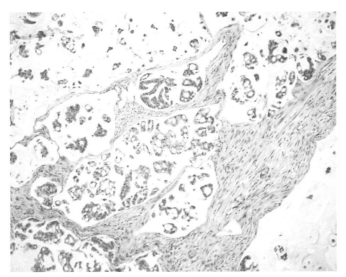

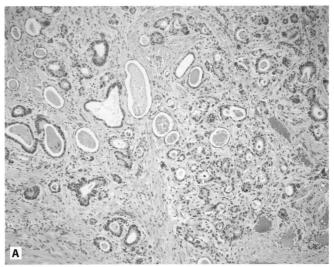

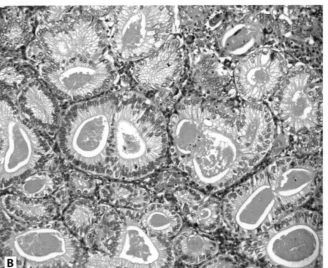

FIGURE 22-5. Mucinous carcinoma. Large mucin pools dissect the intestinal wall, with highly atypical tumor cell clusters.

of tubules and small glands lined by cuboidal-to-columnar epithelium with pale pink, granular, eosinophilic cytoplasm and round nuclei, resembling foveolar epithelium. This is most often present in association with Crohn enteritis in which there is gastric metaplasia (pyloric gland and foveolar types)[9]; however, we have also seen this gastric morphology in sporadic small-bowel adenocarcinoma as a part of a mixed pattern (intestinal or mucinous).

■ SMALL-BOWEL ADENOCARCINOMAS IN SPECIFIC CLINICAL SETTINGS

There are well-known clinical scenarios in which the relative risk of small-bowel adenocarcinoma is increased, including hereditary syndromes such as familial adenomatous polyposis

FIGURE 22-6. Small-bowel adenocarcinoma, signet-ring type. The infiltrating malignant cells have peripheral nuclei compressed by cytoplasmic mucin (signet-ring cells).

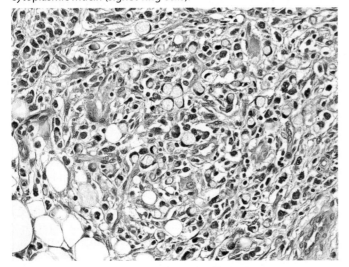

FIGURE 22-7. Ileal adenocarcinoma, gastric tubular type, from a patient with Crohn enteritis. **A.** Highly infiltrative tumor consists of simple glands. **B.** The malignant glands are composed of cuboidal cells with pale pink cytoplasm and large, rounded nuclei, similar to gastric tubular adenocarcinoma.

(FAP), hereditary nonpolyposis colon cancer (HNPCC) syndrome, and Peutz-Jeghers syndrome, as well as inflammatory diseases such as Crohn disease and celiac disease. In these settings, small-bowel adenocarcinomas may exhibit unique histomorphologic, immunophenotypic, and molecular features. For pathologists, awareness of these genetic and inflammatory diseases and their unique clinicopathologic features can be of diagnostic utility. In addition, raising the possibility of a previously undiagnosed genetic or inflammatory predisposition can have significant impact on patient care.

Familial Adenomatous Polyposis

Classic FAP syndrome is underlined by a germline mutation in the adenomatous polyposis coli (*APC*) gene. The syndrome is characterized by the development of hundreds of adenomatous polyps in the colon and rectum and near-inevitable

PART FOUR

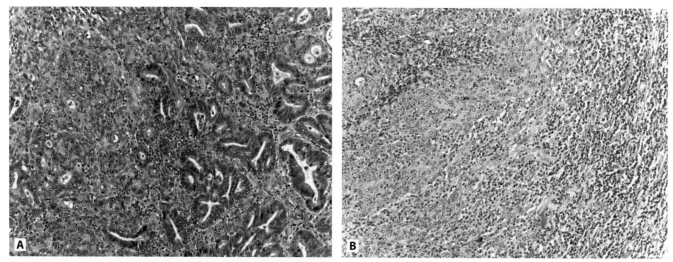

FIGURE 22-8. Ampullary adenocarcinoma with MSH6 loss. This was from a 47-year-old male patient with an ampullary mass. **A.** Well-differentiated adenocarcinoma mixed with poorly differentiated carcinoma. **B.** The poorly differentiated adenocarcinoma exhibiting a syncytial (medullary) pattern. Immunostain demonstrated loss of MSH6. The tumor was negative EBER (Epstein-Barr virus early RNA; not shown).

development of colonic adenocarcinoma if early prophylactic total colectomy is not performed. A majority of patients with FAP also develop small-bowel adenomas, and the reported incidence of small-bowel adenocarcinoma ranges from 1% to 12%, a relative risk over 100-fold above the general population.[10] Approximately 75% of these adenomas and adenocarcinomas arise in the duodenum and ampulla.[11]

Today, small-bowel adenocarcinoma in patients with FAP is a leading cause of cancer-related death in patients following proctocolectomy.[12,13] For this reason, upper endoscopy is routinely performed every 1–5 years in these patients, the frequency depending on duodenal polyp burden.[14,15] Recent endoscopic studies have demonstrated that the degree of duodenal polyposis detected on upper gastrointestinal endoscopy correlates with the degree of polyposis in the jejunum and ileum,[16] and it has been suggested that high-risk patients undergo periodic surveillance of the more distal small bowel using advanced endoscopic techniques.[17]

Hereditary Nonpolyposis Colon Cancer Syndrome

Also known as Lynch syndrome, HNPCC is caused by a germline mutation in one of the four mismatch repair (MMR) genes, usually MSH2 or MLH1 and less often MSH6 or PMS2. Epidemiologic studies of HNPCC consistently demonstrated an increased relative risk for small-bowel adenocarcinoma, ranging from the tens to hundreds, varying on the type of mutation.[18,19] Currently, routine screening for small-bowel neoplasms is not practiced on patients with HNPCC. However, testing for the MMR phenotype is recommended on small-bowel adenocarcinomas with suggestive features because they can be the first manifestation of the syndrome.[20,21]

Approximately 50% of HNPCC-related small-bowel adenocarcinomas are located in the duodenum.[21] Similar to the colorectal adenocarcinomas seen in HNPCC, the small-bowel adenocarcinomas are often poorly differentiated, occasionally with mucinous or medullary features (Figure 22-8). A characteristic feature is the prominent intratumoral and peritumoral lymphocytic infiltrate, which is present in approximately 75% of cases. In addition, the growth pattern is often characterized by a pushing, expansile border rather than infiltrative growth.

Peutz-Jeghers Syndrome

The hamartomatous polyps of Peutz-Jeghers syndrome occur most commonly in the jejunum and ileum, distinguishing this from other polyposis syndromes. While the polyps in Peutz-Jeghers syndrome are considered hamartomas, there is a marked increase in relative risk of small-bowel adenocarcinomas in this syndrome, reportedly[22,23] as high as 520. Thus, endoscopic surveillance of the small bowel is suggested at 2- to 3-year intervals.[15] The carcinomas most often arise from adenomatous areas within the typical Peutz-Jeghers polyp; however, they morphologically resemble sporadic small-bowel adenocarcinomas.

Crohn Disease

Crohn enteritis is a well-documented risk factor for the development of small-bowel adenocarcinoma, putatively due to the carcinogenic consequence of chronic inflammation. The cumulative risk increases with duration of disease: It is estimated at 0.2% in patients with Crohn enteritis of over 10 years' duration and 2.2% in patients with Crohn enteritis of over 25 years' duration.[24] The reported relative risk ranges from 17- to 80-fold greater than the general population.[25–28] Despite this fact, to date there is no agreed-on screening strategy for small-bowel adenocarcinoma in patients with Crohn enteritis.[28]

Crohn-associated small-bowel adenocarcinoma typically arises in areas of active inflammation and, uniquely, is most often located in the terminal ileum. In contrast to sporadic small-bowel adenocarcinoma, adenocarcinomas in the setting of Crohn disease are thought to arise from dysplasia rather than adenoma.[29-31] Dysplasia in Crohn enteritis can be flat or polypoid and in some cases is cytologically identical to adenomatous dysplasia.

In patients with Crohn disease, it is common for the adenocarcinoma to be diagnosed incidentally at the time of surgery. This is because the obstructive symptoms and imaging findings in small-bowel adenocarcinoma are often clinically indistinguishable from a Crohn enteritis flare or benign stricture.[32] The histomorphology of Crohn-associated small-bowel adenocarcinoma can be typical intestinal-type adenocarcinoma, although a number of other tumor morphologies are described with relative frequency, including signet-ring cell, mucinous, undifferentiated, and gastric tubular type[9,31] (Figure 22-7).

Celiac Disease

Malignancy is the primary cause of mortality in patients with celiac disease.[33] While small-intestinal lymphoma, specifically enteropathy-associated T-cell lymphoma (EATL), is the most common malignancy in celiac disease (see also Chapter 18), patients with celiac disease are also at risk for small-bowel adenocarcinoma, with some estimating a relative risk of 60–80.[5,34,35] There is currently no consensus on screening for small-bowel malignancy in celiac disease.[36]

The most common reported location for celiac-associated small-bowel adenocarcinoma is the jejunum, followed by the duodenum. Tumors may be multifocal.[37,38] A handful of reports described celiac-associated small-bowel adenocarcinomas arising in typical intestinal-type adenomas, suggesting a similar adenoma-carcinoma progression sequence rather than flat dysplasia.[38,39] Occasionally, the diagnosis of celiac disease occurs at the same time as the diagnosis of small-bowel adenocarcinoma, in which the typical features of celiac disease are present adjacent to the tumor[40] in biopsy or resected specimens.

■ AMPULLARY ADENOCARCINOMAS

The majority of tumors arising at the ampulla are of either intestinal or pancreatobiliary histologic type; some are of mixed type.[41] Other rare tumor types arising in the ampulla include mucinous, signet-ring cell, undifferentiated, and mixed adenoendocrine carcinoma. Ampullary carcinomas form masses that usually lead to obstruction of the common bile duct, pancreatic duct, or both, depending on the location (Figure 22-9).

Intestinal-type ampullary adenocarcinoma is the most common histologic type. These tumors arise from the duodenal mucosa that forms the papilla and histologically resemble small-bowel adenocarcinomas at other sites (Figure 22-10). Pancreatobiliary-type carcinomas arise from the common

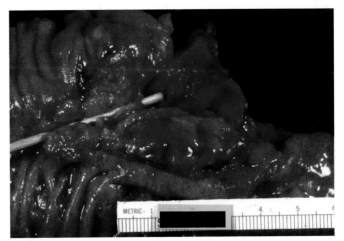

FIGURE 22-9. Ampullary carcinoma arising from an adenoma. A polypoid mass with multiple papillae arising in the most terminal portion of the ampulla caused marked dilation of the pancreatic duct.

channel in the ampulla lined by pancreatobiliary-type epithelium (Figure 22-11). Both the intestinal- and pancreatobiliary-type carcinomas may have a protruding luminal growth overlying an invasive component. The pancreatobiliary type may have a papillary tumor, with deeper infiltrating angulated glands lined by simple cuboidal-to-low-columnar cells in a desmoplastic stroma, similar to pancreatic ductal adenocarcinomas or cholangiocarcinomas (Figure 22-12). However, in resected specimens, the surface portion to the tumor often becomes unrecognizable due to the placement of a stent preoperatively. In multiple studies, ampullary carcinomas of the pancreaticobiliary type have shown a worse prognosis and more frequent nodal metastasis when compared to the

FIGURE 22-10. Ampullary carcinoma, intestinal type. This is a polypoid tumor in the ampulla consisting of well-formed glands and with a brush border of absorptive cells focally seen (arrowheads). Immunohistochemical stains demonstrated the tumor was positive for CK20, CDX2, and negative for CK7 (not shown).

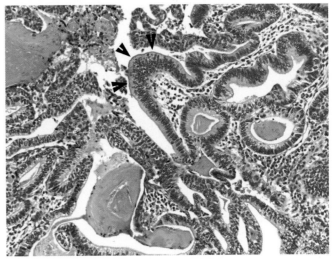

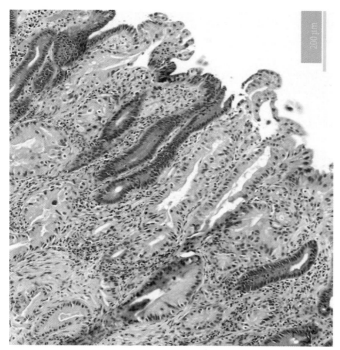

FIGURE 22-11. Ampullary carcinoma, pancreatobiliary type. There is marked cytological atypia in surface as well as glandular epithelia.

intestinal type.[41-43] In addition, the chemotherapy regimens differ. Thus, differentiating between these two histologic types is recommended. As there may be difficulty in morphologic distinction or interobserver discrepancy, typing is best achieved using a panel of immunostains. We routinely include CDX2, MUC2, and CK20, which are positive for intestinal type (Figure 22-13). In contrast, pancreatobiliary-type tumors are negative for these markers but positive for CK7 and MUC1[44,45] (Figure 22-14).

Rarely, both a typical adenocarcinoma component and a high-grade neuroendocrine carcinoma can be seen in the same ampullary tumor (Figure 22-15).

FIGURE 22-12. Ampullary carcinoma, pancreatobiliary type. Irregular and angulated glands infiltrating the desmoplastic stroma.

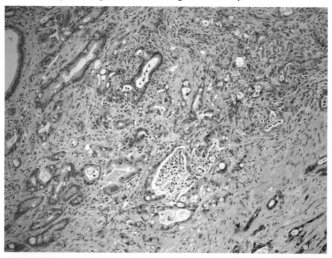

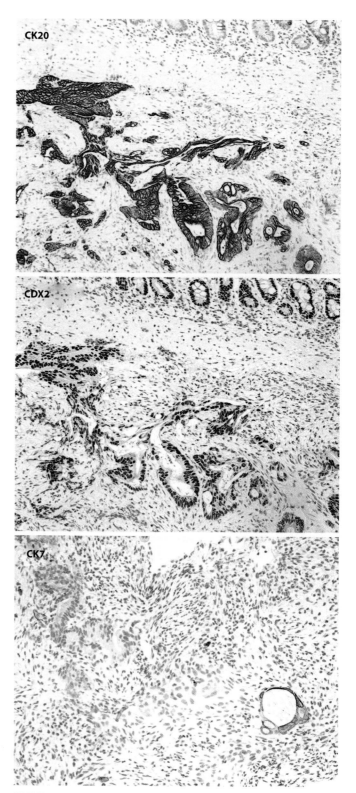

FIGURE 22-13. Immunohistochemistry of an ampullary carcinoma, intestinal type, showing strong positivity for CK20 and CDX2 and only focal positivity for CK7.

Another challenge with carcinomas present in the ampulla is to determine if the site of origin is indeed the ampulla of Vater or carcinoma arising from the distal pancreatic/bile ducts and extending into the ampulla. This distinction is

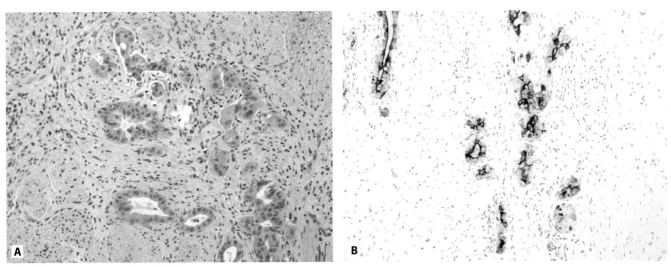

FIGURE 22-14. Immunohistochemistry of an ampullary carcinoma, pancreatobiliary type. **A.** The invasive carcinoma glands. **B.** The tumor cells show positivity for MUC1, a marker normally expressed by small intralobular ductules, and CK7 (not shown).

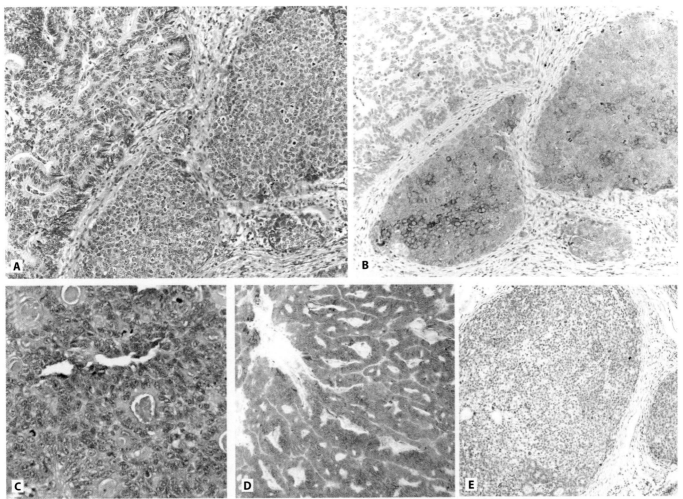

FIGURE 22-15. Mixed adenoendocrine carcinoma of ampulla. **A.** Gland-forming adenocarcinoma on the left and poorly differentiated neuroendocrine carcinoma on the right. **B.** The latter is positive for synaptophysin by immunostain. **C.** Adenocarcinoma exhibits focal mucin production (mucicarmine stain) and MOC31 (**D**). **E.** The neuroendocrine component is negative for MOC31.

PART FOUR

important because of difference in TNM tumor staging. Furthermore, ampullary carcinoma can occasionally be managed with the less-invasive ampullectomy rather than a pancreaticoduodenectomy (Whipple procedure). In addition, pancreatobiliary-type ampullary carcinoma in general has a better prognosis than pancreatic adenocarcinoma or cholangiocarcinoma.[46] Thus, whenever possible, determining the site of origin for these tumors should be attempted. When the tumor is small, the origin can be determined based on the presence and location of mucosal surface precursor lesions, location of bulk of the tumor, and direction of invasive growth. Often, the picture is increasingly obscured as the tumor becomes larger and involves more than one potential site of origin, and the presence of surface dysplasia may be multifocal.[46]

■ IMMUNOHISTOCHEMISTRY IN SMALL-BOWEL ADENOCARCINOMA

The relatively few immunohistochemical studies of adenocarcinoma of the small bowel suggest an immunophenotype that deviates from the epithelium where it arises and is distinctive from colonic adenocarcinoma. Overall, small-bowel adenocarcinomas are most consistently positive for CDX2 and CEA.[9,47,48] Cytokeratins CK20 and CK7 are often positive and coexpressed in the same tumor.[9,48–50] Expression of villin and MUC2 is reported in over half of cases, and MUC5AC and MUC6 are reported in approximately a third of cases,[9,49] depending on the histologic type. The highly variable immunophenotype seen in small-bowel adenocarcinoma is likely related to the frequent multilineage differentiation and association with genetic and inflammatory conditions,[9] as discussed previously. Therefore, it is advised to always keep an open mind when concluding the origin of a tumor (see the following discussion; Figures 22-16 to 22-18).

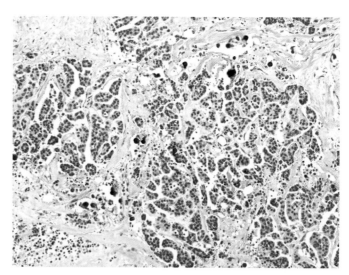

FIGURE 22-17. Ovarian papillary serous carcinoma metastasized to small-bowel wall.

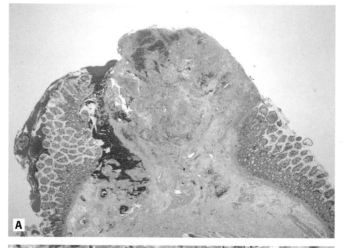

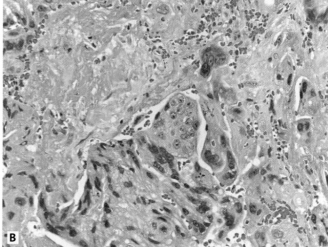

FIGURE 22-18. Metastatic choriocarcinoma to small bowel. **A.** The tumor forms a polypoid mucosal lesion and involves the mucosa and submucosa. **B.** Malignant syncytial trophoblasts.

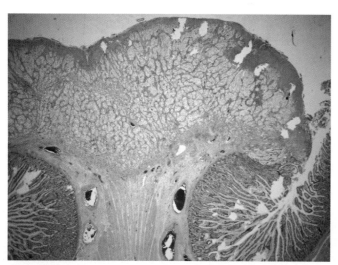

FIGURE 22-16. Metastatic renal cell carcinomas to small bowel (clear cells).

DIFFERENTIAL DIAGNOSIS

A number of benign and malignant tumors enter the differential diagnosis of small-bowel adenocarcinoma clinically or endoscopically, but they rarely present as a diagnostic challenge pathologically. The more common benign tumors include lipomas, leiomyomas, and hamartomas. Gastrointestinal stromal tumors are also relatively common. Besides adenocarcinoma, carcinoid tumors and lymphomas represent the second and third most common primary malignant tumors of the small bowel.[1]

Given the rarity of primary small-bowel adenocarcinoma, metastatic tumors must always be considered in the differential. While virtually any type of adenocarcinoma has been reported to metastasize to the small intestine, the most frequent sites of origin include colon, kidney (Figure 22-16), ovary (Figure 22-17), uterus, stomach, breast, lung, and germ cell tumors (Figure 22-18). Melanomas also notoriously metastasize to the small intestine. The presence of surface dysplasia is supportive of a small-bowel primary; however, occasionally cancerization of the surface epithelium can occur in metastatic lesions, and reactive surface changes overlying a metastatic mass may mimic dysplasia. Most metastatic candidates in the differential can be ruled out or in with a limited panel of immunohistochemical stains. However, in a few scenarios, immunohistochemistry is not useful due to the varied staining pattern of small-bowel adenocarcinoma (see previous discussion) and the overlap with other primaries, such as stomach, colon, and pancreas. In these cases, careful correlation with imaging studies is required for definitive determination of the primary site.

MOLECULAR ALTERATIONS IN SMALL-BOWEL ADENOCARCINOMA

Due to the rarity of small-bowel adenocarcinoma, data on the molecular alterations are limited and often variable from study to study. Some authors have suggested that these tumors also mirror the progressive molecular alterations demonstrated in colorectal adenocarcinoma through the adenoma-carcinoma sequence.

The two well-defined molecular pathways in colorectal adenocarcinoma tumorigenesis include the *APC*, *KRAS*, p53 pathway and the MMR pathway, and mutations in the primary genes involved in these pathways have all been reported in small-bowel adenocarcinomas.[5,51] Regarding the first pathway, the prevalence of mutations in the *KRAS* gene is similar between colorectal and small-bowel adenocarcinomas, typically ranging from 30% to 60%.[52–56] Similarly, the prevalence of p53 mutations is also comparable, ranging from 20% to 50% in both.[52–54,57] The abnormality of p53 in a subset of tumors may be detected immunohistochemically, which can be used to support or confirm a malignant diagnosis of carcinoma in biopsies with limited tumor cells (Figure 22-19). In contrast, while up to 80% of colorectal carcinomas are shown to have mutations in the *APC* gene,

less than 20% of small-bowel adenocarcinomas have these mutations.[52,54,55,58] This is an important molecular difference and has led some to suggest that small-bowel adenocarcinomas have a somewhat distinct pathogenesis.

Inactivation of MMR genes, either by germline mutations (HNPCC syndrome) or promoter hypermethylation (sporadic), occurs in approximately 15% of colorectal adenocarcinomas.[5] Although limited, current data suggest that the deficient MMR phenotype is slightly more frequent in small-bowel adenocarcinoma, with a reported prevalence up to 35%[48,54,59] (Figure 22-8).

A number of other genetic alterations have been reported in small-bowel adenocarcinomas, including mutations in E-Cadherin, SMAD4, VEGF-A, and HER-2, but their significance has not been fully studied.[5,51] In addition, molecular changes in small-bowel adenocarcinomas arising in the various predisposing inflammatory conditions are largely unknown.

SUMMARY

Small-bowel adenocarcinomas are rare; thus, scientific understanding of these tumors is limited. Whenever adenocarcinoma is encountered in the small intestine, potential metastasis from another site must be considered. In general, primary sporadic small-bowel adenocarcinoma is thought to evolve through an adenoma-carcinoma sequence similar to colorectal adenocarcinoma. Likewise, the histomorphology of these tumors often resembles colorectal adenocarcinoma; however, they deviate slightly in their immunohistochemical and molecular features. Awareness of the hereditary and inflammatory clinical settings that place patients at increased risk for small-bowel adenocarcinoma, and an appreciation of their unique pathologic features, is useful diagnostically and can have a significant impact on patient care.

REFERENCES

1. Gill SS, Heuman DM, Mihas AA. Small intestinal neoplasms. *J Clin Gastroenterol.* 2001;33(4):267–282. PMID: 11588539.
2. Lowenfels AB. Why are small-bowel tumours so rare? *Lancet.* 1973;1(7793):24–26. PMID: 4118541.
3. Wattenberg LW. Studies of polycyclic hydrocarbon hydroxylases of the intestine possibly related to cancer. Effect of diet on benzpyrene hydroxylase activity. *Cancer.* 1971;28(1):99–102. PMID: 5110649.
4. Halfdanarson TR, McWilliams RR, Donohue JH, Quevedo JF. A single-institution experience with 491 cases of small bowel adenocarcinoma. Am J Surg. 2010;199(6):797–803. PMID: 20609724.
5. Aparicio T, Zaanan A, Svrcek M, et al. Small bowel adenocarcinoma: epidemiology, risk factors, diagnosis and treatment. *Dig Liver Dis.* 2014;46(2):97–104. PMID: 23796552.
6. Talamonti MS, Goetz LH, Rao S, Joehl RJ. Primary cancers of the small bowel: analysis of prognostic factors and results of surgical management. *Arch Surg.* 2002;137(5):564–570; discussion 570–571. PMID: 11982470.
7. Dabaja BS, Suki D, Pro B, Bonnen M, Ajani J. Adenocarcinoma of the small bowel: presentation, prognostic factors, and outcome of 217 patients. *Cancer.* 2004;101(3):518–526. PMID: 15274064.

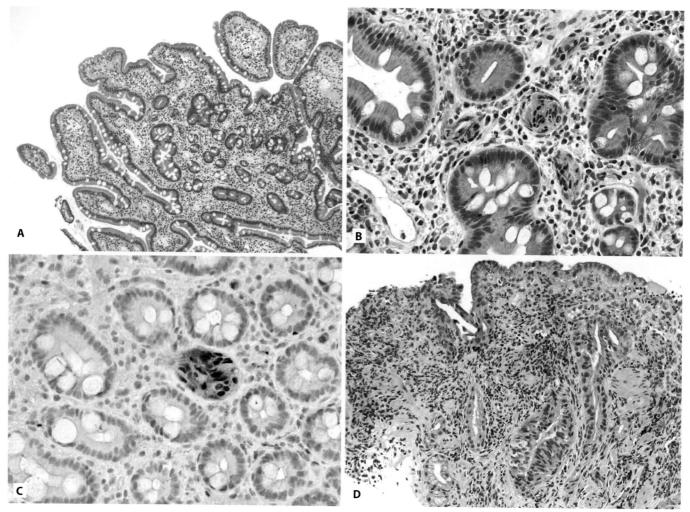

FIGURE 22-19. Biopsy with limited atypical cells. The biopsy from the ampulla consists mostly of intestinal-type mucosa, but with rare small clusters of atypical cells among normal glands, which may represent "crushed" glands (**A**). But, a higher-magnification view raises the possibility of these representing infiltrating carcinoma (**B**). Immunohistochemically, the suspected cell clusters exhibit discretely strong nuclear p53 staining (**C**). Rebiopsy confirmed the presence of an invasive ampullary carcinoma (**D**).

8. Verhulst J, Ferdinande L, Demetter P, Ceelen W. Mucinous subtype as prognostic factor in colorectal cancer: a systematic review and meta-analysis. *J Clin Pathol.* 2012;65(5):381–388. PMID: 22259177.

9. Whitcomb E, Liu X, Xiao SY. Crohn enteritis-associated small bowel adenocarcinomas exhibit gastric differentiation. *Hum Pathol.* 2014;45(2):359–367. PMID: 24331840.

10. Kadmon M, Tandara A, Herfarth C. Duodenal adenomatosis in familial adenomatous polyposis coli. A review of the literature and results from the Heidelberg Polyposis Register. *Int J Colorectal Dis.* 2001;16(2):63–75. PMID: 11355321.

11. Jagelman DG, DeCosse JJ, Bussey HJ. Upper gastrointestinal cancer in familial adenomatous polyposis. *Lancet.* 1988;1(8595):1149–1151. PMID: 2896968.

12. Offerhaus GJ, Giardiello FM, Krush AJ, et al. The risk of upper gastrointestinal cancer in familial adenomatous polyposis. *Gastroenterology.* 1992;102(6):1980–1982. PMID: 1316858.

13. Offerhaus GJ, Entius MM, Giardiello FM. Upper gastrointestinal polyps in familial adenomatous polyposis. *Hepatogastroenterology.* 1999;46(26):667–669. PMID: 10370594.

14. Koornstra JJ. Small bowel endoscopy in familial adenomatous polyposis and Lynch syndrome. *Best Pract Res Clin Gastroenterol.* 2012; 26(3):359–368. PMID: 22704577.

15. Arber N, Moshkowitz M. Small bowel polyposis syndromes. *Curr Gastroenterol Rep.* 2011;13(5):435–441. PMID: 21800071.

16. Plum N, May A, Manner H, Ell C. Small-bowel diagnosis in patients with familial adenomatous polyposis: comparison of push enteroscopy, capsule endoscopy, ileoscopy, and enteroclysis. *Z Gastroenterol.* 2009;47(4):339–346. PMID: 19358059.

17. Genta RM, Feagins LA. Advanced precancerous lesions in the small bowel mucosa. *Best Pract Res Clin Gastroenterol.* 2013;27(2):225–233. PMID: 23809242.

18. Vasen HF, Wijnen JT, Menko FH, et al. Cancer risk in families with hereditary nonpolyposis colorectal cancer diagnosed by mutation analysis. *Gastroenterology.* 1996;110(4):1020–1027. PMID: 8612988.

19. Watson P, Lynch HT. Extracolonic cancer in hereditary nonpolyposis colorectal cancer. *Cancer.* 1993;71(3):677–685. PMID: 8431847.

20. Babba T, Schischmanoff O, Lagorce C, et al. Small bowel carcinoma revealing HNPCC syndrome. *Gastroenterol Clin Biol.* 2010;34(4–5): 325–328. PMID: 20627638.

21. Schulmann K, Brasch FE, Kunstmann E, et al. HNPCC-associated small bowel cancer: clinical and molecular characteristics. *Gastroenterology*. 2005;128(3):590–599. PMID: 15765394.

22. Lim W, Olschwang S, Keller JJ, et al. Relative frequency and morphology of cancers in STK11 mutation carriers. *Gastroenterology*. 2004;126(7):1788–1794. PMID: 15188174.

23. Giardiello FM, Brensinger JD, Tersmette AC, et al. Very high risk of cancer in familial Peutz-Jeghers syndrome. *Gastroenterology*. 2000;119(6):1447–1453. PMID: 11113065.

24. Palascak-Juif V, Bouvier AM, Cosnes J, et al. Small bowel adenocarcinoma in patients with Crohn's disease compared with small bowel adenocarcinoma de novo. *Inflamm Bowel Dis*. 2005;11(9):828–832. PMID: 16116317.

25. Greenstein AJ, Sachar DB, Smith H, Janowitz HD, Aufses AH Jr. A comparison of cancer risk in Crohn's disease and ulcerative colitis. *Cancer*. 1981;48(12):2742–2745. PMID: 7306930.

26. Bernstein CN, Blanchard JF, Kliewer E, Wajda A. Cancer risk in patients with inflammatory bowel disease: a population-based study. *Cancer*. 2001;91(4):854–862. PMID: 11241255.

27. Canavan C, Abrams KR, Mayberry J. Meta-analysis: colorectal and small bowel cancer risk in patients with Crohn's disease. *Aliment Pharmacol Ther*. 2006;23(8):1097–1104. PMID: 16611269.

28. Elriz K, Carrat F, Carbonnel F, Marthey L, Bouvier AM, Beaugerie L. Incidence, presentation, and prognosis of small bowel adenocarcinoma in patients with small bowel Crohn's disease: a prospective observational study. *Inflamm Bowel Dis*. 2013;19(9):1823–1826. PMID: 23702807.

29. Simpson S, Traube J, Riddell RH. The histologic appearance of dysplasia (precarcinomatous change) in Crohn's disease of the small and large intestine. *Gastroenterology*. 1981;81(3):492–501. PMID: 7250636.

30. Cuvelier C, Bekaert E, De Potter C, Pauwels C, De Vos M, Roels H. Crohn's disease with adenocarcinoma and dysplasia. Macroscopical, histological, and immunohistochemical aspects of two cases. *Am J Surg Pathol*. 1989;13(3):187–196. PMID: 2465699.

31. Sigel JE, Petras RE, Lashner BA, Fazio VW, Goldblum JR. Intestinal adenocarcinoma in Crohn's disease: a report of 30 cases with a focus on coexisting dysplasia. *Am J Surg Pathol*. 1999;23(6):651–655. PMID: 10366146.

32. Dossett LA, White LM, Welch DC, et al. Small bowel adenocarcinoma complicating Crohn's disease: case series and review of the literature. *Am Surg*. 2007;73(11):1181–1187. PMID: 18092659.

33. Corrao G, Corazza GR, Bagnardi V, et al. Mortality in patients with coeliac disease and their relatives: a cohort study. *Lancet*. 2001;358(9279):356–361. PMID: 11502314.

34. Askling J, Linet M, Gridley G, Halstensen TS, Ekstrom K, Ekbom A. Cancer incidence in a population-based cohort of individuals hospitalized with celiac disease or dermatitis herpetiformis. *Gastroenterology*. 2002;123(5):1428–1435. PMID: 12404215.

35. Howdle PD, Jalal PK, Holmes GK, Houlston RS. Primary small-bowel malignancy in the UK and its association with coeliac disease. *QJM*. 2003;96(5):345–353. PMID: 12702783.

36. Daveson AJ, Anderson RP. Small bowel endoscopy and coeliac disease. *Best Pract Res Clin Gastroenterol*. 2012;26(3):315–323. PMID: 22704573.

37. Straker RJ, Gunasekaran S, Brady PG. Adenocarcinoma of the jejunum in association with celiac sprue. *J Clin Gastroenterol*. 1989;11(3):320–323. PMID: 2754219.

38. Bruno CJ, Batts KP, Ahlquist DA. Evidence against flat dysplasia as a regional field defect in small bowel adenocarcinoma associated with celiac sprue. *Mayo Clin Proc*. 1997;72(4):320–322. PMID: 9121177.

39. Rampertab SD, Forde KA, Green PH. Small bowel neoplasia in coeliac disease. *Gut*. 2003;52(8):1211–1214. PMID: 12865284. PMCID: PMC1773745.

40. Green PH, Rampertab SD. Small bowel carcinoma and coeliac disease. *Gut*. 2004;53(5):774. PMID: 15082608. PMCID: PMC1774047.

41. Kimura W, Futakawa N, Yamagata S, et al. Different clinicopathologic findings in two histologic types of carcinoma of papilla of Vater. *Jpn J Cancer Res*. 1994;85(2):161–166. PMID: 7511574.

42. Howe JR, Klimstra DS, Moccia RD, Conlon KC, Brennan MF. Factors predictive of survival in ampullary carcinoma. *Ann Surg*. 1998;228(1):87–94. PMID: 9671071. PMCID: PMC1191432.

43. Zhou H, Schaefer N, Wolff M, Fischer HP. Carcinoma of the ampulla of Vater: comparative histologic/immunohistochemical classification and follow-up. *Am J Surg Pathol*. 2004;28(7):875–882. PMID: 15223956.

44. Chu PG, Schwarz RE, Lau SK, Yen Y, Weiss LM. Immunohistochemical staining in the diagnosis of pancreatobiliary and ampulla of Vater adenocarcinoma: application of CDX2, CK17, MUC1, and MUC2. *Am J Surg Pathol*. 2005;29(3):359–367. PMID: 15725805.

45. Kumari N, Prabha K, Singh RK, Baitha DK, Krishnani N. Intestinal and pancreatobiliary differentiation in periampullary carcinoma: the role of immunohistochemistry. *Hum Pathol*. 2013;44(10):2213–2219. PMID: 23834763.

46. Westgaard A, Tafjord S, Farstad IN, et al. Pancreatobiliary versus intestinal histologic type of differentiation is an independent prognostic factor in resected periampullary adenocarcinoma. *BMC Cancer*. 2008;8:170. PMID: 18547417. PMCID: PMC2430209.

47. Blackman E, Nash SV. Diagnosis of duodenal and ampullary epithelial neoplasms by endoscopic biopsy: a clinicopathologic and immunohistochemical study. *Hum Pathol*. 1985;16(9):901–910. PMID: 4029945.

48. Overman MJ, Pozadzides J, Kopetz S, et al. Immunophenotype and molecular characterisation of adenocarcinoma of the small intestine. *Br J Cancer*. 2010;102(1):144–150. PMID: 19935793. PMCID: PMC2813754.

49. Lee MJ, Lee HS, Kim WH, Choi Y, Yang M. Expression of mucins and cytokeratins in primary carcinomas of the digestive system. *Mod Pathol*. 2003;16(5):403–410. PMID: 12748245.

50. Chen ZM, Wang HL. Alteration of cytokeratin 7 and cytokeratin 20 expression profile is uniquely associated with tumorigenesis of primary adenocarcinoma of the small intestine. *Am J Surg Pathol*. 2004;28(10):1352–1359. PMID: 15371952.

51. Delaunoit T, Neczyporenko F, Limburg PJ, Erlichman C. Pathogenesis and risk factors of small bowel adenocarcinoma: a colorectal cancer sibling? *Am J Gastroenterol*. 2005;100(3):703–710. PMID: 15743371.

52. Arai M, Shimizu S, Imai Y, et al. Mutations of the Ki-ras, p53 and APC genes in adenocarcinomas of the human small intestine. *Int J Cancer*. 1997;70(4):390–395. PMID: 9033644.

53. Arber N, Shapira I, Ratan J, et al. Activation of c-K-ras mutations in human gastrointestinal tumors. *Gastroenterology*. 2000;118(6):1045–1050. PMID: 10833479.

54. Wheeler JM, Warren BF, Mortensen NJ, et al. An insight into the genetic pathway of adenocarcinoma of the small intestine. *Gut*. 2002;50(2):218–223. PMID: 11788563. PMCID: PMC1773117.

55. Blaker H, Helmchen B, Bonisch A, et al. Mutational activation of the RAS-RAF-MAPK and the Wnt pathway in small intestinal adenocarcinomas. *Scand J Gastroenterol*. 2004;39(8):748–753. PMID: 15513360.

56. Fu T, Guzzetta AA, Jeschke J, et al. KRAS G>A mutation favors poor tumor differentiation but may not be associated with prognosis in patients with curatively resected duodenal adenocarcinoma. *Int J Cancer*. 2013;132(11):2502–2509. PMID: 23065691. PMCID: PMC3579006.

57. Zhu L, Kim K, Domenico DR, Appert HE, Howard JM. Adenocarcinoma of duodenum and ampulla of Vater: clinicopathology study and expression of p53, c-neu, TGF-alpha, CEA, and EMA. *J Surg Oncol*. 1996;61(2):100–105. PMID: 8606540.

58. Blaker H, von Herbay A, Penzel R, Gross S, Otto HF. Genetics of adenocarcinomas of the small intestine: frequent deletions at chromosome 18q and mutations of the SMAD4 gene. *Oncogene*. 2002;21(1):158–164. PMID: 11791187.

59. Planck M, Ericson K, Piotrowska Z, Halvarsson B, Rambech E, Nilbert M. Microsatellite instability and expression of MLH1 and MSH2 in carcinomas of the small intestine. *Cancer*. 2003;97(6):1551–1557. PMID: 12627520.

PART FOUR

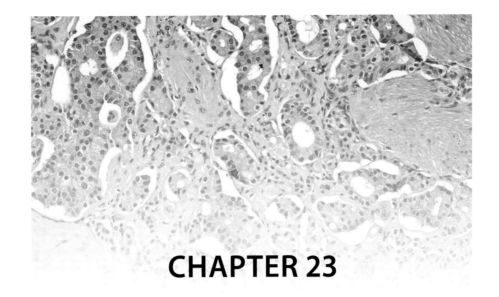

CHAPTER 23

Other Small-Bowel Tumors

H. Aimee Kwak and Shu-Yuan Xiao

◼ INTRODUCTION

In this chapter, neuroendocrine tumors (NETs) and tumors of the mesenchymal components and lymphoid tissue, are discussed. General features of NETs and gastrointestinal stroma tumors (GISTs) have been described in previous chapters as part of general topics. Features unique to the small bowel are emphasized here.

◼ NEUROENDOCRINE TUMORS OF THE SMALL BOWEL

Although adenocarcinoma previously comprised the majority of small-bowel cancers, carcinoid tumors have been the most reported to the National Cancer Data Base (NCDB) since 2000. A review of small-intestinal cancers in the NCDB over 20 years showed that 37.4% were carcinoid tumors, with a slight predominance in males and a median age of occurrence of 66 years. The most common location of carcinoids is in the ileum, followed by the duodenum and jejunum.[1] The World Health Organization (WHO) classification for NETs is divided into 3 categories: NET grade 1, NET grade 2, and neuroendocrine carcinoma (NEC) grade 3.

Duodenal NETs

Duodenal NETs are mostly found in the first and second parts of the duodenum and may be categorized into 5 types: gastrin-producing tumors, somatostatin-producing tumors, gangliocytic paragangliomas, nonfunctional NETs, and NECs.

Gastrinomas can be associated with Zollinger-Ellison syndrome (ZES) and present with peptic ulcer disease, gastroesophageal reflux, or diarrhea from excess gastric acid production. Approximately 22%–26% of gastrinomas are associated with type I multiple endocrine neoplasia (MEN 1), while the rest arise sporadically.[2,3] Somatostatinomas are usually periampullary. Compared to their pancreatic counterpart, most duodenal somatostatin-producing tumors do not present with recognizable "somatostatinoma syndrome" (diabetes mellitus, cholelithiasis, and steatorrhea). In addition, duodenal somatostatinomas are more commonly associated with von Recklinghausen's disease (neurofibromatosis type I) than pancreatic somatostatinomas and are more likely to have glandular architecture and psammoma bodies.[4-6] Gangliocytic paragangliomas are usually periampullary. Nonfunctional NETs typically are immunoreactive with serotonin or calcitonin antibodies. Finally, NECs are often periampullary, high-grade, invasive tumors.

The majority of duodenal NETs are nonfunctioning and do not cause symptoms. However, when symptomatic, the symptoms include abdominal pain, dyspepsia, or gastrointestinal (GI) bleeding. The tumors are polypoid or sessile, submucosal lesions[7,8] endoscopically. Duodenal NETs are usually single lesions restricted to the submucosa, although many also involve the mucosa. The average size of the tumor ranges from 1.2 to 1.8 cm. Histologically, the tumors are characterized by uniform cells that form insular, solid, or glandular architecture (Figure 23-1). The tumor cells usually have a medium amount of granular cytoplasm, round nuclei,

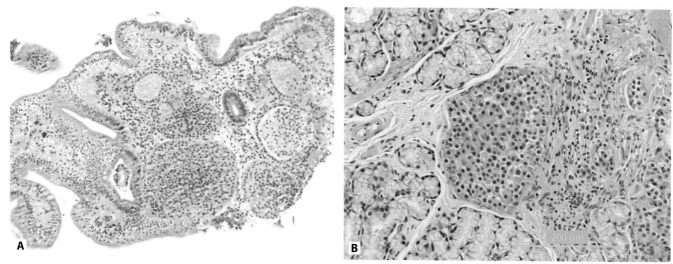

FIGURE 23-1. Duodenal neuroendocrine tumor. The mucosal biopsy reveals nests of well-differentiated neuroendocrine tumor cells infiltrating the mucosa (**A**) and submucosa (**B**).

and stippled chromatin (Figure 23-2). Immunohistochemistry (IHC) typically shows positive staining for chromogranin, neuron-specific enolase (NSE), and synaptophysin. Specific hormones such as gastrin, somatostatin, or serotonin may also be detected through IHC and if positive, may be assessed in the serum along with chromogranin A.[9] Gastrinomas, most of which are duodenal, can be seen in 75% of patients with ZES. The tumors can be single or multiple. In about 30% of tumors, there is metastasis.[10] There are no unique histologic features for gastrinomas (Figure 23-3), but positive immunostain for gastrin is diagnostic (Figure 23-4). Somatostinoma is characterized by glandular formation, often with psammoma bodies (Figure 23-5).

The most sensitive method of detection of duodenal NETs is endoscopy with endoscopic ultrasound. After initial diagnosis, imaging with computed tomography (CT) or magnetic resonance imaging (MRI) is helpful in determining the extent of the disease. Although duodenal NETs have a 40%–60% rate of lymph node metastases, the distant metastasis rate is less than 10%. Curative resection is the treatment of choice for most NETs because duodenal NETs are usually indolent and low grade. One study associated the risk of metastases with tumor size greater than 2 cm, tumor invading the muscularis propria, and the presence of mitotic figures.[6] In cases with nonresectable disease or distant metastases, palliative resection or ablative therapy may be used.[9]

FIGURE 23-2. Well-differentiated neuroendocrine tumor. Monotonous population of small endocrine cells with a medium amount of cytoplasm and round nuclei without prominent nucleoli. There is no mitosis.

FIGURE 23-3. Gastrinoma exhibiting a well-circumscribed submucosal mass. The overlying duodenal mucosa exhibits mild peptic injury.

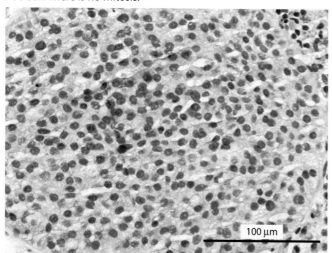

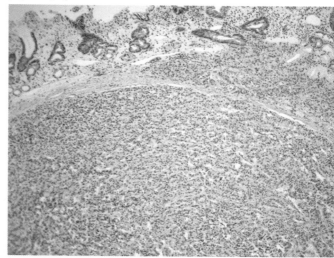

Chemotherapy may be considered in poorly differentiated NECs.[11] The 5-year overall survival (OS) rate for well-differentiated duodenal NETs is 85%.[12]

Gangliocytic Paraganglioma

First described by Dahl in 1957, gangliocytic paragangliomas are uncommon tumors most often found in the second portion of the duodenum near the periampullary region.[13] These tumors are characterized by having three cell types: epithelioid cells, spindle cells, and ganglion-like cells (Figure 23-6). The histogenesis of the tumor remains unclear, with hypotheses including beginnings as a pluripotent stem cell of the neural crest and hamartomatous lesions derived from endodermal and neuroectodermal origin.[13,14]

A recent literature review of gangliocytic paragangliomas demonstrated a wide age range at presentation, with a mean age of 52 years and a male-to-female ratio of 1.5:1. Patients usually present with bleeding or abdominal pain with occasional cases of biliary obstruction.[15,16] On gross examination, the tumor forms a polypoid or pedunculated, white-tan and yellow, solid mass, which can cause mucosal ulceration. Tumor size ranges from 0.5 to 10 cm (mean of 2.5 cm), and the tumor usually arises from the submucosal or muscular layers.

Histology reveals a triphasic tumor resembling a blend of paraganglioma, NET, and ganglioneuroma. The epithelioid cells are arranged in nests or trabeculae and contain amphophilic to eosinophilic, granular cytoplasm, stippled chromatin, and inconspicuous nucleoli (Figure 23-6). Ganglion-like cells have abundant eosinophilic cytoplasm with round nuclei and prominent nucleoli. The spindle cells form slender fascicles, which wrap around the epithelioid nests or ganglion-like cells (Figure 23-6). IHC stains can be helpful in highlighting the different cell types. Epithelioid cells react positively for neuroendocrine markers chromogranin A, synaptophysin, and NSE. Ganglion-like cells express synaptophysin and NSE, while spindle cells show positivity for S100 and neurofilament.[14,15,17]

Although there have been reports of metastases of gangliocytic paraganglioma to the lymph nodes with rare spread to the liver,[18–20] these tumors generally have a benign outcome. Given the good prognosis of this tumor and no consensus on adjuvant therapy, patients are usually treated with local excision and observation without adjuvant therapy.[15]

Jejunoileal NETs

The ileal NETs comprise 45% of all small-intestinal NETs, whereas NETs in the jejunum are rare.[21,22] Although most jejunoileal NETs have positive immunoreactivity for serotonin by IHC, these tumors are usually detected on onset of nonspecific abdominal pain, during workup for metastatic NETs, or incidentally on colonoscopy. Carcinoid syndrome is seen in metastatic disease to the liver, which is characterized by flushing, diarrhea, bronchial wheezing, and carcinoid heart disease (Hedinger syndrome).[23] It has been demonstrated that the first 50 cm of jejunum or "upper jejunum" has a heterogeneous group of NETs expressing gastrin or

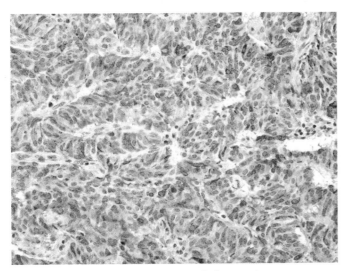

FIGURE 23-4. Gastrinoma: immunostain for gastrin.

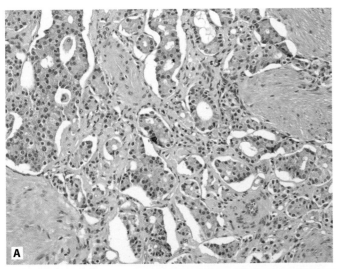
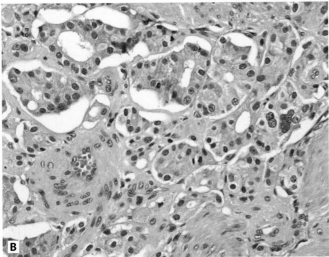

FIGURE 23-5. Duodenal somatostinoma. The tumor forms an anastomosing glandular pattern (**A**), but otherwise shows typical endocrine features cytologically (**B**). Rarely, psammoma bodies may be seen as well.

PART FOUR

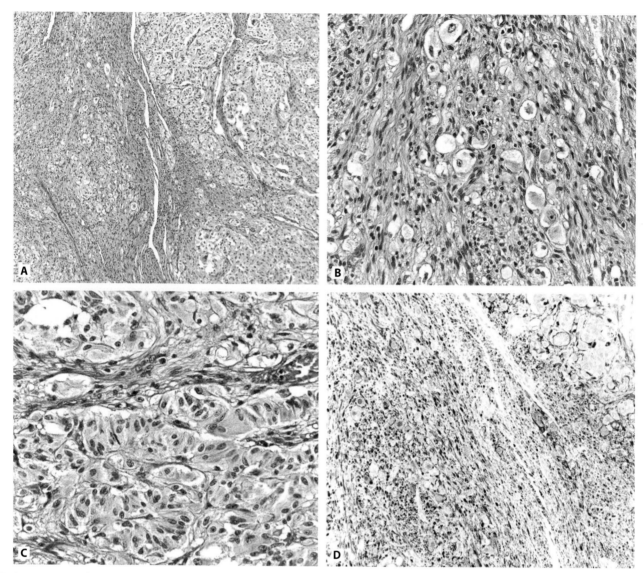

FIGURE 23-6. Gangliocytic paraganglioma. Duodenal submucosal mass. **A.** Heterologous components of neuroendocrine cells form trabeculli and nests to the right and a mixed spindle cell and ganglion cells to the left. **B.** The gangliocytic component with interspersed spindle cells is seen. **C.** The epithelioid endocrine tumor component is shown. **D.** Immunostain for S100 highlights the sustentacular cells.

glucagon or no hormone expression; the "lower jejunum" and ileum are enterochromaffin tumors with serotonin expression.[22]

Jejunoileal NETs have a male predominance, with a male-to-female ratio of 2.2 and a median age of presentation of 62 years. The tumors are usually single, and 47% are 2 cm or larger. Histologically, the majority of jejunoileal tumors have an insular pattern (Figure 23-7), with expression of chromogranin A and NSE by IHC. Over 75% of the NETs have transmural invasion, 31% have nodal metastases, and 32% have distant metastases. The prognosis of jejunoileal NETs is dependent on stage; the 5-year OS is 58%–85% for stage IV disease and 91%–100% for stage I–III tumors.[24,25] In a multivariate analysis, Ki-67 was an independent risk factor for an unfavorable outcome.[25]

Cancer located in the Meckel diverticulum (MDC) can occur but is extremely rare[26]; over 75% of these are malignant. The patients are diagnosed at a mean age of 61 years, with a male predominance of 2:1.

According to the European Neuroendocrine Tumor Society guidelines, histology is necessary for diagnosing jejunoileal NETs, with the help of IHC for chromogranin A and synaptophysin. In addition, lab tests to measure plasma levels of chromogranin A and urinary 5-hydroxyindoleacetic acid (5-HIAA) should be performed to determine if the tumor is functional. Imaging modalities after initial diagnosis include CT or MRI with positron emission tomography (PET) or somatostatin receptor imaging, if applicable. Treatment should aim for cure, with segmental resection and lymph node dissection.[27] In nonresectable disease, surgery

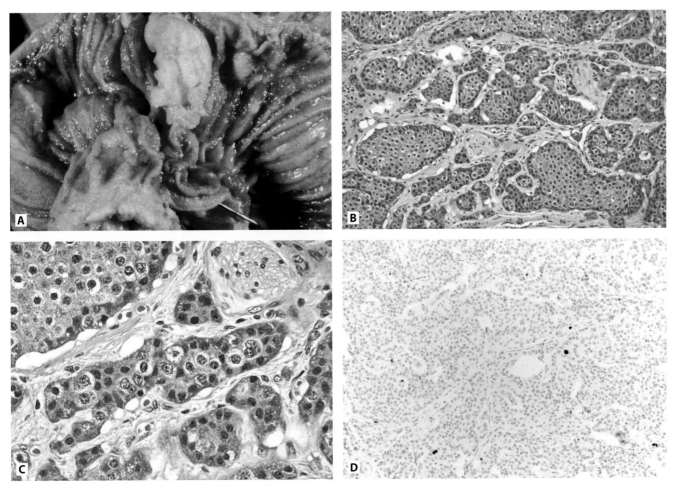

FIGURE 23-7. Ileal carcinoid. **A.** Carcinoid tumor of the ileum, with yellow color and homogeneous texture. **B.** The tumor focally assumes an insular pattern. **C.** High-power view of nuclei demonstrating a mixture of fine and coarse chromatin, imparting a "salt-and-pepper" appearance. **D.** Ki-67 index by immunostain.

can be performed for palliative purposes. Other treatment modalities for nonresectable disease include somatostatin analogues, ablation, chemotherapy, and radiotherapy.[28,29]

GASTROINTESTINAL STROMAL TUMORS

Small-bowel GISTs have an equal gender distribution, with a median age of 53 years for male and 59 years for female. Patients usually present with anemia or acute abdomen. The tumors range from 4.5 to 7 cm in median size, with duodenal tumors being smaller.[30,31] Small-bowel GISTS can be sessile, pedunculated to round, or hourglass shaped (Chapter 5, Figure 5-1) and can form a small intraluminal or large external mass, commonly seen with ulceration (Figure 23-8). The larger lesions can have central necrosis with cavitation. As discussed in Chapter 5, GISTs arise from interstitial cells of Cajal (ICC), some of which are associated with the myenteric neural plexus located between the two layers of muscularis propria. Occasionally, the origin of GISTs from this location can be easily discernible (Figure 23-9).

Histologically, the tumor can have single or multiple nodules (Figure 23-10). Small-intestinal GISTs have

FIGURE 23-8. Gastrointestinal stromal tumor. This large tumor manifests as an intraluminal protrusion with central ulceration.

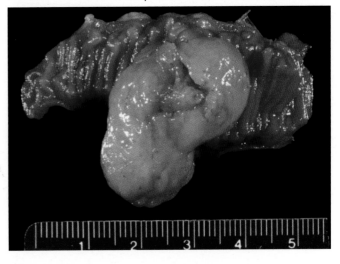

PART FOUR

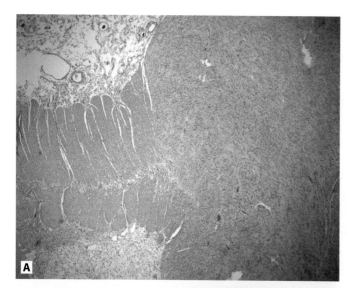

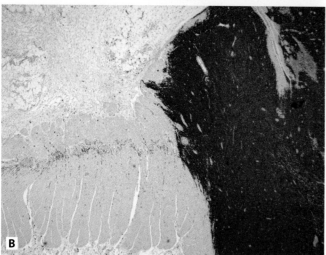

FIGURE 23-9. A gastrointestinal stromal tumor (GIST) arising from the same location as the myenteric plexus. **A.** A large tumor arising between the 2 layers of muscularis propria. **B.** Immunostain for DOG-1 (anoctamin 1) demonstrates diffuse staining of the tumor.

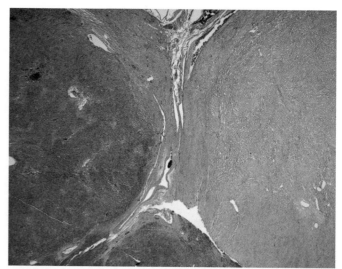

FIGURE 23-10. Gastrointestinal stromal tumor (GIST) with multiple nodules. This small-bowel GIST consists of multiple well-circumscribed nodules with distinctive features, with markedly hypercellular ones and nearly hyalinized hypocellular ones.

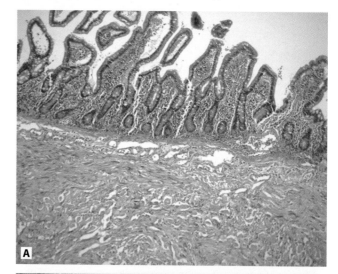

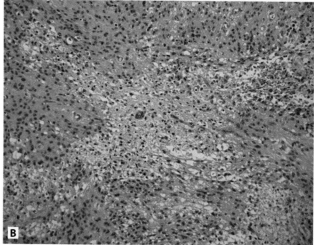

FIGURE 23-11. Gastrointestinal stromal tumor. **A.** Submucosal mass of small bowel, spindle cell type, with thick skeinoid fibers. **B.** Epithelioid type with necrosis.

a relatively monotypic spindled cell morphology, with a reported 44%–52% demonstrating eosinophilic stromal globules designated as skenoid fibers (Chapter 5, Figure 5-7) (Figure 23-11), which represent tangles of curvilinear fibers with fluffy borders on electron microscopy.[30,32,33] Occasionally, small-intestinal GISTs have an epithelioid morphology (Figure 23-11B), which has been associated with malignant behavior. Other high-risk features include tumor necrosis (Figure 23-11B). However, intratumoral degeneration is common (Figure 23-12), which should not be confused with necrosis. The tumor cells usually express KIT (CD117) and DOG-1 (anoctamin 1) and have variable coexpression of CD34, smooth muscle actin (SMA), and S100 (40%–79%, 23%–34%, and 14%–37% of cases, respectively). Clinicopathologic studies of small-intestinal GISTs have shown that

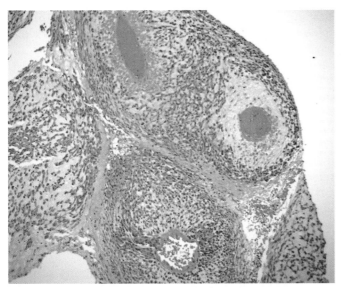

FIGURE 23-12. A jejunal gastrointestinal stromal tumor with degenerative changes.

prognosis is dependent on size and mitotic count, with an overall two-fold increase of tumor-related mortality compared to gastric GISTs. Duodenal GISTs greater than 5 cm or with more than 5 mitoses per 50 high-power fields (HPF) had increased mortality, and jejunal and ileal GISTs greater than 10 cm or with more than 5 mitoses per 50 HPF had a greater likelihood of metastasizing.[30,33]

CLEAR CELL SARCOMA-LIKE GASTROINTESTINAL TUMOR

Clear cell sarcoma (CSS) is a rare soft tissue neoplasm formerly known as malignant melanoma of soft parts due to its melanocytic differentiation appreciated on light and electron microscopy. First described by Enzinger in 1965, CSS usually affects young adults and involves the tendons and aponeuroses of the lower extremities.[34] The clear cell sarcoma-like gastrointestinal tumor (CCSLGT) is also known as an osteoclast-rich tumor of the GI tract, with features resembling CSS of soft parts and is a rare neoplasm primarily seen in the ileum (see also Chapter 5). Unlike melanoma, which frequently exhibits mutations in BRAF, CSS and CCSLGT have the characteristic translocations t(12;22)(q13q12)(EWS-ATF1) and t(2;22)(q34q12)(EWS-CREB1), respectively.[35–38]

Although CSS and CCSLGT share a common EWS rearrangement and are positive for S100 on IHC, CCSLGT tends to behave more aggressively and is unlikely to express melanocytic markers HMB45, MITF, or Melan A.[37,39] The median age of those affected is 37 years, and there is no gender predilection. Patients often present with obstructive symptoms and anemia. Endoscopic examination or CT imaging may detect thickening of the small-intestinal wall or a mass with overlying ulceration.[40,41] The tumor is solid

with a cut surface that is gray to white-tan; the median size is approximately 4 cm.

Histologically, the tumor demonstrates monomorphic cells in solid sheets, nests, or fascicles separated by fibrous septa. The cells are medium size and polygonal, with clear or pale eosinophilic cytoplasm, vesicular chromatin, and prominent nucleoli. Scattered CD68+ osteoclast-type multinucleated giant cells may be seen. IHC consistently demonstrates positivity for S100, with variable immunoreactivity seen with vimentin, CD56, NSE, and synaptophysin. The tumor cells are negative for HMB45 and CD117. Differential diagnosis includes GIST, metastatic melanoma, epithelioid malignant peripheral nerve sheath tumor (MPNST), and perivascular epithelioid cell neoplasm (PEComa, discussed in a following section).

Treatment includes resection of the tumor with local lymph node resection as approximately 60% of cases have metastases to the lymph nodes. Distant metastases occur in the liver. A beneficial role of chemotherapy has not been documented. CCSLGT is an aggressive neoplasm; one study of 12 cases and another report based on review of the literature reported a 50% mortality rate.[41,42]

LEIOMYOMA AND LEIOMYOSARCOMA

Leiomyoma (LM) and leiomyosarcoma (LMS) are rare in the small intestine.[43–45] A case series[46] of small-intestinal smooth muscle tumors had 9 LM and 16 LMS occurring in 15 men and 10 women with a median age of 62 years. Patients with clinical symptoms most often presented with intestinal obstruction or GI bleeding. LMS ranges from endophytic to polypoid and solid to cystic with a cut surface that is grayish-white to tan. LM has fascicles or bundles of uniform, spindled, smooth muscle cells with eosinophilic cytoplasm (Figure 23-13). Cytoplasmic eosinophilic globules are seen in some of the cases. There should be no nuclear atypia, and mitoses are rare (<1–3/50 HPF). Histologic features of LMS include the presence of significant nuclear atypia, increased mitoses (15 of 16 cases ≥ 35/50 HPF), and coagulative necrosis (Figure 23-14). By definition, LM and LMS are positive for SMA and desmin, and negative for CD117/c-kit. Like its uterine counterpart, small-bowel LMS can also exhibit increased p16 expression (Figure 23-14D).

It is not usual to find scattered ICC in smooth muscle tumors when sections are evaluated with immunostain for CD117 or DOG-1 (Figure 23-15). This staining pattern should not be confused with GIST.

Leiomyosarcoma has high recurrence and mortality rates. High histological grade (based on degree of cellularity, differentiation, number of mitoses, and amount of tumor necrosis) and size greater than 5 cm predict recurrence.[47] Due to the rarity of cases, treatment guidelines for LM and LMS are not well established. Surgical resection of the tumor is usually performed with long-term follow-up due to the risk of late recurrence (defined as recurrence occurring 5 years after surgical resection).[48]

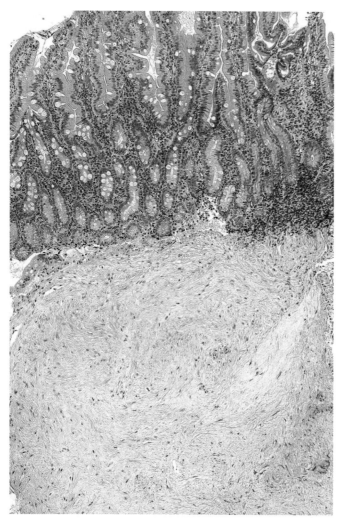

FIGURE 23-13. Duodenal leiomyoma. This well-circumscribed tumor is rather hypocellular, consisting of spindle cells with bland nuclei.

▉ PERIVASCULAR EPITHELIOID CELL TUMORS

Perivascular epithelioid cell tumors are a family of mesenchymal tumors that express melanocytic and smooth muscle markers. The cell of origin is unknown. PEComas are rare in the GI tract, with the largest cohort study consisting of 35 patients.[49] The most frequent location for GI PEComas was in the colon, followed by one-third of cases reported in the small intestine. The patients usually have abdominal pain, GI bleeding, and weight loss. The median tumor size is 6.2 cm, and the tumor usually involves all layers of the bowel wall and even mesentery. Gross or endoscopic examination showed either a polypoid lesion or a mass.[49]

Histologically, PEComas in the GI tract are variably circumscribed and form nests, trabeculae, or sheets of tumor cells that are separated by delicate vasculature (Figure 23-16). The tumor cells are usually purely epithelioid or predominantly epithelioid mixed with a spindled cell component and rarely are purely spindled. The epithelioid cells are round, ovoid, or polygonal with abundant granular eosinophilic or clear cytoplasm and prominent nucleoli (Figure 23-16). The spindled cells have pale eosinophilic cytoplasm that is somewhat granular.

The differential diagnosis for PEComas is vast. IHC stains are needed in distinguishing PEComas from an epithelioid GI stromal tumor, paraganglioma, metastatic renal cell carcinoma, or CSS-like tumor. The tumor cells either focally or diffusely react for at least one melanocytic marker (HMB45, Melan A, MITF, or TFE3) and also express smooth muscle markers such as SMA, caldesmon, or desmin. The tumor cells are negative for cytokeratins, chromogranin A, CD10, and CD34. S100 is positive in a subset of tumors, with up to 18% in one study, although the immunoreactivity is usually focal or weak, in contrast to diffuse, nuclear positivity in melanomas. In addition, a careful clinical history should be acquired to rule out metastatic melanoma.

Doyle et al. reported that increased mitoses of more than 2/10 HPF, marked nuclear atypia, and diffuse pleomorphism are associated with metastases. PEComas of the GI tract demonstrate broad biological behavior, from benign to aggressive, as seen in high-grade sarcomas. In the GI case series, 37% of patients with follow-up had metastases, and 16% died of the disease. In addition to excision of the primary lesion, 10 patients with metastases also received adjuvant chemotherapy.[49] PEComas in the GI tract are not associated with patients with tuberous sclerosis (TSC), who have germline mutations in *TSC1* and *TSC2* genes; however, sporadic PEComas have been shown to have mutations in *TSC2*. Mutations in *TSC1* and *TSC2* lead to activation of the mTOR signaling pathway. Thus, chemotherapy regimens can include mTOR inhibitors, with some efficacy also shown in patients without TSC.[50]

▉ DESMOID TUMOR/MESENTERIC FIBROMATOSIS

Desmoid tumors are rare mesenchymal tumors composed of monoclonal proliferations of myofibroblasts; they are known to be locally aggressive without potential of metastasis. They are classified as extra-abdominal and abdominal fibromatosis, with the designations further subdivided into superficial abdominal and intra-abdominal fibromatosis. Superficial abdominal fibromatosis involves the abdominal wall muscles, whereas intra-abdominal fibromatosis most often occurs within the mesentery and can have extension into the retroperitoneum. This entity is also referred to as mesenteric fibromatosis.

Desmoid tumors are usually sporadic. Patients are diagnosed at an average age of 31–40 years, with a female-to-male ratio of 1.6:1. About 13%–16% of tumors occur in association with familial adenomatous polyposis (FAP).[51,52] Both sporadic and FAP-related desmoid tumors tend to be associated with previous abdominal surgery, trauma, and high estrogen levels. Furthermore, FAP-associated desmoid tumors are predominantly abdominal with intra-abdominal tumors and have a poor outcome due to complications such

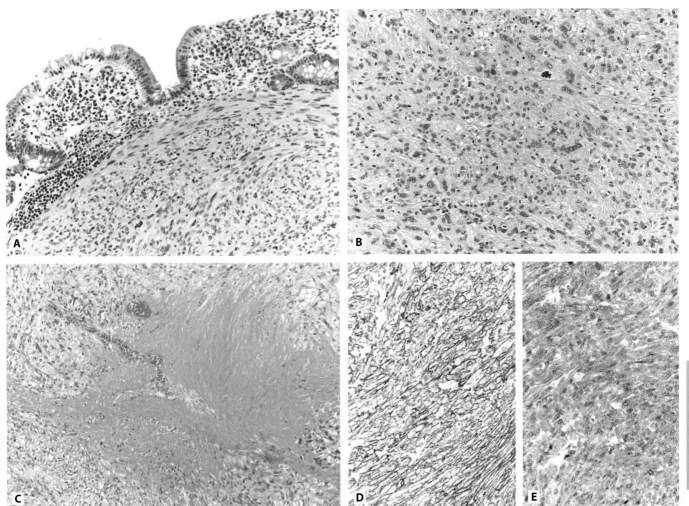

FIGURE 23-14. Leiomyosarcoma. This was from a 79-year-old woman who presented with abdominal pain. A 5.1-cm fungating ileal mass was identified. The tumor is intramural but focally extends to the mucosa, causing flattening of villi (**A**). It is mainly spindle cells but with a focal epithelioid cell component with marked nuclear atypia and frequent mitosis (**B**). Foci of necrosis are evident as well (**C**). Immunohistochemically, the tumor was focally positive for desmin, diffusely positive for smooth muscle actin (SMA) (**D**), but negative for CD117 and DOG-1. Tumor cells also exhibited p16 overexpression (**E**), but staining for EBER was negative.

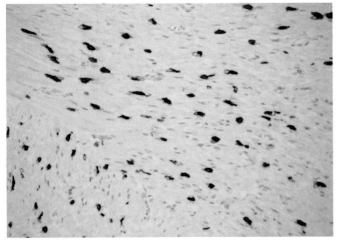

FIGURE 23-15. Smooth muscle tumor with scattered CD117-positive cells.

as ureteral or intestinal obstruction with perforation, fistula formation, and hemorrhage.[51,53,54]

Patients with mesenteric fibromatosis most often present with abdominal pain or a painless abdominal mass. Mesenteric fibromatosis forms solitary or multiple, firm, well-to-poorly circumscribed masses with a wide range in size, from less than 1 cm to 30 cm and a median size of 5 cm to 7 cm.[55,56] The cut surface of these tumors is glistening and white and can resemble a scar[57] (Figure 23-17).

Diagnosis is made by histologic examination demonstrating bundles of uniform, elongated, spindled cells in a collagenous stroma (Figure 23-18). The nuclei contain minute nucleoli and are without cytologic atypia. The borders of the lesion demonstrate infiltration of the surrounding tissue, including extension into the small-intestinal wall. Inflammation is usually scant, and myxoid change, keloid collagen fibers, and muscular hyperplasia of the small arteries

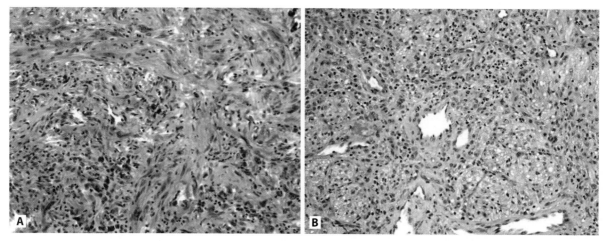

FIGURE 23-16. Small-bowel perivascular epithelioid cell neoplasm (PEComa). **A.** Spindle area. **B.** Epithelioid area.

may be present. The tumor cells are often positive for SMA and have nuclear positivity for β-catenin (Figure 23-18B), but typically are negative for desmin.[58]

Desmoid tumors are locally aggressive with a high recurrence rate of 20%–29% or higher. The 5-year local recurrence-free survival ranges from 50% to 80%, and factors associated with recurrence are young age and a history of a prior recurrence.[56,59–61] Tumor location and margin status have variable prognostic value for recurrence. The mainstay of treatment is surgical resection. Although controversial, patients may receive systemic or radiation therapy if they present with recurrence, have unresectable disease, or have positive tumor resection margins. Even with a high recurrence rate, deaths due to desmoid tumors are uncommon.[56,59,60]

ANGIOSARCOMA

An angiosarcoma is a high-grade vascular tumor that rarely occurs as a primary malignancy of the small intestine. Historically, cases in the GI tract were associated with exposure

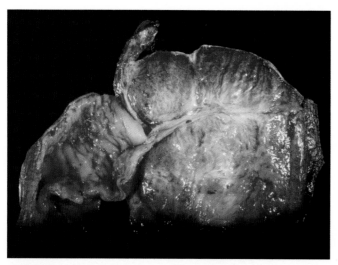

FIGURE 23-17. Desmoid tumor. This large fibrotic tumor encroached on the small bowel, causing severe narrowing.

to radiation therapy for treatment of a gynecologic malignancy, toxins (ie, vinyl chloride, arsenic), or foreign bodies.[62] Patients typically present with abdominal pain, GI bleeding, or anemia and occasionally with obstruction.[63] Clinical diagnosis is difficult due to the nonspecific symptoms. CT, nuclear RBC (red blood cell) tagged scan, barium study, and endoscopy may be used in an extensive search for a source of bleeding.

Angiosarcomas can be single or multifocal.[64] Histologic examination demonstrates a vasoformative, solid, or dimorphic pattern. The vasoformative pattern consists of delicate vascular channels lined by atypical endothelial cells with enlarged and hyperchromatic nuclei, whereas the solid pattern contains sheets of spindle or epithelioid cells with occasional intracytoplasmic lumina or slit-like spaces. The tumor cells can express cytokeratins, which may mimic a carcinoma; however, IHC with vascular markers CD31, CD34, and factor VIII help make the diagnosis of angiosarcoma.[65,66]

Treatment is usually surgical resection. Chemotherapy and radiation therapy may be used, although efficacy and standardization of treatment are not well established. Prognosis is poor, with approximately 75% of patients dying 6 months to 1 year after initial presentation.[64]

LYMPHOMA

The GI tract is the most common site for extranodal non-Hodgkin lymphoma (NHL), comprising 25%–46% of cases[67,68]; the small intestine is the second most common location (10%–35%) (Figure 23-19). Diffuse large B-cell lymphoma (DLBCL) is the most common primary small-intestinal NHL. Other NHLs include low-grade B-cell lymphomas: extranodal mucosa-associated lymphoid tissue (MALT) lymphoma, follicular lymphoma, and mantle cell lymphoma. A recent North American study of primary GI NHLs reported an incidence in those with a median age of 64 years and a slight predominance in males (1.5:1).[69] In the pediatric population, the small intestine is the most common tumor site, and Burkitt lymphoma is the most prevalent NHL.[70]

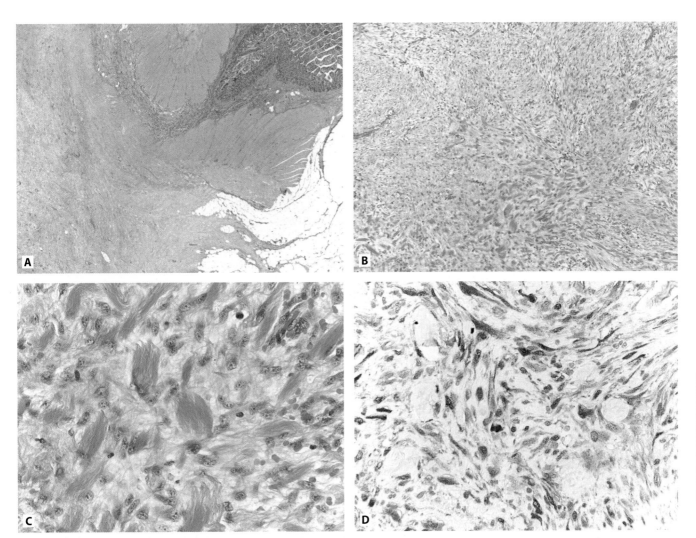

FIGURE 23-18. Desmoid tumor histology. **A.** The tumor involves both the mesentery and the small-bowel wall, focally infiltrating the muscularis propria. **B.** The tumor is hypercellular, consisting of bland spindle cells in fascicles with interspersed thick collagen bundles. **C.** High-power view of the thick collagen bundles cut in short "strokes" due to a highly curved configuration. **D.** Immunostain for β-catenin.

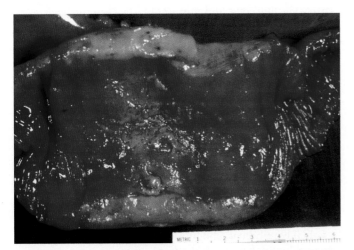

FIGURE 23-19. Lymphoma involving the terminal ileum. The infiltrative process caused marked thickening of the bowel wall and mucosa, with loss of mucosal folds, hemorrhage, and erosions.

In addition, Burkitt lymphoma is often seen in patients with HIV in the United States. T-cell lymphomas of the small intestine are mainly enteropathy-associated T-cell lymphomas, discussed in Chapter 18.

Clinical symptoms are vague and usually include abdominal pain followed less frequently by nausea, weight loss, obstruction, and perforation. Imaging with CT or endoscopic examination may demonstrate multiple nodular or polypoid lesions, also known as multiple lymphomatous polyposis (MLP). Although MLP was initially associated with mantle cell lymphoma, it has also been seen with MALT lymphoma, follicular lymphoma, and DLBCL.[71,72] NHL can also appear annular or as a single mass with or without ulceration.

Diffuse Large B-Cell Lymphoma

Diffuse large B-cell lymphoma is the dominant primary small-intestinal NHL. Histologically, there are diffuse sheets of infiltrative, atypical lymphoid cells, which are 2–4 times

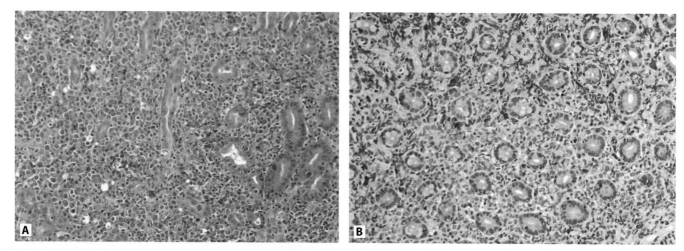

FIGURE 23-20. Diffuse large B-cell lymphoma of the duodenum. **A.** Diffuse infiltration by monotonous, large, atypical lymphocytes, expanding the lamina propria with separation of the glands; a lymphoepithelial lesion is not evident. **B.** One of the common features of lymphocytes is nuclear streaming artifact (upper left corner), particularly in frozen sections.

larger than a normal lymphocyte (Figure 23-20). Immunophenotype will show pan B-cell markers (CD19, CD20, CD22, CD79a), although the neoplastic cells may lose expression of a B-cell marker. Molecular studies demonstrate rearrangements between the immunoglobulin heavy-chain gene and *BCL6*, *BCL2*, or *MYC*. DLBCL may occur de novo or be secondary to transformation of a MALT lymphoma, with the latter demonstrating MALT lymphoma within the lesion.[73] Rarely, the lymphoma can occur as a long-term complication of organ transplantation, in the form of posttransplant lymphoproliferative disorder (Figure 23-21).

MALT Lymphoma

Mucosa-associated lymphoid tissue (MALT) lymphoma is the second most common primary NHL in the small intestine. It is histologically similar to gastric MALT lymphoma, but the lymphoepithelial lesions are less prominent. Morphologically, MALT lymphoma forms a heterogeneous population consisting of small B cells—marginal zone cells, monocytoid cells, centrocyte-like cells, and small lymphocytes—with a dispersed smaller population of immunoblasts. IHC shows an immunophenotype similar to marginal zone B cells (CD20+, CD79a+, CD19+, CD5−, CD10−, CD23−, cyclin D1−). The most common cytogenetic abnormalities include translocations t(11;18)(q21;q21) and t(1;14)(p22;q32) as well as trisomy 3 or 8. If MALT lymphoma has extensive plasmacytic differentiation, the lymphoma cells will demonstrate immunoglobulin light-chain restriction by in situ hybridization.

Immunoproliferative Small-Intestinal Disease (α-Heavy-Chain Disease)

Immunoproliferative small-intestinal disease (IPSID) is a unique type of MALT lymphoma and includes α-heavy-chain disease, which could represent a different phase of the same disease process. Most commonly occurring in the Mediterranean, Africa, and the Middle East, IPSID usually

affects young adults of low socioeconomic status. Clinical presentation includes colicky abdominal pain, chronic intermittent diarrhea, and symptoms due to malabsorption: weight loss, clubbing, and peripheral edema.[74-76] Imaging and endoscopy may show an unremarkable examination or mucosal thickening and nodularity in the duodenum and jejunum. Serum or intestinal secretions may show the presence of elevated immunoglobulin (Ig) A and α-heavy-chain protein.[77,78]

Immunoproliferative small-intestinal disease is divided into 3 stages. Stage A demonstrates a plasmacytic or lymphoplasmacytic infiltrate confined to the mucosa and mesenteric lymph nodes. Stage B shows an infiltrate of CD20+ centrocyte-like B cells forming nodular lymphoepithelial lesions and extends beyond the muscularis mucosa. Stage C has lymphomatous masses with transformation to DLBCL. Immunoblasts and plasmablasts are present and marked cytologic atypia is seen. IHC demonstrates the presence of α-heavy chains without light-chain synthesis in the plasmacytic cells, centrocyte-like cells, and immunoblasts, seen in stages A, B, and C, respectively.[79,80] No consistent cytogenetic abnormalities have been identified.

There has been association of IPSID with *Campylobacter jejuni* infections, and patients with early disease (stage A) may obtain clinical remission with antibiotic treatment.[74,77,81] Two separate studies suggested that early disease should be treated with antibiotics, and intermediate or advanced disease with combined antibiotics and chemotherapy. The 5-year OS rate ranges from 40% to 70%.[74,77] Surgery is generally reserved for palliation or staging and diagnostic purposes.

Follicular Lymphoma

Follicular lymphoma in the GI tract is rare, making up 5% or less of GI lymphomas, and most often involves the duodenum, followed by the ileum.[82,83] The tumors manifest as transmural nodular masses, often causing bowel obstruction (Figure 23-22). The microscopic morphology is indistinguishable from nodal

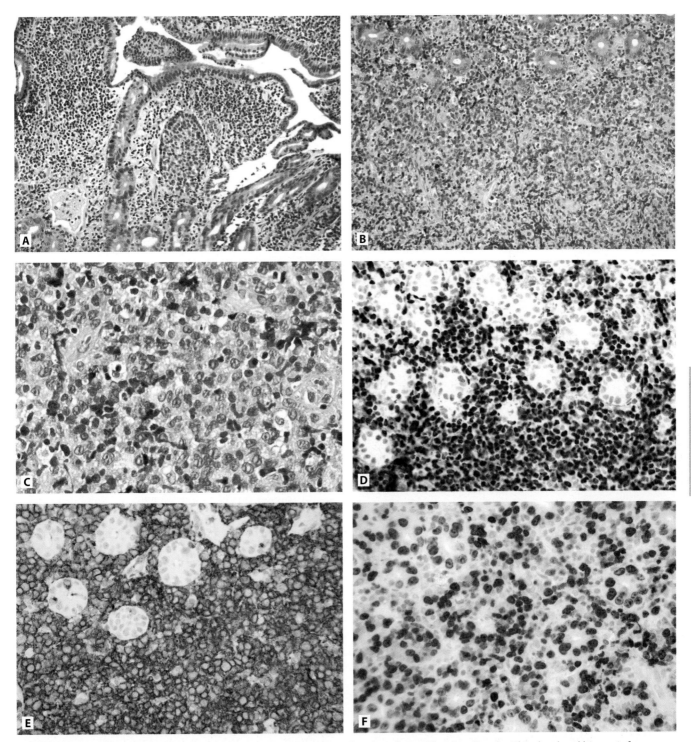

FIGURE 23-21. Diffuse large B-cell lymphoma as a remote posttransplant lymphoproliferative disorder. This duodenal biopsy is from a 37-year-old woman who had a remote history of kidney-pancreas transplantation. There is marked expansion of the small-bowel villi by clusters of large atypical lymphocytes in a background of reactive lymphoplasmacytic infiltration (**A, B**). The tumor cells contain relatively abundant cytoplasm, large nuclei, and one or two small nucleoli in each (**C**). Immunohistochemically, the cells are positive for BCL6 (**D**), CD10 (**E**), CD19, and CD20 and negative for CD3. Ki-67 nuclear stain is noted in over 80% of tumor cells (**F**). In situ hybridization for EBER was negative.

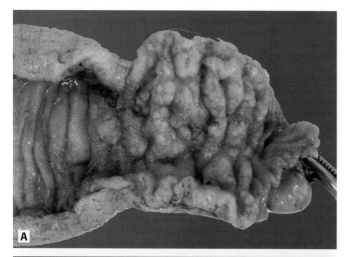

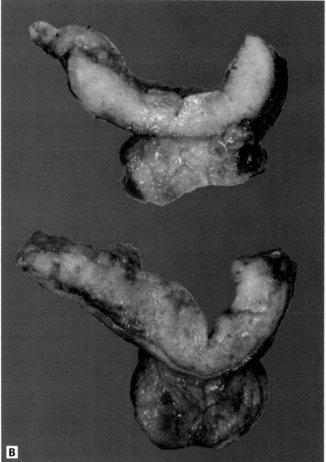

FIGURE 23-22. Follicular lymphoma of jejunum in a patient with small-bowel obstruction. **A.** The circumferential multinodular mass (4.5 cm) is raised on the mucosa. **B.** Cross sectioning showing transmural involvement, with a light-tan, fleshy cut surface.

follicular lymphoma. The neoplastic follicles have germinal centers composed of a monotonous population of centrocytes with cleaved nuclei and larger centroblasts (Figure 23-23). Histologic grading, such as for nodal follicular lymphoma, relies on the number of centroblasts per high-power field (Figure 23-23). The immunophenotypes of the tumor cells are

CD20+, CD10+, Bcl2+, and CD5−, whereas normal germinal centers are Bcl2− and CD10+. The tumor is characterized by t(14;18)(q34;q21) translocation and *BCL2* gene rearrangement.

Mantle Cell Lymphoma

Most commonly associated with MLP, mantle cell lymphoma of the small intestine is histologically identical to its nodal counterpart. Histology usually demonstrates a diffuse or nodular monotonous population of small lymphocytes with angulated nuclei admixed with epithelioid histiocytes and hyalinized small blood vessels. The lymphoma cells express B-cell markers CD19 and CD20. In addition, there is characteristic weak coexpression of CD5, FMC7, and CD43 and expression of cyclinD1. Cytogenetic studies show a t(11;14)(q13;q32) translocation between genes *CCND1* and *IGH*.

Burkitt Lymphoma

The most common small-intestinal malignancy in the pediatric population in the United States, sporadic Burkitt lymphoma, is usually located in the ileocecal region. Histologically, Burkitt lymphoma has appeared as a diffuse infiltrate of monotonous, medium-size cells with frequent mitoses and apoptosis (Figure 23-24). Benign phagocytic histiocytes engulfing apoptotic debris give the lymphoma its characteristic "starry sky" appearance. The cells have a pan B-cell immunophenotype (CD19, CD20, CD22, CD79a) and coexpress CD10 but are negative for CD5. Cytogenetic studies most often show the characteristic translocation t(8;14)(q24;q32) between genes *MYC* and *IGH*. The overall 5- and 10-year survival rates are 87% and 86%, respectively. Surgical resection is recommended for localized disease, whereas surgery, chemotherapy, and radiation are used for metastatic disease.

■ REFERENCES

1. Bilimoria KY, Bentrem DJ, Wayne JD, Ko CY, Bennett CL, Talamonti MS. Small bowel cancer in the United States: changes in epidemiology, treatment, and survival over the last 20 years. *Ann Surg.* 2009;249:63–71.
2. Roy PK, Venzon DJ, Shojamanesh H, et al. Zollinger-Ellison syndrome. Clinical presentation in 261 patients. *Medicine.* 2000;79:379–411.
3. Ruszniewski P, Podevin P, Cadiot G, et al. Clinical, anatomical, and evolutive features of patients with the Zollinger-Ellison syndrome combined with type I multiple endocrine neoplasia. *Pancreas.* 1993;8:295–304.
4. Mao C, Shah A, Hanson DJ, Howard JM. Von Recklinghausen's disease associated with duodenal somatostatinoma: contrast of duodenal versus pancreatic somatostatinomas. *J Surg Oncol.* 1995;59:67–73.
5. Soga J, Yakuwa Y. Somatostatinoma/inhibitory syndrome: a statistical evaluation of 173 reported cases as compared to other pancreatic endocrinomas. *J Exp Clin Cancer Res.* 1999;18:13–22.
6. Burke AP, Sobin LH, Federspiel BH, Shekitka KM, Helwig EB. Carcinoid tumors of the duodenum. A clinicopathologic study of 99 cases. *Arch Pathol Lab Med.* 1990;114:700–704.
7. Waisberg J, Joppert-Netto G, Vasconcellos C, Sartini GH, Miranda LS, Franco MI. Carcinoid tumor of the duodenum: a rare tumor at an unusual site. Case series from a single institution. *Arq Gastroenterol.* 2013;50:3–9.

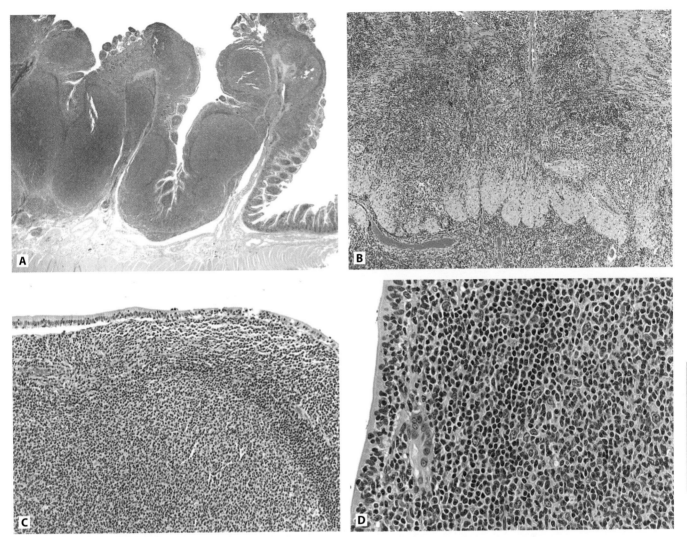

FIGURE 23-23. Follicular lymphoma (same case as in Figure 23-22). **A.** At the edge of the tumor, there are multiple prominent nodular lymphoid follicles in the mucosa and submucosa. **B.** Transmural infiltration of the lymphoid cells with focal disruption of muscularis propria. **C.** The lymphoid nodule composed of a monotonous population of centrocyte-like cells. **D.** There are rare centroblasts (2–3 per HPF). In addition, immunostains demonstrated the B-cell phenotype with staining for CD10, BCL6, BCL2, and a Ki-67 proliferative index of 20% (not shown).

8. Mullen JT, Wang H, Yao JC, et al. Carcinoid tumors of the duodenum. *Surgery.* 2005;138:971–977; discussion 977–978.

9. Jensen RT, Rindi G, Arnold R, et al. Well-differentiated duodenal tumor/carcinoma (excluding gastrinomas). *Neuroendocrinology.* 2006;84:165–172.

10. Donow C, Pipeleers-Marichal M, Schroder S, Stamm B, Heitz PU, Kloppel G. Surgical pathology of gastrinoma. Site, size, multicentricity, association with multiple endocrine neoplasia type 1, and malignancy. *Cancer.* 1991;68:1329–1334.

11. Kloppel G, Couvelard A, Perren A, et al. ENETS consensus guidelines for the standards of care in neuroendocrine tumors: towards a standardized approach to the diagnosis of gastroenteropancreatic neuroendocrine tumors and their prognostic stratification. *Neuroendocrinology.* 2009;90:162–166.

12. Soga J. Endocrinocarcinomas (carcinoids and their variants) of the duodenum. An evaluation of 927 cases. *J Exp Clin Cancer Res.* 2003; 22:349–363.

13. Dahl EV, Waugh JM, Dahlin DC. Gastrointestinal ganglioneuromas; brief review with report of a duodenal ganglioneuroma. *Am J Pathol.* 1957;33:953–965.

14. Perrone T, Sibley RK, Rosai J. Duodenal gangliocytic paraganglioma. An immunohistochemical and ultrastructural study and a hypothesis concerning its origin. *Am J Surg Pathol.* 1985;9:31–41.

15. Okubo Y, Wakayama M, Nemoto T, et al. Literature survey on epidemiology and pathology of gangliocytic paraganglioma. *BMC Cancer.* 2011;11:187.

16. Witkiewicz A, Galler A, Yeo CJ, Gross SD. Gangliocytic paraganglioma: case report and review of the literature. *J Gastrointest Surg.* 2007;11:1351–1354.

17. Barbareschi M, Frigo B, Aldovini D, Leonardi E, Cristina S, Falleni M. Duodenal gangliocytic paraganglioma. Report of a case and review of the literature. *Virchows Arch A Pathol Anat Histopathol.* 1989;416:81–89.

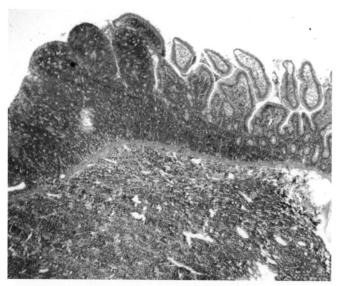

FIGURE 23-24. Burkitt lymphoma of small bowel. The tumor is mainly in the submucosa with focal extension to the mucosa, causing focal villous blunting.

18. Rowsell C, Coburn N, Chetty R. Gangliocytic paraganglioma: a rare case with metastases of all 3 elements to liver and lymph nodes. *Ann Diagn Pathol.* 2011;15:467–471.

19. Inai K, Kobuke T, Yonehara S, Tokuoka S. Duodenal gangliocytic paraganglioma with lymph node metastasis in a 17-year-old boy. *Cancer.* 1989;63:2540–2545.

20. Dookhan DB, Miettinen M, Finkel G, Gibas Z. Recurrent duodenal gangliocytic paraganglioma with lymph node metastases. *Histopathology.* 1993;22:399–401.

21. Lawrence B, Gustafsson BI, Chan A, Svejda B, Kidd M, Modlin IM. The epidemiology of gastroenteropancreatic neuroendocrine tumors. *Endocrinol Metab Clin North Am.* 2011;40:1–18, vii.

22. Burke AP, Thomas RM, Elsayed AM, Sobin LH. Carcinoids of the jejunum and ileum: an immunohistochemical and clinicopathologic study of 167 cases. *Cancer.* 1997;79:1086–1093.

23. Lundin L, Norheim I, Landelius J, Oberg K, Theodorsson-Norheim E. Carcinoid heart disease: relationship of circulating vasoactive substances to ultrasound-detectable cardiac abnormalities. *Circulation.* 1988;77:264–269.

24. Strosberg JR, Weber JM, Feldman M, Coppola D, Meredith K, Kvols LK. Prognostic validity of the American Joint Committee on Cancer staging classification for midgut neuroendocrine tumors. *J Clin Oncol.* 2013;31:420–425.

25. Panzuto F, Campana D, Fazio N, et al. Risk factors for disease progression in advanced jejunoileal neuroendocrine tumors. *Neuroendocrinology.* 2012;96:32–40.

26. Thirunavukarasu P, Sathaiah M, Sukumar S, et al. Meckel's diverticulum—a high-risk region for malignancy in the ileum. Insights from a population-based epidemiological study and implications in surgical management. *Ann Surg.* 2011;253:223–230.

27. Pape UF, Perren A, Niederle B, et al. ENETS Consensus Guidelines for the management of patients with neuroendocrine neoplasms from the jejuno-ileum and the appendix including goblet cell carcinomas. *Neuroendocrinology.* 2012;95:135–156.

28. Pavel M, Baudin E, Couvelard A, et al. ENETS consensus guidelines for the management of patients with liver and other distant metastases from neuroendocrine neoplasms of foregut, midgut, hindgut, and unknown primary. *Neuroendocrinology.* 2012;95:157–176.

29. Ramage JK, Ahmed A, Ardill J, et al. Guidelines for the management of gastroenteropancreatic neuroendocrine (including carcinoid) tumours (NETs). *Gut.* 2012;61:6–32.

30. Miettinen M, Kopczynski J, Makhlouf HR, et al. Gastrointestinal stromal tumors, intramural leiomyomas, and leiomyosarcomas in the duodenum: a clinicopathologic, immunohistochemical, and molecular genetic study of 167 cases. *Am J Surg Pathol.* 2003;27:625–641.

31. Miettinen M, Lasota J. Gastrointestinal stromal tumors: review on morphology, molecular pathology, prognosis, and differential diagnosis. *Arch Pathol Lab Med.* 2006;130:1466–1478.

32. Min KW. Small intestinal stromal tumors with skeinoid fibers. Clinicopathological, immunohistochemical, and ultrastructural investigations. *Am J Surg Pathol.* 1992;16:145–155.

33. Miettinen M, Makhlouf H, Sobin LH, Lasota J. Gastrointestinal stromal tumors of the jejunum and ileum: a clinicopathologic, immunohistochemical, and molecular genetic study of 906 cases before imatinib with long-term follow-up. *Am J Surg Pathol.* 2006;30:477–489.

34. Enzinger FM. Clear-cell sarcoma of tendons and aponeuroses. An analysis of 21 cases. Cancer. 1965;18:1163–1174.

35. Panagopoulos I, Mertens F, Isaksson M, Mandahl N. Absence of mutations of the BRAF gene in malignant melanoma of soft parts (clear cell sarcoma of tendons and aponeuroses). *Cancer Genet Cytogenet.* 2005;156:74–76.

36. Panagopoulos I, Mertens F, Debiec-Rychter M, et al. Molecular genetic characterization of the EWS/ATF1 fusion gene in clear cell sarcoma of tendons and aponeuroses. *Int J Cancer.* 2002;99:560–567.

37. Hisaoka M, Ishida T, Kuo TT, et al. Clear cell sarcoma of soft tissue: a clinicopathologic, immunohistochemical, and molecular analysis of 33 cases. *Am J Surg Pathol.* 2008;32:452–460.

38. Antonescu CR, Nafa K, Segal NH, Dal Cin P, Ladanyi M. EWS-CREB1: a recurrent variant fusion in clear cell sarcoma—association with gastrointestinal location and absence of melanocytic differentiation. *Clin Cancer Res.* 2006;12:5356–5362.

39. Yegen G, Gulluoglu M, Mete O, Onder S, Kapran Y. Clear cell sarcoma-like tumor of the gastrointestinal tract: a case report and review of the literature. *Int J Surg Pathol.* 2015;23(1):61–67.

40. Zambrano E, Reyes-Mugica M, Franchi A, Rosai J. An osteoclast-rich tumor of the gastrointestinal tract with features resembling clear cell sarcoma of soft parts: reports of 6 cases of a GIST simulator. *Int J Surg Pathol.* 2003;11:75–81.

41. D'Amico FE, Ruffolo C, Romeo S, Massani M, Dei Tos AP, Bassi N. Clear cell sarcoma of the ileum: report of a case and review of the literature. *Int J Surg Pathol.* 2012;20:401–406.

42. Stockman DL, Miettinen M, Suster S, et al. Malignant gastrointestinal neuroectodermal tumor: clinicopathologic, immunohistochemical, ultrastructural, and molecular analysis of 16 cases with a reappraisal of clear cell sarcoma-like tumors of the gastrointestinal tract. *Am J Surg Pathol.* 2012;36:857–868.

43. Sarlomo-Rikala M, Kovatich AJ, Barusevicius A, Miettinen M. CD117: a sensitive marker for gastrointestinal stromal tumors that is more specific than CD34. *Mod Pathol.* 1998;11:728–734.

44. Agaimy A, Wunsch PH. True smooth muscle neoplasms of the gastrointestinal tract: morphological spectrum and classification in a series of 85 cases from a single institute. *Langenbeck's Arch Surg.* 2007;392:75–81.

45. Miettinen M, Sobin LH, Sarlomo-Rikala M. Immunohistochemical spectrum of GISTs at different sites and their differential diagnosis with a reference to CD117 (KIT). *Mod Pathol.* 2000;13:1134–1142.

46. Yamaguchi U, Hasegawa T, Masuda T, et al. Differential diagnosis of gastrointestinal stromal tumor and other spindle cell tumors in the gastrointestinal tract based on immunohistochemical analysis. *Virchows Arch.* 2004;445:142–150.

47. Yamamoto H, Handa M, Tobo T, et al. Clinicopathological features of primary leiomyosarcoma of the gastrointestinal tract following recognition of gastrointestinal stromal tumours. *Histopathology.* 2013;63:194–207.

48. Gladdy RA, Qin LX, Moraco N, Agaram NP, Brennan MF, Singer S. Predictors of survival and recurrence in primary leiomyosarcoma. *Ann Surg Oncol.* 2013;20:1851–1857.

49. Doyle LA, Hornick JL, Fletcher CD. PEComa of the gastrointestinal tract: clinicopathologic study of 35 cases with evaluation of prognostic parameters. *Am J Surg Pathol.* 2013;37:1769–1782.

50. Dickson MA, Schwartz GK, Antonescu CR, Kwiatkowski DJ, Malinowska IA. Extrarenal perivascular epithelioid cell tumors (PEComas) respond to mTOR inhibition: clinical and molecular correlates. *Int J Cancer.* 2013;132:1711–1717.

51. Fallen T, Wilson M, Morlan B, Lindor NM. Desmoid tumors - a characterization of patients seen at Mayo Clinic 1976–1999. *Fam Cancer.* 2006;5:191–194.

52. Burke AP, Sobin LH, Shekitka KM, Federspiel BH, Helwig EB. Intra-abdominal fibromatosis. A pathologic analysis of 130 tumors with comparison of clinical subgroups. *Am J Surg Pathol.* 1990;14:335–341.

53. Gurbuz AK, Giardiello FM, Petersen GM, et al. Desmoid tumours in familial adenomatous polyposis. *Gut.* 1994;35:377–381.

54. Clark SK, Neale KF, Landgrebe JC, Phillips RKS. Desmoid tumours complicating familial adenomatous polyposis. *Br J Surg.* 1999;86:1185–1189.

55. Zeng WG, Zhou ZX, Liang JW, et al. Prognostic factors for desmoid tumor: a surgical series of 233 patients at a single institution. *Tumour Biol.* 2014;35(8):7513–7521.

56. Peng PD, Hyder O, Mavros MN, et al. Management and recurrence patterns of desmoids tumors: a multi-institutional analysis of 211 patients. *Ann Surg Oncol.* 2012;19:4036–4042.

57. World Health Organization. *WHO Classification of Tumors of Soft Tissue and Bone.* 4th ed. Lyon, France: International Agency for Research on Cancer; 2013.

58. Carlson JW, Fletcher CD. Immunohistochemistry for beta-catenin in the differential diagnosis of spindle cell lesions: analysis of a series and review of the literature. *Histopathology.* 2007;51:509–514.

59. Crago AM, Denton B, Salas S, et al. A prognostic nomogram for prediction of recurrence in desmoid fibromatosis. *Ann Surg.* 2013;258:347–353.

60. Huang K, Wang CM, Chen JG, et al. Prognostic factors influencing event-free survival and treatments in desmoid-type fibromatosis: analysis from a large institution. *Am J Surg.* 2014;207:847–854.

61. Mullen JT, Delaney TF, Kobayashi WK, et al. Desmoid tumor: analysis of prognostic factors and outcomes in a surgical series. *Ann Surg Oncol.* 2012;19:4028–4035.

62. El-Zohairy M, Khalil el SA, Fakhr I, El-Shahawy M, Gouda I. Gastrointestinal stromal tumor (GIST)'s surgical treatment, NCI experience. *J Egypt Natl Cancer Inst.* 2005;17:56–66.

63. Ni Q, Shang D, Peng H, et al. Primary angiosarcoma of the small intestine with metastasis to the liver: a case report and review of the literature. *World J Surg Oncol.* 2013;11:242.

64. Grewal JS, Daniel AR, Carson EJ, Catanzaro AT, Shehab TM, Tworek JA. Rapidly progressive metastatic multicentric epithelioid angiosarcoma of the small bowel: a case report and a review of literature. *Int J Colorectal Dis.* 2008;23:745–756.

65. Allison KH, Yoder BJ, Bronner MP, Goldblum JR, Rubin BP. Angiosarcoma involving the gastrointestinal tract: a series of primary and metastatic cases. *Am J Surg Pathol.* 2004;28:298–307.

66. Ohsawa M, Naka N, Tomita Y, Kawamori D, Kanno H, Aozasa K. Use of immunohistochemical procedures in diagnosing angiosarcoma. Evaluation of 98 cases. *Cancer.* 1995;75:2867–2874.

67. Freeman C, Berg JW, Cutler SJ. Occurrence and prognosis of extranodal lymphomas. *Cancer.* 1972;29:252–260.

68. Otter R, Bieger R, Kluin PM, Hermans J, Willemze R. Primary gastrointestinal non-Hodgkin's lymphoma in a population-based registry. *Br J Cancer.* 1989;60:745–750.

69. Howell JM, Auer-Grzesiak I, Zhang J, Andrews CN, Stewart D, Urbanski SJ. Increasing incidence rates, distribution and histological characteristics of primary gastrointestinal non-Hodgkin lymphoma in a North American population. *Can J Gastroenterol.* 2012;26:452–456.

70. Kassira N, Pedroso FE, Cheung MC, Koniaris LG, Sola JE. Primary gastrointestinal tract lymphoma in the pediatric patient: review of 265 patients from the SEER registry. *J Pediatr Surg.* 2011;46:1956–1964.

71. Hirata N, Tominaga K, Ohta K, et al. A case of mucosa-associated lymphoid tissue lymphoma forming multiple lymphomatous polyposis in the small intestine. *World J Gastroenterol.* 2007;13:1453–1457.

72. Cheung MC, Zhuge Y, Yang R, Koniaris LG. Disappearance of racial disparities in gastrointestinal stromal tumor outcomes. *J Am Coll Surg.* 2009;209:7–16.

73. Ghimire P, Wu GY, Zhu L. Primary gastrointestinal lymphoma. *World J Gastroenterol.* 2011;17:697–707.

74. Akbulut H, Soykan I, Yakaryilmaz F, et al. Five-year results of the treatment of 23 patients with immunoproliferative small intestinal disease: a Turkish experience. *Cancer.* 1997;80:8–14.

75. Al-Bahrani ZR, Al-Mondhiry H, Bakir F, Al-Saleem T. Clinical and pathologic subtypes of primary intestinal lymphoma. Experience with 132 patients over a 14-year period. *Cancer.* 1983;52:1666–1672.

76. Khojasteh A, Haghighi P. Immunoproliferative small intestinal disease: portrait of a potentially preventable cancer from the Third World. *Am J Med.* 1990;89:483–490.

77. Ben-Ayed F, Halphen M, Najjar T, et al. Treatment of alpha chain disease. Results of a prospective study in 21 Tunisian patients by the Tunisian-French intestinal Lymphoma Study Group. *Cancer.* 1989;63:1251–1256.

78. Gilinsky NH, Novis BH, Wright JP, Dent DM, King H, Marks IN. Immunoproliferative small-intestinal disease: clinical features and outcome in 30 cases. *Medicine.* 1987;66:438–446.

79. Isaacson PG, Dogan A, Price SK, Spencer J. Immunoproliferative small-intestinal disease. An immunohistochemical study. *Am J Surg Pathol.* 1989;13:1023–1033.

80. Ramot B, Levanon M, Hahn Y, Lahat N, Moroz C. The mutual clonal origin of the lymphoplasmocytic and lymphoma cell in alpha-heavy chain disease. *Clin Exp Immunol.* 1977;27:440–445.

81. Lecuit M, Abachin E, Martin A, et al. Immunoproliferative small intestinal disease associated with *Campylobacter jejuni.* *N Engl J Med.* 2004;350:239–248.

82. Yoshino T, Miyake K, Ichimura K, et al. Increased incidence of follicular lymphoma in the duodenum. *Am J Surg Pathol.* 2000;24:688–693.

83. d'Amore F, Brincker H, Gronbaek K, et al. Non-Hodgkin's lymphoma of the gastrointestinal tract: a population-based analysis of incidence, geographic distribution, clinicopathologic presentation features, and prognosis. Danish Lymphoma Study Group. *J Clin Oncol.* 1994;12:1673–1684.

PART FOUR

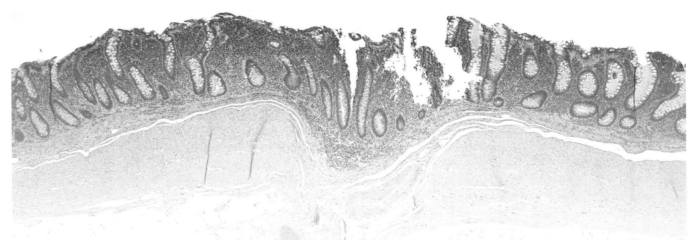

PART FIVE

APPENDIX

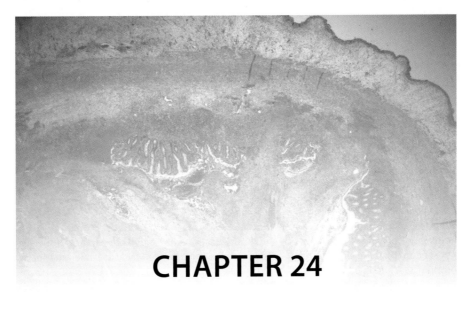

CHAPTER 24

Appendicitis

Michael S. Landau and Reetesh K. Pai

◼ ACUTE APPENDICITIS

Clinical Features

Acute appendicitis is one of the most common indications for abdominal surgery in the Western world. It occurs in 7% to 12% of the general population, and although it can affect patients of any age, it is typically seen in children and young adults.[1] Classically, patients present with colicky abdominal pain of gradual onset and increasing severity that is typically localized to the right lower quadrant. Guarding and rebound tenderness may also be observed. Complications include gangrenous or perforated appendicitis with peritonitis, which occurs more frequently in patients with delayed diagnosis, young children, and the elderly.[2] Most cases of acute appendicitis are thought to be the result of obstruction of the appendiceal lumen by a fecalith, lymphoid hyperplasia, foreign bodies, infection, or neoplasia.[3] Obstruction leads to mixed bacterial infection that spreads from the mucosa into the wall.[4] Diagnostic imaging studies, including ultrasound and computed tomography (CT), are useful in the clinical diagnosis of acute appendicitis.[5]

Pathologic Features

Macroscopic examination of uncomplicated acute suppurative appendicitis is characterized by a dull appearance of the typically glistening serosal surface and dilation and congestion of the serosal vessels (Figure 24-1). Purulent exudate can also be seen when the serosa is affected. Thickening of the appendiceal wall by inflammation and intramural edema is often observed, along with dilation of the lumen and intraluminal pus. Gangrenous appendicitis occurs when the mural inflammation leads to appendiceal ischemia, transmural necrosis, and serosal exudate (Figure 24-2). Perforation can occur and may lead to abscess formation or an indurated inflammatory mass (phlegmon) in the right lower quadrant.

The minimal histologic criteria for a diagnosis of acute suppurative appendicitis are controversial. Most patients with clinical symptoms will demonstrate neutrophilic inflammation within the muscularis propria (Figure 24-1). Thus, the diagnosis of acute suppurative appendicitis should probably be reserved for appendices with neutrophilic infiltration of the muscularis propria. Some patients with very early acute appendicitis may only exhibit mucosal or submucosal neutrophilic inflammation, although extensive histologic sampling will often demonstrate some degree of mural neutrophilic inflammation. Neutrophilic inflammation limited to the mucosa/submucosa is nonspecific and can be seen in association with fecaliths and enteric infections. In clinical practice, in those rare cases when the initial sections of the appendix show neutrophilic inflammation limited to the mucosa/submucosa, additional sections of the appendix should be submitted for histologic examination. If the acute inflammation is still limited to the mucosa/submucosa, then a diagnosis of mucosal/submucosal acute appendicitis should be rendered with a comment discussing the differential diagnosis.[4]

In some patients, a clinical diagnosis of acute appendicitis cannot be confirmed by histologic assessment of the

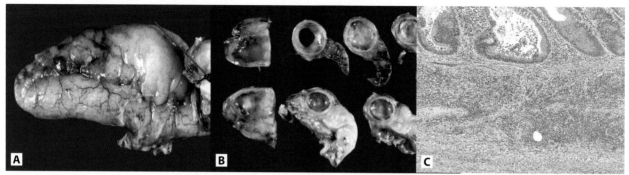

FIGURE 24-1. A. Gross appearance of acute suppurative appendicitis typically reveals a dull appearance of the serosa with serosal exudate and intraluminal pus on cut section (**B**). **C.** Acute suppurative appendicitis is characterized by acute inflammation within the lumen and appendiceal muscularis propria associated with wall thickening.

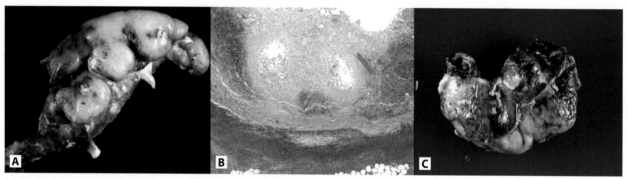

FIGURE 24-2. A. Gangrenous appendicitis with bluish-black discoloration with edema of the mesoappendix with fat necrosis. **B.** Gangrenous appendicitis is associated with mucosal necrosis and full-thickness neutrophilic inflammation of the muscularis propria and periappendiceal soft tissue. **C.** Gross appearance of perforated appendicitis with black discoloration at the necrotic tip of the appendix.

resected appendix. In such cases, the entire appendix should be submitted for histologic examination to ensure that focal, microscopic areas of inflammation or lesions are detected.

Occasionally, appendiceal diverticular disease can present with clinical symptoms similar to those of acute suppurative appendicitis.[6] Diverticula can rupture and be associated with serosal mucinous deposits and inflammation (Figure 24-3). Importantly, the epithelium lining the diverticula shows no evidence of dysplasia. Thus, these cases should not be misinterpreted as a low-grade appendiceal mucinous neoplasm (LAMN).

Treated "Interval" Appendicitis

In patients with uncomplicated acute suppurative appendicitis, surgical intervention is the standard of care. The identification of perforation and abscess formation is an indication for antibiotic therapy and drainage followed by delayed or "interval" appendectomy. Interval appendectomy specimens often demonstrate mural fibrosis/thickening associated with chronic inflammation with lymphoid aggregates, granulomas, and xanthogranulomatous inflammation. Serosal fibrosis and

FIGURE 24-3. Appendiceal diverticulum in a patient with a clinical diagnosis of acute appendicitis (MP, muscularis propria). The mucosal lining of the diverticulum shows no evidence of dysplasia, providing no support for involvement by low-grade mucinous neoplasm.

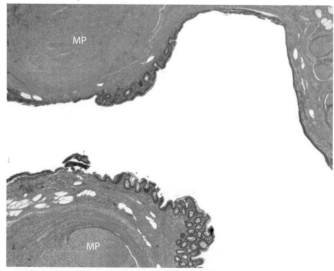

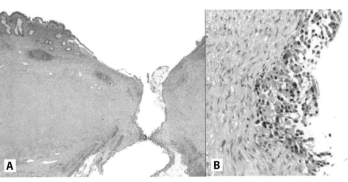
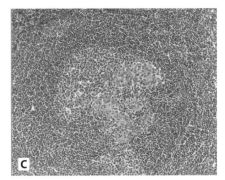

FIGURE 24-4. **A.** Delayed, "interval," appendectomy showing mural fibrosis and evidence of prior perforation with a full-thickness disruption of the muscularis propria lined by histiocytes and giant cells (**B**). **C.** Tight epithelioid granulomas were focally present in this case of delayed, interval appendectomy.

adhesions may also be observed. Acute neutrophilic inflammation is typically not identified. Granulomas are found in approximately 60% of cases and can be either tight epithelioid granulomas or loose aggregates of histiocytes (Figure 24-4).[7] The granulomas are often closely associated with lymphoid follicles and may be associated with giant cells. The presence of granulomas may raise concern for the possibility of chronic idiopathic inflammatory bowel disease, specifically Crohn disease, if the clinical setting is unknown. Thus, careful review of the medical record for a history of delayed or interval appendectomy is necessary when granulomatous appendicitis is identified.

GRANULOMATOUS APPENDICITIS

Granulomatous appendicitis accounts for 2% of all cases of appendicitis.[8] The most common cause of granulomatous appendicitis is delayed or interval appendicitis (see preceding discussion). If after review of the clinical history the possibility of delayed or interval appendicitis is excluded, the differential diagnostic considerations for granulomatous appendicitis include bacterial infection with pathogenic *Yersinia* species, Crohn disease (discussed in the next section), sarcoidosis, foreign body reaction, and other infectious agents (mycobacteria, fungi, or parasites). Infectious causes of granulomatous appendicitis should especially be considered if a significant number of granulomas are identified, if the granulomas are large (>200 μm) or confluent, or if a central microabscess or caseous necrosis is identified.[8] Acid fast, silver, and Gram stains should be performed to evaluate for organisms in such cases. Lamps and colleagues identified pathogenic *Yersinia* species by polymerase chain reaction (PCR) in 25% of cases of granulomatous appendicitis,[9] providing support for an etiologic role of *Yersinia* species in appendicitis with prominent granulomatous inflammation (Figure 24-5). Typically, mucosal ulceration is identified in association with granulomas in *Yersinia*-associated appendicitis. The granulomas can be transmural and are often associated with central microabscess and a prominent lymphoid cuff.[9] Unfortunately,

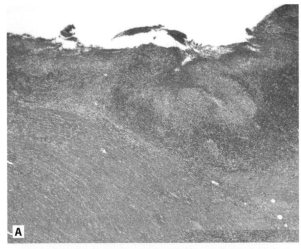

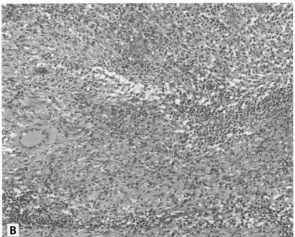

FIGURE 24-5. **A.** *Yersinia*-associated appendicitis characterized by mucosal ulceration and chronic inflammation with lymphoid aggregates. **B.** Transmural granulomas with central microabscesses are present and should raise concern for infection as they are often seen in *Yersinia*-associated appendicitis.

Yersinia organisms are not readily identified with special histochemical stains or by microbiologic culture studies. Finally, sarcoidosis, a diagnosis of exclusion, can involve any organ of the body, including the appendix.

■ INFLAMMATORY BOWEL DISEASE INVOLVING THE APPENDIX

Much discussion in the literature has centered on the relationship between appendiceal inflammation and inflammatory bowel disease. In colectomy specimens of ulcerative pancolitis, the appendix is involved in approximately 60% of cases.[10] Interestingly, the appendix is also often involved in ulcerative colitis (UC) that otherwise spares the proximal colon.[11] Pathologic features of UC involving the appendix are identical to those of UC involving the colon and include a combination of basal lymphoplasmacytosis, crypt distortion, ulceration, neutrophilic cryptitis, and crypt abscesses.[10,11]

Similarly, the area of the cecum around the appendiceal orifice shows endoscopic and histologic involvement in up to 75% of cases of distal UC[12] (Figure 24-6) (see also Chapter 26). Endoscopically, appendiceal orifice inflammation appears as periappendiceal erythema, friability, erosions, and sometimes ulcers and has been termed a "cecal patch" or a "periappendiceal red patch." Biopsies of the appendiceal orifice in these cases typically show classic features of UC; intervening biopsies taken between the appendiceal orifice and the more distal area of disease may be histologically normal.[12] Thus, in cases of UC that otherwise spare the proximal colon, appendiceal and appendiceal orifice involvement constitute a "skip lesion" which should not be interpreted as evidence for Crohn disease in the absence of other clinical, radiologic, or pathologic features that suggest Crohn disease.

The cause of the appendiceal skip lesion in UC is not known, but its frequent occurrence suggests that the appendix may play a role in the pathogenesis of UC.[13] Further support for this hypothesis comes from several epidemiological studies that showed that appendectomy decreased the risk of later development of UC.[14–16] Appendiceal involvement in UC has been shown to have clinical significance in that appendiceal ulceration in UC proctocolectomies is highly specific (100%) for the subsequent development of pouchitis, although its sensitivity is low (41%).[17]

Regarding Crohn disease, acute inflammation is seen in approximately 50% of appendices resected in contiguity with typical small-bowel or colonic Crohn disease[18]; of these, approximately 40% show granulomas.[19] When granulomas are seen in the appendix in the setting of Crohn disease (Figure 24-7), they tend to be sparse, with a maximum of 3 granulomas per tissue section according to one study.[19] On the other hand, idiopathic granulomatous appendicitis from patients who do not develop Crohn disease elsewhere in the gastrointestinal tract usually shows numerous granulomas, with an average of 19.7 and a maximum of 71 granulomas per tissue section.[19]

For many years, the finding of granulomatous appendicitis in an appendectomy specimen with negative fungal and mycobacterial stains was considered to represent involvement by Crohn disease. However, more recent studies that included clinical follow-up found that only 0% to 13% of these patients developed Crohn disease elsewhere in the gastrointestinal tract.[19–21] Therefore, granulomatous appendicitis in an appendectomy with negative fungal and mycobacterial stains is much more likely to represent delayed or interval appendicitis (see previous discussion) than Crohn disease. In the absence of a history of delayed appendectomy, other etiologies including Crohn disease, sarcoidosis, and other infections such as parasites or Yersinia should be explored.

As for the association of inflammatory bowel disease (IBD) with appendiceal neoplasms, a study showed that the prevalence of LAMNs are not significantly different between patients with IBD (either UC or Crohn disease) and those without IBD. However, LAMNs are 15-fold more prevalent among patients with IBD with synchronous colorectal neoplasia (5.8%) compared to patients without IBD (0.4%) and

FIGURE 24-6. Ulcerative colitis (UC) involving the appendix. **A.** In this colectomy specimen of UC, the proximal ascending colon is uninvolved. (The small area of uninvolved mucosa in the distal colon likely represents partial healing induced by medical treatment.) **B.** The appendix shows ulceration with neutrophilic exudate, indicating involvement by UC as an "appendiceal skip lesion."

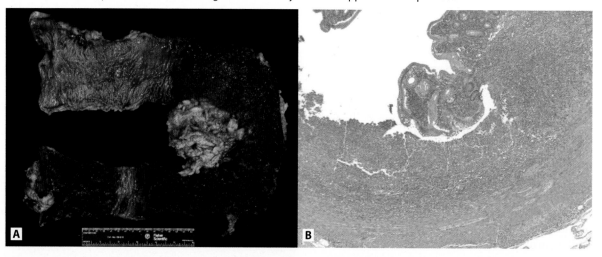

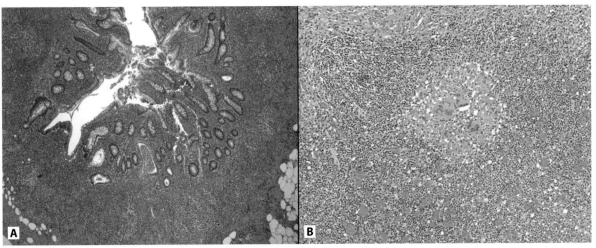

FIGURE 24-7. Crohn disease involving the appendix. **A.** A crypt abscess is seen in this appendix resected as part of a total colectomy, which showed other features of Crohn disease. **B.** Rare nonnecrotizing granulomas also were seen in the appendix in this case.

8-fold more prevalent compared to patients with IBD without synchronous colorectal neoplasia (0.8%).[22] Despite the case-control design of the study, it seems likely that IBD-related appendiceal inflammation predisposes to LAMN similarly to the way in which IBD-related inflammation predisposes to neoplasia in the colon and small bowel. The much lower occurrence of LAMN in IBD compared to colorectal dysplasia or carcinoma most likely reflects the much smaller area of mucosa at risk in the appendix compared to that of the colon. Finally, although rare cases of appendiceal adenocarcinoma arising in IBD have been described in case reports,[23–25] a definite association has not been demonstrated.

■ SPECIFIC INFECTIOUS TYPES OF APPENDICITIS

Bacterial cultures in acute suppurative appendicitis almost always reveal a mixture of aerobic and anaerobic bacterial organisms. Aside from nonspecific acute suppurative appendicitis, other specific bacterial organisms can also give rise to appendicitis. As mentioned, pathogenic *Yersinia* species may be a common cause of appendicitis, particularly in cases with transmural granulomatous inflammation associated with prominent lymphoid cuffs. *Actinomyces israelii* may be a rare cause of appendicitis; however, the appendix is the most common intra-abdominal organ involved by actinomycosis.[26] Characteristic sulfur granules, consisting of irregular clusters of bacteria, are identified within the appendiceal wall of

FIGURE 24-8. **A.** *Enterobius vermicularis* involving the lumen of the appendix. This organism is characterized by lateral alae and easily visible internal organs. **B.** Remote *Schistosoma haematobium* appendicitis is characterized by numerous calcified eggs involving the muscularis propria and submucosa. The calcified eggs have internal structure and are not associated with an inflammatory reaction (inset).

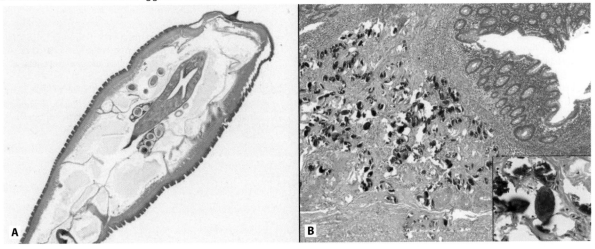

cases of *Actinomyces*-associated appendicitis. Importantly, the presence of *Actinomyces* within the appendiceal lumen is not sufficient for a diagnosis of invasive actinomycosis as commensal *Actinomyces* can be present within the appendiceal lumen. *Mycobacterium tuberculosis* rarely involves the appendix and when it does is almost always associated with infection elsewhere. Similarly, *Clostridium difficile* can involve the appendix but is typically associated with widespread pseudomembranous colitis.

Fungal causes of appendicitis are rare and when identified are usually seen as a part of a generalized systemic infection, often in immunocompromised patients.

Parasitic organisms can be found in the lumen of the appendix. The most common parasite seen in the appendix is *Enterobius vermicularis* (pinworm); however, the organisms are usually not invasive, and it is unclear if they cause mucosal damage. Histologically, pinworms are characterized by prominent lateral alae and easily visible internal organs (Figure 24-8). *Strongyloides stercoralis* can cause appendicitis that often has a prominent eosinophilic and neutrophilic infiltrate and may be granulomatous. Larvae and adult worms may be found in the crypts of the appendix or transmurally in the case of severe infection.[26] Finally, *Schistosoma haematobium* can rarely cause appendicitis. Ova induce a granulomatous reaction with inflammation rich in eosinophils. Older infections are characterized by fibrosis and numerous calcified eggs (Figure 24-8).

Viral infections of the appendix are not common. Adenovirus infection can lead to lymphoid hyperplasia of the ileum and ileocecal area, resulting in intussusception and prompting segmental resection and incidental appendectomy. In such cases, lymphoid hyperplasia is seen in the ileum and appendix, and the overlying mucosal epithelium demonstrates an adenovirus cytopathic effect characterized by enlarged basophilic nuclei, also known as "smudge" cells.

■ REFERENCES

1. Addiss DG, Shaffer N, Fowler BS, Tauxe RV. The epidemiology of appendicitis and appendectomy in the United States. *Am J Epidemiol.* 1990;132(5):910–925.
2. Livingston EH, Woodward WA, Sarosi GA, Haley RW. Disconnect between incidence of nonperforated and perforated appendicitis: implications for pathophysiology and management. *Ann Surg.* 2007;245(6):886–892.
3. Birnbaum BA, Wilson SR. Appendicitis at the millennium. *Radiology.* 2000;215(2):337–348.
4. Lamps LW. Appendicitis and infections of the appendix. *Semin Diagn Pathol.* 2004;21(2):86–97.
5. Chan L, Shin LK, Pai RK, Jeffrey RB. Pathologic continuum of acute appendicitis: sonographic findings and clinical management implications. *Ultrasound Q.* 2011;27(2):71–79.
6. Hsu M, Young RH, Misdraji J. Ruptured appendiceal diverticula mimicking low-grade appendiceal mucinous neoplasms. *Am J Surg Pathol.* 2009;33(10):1515–1521.
7. Guo G, Greenson JK. Histopathology of interval (delayed) appendectomy specimens: strong association with granulomatous and xanthogranulomatous appendicitis. *Am J Surg Pathol.* 2003;27(8):1147–1151.
8. Bronner MP. Granulomatous appendicitis and the appendix in idiopathic inflammatory bowel disease. *Semin Diagn Pathol.* 2004;21(2):98–107.
9. Lamps LW, Madhusudhan KT, Greenson JK, et al. The role of *Yersinia enterocolitica* and *Yersinia pseudotuberculosis* in granulomatous appendicitis: a histologic and molecular study. *Am J Surg Pathol.* 2001;25(4):508–515.
10. Goldblum JR, Appelman HD. Appendiceal involvement in ulcerative colitis. *Mod Pathol.* 1992;5(6):607–610.
11. Groisman GM, George J, Harpaz N. Ulcerative appendicitis in universal and nonuniversal ulcerative colitis. *Mod Pathol.* 1994;7(3):322–325.
12. D'Haens G, Geboes K, Peeters M, Baert F, Ectors N, Rutgeerts P. Patchy cecal inflammation associated with distal ulcerative colitis: a prospective endoscopic study. *Am J Gastroenterol.* 1997;92(8):1275–1279.
13. Park SH, Loftus EV Jr, Yang SK. Appendiceal skip inflammation and ulcerative colitis. *Dig Dis Sci.* 2014;59(9):2050–2057.
14. Rutgeerts P, D'Haens G, Hiele M, Geboes K, Vantrappen G. Appendectomy protects against ulcerative colitis. *Gastroenterology.* 1994;106(5):1251–1253.
15. Andersson RE, Olaison G, Tysk C, Ekbom A. Appendectomy and protection against ulcerative colitis. *N Engl J Med.* 2001;344(11):808–814.
16. Russel MG, Dorant E, Brummer RJ, et al. Appendectomy and the risk of developing ulcerative colitis or Crohn's disease: results of a large case-control study. South Limburg Inflammatory Bowel Disease Study Group. *Gastroenterology.* 1997;113(2):377–382.
17. Yantiss RK, Sapp HL, Farraye FA, et al. Histologic predictors of pouchitis in patients with chronic ulcerative colitis. *Am J Surg Pathol.* 2004;28(8):999–1006.
18. Scott IS, Sheaff M, Coumbe A, Feakins RM, Rampton DS. Appendiceal inflammation in ulcerative colitis. *Histopathology.* 1998;33(2):168–173.
19. Dudley TH Jr, Dean PJ. Idiopathic granulomatous appendicitis, or Crohn's disease of the appendix revisited. *Hum Pathol.* 1993;24(6):595–601.
20. Huang JC, Appelman HD. Another look at chronic appendicitis resembling Crohn's disease. *Mod Pathol.* 1996;9(10):975–981.
21. Richards ML, Aberger FJ, Landercasper J. Granulomatous appendicitis: Crohn's disease, atypical Crohn's or not Crohn's at all? *J Am Coll Surg.* 1997;185(1):13–17.
22. Orta L, Trindade AJ, Luo J, Harpaz N. Appendiceal mucinous cystadenoma is a neoplastic complication of IBD: case-control study of primary appendiceal neoplasms. *Inflamm Bowel Dis.* 2009;15(3):415–421.
23. Odze RD, Medline P, Cohen Z. Adenocarcinoma arising in an appendix involved with chronic ulcerative colitis. *Am J Gastroenterol.* 1994;89(10):1905–1907.
24. Villanueva Saenz E, Perez-Aguirre J, Belmonte MC, Martinez PH, Marquez RM, Carranza RJ. Appendix adenocarcinoma associated with ulcerative colitis: a case report and literature review. *Tech Coloproctol.* 2006;10(1):54–56.
25. Zannoni U, Masci C, Bazzocchi R, et al. Cancer of the appendix in long-standing ulcerative colitis: a case report. *Tumori.* 1997;83(6):958–959.
26. Lamps LW. Infectious causes of appendicitis. *Infect Dis Clin North Am.* 2010;24(4):995–1018, ix–x.

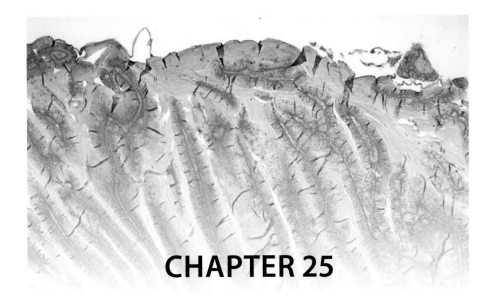

CHAPTER 25

Neoplasms of the Appendix

Reetesh K. Pai

■ MUCINOUS NEOPLASMS

General Considerations on Diagnostic Terminology

Despite advances in our understanding of appendiceal mucinous neoplasms and their relationship to the pseudomyxoma peritonei syndrome, the classification of mucinous tumors of the appendix is still confusing. Most cases of pseudomyxoma peritonei, a clinical entity characterized by grossly evident, diffuse, intra-abdominal mucinous ascites involving the peritoneal surfaces, develop as a result of a mucinous neoplasm arising in the appendix.[1-5] Several studies have demonstrated that disseminated appendiceal mucinous neoplasms exhibit a wide spectrum of clinical behavior, including neoplasms that are relatively slow growing but with considerable risk for recurrence and eventual death and those that are highly aggressive with increased likelihood of early death.[6-11]

In an attempt to simplify the diagnostic terminology of appendiceal mucinous neoplasms, both the fourth edition of the World Health Organization (WHO) *Classification of Tumors of the Digestive System* and the seventh edition of the American Joint Committee on Cancer (AJCC) staging manual differentiate low-grade from high-grade mucinous neoplasms (mucinous adenocarcinoma). The WHO identifies morphologic characteristics (architecture, cytology, presence of signet-ring cells, and mitotic activity) that can be used to classify low- and high-grade tumors.[12] The three-tier

approach adopted by the AJCC (low-grade tumors are classified as grade G1, and high-grade tumors may be classified as grade G2 or G3) would appear to offer a necessary refinement.[13] The AJCC system also uses the descriptive terminology well-, moderately, and poorly differentiated in parallel with the alphanumeric grades (G1, G2, G3, respectively). These descriptive terms are widely used to grade other gastrointestinal cancers but can be particularly confusing and difficult to apply to mucinous tumors of the appendix. Therefore, they should be avoided. A simplified approach to diagnostic reporting of appendiceal mucinous neoplasms based on the three-tier AJCC grading scheme is detailed next and summarized in Tables 25-1, 25-2, and 25-3.

Clinical Features

The majority of patients with mucinous neoplasms of the appendix present with acute pain that is often similar to that identified in acute appendicitis. For those patients with peritoneal dissemination, other common clinical presentations include progressive abdominal distention, new onset of a hernia, or palpable mass on abdominal or pelvic examination. Patients with disseminated low-grade neoplasms usually remain asymptomatic for years and present with compressive effects from slow accumulation of mucinous deposits. In contrast, patients with high-grade mucinous adenocarcinomas typically present early in the disease course due to

TABLE 25-1. Risk stratification of low-grade appendiceal epithelial neoplasms by pathologic findings.

Diagnostic terminology	Pathologic features	Risk of disseminated disease (pseudomyxoma peritonei)
Mucinous adenoma	• Cytologically low-grade mucinous columnar epithelium with flattened or villous architecture • Absence of extra-appendiceal epithelium, extra-appendiceal mucin, and invasion • Acellular mucin within appendiceal wall is acceptable	• No risk of recurrence
Low-grade appendiceal mucinous neoplasm with extra-appendiceal acellular mucin	• Cytologically low-grade mucinous columnar epithelium with flattened or villous architecture • Extra-appendiceal *acellular* mucin present on visceral peritoneal surface • Absence of extra-appendiceal epithelium and invasion	• ~4% risk of recurrence and peritoneal dissemination in neoplasms localized to the right lower quadrant at initial presentation • Close clinical follow-up is recommended
Low-grade appendiceal mucinous neoplasm with extra-appendiceal neoplastic epithelium	• Cytologically low-grade mucinous columnar epithelium with flattened or villous architecture • Presence of any extra-appendiceal epithelium • Absence of invasion	• ~40% risk of recurrence and peritoneal dissemination in neoplasms localized to the right lower quadrant at initial presentation • Close clinical follow-up is recommended with uncertain role for additional surgery or hyperthermic intraperitoneal chemoperfusion therapy

the destructive invasion of the adenocarcinoma, resulting in bowel obstruction, ureteral obstruction, and enteric fistulas.

Low-Grade Appendiceal Mucinous Neoplasms

Pathologic Features

Most appendices involved by mucinous neoplasms demonstrate dilation of the appendiceal lumen as a result of abnormal accumulation of mucin within the lumen. The gross examination of these neoplasms should include the location of the tumor within the appendix (tip vs body vs base), the distance of the tumor from the proximal resection margin, the presence or absence of mucin deposits on the serosal surface or in the wall of the appendix, the

presence or absence of perforation, and the presence of any solid areas. The entire appendix should be submitted for histologic examination, with the margin of resection separately designated.

To classify as a mucinous neoplasm, circumferential involvement of the mucosa by a mucin-rich epithelium must be identified involving at least one segment of the appendix. The distinction between low-grade and high-grade tumors is of critical importance in guiding patient therapy. Evaluation for a limited set of adverse histologic features, including cytologic grade, destructive invasion, signet-ring cells, angiolymphatic invasion, and perineural invasion, allows for separation of mucinous neoplasms into prognostically relevant groups. Low-grade appendiceal mucinous neoplasms

TABLE 25-2. Summary of pathologic features of high-grade appendiceal neoplasms.

High-grade mucinous adenocarcinoma	• Presence of destructive invasion into appendiceal wall, often with small clusters of epithelium present within small dissecting mucin pools • Presence of *any* high-grade cytology • High cellularity, with epithelium accounting for > 20% of the tumor • Angiolymphatic and perineural invasion may be seen but are infrequent	• Most patients develop disseminated peritoneal disease
High-grade invasive mucinous/signet-ring cell adenocarcinoma	• Presence of signet-ring cell component • Includes both pure signet-ring cell adenocarcinoma or mixed mucinous/signet-ring cell adenocarcinoma • Presence of destructive invasion into appendiceal wall • High cellularity with epithelium accounting for > 20% of the tumor • Angiolymphatic and perineural invasions are frequently identified	• Most patients develop disseminated peritoneal disease
Nonmucinous invasive adenocarcinoma	• Morphologically resembles conventional colorectal adenocarcinoma • Lacks mucinous component to the tumor • Much less commonly encountered compared to mucinous adenocarcinoma	• Limited literature experience but natural history likely similar to that of conventional colorectal adenocarcinoma

TABLE 25-3. Summary of grade assessment in pseudomyxoma peritonei of appendiceal origin.

Diagnostic terminology	Histologic criteria and molecular features	Treatment and prognosis
Acellular mucin only	• Copious mucin without evidence of neoplastic epithelium • Requires extensive sampling to identify epithelium	• Typically treated with cytoreductive surgery and hyperthermic intraperitoneal chemoperfusion (CRS/HIPEC) • Low risk of disease recurrence

Disseminated low-grade appendiceal mucinous neoplasm, grade G1	• Copious mucinous deposits containing strips of cytologically low-grade mucinous columnar epithelium
	• *Must lack all* of the following features:
	  ○ Destructive invasion into subjacent tissues
	  ○ Angiolymphatic or perineural invasion
	  ○ Lymph node metastasis
	  ○ Signet-ring cell component
	  ○ High cellularity
		• Typically treated with CRS/HIPEC
		• Frequent intraabdominal peritoneal recurrences common
		• Distant metastatic spread not seen
		• Overall 5-year survival ~ 90% and 10-year survival 45-68%

High-grade mucinous adenocarcinoma, grade G2	• Presence of *any* of the following features:
	  ○ High-grade mucinous epithelium
	  ○ Destructive invasion into subjacent tissues
	  ○ Angiolymphatic or perineural invasion
	  ○ Lymph node metastasis
	  ○ High cellularity
	• Lacks a signet-ring cell component
		• Typically treated with systemic chemotherapy using 5-fluorouracil-based regimens similar to those used in colorectal carcinoma with option of CRS/HIPEC in patients with therapeutic response
		• Frequent intra-abdominal peritoneal recurrences common
		• Distant metastatic spread may be seen
		• Overall 5-year survival ~ 60%

High-grade mucinous/signet-ring cell adenocarcinoma, grade G3	• Presence of a signet-ring cell component
	• Typically also demonstrates the following:
	  ○ Destructive invasion into subjacent tissues
	  ○ Angiolymphatic or perineural invasion
	  ○ Lymph node metastasis
	  ○ High cellularity
		• Typically treated with systemic chemotherapy using 5-fluorouracil-based regimens similar to those used in colorectal carcinoma with option of CRS/HIPEC in patients with therapeutic response
		• Frequent intra-abdominal peritoneal recurrences common
		• Distant metastatic spread may be seen
		• Overall 5-year survival ~ 25%

(LAMNs) lack all these adverse histologic features. These neoplasms are characterized by low cytologic grade, defined as mildly enlarged hyperchromatic nuclei with nuclear stratification but with maintenance of cell polarity (Figure 25-1). The tumor may manifest as a dilated appendiceal lumen with a flat mucinous epithelial lining. Alternatively, the mucinous epithelium may be arranged in uniform slender villi. In most cases, the appendiceal wall will exhibit fibrosis, lymphoid follicle atrophy, and chronic inflammation. Dystrophic calcifications may also be seen.

Intramural glandular epithelium protruding through a defect in the muscular wall and exhibiting a rounded, "pushing" border without irregular, jagged neoplastic glands should be classified as diverticula or herniations rather than true invasion (Figure 25-2). Diverticula may be associated with extruded mucin within the appendiceal wall or on the visceral peritoneal surface of the appendix. Assessment for the presence of mucinous deposits on the visceral peritoneal surface of the appendix is necessary for assessment of risk of recurrent disease. True mucinous deposits of the appendiceal serosal surface are associated with a granulation tissue-like response or neovascularization (Figure 25-3).

The presence of granulation tissue or neovascularization is indicative of tissue response to the mucinous deposits and ensures that the mucin deposits are not the result of artifactual "carryover" contamination from tissue sectioning or processing. Mucinous deposits may also be accompanied by mesothelial hyperplasia and chronic inflammation.

Disseminated LAMNs would encompass those cases previously classified as disseminated peritoneal adenomucinosis (DPAM)[10,11] and those cases classified as low-grade mucinous carcinoma peritonei.[7] Disseminated low-grade mucinous neoplasm and low-grade mucinous adenocarcinoma are equally acceptable and interchangeable diagnostic terms. Many institutions have elected to employ low-grade mucinous neoplasm as the preferred diagnostic terminology to avoid confusion with gland-forming high-grade adenocarcinomas.

Disseminated low-grade mucinous neoplasms are characterized by a predominance of copious mucin pools within the peritoneal cavity (Figure 25-4). Typically, most tumors contain strips and clusters of mucinous epithelium with low cytologic atypia. Rare cases are composed entirely of acellular mucin. Lymph node involvement is not identified and,

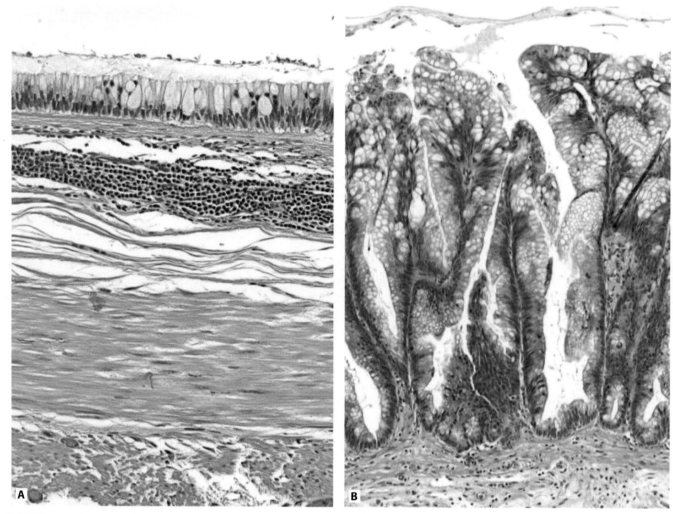

FIGURE 25-1. A. Low-grade appendiceal mucinous neoplasm with flat mucinous epithelium involving the mucosa and associated with fibrosis of the appendiceal wall. **B.** Low-grade appendiceal mucinous neoplasm with undulating/villiform mucinous epithelial growth involving the mucosa.

FIGURE 25-2. Low-grade appendiceal mucinous neoplasm involving an appendiceal diverticulum extending into the muscularis propria of the appendix.

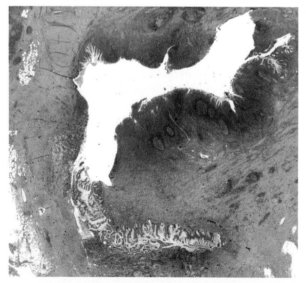

if present, should prompt consideration for a high-grade adenocarcinoma. Importantly, destructive invasion, signet-ring cells, angiolymphatic invasion, and perineural invasion should not be identified. Disseminated low-grade neoplasms frequently dissect into the wall of intestinal organs and involve the spleen, pancreas, ovaries, omentum, and liver parenchyma. However, the presence of neoplastic mucinous epithelium and mucin within these organs is not sufficient for a diagnosis of destructive invasion as these tumors typically display a "pushing" border without unequivocal, haphazard infiltration.

Molecular Features
KRAS exon 2 mutations are identified in between 50% and 60% of low-grade mucinous neoplasms of the appendix.[14] *GNAS* mutations are seen in approximately 30% to 40% of low-grade mucinous neoplasms. In contrast, *BRAF* V600E mutations are rarely, if ever, identified.[15] High levels of microsatellite instability (MSI-H) have not been identified in LAMNs.[16]

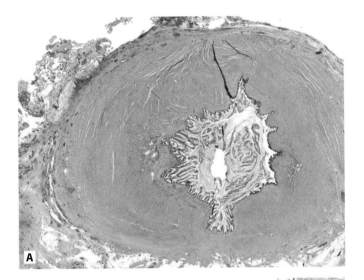

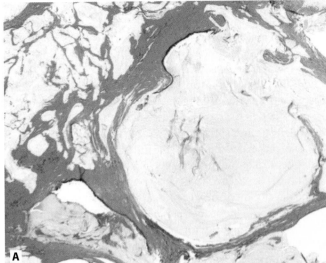

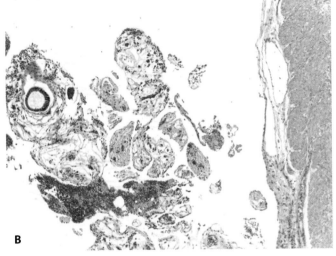

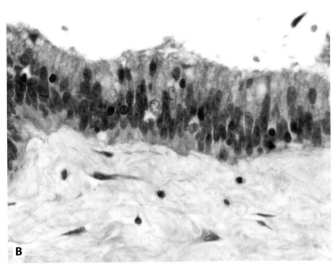

FIGURE 25-3. **A.** Low-grade appendiceal mucinous neoplasm with mucinous deposits associated with a tissue reaction present on appendiceal serosal surface. Acellular mucinous deposits are associated with a low risk of development of peritoneal dissemination. **B.** The presence of neoplastic mucinous epithelium within mucinous deposits on the visceral peritoneal surface of the appendix is associated with a high risk of development of full-blown peritoneal dissemination.

FIGURE 25-4. Disseminated low-grade appendiceal mucinous neoplasm (ie, classic pseudomyxoma peritonei) typically displays copious mucin pools within the peritoneal deposits (**A**), which harbor strips of mucinous epithelium with low cytologic grade (**B**).

Prognosis and Treatment

At the low end of the spectrum are those tumors that may be labeled mucinous adenoma (cystadenoma) (Table 25-1). This diagnosis should be strictly reserved for those LAMNs confined to the appendix without any deposits of mucin or neoplastic epithelium on the appendiceal visceral peritoneal surface or within the abdominal cavity. The entire appendix must be submitted for histologic evaluation for microscopic evidence of disease outside the appendix. This diagnosis also requires correlation with the intraoperative findings and a diligent search by the surgeon for any evidence of disease outside the appendix. Mucinous adenomas, so defined, are cured by complete resection, with essentially no risk for recurrent disease. A diagnosis of mucocele is discouraged as

this term is a macroscopic description and not a histopathologic diagnosis.

Low-grade mucinous neoplasms associated with acellular mucin present on the visceral appendiceal surface of the appendix are associated with a small, but definite, risk for the development of recurrent neoplasm (Table 25-1). The accumulated literature experience with patients with low-grade mucinous neoplasms of the appendix with acellular mucin on the visceral peritoneal surfaces indicates an approximately 4% risk of development of recurrent disease.[8,17] This likely reflects the difficulty in identifying microscopic foci of neoplastic epithelium within the acellular mucin pools. As for all mucinous neoplasms of the appendix, the entire appendix must be submitted for histologic evaluation for extra-appendiceal neoplastic epithelium, and deeper-level sections should also be performed of acellular mucinous deposits. This diagnosis also requires correlating with the intraoperative findings and a diligent search by the surgeon for any evidence of disease outside the right lower quadrant. For purposes of diagnostic reporting, the tumors should be labeled as low-grade mucinous neoplasms with acellular mucin involving the visceral peritoneal surface, with a diagnostic comment describing the low risk (~4%) of subsequent development of recurrent disease and with the recommendation of close clinical follow-up.

The presence of neoplastic mucinous epithelium with periappendiceal mucin deposits localized to the right lower quadrant is associated with a significant risk for the subsequent development of full-blown disseminated disease (ie, pseudomyxoma peritonei) (Table 25-1). The accumulated literature experience with patients with low-grade mucinous neoplasms of the appendix with cellular periappendiceal mucin localized to the right lower quadrant indicates an approximately 40% risk of development of recurrent disease.[8,17] For purposes of diagnostic reporting, the tumors should be labeled as low-grade mucinous neoplasms with cellular mucin deposits involving the appendiceal visceral peritoneal surface with a diagnostic comment describing the high risk (~40%) of subsequent development of recurrent disease. The management of these patients and the role of additional surgery or HIPEC (hyperthermic intraperitoneal chemoperfusion) are uncertain.

Disseminated low-grade mucinous neoplasms are those cases that present with full-blown peritoneal dissemination (ie, classic pseudomyxoma peritonei) (Table 25-3). These neoplasms are typically treated with cytoreductive surgery (CRS) and HIPEC. Patients typically have a prolonged clinical course with multiple episodes of tumor recurrence, which may be treated with CRS with or without HIPEC. Systemic chemotherapy is typically not effective with disseminated low-grade mucinous neoplasms. The overall 5-year survival for patients with disseminated low-grade mucinous neoplasms ranges from 60% to 90%.[6,7,9–11] The 10-year survival ranges from 45% to 68%.[9,10,18] Rare cases of disseminated mucinous neoplasms are composed entirely of acellular mucinous deposits within the peritoneal cavity despite extensive histologic sampling and evaluation for neoplastic mucinous epithelium. The limited literature data suggest that patients with acellular peritoneal mucin have a much lower risk of disease recurrence and have an improved overall survival compared to those patients with cellular low-grade disease.[5,14]

High-Grade Mucinous Adenocarcinoma

Pathologic Features

Circumferential involvement of the mucosa by a mucin-rich epithelium involving at least 1 segment of the appendix must be identified. In contrast to low-grade mucinous neoplasms, the mucinous epithelium demonstrates high-grade cytologic features characterized by the presence of enlarged, vesicular nuclei with full-thickness stratification, loss of nuclear polarity, prominent nucleoli, cribriform or micropapillary

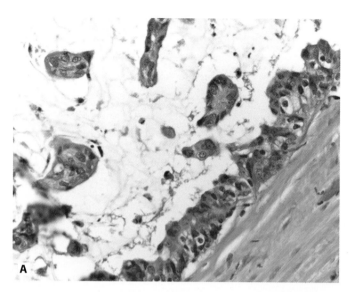

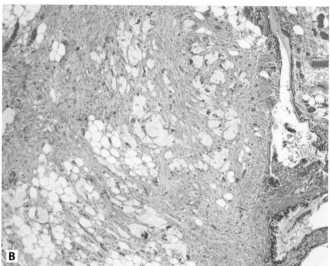

FIGURE 25-5. High-grade mucinous adenocarcinoma (grade G2) displays high cytologic grade with nuclear enlargement, nuclear pleomorphism, and prominent nucleoli (**A**). The most common pattern of destructive invasion is small mucin pools containing small clusters of neoplastic epithelium dissecting into subjacent tissues (**B**).

growth, and increased mitotic figures, which often extend to the luminal aspect of the epithelial cell (Table 25-2 and Figure 25-5). These neoplasms often display a complex architecture composed of papillary fronds, with confluent, cribriform epithelial growth often filling the appendiceal lumen. However, some cases may lack complex architecture and be composed of a flat or undulating mucinous epithelial lining exhibiting high-grade cytology. Cytologic grade within an appendiceal mucinous neoplasm can be heterogeneous, with areas of low cytologic grade admixed with areas of unequivocal high cytologic grade. This heterogeneity highlights the need for generous sampling of both the primary appendix and the peritoneal tumor deposits for histologic evaluation.

Most high-grade mucinous adenocarcinomas demonstrate unequivocal destructive invasion into the wall of the appendix. Histologic patterns of invasion seen in high-grade mucinous adenocarcinoma are (1) infiltrating, haphazard, irregular, jagged neoplastic glands or single cells associated with desmoplastic stromal reaction; (2) expansile and confluent cribriform glandular growth in peritoneal tumor deposits; or (3) small pools of mucin containing floating nests, glands, or single neoplastic cells with or without desmoplastic stromal reaction (Figure 25-5). The unique small mucin pool pattern of invasion is the most common pattern of destructive invasion in appendiceal mucinous adenocarcinoma and is often overlooked. Typically, these adenocarcinomas are cellular, with neoplastic epithelium accounting for more than 20% of the mucinous component of the tumor. Angiolymphatic invasion and perineural invasion may be seen but are only identified in 5%–15% of cases. Lymph node metastasis is seen in about 20% of cases.

Compared with high-grade mucinous adenocarcinoma, nonmucinous adenocarcinomas of the appendix are rare; these resemble their colorectal counterparts and should be graded using the colorectal adenocarcinoma grading scheme.

Molecular Features

Similar to low-grade mucinous neoplasms, high-grade mucinous adenocarcinomas typically harbor *KRAS* exon 2 mutations in between 60% and 70% of cases.[14] *GNAS* mutations are seen in approximately 30%–40% of high-grade mucinous adenocarcinomas. In contrast, *BRAF* V600E mutations are rarely, if ever, identified.[15] MSI-H have been identified in up to 3% of appendiceal adenocarcinoma.[19] High-grade mucinous adenocarcinomas accumulate allelic loss of mutational damage manifested by high-frequency loss of heterozygosity compared with low-grade mucinous neoplasms.[14] SMAD4 immunohistochemical expression is also frequently lost in high-grade mucinous adenocarcinoma and is associated with worse survival.[20]

Prognosis and Treatment

There are multiple clinical factors that influence survival in patients with disseminated mucinous appendiceal neoplasms, but pathologic grade has repeatedly been shown to be an independent prognostic factor.[6–9,11,21] Patients with high-grade mucinous adenocarcinoma have a significantly worse overall survival in comparison to patients with disseminated low-grade mucinous neoplasms. The overall 5-year survival for patients with high-grade mucinous adenocarcinoma is approximately 60%. Patients with high-grade mucinous adenocarcinomas are often given systemic neoadjuvant chemotherapy in an attempt to reduce tumor volume with the option for CRS and HIPEC after assessment of tumor response to systemic chemotherapy.[22]

Rarely, a primary appendiceal mucinous neoplasm will harbor high-grade cytology but lack destructive invasion with the appendix and will not be associated with metastatic disease at presentation. For diagnostic reporting purposes, such neoplasms are best classified as noninvasive high-grade appendiceal mucinous neoplasms (Table 25-2). There is limited literature data regarding these noninvasive high-grade appendiceal mucinous neoplasms. However, of those cases reported in the literature, some tumors exhibiting high-grade cytology but lacking obvious invasion within the appendix did pursue a highly aggressive clinical course.[8,9]

High-Grade Mucinous/Signet-Ring Cell Adenocarcinoma

Pathologic Features

The high-grade mucinous/signet-ring cell adenocarcinoma group represents a heterogeneous group of appendiceal adenocarcinomas that have in common the presence of a signet-ring cell component (Table 25-2). Signet-ring cells are characterized by infiltrating tumor cells with prominent intracytoplasmic mucin displacing and indenting the nucleus (Figure 25-6). Most tumors are composed almost entirely of signet-ring cells, while a minority of cases display mixed mucinous and signet-ring cell morphology. Isolated degenerating mucinous neoplastic epithelial cells floating within mucin pools may mimic signet-ring cells. The presence of focal areas (<10% of the tumor area) with signet-ring cell-like morphology often floating in mucin pools is a frequent reason for a discordant grade assessment. It may be helpful for the purpose of diagnostic reproducibility to require more than focal (eg, > 10%) signet-ring cells to qualify as a high-grade mucinous/signet-ring cell adenocarcinoma. Although there is limited literature experience, a subset of high-grade mucinous/signet-ring cell adenocarcinomas is likely derived from precursor goblet cell carcinoids of the appendix.

Molecular Features

The molecular biology of high-grade mucinous/signet-ring cell adenocarcinoma is still largely unknown. Relatively few

FIGURE 25-6. High-grade mucinous/signet-ring cell carcinoma composed of signet-ring cells floating in pools of mucin.

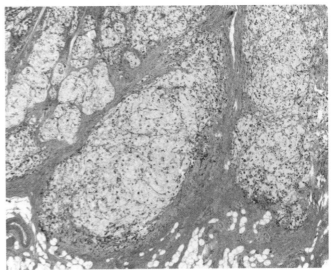

adenocarcinomas with signet-ring cells harbor mutations in *KRAS*, *GNAS*, or *BRAF*.[14] MSI-H are also not present.[19]

Prognosis and Treatment

Compared to patients with high-grade mucinous adenocarcinoma without a signet-ring cell component, patients with high-grade mucinous adenocarcinoma with signet-ring cells typically have a slightly worse overall survival, although both high-grade tumor subtypes have a dismal prognosis. Patients with high-grade mucinous/signet-ring cell adenocarcinomas are often given systemic neoadjuvant chemotherapy in an attempt to reduce tumor volume with the option for CRS and HIPEC after assessment of tumor response to systemic chemotherapy.[22]

■ NEUROENDOCRINE NEOPLASMS

Neuroendocrine Tumors

General Considerations

While alternative terms, such as neuroendocrine neoplasm and endocrine neoplasm, are also acceptable and strongly advocated by some authors, for the sake of clarity and in keeping with the WHO classification, the term *neuroendocrine tumor* (NET) is used in this chapter.[23] The gastrointestinal tract is a common location for NETs, where they commonly occur in the appendix. NETs of the appendix are further classified using the criteria applicable to all gastrointestinal and pancreatic NETs published by the WHO.[23] Grading is performed primarily by the assessment of mitotic activity and Ki-67 proliferation index (Table 25-4). An NET is defined as a well-differentiated neuroendocrine neoplasm expressing general markers of neuroendocrine differentiation (such as chromogranin A and synaptophysin) with a low number of mitoses (<20 per 10 high-power fields) and low Ki-67 proliferation index (<20%) and encompasses G1 (<2 mitoses per 10 high-power fields and ≤ 2% Ki-67 index) and G2 (2–20 mitoses per 10 high-power fields or 3%–20% Ki-67 index) NETs.

TABLE 25-4. World Health Organization (WHO) 2010 classification of neuroendocrine neoplasms.

WHO grade	Mitotic count[a]	Ki-67 index[b]	Terminology
G1	<2 per 10 HPF	≤2%	Neuroendocrine tumor
G2	2–20 per 10 HPF	3%–20%	Neuroendocrine tumor
G3	>20 per 10 HPF	>20%	Neuroendocrine carcinoma (small-cell or large-cell type)

Abbreviation: HPF, high-power field.

[a]The grading requires mitotic count in at least 50 HPF.

[b]Ki-67 index using the MIB1 antibody as a percentage of 500–2000 cells counted in areas of strongest nuclear labeling. If grade differs for mitotic count compared with Ki-67 index, then the higher grade should be used.

Clinical Features

Appendiceal NETs are not associated with clinical syndromes due to hormone hypersecretion, with the exception of the carcinoid syndrome due to serotonin secretion in the metastatic setting.[24] They are typically identified incidentally in appendices removed for the clinical diagnosis of appendicitis. The incidence of appendiceal NETs identified in appendectomy specimens is approximately 0.5%,[25-27] with a 2:1 female predominance.[28]

Pathologic Features

Most appendiceal NETs are located in the tip. They have a variable gross appearance but are often oval or round with a tan-yellow appearance. The NETs are composed of uniform cells with lightly eosinophilic cytoplasm arranged in rounded nests or a trabecular growth pattern (Figure 25-7). Pleomorphism and mitotic activity are usually not identified, and a Ki-67 proliferation index is typically less than 2% (corresponding to WHO G1 NET). The tumor may invade through the muscular wall into the subserosal and mesoappendiceal adipose tissue. Angiolymphatic invasion and perineural invasion may also be seen. By immunohistochemistry, the tumor cells are positive for synaptophysin, chromogranin, and CDX2.

The tubular carcinoid is a distinct histologic variant of appendiceal NETs. Tubular carcinoids are characterized by tubular gland-like structures that may contain inspissated mucin in their lumens but lack intracytoplasmic mucin within the neoplastic cells (Figure 25-7). This neoplasm may be misdiagnosed as metastatic adenocarcinoma given its tubular/glandular architecture and its lack of connection to the overlying mucosa. Tubular carcinoids are strongly positive for synaptophysin and glucagon and may be negative for chromogranin.[29]

Prognosis and Treatment

A number of clinical and pathologic features have an impact on the prognosis in NETs of the appendix. Using the seventh edition of the AJCC staging scheme, tumor stage in appendiceal NETs is based on tumor size and extent of invasion.[13] Recent studies have identified that AJCC pT3 (tumor > 4 cm or with extension into the ileum) and pT4 (tumor has directly invaded other adjacent organs or structure) tumors are significantly associated with worse overall survival.[30] Historically, tumor size has been considered to be the most important predictor of prognosis.[28] Patients with tumors less than 1 cm in size have a favorable prognosis and generally are treated with appendectomy alone. Most literature supports a right hemicolectomy in patients with tumors greater than 2 cm in size and those with a positive resection margin.[28] Some authors also suggest consideration for right hemicolectomy for patients with deep invasion of the mesoappendix and the presence of angiolymphatic invasion,[31] although not all studies have found these features to be associated with worse prognosis.[13,30] The impact of WHO grade on prognosis in NETs of the appendix is also controversial, with a recent

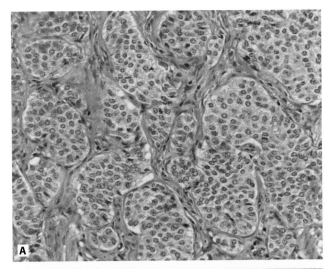

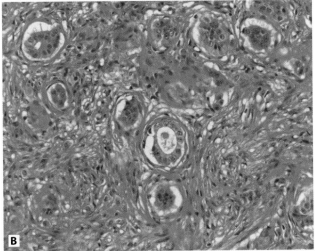

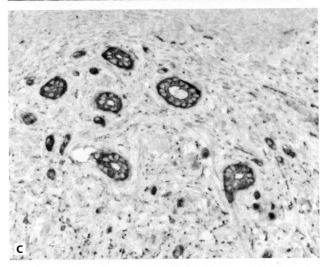

FIGURE 25-7. Typical neuroendocrine tumor (carcinoid tumor) of the appendix composed of rounded aggregates of neuroendocrine cells with bland cytology (**A**). Tubular carcinoid tumors of the appendix are a distinct histologic variant of appendiceal neuroendocrine tumors characterized by tubular gland-like structures that may contain inspissated mucin in their lumens but lack intracytoplasmic mucin within the neoplastic cells (**B**). Tubular carcinoid tumors of the appendix are typically strongly positive for synaptophysin (**C**) but may be negative for chromogranin.

study identifying no difference in survival between G1 and G2 NETs of the appendix.[30] NETs in the pediatric population are typically indolent, with excellent prognosis after appendectomy; the role of right hemicolectomy in pediatric patients is still uncertain.[32–34] Tubular carcinoids do not metastasize and may be treated with appendectomy alone.[35]

Neuroendocrine Carcinoma

Neuroendocrine carcinomas are defined by the presence of either a high mitotic rate (>20 per 10 high-power fields) or greater than 20% Ki-67 index (Table 25-4). Neuroendocrine carcinomas can be further subdivided into small-cell and large-cell types. Primary neuroendocrine carcinomas of the appendix are extraordinarily rare and are clinically aggressive.

Goblet Cell Carcinoid

Clinical Features

Similar to typical appendiceal NETs, goblet cell carcinoids of the appendix are not associated with clinical syndromes due to hormone hypersecretion and are typically identified incidentally in appendices removed for appendicitis. However, some patients may present with disseminated peritoneal disease.

Pathologic Features

Goblet cell carcinoids are often not identified on macroscopic examination because these tumors typically diffusely infiltrate into the wall of the appendix and do not form a mass (Table 25-5). The neoplastic cells are characterized by a concentric infiltration by small clusters and nests of goblet cells with signet-ring cell morphology (Figure 25-8). Paneth cells may be seen admixed with the goblet cells. The tumor cells may also be arranged in a cohesive linear pattern, but this morphology typically only comprises a minority of the tumor. Lakes of mucin may be seen surrounding the nests or in the stroma adjacent to tumor cells. To be included as a typical goblet cell carcinoid, the tumor cells should exhibit minimal cytologic atypia.[36] Typical goblet cell carcinoids are infiltrative but are associated with minimal-to-no desmoplasia and minimal distortion of the appendiceal wall. Perineural invasion is frequent, and angiolymphatic invasion may be observed. Goblet cell carcinoids typically demonstrate immunoreactivity with markers of neuroendocrine differentiation, including chromogranin and synaptophysin. Most tumors display focal staining of 5%–25% of tumor cells, in contrast to the diffuse staining observed in classic appendiceal NETs. The tumor cells are also positive for CEA, cytokeratin 20, and MUC2.[36]

Prognosis and Treatment

Goblet cell carcinoids are characterized by unpredictable behavior. Lymph node metastasis is common in goblet cell carcinoids, and metastasis to the peritoneum, omentum, and pelvic organs, particularly the ovaries, is especially common.

TABLE 25-5. Pathologic features of goblet cell carcinoid and mixed adenoneuroendocrine carcinoma (MANEC).

WHO (2010) terminology	Alternative terminology	Pathologic features
Goblet cell carcinoid	Typical goblet cell carcinoid	• Goblet cells arranged in well-defined clusters or in a cohesive linear pattern • Minimal cytologic atypia, desmoplasia, or distortion of the appendiceal wall • Extracellular mucin often seen
MANEC, signet-ring cell type	Adenocarcinoma ex goblet cell carcinoid, signet-ring cell type	• At least focal evidence of typical goblet cell carcinoid • Discohesive single-cell infiltrating pattern or irregular large clusters of signet-ring cells • Cytologic atypia present • Desmoplasia and destruction of the appendiceal wall present
MANEC, poorly differentiated type	Adenocarcinoma ex goblet cell carcinoid, poorly differentiated type	• At least focal evidence of typical goblet cell carcinoid • >1 low-power field (1 mm²) with poorly differentiated adenocarcinoma with the following: ○ High-grade gland-forming adenocarcinoma ○ Confluent sheets of signet-ring cells ○ Undifferentiated carcinoma

The optimal management approach for goblet cell carcinoids incidentally discovered within an appendectomy is still uncertain but depends on the stage of the tumor. Goblet cell carcinoids are staged according to the appendiceal adenocarcinoma scheme. Most goblet cell carcinoids will demonstrate invasion through the appendiceal wall, corresponding to a pT3 or pT4 designation, and in this setting right hemicolectomy and bilateral oophorectomy in peri- or postmenopausal women should be considered.[36] The appropriate management for goblet cell carcinoids localized and confined to the appendix (pT1 and pT2) is not well established. Patients with peritoneal dissemination of goblet cell carcinoid may be treated with CRS/HIPEC. Adjuvant systemic chemotherapy is often considered in patients with stage 3 or 4 disease.

Mixed Adenoneuroendocrine Carcinoma

Pathologic Features

Mixed adenoneuroendocrine carcinoma (MANEC) in the appendix refers to adenocarcinomas that arise from a pre-existing goblet cell carcinoid. MANEC is synonymous with adenocarcinoma ex goblet cell carcinoid. Two types of MANEC have been characterized in the appendix: signet-ring cell carcinoma type and poorly differentiated adenocarcinoma type.[36] MANEC of the signet-ring cell carcinoma

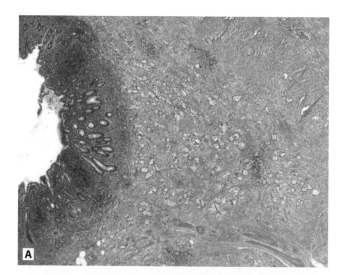

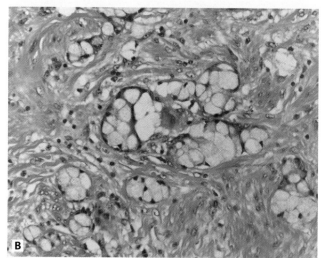

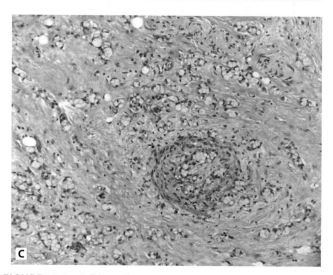

FIGURE 25-8. Goblet cell carcinoid of the appendix present within the wall of the appendix without involvement of the mucosa (**A**). Goblet cell carcinoids are composed of small clusters and nests of goblet cells with signet-ring cell morphology that lack significant nuclear atypia (**B**). In contrast, mixed adenoneuroendocrine carcinoma (MANEC), signet-ring cell type, contains many infiltrating single cells with signet-ring cell morphology and nuclear atypia (**C**).

type is more frequent and demonstrates signet-ring cells with significant cytologic atypia infiltrating in discohesive single-file arrangement or as single cells and associated with stromal desmoplasia and destruction of the appendiceal wall. The poorly differentiated adenocarcinoma type is defined by a component (>1 low-power field) of poorly differentiated adenocarcinoma that may be (1) gland forming, (2) confluent sheets of signet-ring cells, or (3) undifferentiated carcinoma.[36] Both types frequently demonstrate lymph node metastasis and are often stage 4 at presentation. Immunoreactivity with neuroendocrine markers may be diminished or absent in the infiltrating carcinoma components of MANEC but is identified within the preexisting goblet cell carcinoid.

Rarely, a primary appendiceal mucinous neoplasm will coexist with a classic appendiceal NET.[8] The tumors in these cases are separate neoplasms, and the designation of MANEC should not be employed in this setting.

Prognosis and Treatment

Patients with MANEC of the signet-ring cell carcinoma type have an improved prognosis over those with MANEC of the poorly differentiated carcinoma type, although both types have a poor prognosis.[36] Systemic chemotherapy is typically given with the option of CRS/HIPEC.

POLYPS OF THE APPENDIX

Serrated Polyps

A simplified diagnostic approach to appendiceal polyps is detailed in Table 25-6. Appendiceal serrated polyps morphologically resemble their colorectal counterparts. However, serrated polyps of the appendix that resemble hyperplastic polyps and sessile serrated adenomas often harbor *KRAS* mutations and infrequently display *BRAF* mutations, indicating the serrated pathway in the appendix is different from the serrated pathway in the colon/rectum.[15] Serrated polyps are divided into two groups based on the presence or absence of cytological dysplasia.

Serrated polyps without cytological dysplasia may be either discrete or circumferentially involve the appendiceal mucosa (Figure 25-9). Serrated luminal architecture similar to that seen in hyperplastic polyps and sessile serrated adenomas of the colon is identified. These polyps are incidentally identified in appendectomy specimens or in right hemicolectomy specimens performed for other clinical reasons. Once removed by appendectomy, serrated polyps without cytological dysplasia have no risk of progression to invasive adenocarcinoma or disseminated peritoneal disease.

Serrated polyps with cytological dysplasia often result in gross dilation of the appendix and circumferentially involve the appendiceal mucosa. Serrated luminal architecture similar to that seen in sessile serrated adenomas or traditional serrated adenomas of the colon is identified. These polyps may be associated with invasive adenocarcinoma, which can exhibit a nonmucinous histology. If a serrated polyp with cytological dysplasia is identified, the entire appendix should

TABLE 25-6. Diagnostic approach to appendiceal polyps and adenomas.

Diagnostic terminology	Clinicopathologic and molecular features
Serrated polyp without cytological dysplasia	• May be a discrete polyp (~30%) or circumferentially involve the appendiceal lumen (~70%) • Serrated luminal architecture present • Less frequently cystically dilated on gross examination • Cytological dysplasia not present • No risk of progression to disseminated appendiceal neoplasia or invasive adenocarcinoma
Serrated polyp with cytological dysplasia	• Often circumferentially involves the appendiceal lumen • Serrated luminal architecture present • Often cystically dilated on gross examination • Cytological dysplasia present • At risk for invasive adenocarcinoma, which can exhibit a nonmucinous histology
Mucinous adenoma	• Often circumferentially involves the appendiceal lumen • Prominent intracytoplasmic mucin or gross luminal mucin present • Frequently cystically dilated on gross examination • Cytological dysplasia present • Risk stratification for disseminated mucinous appendiceal neoplasia requires careful evaluation of entire appendix for extra-appendiceal mucin and neoplastic epithelium
Nonmucinous (tubular/tubulovillous) adenoma	• Much less common in the appendix compared to mucinous adenomas • Prominent intracytoplasmic mucin absent • May be cystically dilated on gross examination • Cytological dysplasia present • At risk for invasive adenocarcinoma, which can exhibit a nonmucinous histology

be submitted for histologic review to evaluate for invasive adenocarcinoma. If invasive adenocarcinoma is excluded and the margin of resection is uninvolved, then no further therapy is required.

Adenoma

Mucinous adenomas are discussed in the section on LAMNs. Rarely, an adenoma of the appendix will be nonmucinous and histologically resemble conventional tubular/tubulovillous adenomas of the colon and rectum (Figure 25-9). These adenomas may be associated with invasive adenocarcinoma, which can exhibit a nonmucinous histology. If a tubular/tubulovillous adenoma of the appendix is identified, the entire appendix should be submitted for histologic review

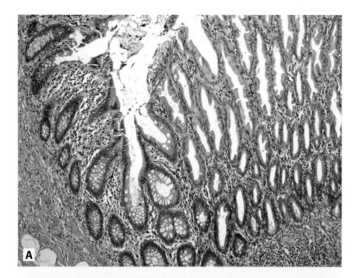

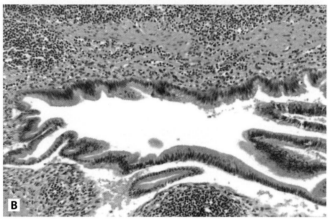

FIGURE 25-9. Nondysplastic serrated polyp of the appendix resembling a colorectal hyperplastic polyp (**A**). Nonmucinous adenoma of the appendix with low-grade cytologic features resembling a tubular adenoma of the colon/rectum (**B**).

to evaluate for invasive adenocarcinoma. If invasive adenocarcinoma is excluded and the margin of resection is uninvolved, then no further therapy is required.

■ MISCELLANEOUS TUMORS

Tumors metastatic to the appendix can be observed and typically involve the serosal surface or periappendiceal adipose tissue. Endometriosis can involve the appendix and may display intestinal metaplasia, mimicking a primary appendiceal mucinous neoplasm.[37] When identified, lymphoma involving the appendix is typically associated with generalized involvement of the intestinal tract; primary lymphoma of the appendix is rare.

■ REFERENCES

1. Chuaqui RF, Zhuang Z, Emmert-Buck MR, et al. Genetic analysis of synchronous mucinous tumors of the ovary and appendix. *Hum Pathol.* 1996;27:165–171.

2. Ronnett BM, Shmookler BM, Diener-West M, Sugarbaker PH, Kurman RJ. Immunohistochemical evidence supporting the appendiceal origin of pseudomyxoma peritonei in women. *Int J Gynecol Pathol.* 1997;16:1–9.

3. Teixeira MR, Qvist H, Giercksky KE, Bohler PJ, Heim S. Cytogenetic analysis of several pseudomyxoma peritonei lesions originating from a mucinous cystadenoma of the appendix. *Cancer Genet Cytogenet.* 1997;93:157–159.

4. Szych C, Staebler A, Connolly DC, Wu R, Cho KR, Ronnett BM. Molecular genetic evidence supporting the clonality and appendiceal origin of Pseudomyxoma peritonei in women. *Am J Pathol.* 1999;154:1849–1855.

5. Young RH, Gilks CB, Scully RE. Mucinous tumors of the appendix associated with mucinous tumors of the ovary and pseudomyxoma peritonei. A clinicopathological analysis of 22 cases supporting an origin in the appendix. *Am J Surg Pathol.* 1991;15:415–429.

6. Carr NJ, Finch J, Ilesley IC, et al. Pathology and prognosis in pseudomyxoma peritonei: a review of 274 cases. *J Clin Pathol.* 2012;65:919–923.

7. Bradley RF, Stewart JHt, Russell GB, Levine EA, Geisinger KR. Pseudomyxoma peritonei of appendiceal origin: a clinicopathologic analysis of 101 patients uniformly treated at a single institution, with literature review. *Am J Surg Pathol.* 2006;30:551–559.

8. Pai RK, Beck AH, Norton JA, Longacre TA. Appendiceal mucinous neoplasms: clinicopathologic study of 116 cases with analysis of factors predicting recurrence. *Am J Surg Pathol.* 2009;33:1425–1439.

9. Misdraji J, Yantiss RK, Graeme-Cook FM, Balis UJ, Young RH. Appendiceal mucinous neoplasms: a clinicopathologic analysis of 107 cases. *Am J Surg Pathol.* 2003;27:1089–1103.

10. Ronnett BM, Yan H, Kurman RJ, Shmookler BM, Wu L, Sugarbaker PH. Patients with pseudomyxoma peritonei associated with disseminated peritoneal adenomucinosis have a significantly more favorable prognosis than patients with peritoneal mucinous carcinomatosis. *Cancer.* 2001;92:85–91.

11. Ronnett BM, Zahn CM, Kurman RJ, Kass ME, Sugarbaker PH, Shmookler BM. Disseminated peritoneal adenomucinosis and peritoneal mucinous carcinomatosis. A clinicopathologic analysis of 109 cases with emphasis on distinguishing pathologic features, site of origin, prognosis, and relationship to "pseudomyxoma peritonei". *Am J Surg Pathol.* 1995;19:1390–1408.

12. Carr NJ SL. Adenocarcinoma of the appendix. In: Bosman FT CF, Hruban RH, Theise ND, ed. *WHO Classification of Tumors of the Digestive System.* Lyon, France: IARC Press; 2010:122–125.

13. Edge SB, Byrd DR, Compton CC, Fritz AG, Greene FL, Trotti A, eds. Appendix. In: *AJCC Cancer Staging Manual.* 7th ed. Chicago, IL: Springer; 2010:143–164.

14. Davison JM, Choudry HA, Pingpank JF, et al. Clinicopathologic and molecular analysis of disseminated appendiceal mucinous neoplasms: identification of factors predicting survival and proposed criteria for a three-tiered assessment of tumor grade. *Mod Pathol.* 2014;27(11):1521–1539.

15. Pai RK, Hartman DJ, Gonzalo DH, et al. Serrated lesion of the appendix frequently harbor KRAS mutations and not BRAF mutations indicating a distinctly different serrated neoplastic pathway in the appendix. *Hum Pathol.* 2014;45:227–235.

16. Misdraji J, Burgart LJ, Lauwers GY. Defective mismatch repair in the pathogenesis of low-grade appendiceal mucinous neoplasms and adenocarcinomas. *Mod Pathol.* 2004;17:1447–1454.

17. Yantiss RK, Shia J, Klimstra DS, Hahn HP, Odze RD, Misdraji J. Prognostic significance of localized extra-appendiceal mucin deposition in appendiceal mucinous neoplasms. *Am J Surg Pathol.* 2008;33:248–255.

18. Chua TC, Moran BJ, Sugarbaker PH, et al. Early- and long-term outcome data of patients with pseudomyxoma peritonei from appendiceal origin treated by a strategy of cytoreductive surgery and hyperthermic intraperitoneal chemotherapy. *J Clin Oncol.* 2012;30:2449–2456.

19. Taggart MW, Galbincea J, Mansfield PF, et al. High-level microsatellite instability in appendiceal carcinomas. *Am J Surg Pathol.* 2013;37:1192–1200.

20. Davison JM, Hartman DA, Singhi AD, et al. Loss of SMAD4 protein expression is associated with high tumor grade and poor prognosis in disseminated appendiceal mucinous neoplasms. *Am J Surg Pathol.* 2014;38:583–592.

21. Baratti D, Kusamura S, Nonaka D, et al. Pseudomyxoma peritonei: clinical pathological and biological prognostic factors in patients treated with cytoreductive surgery and hyperthermic intraperitoneal chemotherapy (HIPEC). *Ann Surg Oncol.* 2008;15:526–534.

22. Bijelic L, Kumar AS, Stuart OA, Sugarbaker PH. Systemic chemotherapy prior to cytoreductive surgery and HIPEC for carcinomatosis from appendix cancer: impact on perioperative outcomes and short-term survival. *Gastroenterol Res Pract.* 2012;2012:163284.

23. Rindi G, Arnold R, Bosman FT, et al. Nomenclature and classification of neuroendocrine neoplasms of the digestive system. In: Bosman FT, Carneiro F, Hruban RH, Theise ND, eds. *WHO Classification of Tumours of the Digestive System.* Lyon, France: IARC Press; 2010:13–14.

24. Komminoth P, Arnold R, Capella C, et al. Neuroendocrine neoplasms of the appendix. In: Bosman FT, Carneiro F, Hruban RH, Theise ND, eds. *WHO Classification of Tumours of the Digestive System.* Lyon, France: IARC Press; 2010:126–128.

25. Blair NP, Bugis SP, Turner LJ, MacLeod MM. Review of the pathologic diagnoses of 2,216 appendectomy specimens. *Am J Surg.* 1993;165:618–620.

26. Chang AR. An analysis of the pathology of 3003 appendices. *Aust N Z J Surg.* 1981;51:169–178.

27. Moertel CG, Dockerty MB, Judd ES. Carcinoid tumors of the vermiform appendix. *Cancer.* 1968;21:270–278.

28. Carr NJ, Sobin LH. Neuroendocrine tumors of the appendix. *Semin Diagn Pathol.* 2004;21:108–119.

29. Pai RK, Longacre TA. Appendiceal mucinous tumors and pseudomyxoma peritonei: histologic features, diagnostic problems, and proposed classification. *Adv Anat Pathol.* 2005;12:291–311.

30. Volante M, Daniele L, Asioli S, et al. Tumor staging but not grading is associated with adverse clinical outcome in neuroendocrine tumors of the appendix: a retrospective clinical pathologic analysis of 138 cases. *Am J Surg Pathol.* 2013;37:606–612.

31. Alexandraki KI, Griniatsos J, Bramis KI, et al. Clinical value of right hemicolectomy for appendiceal carcinoids using pathologic criteria. *J Endocrinol Invest.* 2011;34:255–259.

32. Prommegger R, Obrist P, Ensinger C, Profanter C, Mittermair R, Hager J. Retrospective evaluation of carcinoid tumors of the appendix in children. *World J Surg.* 2002;26:1489–1492.

33. Parkes SE, Muir KR, al Sheyyab M, et al. Carcinoid tumours of the appendix in children 1957–1986: incidence, treatment and outcome. *Br J Surg.* 1993;80:502–504.

34. Pelizzo G, La Riccia A, Bouvier R, Chappuis JP, Franchella A. Carcinoid tumors of the appendix in children. *Pediatr Surg Int.* 2001;17:399–402.

35. Burke AP, Sobin LH, Federspiel BH, Shekitka KM, Helwig EB. Goblet cell carcinoids and related tumors of the vermiform appendix. *Am J Clin Pathol.* 1990;94:27–35.

36. Tang LH, Shia J, Soslow RA, et al. Pathologic classification and clinical behavior of the spectrum of goblet cell carcinoid tumors of the appendix. *Am J Surg Pathol.* 2008;32:1429–1443.

37. Misdraji J, Lauwers GY, Irving JA, Batts KP, Young RH. Appendiceal or cecal endometriosis with intestinal metaplasia: a potential mimic of appendiceal mucinous neoplasms. *Am J Surg Pathol.* 2014;38:698–705.

PART FIVE

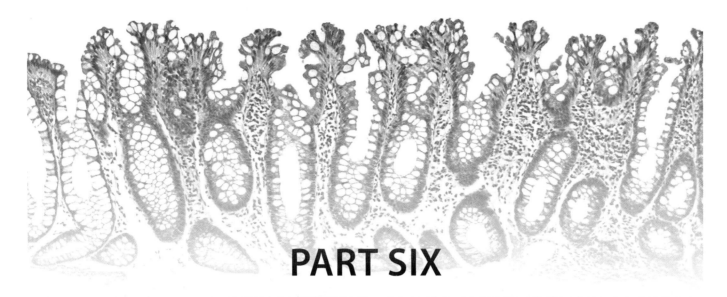

PART SIX

COLON

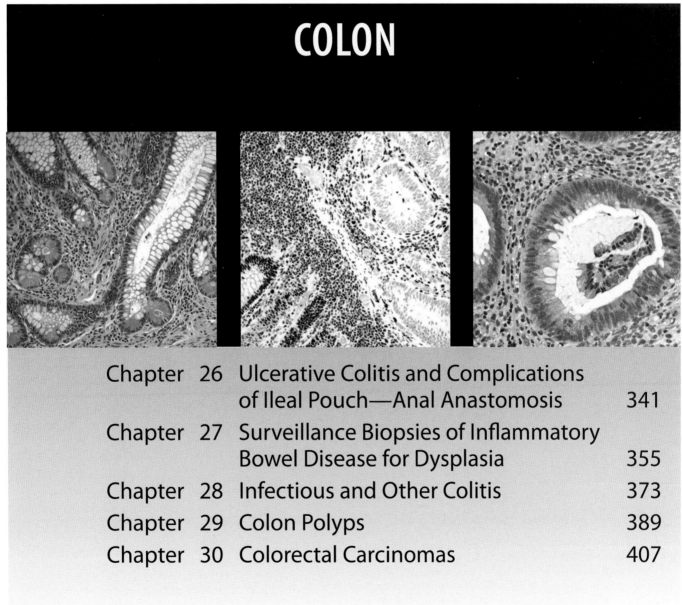

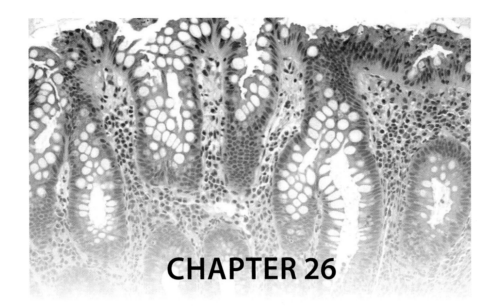

CHAPTER 26

Ulcerative Colitis and Complications of Ileal Pouch–Anal Anastomosis

Xiuli Liu

■ INTRODUCTION

The underlying pathology of ulcerative colitis (UC) is that of a chronic relapsing inflammation of the colon, classically manifesting as a contiguous and superficial mucosal inflammation and injury, with altered crypt architecture microscopically. Rarely, there may be upper gastrointestinal (GI) involvement. Some patients have extra-GI involvement, such as of the skin, oral or genital mucosa, and bile duct (primary sclerosing cholangitis). The rectum is always involved. Depending on the extent of involvement, UC can be termed *ulcerative proctitis*, *left-sided colitis*, *subtotal colitis*, or *pancolitis*.[1] Classic UC should exhibit no stricture, stenosis, segmental sparing, rectal sparing, or fistula tract.

■ MACROSCOPIC FEATURES OF ULCERATIVE COLITIS

Ulcerative colitis is characterized by diffuse and contiguous inflammation of the colonic mucosa. The resected specimen shows diffuse granular, edematous, and erythematous mucosa with or without ulceration (Figure 26-1). The abnormality is more severe distally. There is no fat wrapping, stricture, fistula tract, or bowel wall thickening. However, in long-standing and severe cases, there may be a "cobblestone"-like mucosal appearance. There might also be slight but diffuse narrowing in the distal colon due to submucosal fibrosis subsequent to severe ulceration. Inflammatory polyps or pseudopolyps may also be seen (Figure 26-2).

■ MICROSCOPIC FEATURES OF ULCERATIVE COLITIS

Although some patients present with acute-onset bloody diarrhea and abdominal pain, the histology of UC always shows changes of chronicity as characterized by mucosal architectural distortion (crypt branching, budding, atrophy, or loss); Paneth cell metaplasia of the left colon; basal lymphoplasmacytosis; and rarely pyloric gland metaplasia.

Microscopic Features of Ulcerative Colitis Prior to Medical Treatment

Evaluation of the first set of colonic biopsies prior to medical treatment is essential in establishing the diagnosis of UC in a patient with acute-onset bloody diarrhea. It not only allows distinction between acute self-limited colitis and idiopathic inflammatory bowel disease (IBD) but also provides valuable information for subtyping IBD (between UC and Crohn disease). The key histologic feature of UC is chronicity with a diffuse and uniform distribution and universal involvement of the rectum.

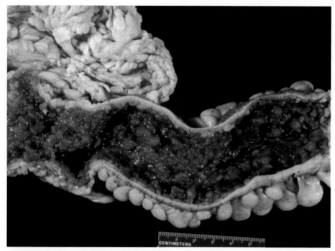

FIGURE 26-1. Ulcerative colitis. The colon demonstrates diffuse, erythematous, hemorrhagic, friable mucosa. There is no wall thickening, fat wrapping, or fistulas.

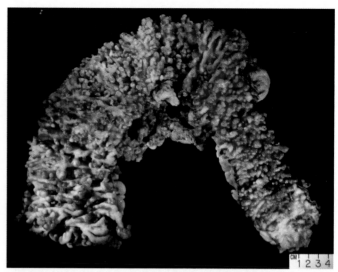

FIGURE 26-2. Ulcerative colitis (UC) with numerous inflammatory polyps. This patient had previous episodes of severely active UC. The intervening mucosa only shows mild granularity.

As described, in addition to obvious crypt branching, crypt architectural distortion may manifest as shortening (ie, presence of space between the bottom of the crypts and the upper edge of the muscularis mucosae) (Figures 26-3A, 26-3B), usually accompanied by basal lymphoplasmacytosis (Figure 26-3B). Occasionally, crypts may be elongated instead due to focal mucosal regenerative hyperplasia, even rendering a "villous" architecture (Figure 26-3C). A Paneth cell is normally present in the right colon, up to the splenic flexure. Its presence in the left colon of adults is a metaplastic process due to chronic crypt injury (Figure 26-3D).

Grade of Activity

The disease severity of UC is primarily evaluated clinically based on symptoms, physical examination, and laboratory tests[1] (Table 26-1). Histological grading of activity is also expected by the treating physician. This is mainly based on neutrophil-mediated epithelial injury, manifested as cryptitis, crypt abscess, infiltration of surface epithelium with or without erosion, and ulceration. Table 26-2 lists a grading scheme from literature.[2] While it may be a useful tool for clinical research purposes, it is difficult for use in daily practice as some information may not be readily available.

For assessment of biopsies in our daily practice, each biopsy is assessed individually and graded as quiescent, mildly active, moderately active, or severely active. Mild activity is defined by infiltration of surface or crypt epithelium by neutrophils (cryptitis) or crypt abscesses present in less than 50% of the crypts (Figure 26-4A). Moderate activity is characterized by cryptitis or crypt abscesses involving more than 50% of crypts (Figure 26-4B). Active ongoing erosions or ulceration qualify for severe activity (Figure 26-4C). The histologic grading likely depends on the sampling, and there may be variation among biopsies from different sites during a

single colonoscopy procedure. Histologic grading of activity is important as it gives the clinician a sense of distribution of disease severity. Discrepancy between biopsy activity grade and that of clinical and endoscopic impressions is acceptable. It should also be pointed out that in some quiescent cases there may be focal or extensive mucosa denudations (healing ulcer) (Figure 26-4D) that lack significant neutrophilic infiltration and thus should not be considered severely active.

Atypical Features of Ulcerative Colitis without Prior Treatment

In some circumstances, the microscopic features of UC may be atypical even without prior treatment and may make the diagnosis of UC uncertain. These are discussed next.

Pretreatment Presentation of Ulcerative Colitis in Children

Several studies showed that endoscopic or histologic rectal sparing may be present at the time of initial assessment in some pediatric patients with UC.[3-6] In the 2004 study by Glickman et al, relative rectal sparing (defined as less-severe inflammation in the rectum as compared to the proximal regions) and absolute rectal sparing (normal histology) occurs in up to 30% of pediatric patients. In addition, patchy inflammation is noted in 21% of pediatric cases.[6]

Cecum or Ascending Colon Inflammation in Left-Sided Colitis

Some patients with otherwise-typical left-sided colitis (distal to the splenic flexure) have inflammation in the cecum or ascending colon (referred to as a "cecal red patch") or appendiceal involvement with complete endoscopic and histologic sparing of the transverse colon.[7-11] Mutinga et al[10] reported that patchy right-sided inflammation is present in 9% of unselected patients with left-sided disease.

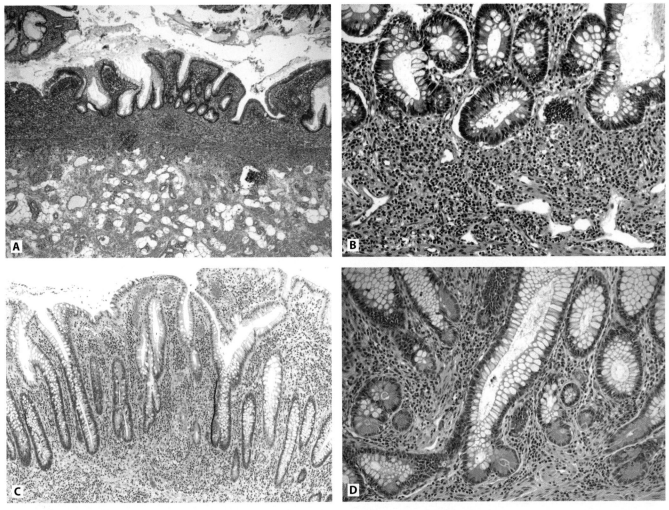

FIGURE 26-3. Microscopic features of ulcerative colitis. **A, B.** Architectural distortion, including shortening of crypts and variation in size and shape of crypts and basal lymphoplasmacytosis. **C.** Elongation of crypts with villiform pattern. **D.** Paneth cell metaplasia in the left colon.

Fulminant Ulcerative Colitis

Patients with fulminant UC and extensive mucosal ulceration may show Crohn-like features, such as relative or absolute rectal sparing and patchiness of disease, or deeper ulceration that may lead to an erroneous diagnosis of Crohn disease (Figure 26-5). An awareness of this clinical presentation is helpful in reaching the correct diagnosis.

Backwash Ileitis

Inflammation of the terminal ileum (up to a few centimeters) is reported to occur in about 20% of UC cases.[12] Histologic study of colectomy specimens revealed that most backwash ileitis had pancolitis (94%) or severe activity (65%). It is believed that mild ileitis may be due to inflammation-induced incompetence of the ileocecal valve and subsequent

TABLE 26-1. Montreal classification of ulcerative colitis severity.

Severity	Term	Criteria
S0	Clinical remission	Asymptomatic
S1	Mild	Passage of 4 or fewer stools/day (with or without blood), absence of any systemic illness, and normal inflammatory markers (ESR)
S2	Moderate	Passage of more than 4 stools/day but with minimal signs of systemic toxicity
S3	Severe	Passage of 6 or more bloody stools daily, pulse rate of at least 90 beats/min, temperature of at least 37.5°C, hemoglobin of less than 10.5 g/dL, and ESR of at least 30 mm/h

Abbreviation: ESR, erythrocyte sedimentation rate.

PART SIX

TABLE 26-2. Histologic evaluation of ulcerative colitis severity.

Term	Clinical scenario	Architectural distortion	Chronic inflammation	Neutrophilic inflammation	Ulceration
				Criteria	
Quiescent ulcerative colitis	Clinical remission	Present	Absent	Absent	Absent
Inactive ulcerative colitis	Recently treated UC	Present	Present	Absent	Absent
Mildly active ulcerative colitis	Symptomatic diarrhea but no systemic toxicity	Present	Present	Present, involving < 50% of crypts	Absent
Moderately active ulcerative colitis	Symptomatic diarrhea, minimal systemic toxicity	Present	Present	Present, involving > 50% of crypts	Absent
Severely active ulcerative colitis	Symptomatic diarrhea, systemic toxicity, increased ESR	Present	Present	Present, involving > 50% of crypts	Present in < 50% of colonic mucosa
Fulminant colitis[a]	Symptomatic diarrhea, systemic toxicity, with or without megacolon or perforation	Present	Present	Present, involving > 50% of crypts	Present in > 50% of colonic mucosa

Abbreviations: ESR, erythrocyte sedimentation rate; UC, ulcerative colitis.

[a]Applies to colectomy specimen only

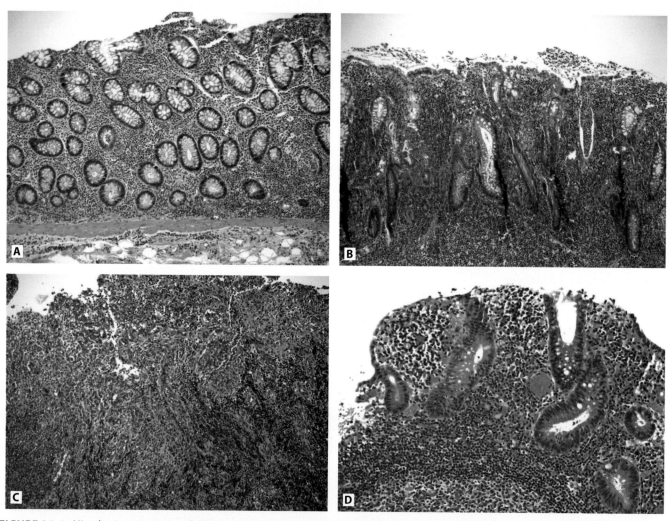

FIGURE 26-4. Histologic assessment of disease activity in UC. **A.** Mildly active UC manifested by infiltration of the lamina propria by a mixture of lymphocytes and plasma cells and infiltration of surface or crypt epithelium by neutrophils (cryptitis) or crypt abscesses are present in less than 50% of crypts. **B.** Moderately active UC is characterized by cryptitis and crypt abscesses involving more than 50% of crypts. **C.** Severely active UC is characterized by ulceration or erosion. **D.** Focal denudation in quiescent phase.

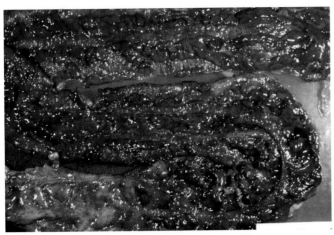

FIGURE 26-5. Fulminant colitis. Total colectomy for toxic megacolon, exhibiting extensive mucosal necrosis and dilation of the colon.

retrograde flow of colonic contents into the distal ileum (thus the term *backwash*), stasis due to inflammation-induced colonic hypomotility, or continuous extension of inflammation from the colon. Backwash ileitis is often mild and consists of patchy neutrophilic inflammation in the lamina propria, focal cryptitis, or crypt abscesses. The presence of backwash ileitis in colectomy specimens has no impact on the prevalence of pouch complications or outcomes.[12,13]

Granulomas

Not uncommonly, small clusters of histiocytes and giant cells containing pale or foamy cytoplasm may be seen in association with a damaged/ruptured crypt or denudated/eroded surface. These should be viewed as a histiocytic response to mucin or fecal material as a result of crypt rupture or surface erosion and thus be termed crypt or mucin granulomas (Figure 26-6A). These can be seen in both UC and Crohn disease. Occasionally, the association with a ruptured crypt is only demonstrated in additional levels of sectioning (Figure 26-6B). However, any discrete, well-formed epithelioid granuloma or isolated giant cells in the lamina propria away from epithelial injury in the setting of chronic colitis should raise the possibility of Crohn disease[14] (see Chapter 4).

Microscopic Features of Treated Ulcerative Colitis

It is recognized that patients with UC may develop endoscopically or histologically discontinuous disease as a result of medical therapy[15–18] due to the limit of sensitivity intrinsically associated with morphology. There may be rectal sparing as well. Thus, evaluation for disease distribution in treated patients is not as reliable as pretreatment biopsies and may not be used for the distinction between UC and Crohn disease. This being said, for most cases of UC, crypt architectural distortion can remain for a long time in the involved segment of the colon, and most cases have typical continuous crypt architectural distortion.

In our practice, recognizing the limited sensitivity of hematoxylin and eosin (H&E) microscopy, if the patient had an established history of UC and had undergone treatment and the biopsy exhibited normal histology, then a diagnosis of normal colonic mucosa or "without pathologic change" is not encouraged. Instead, we prefer using a phrase such as "colonic mucosa, histologically unremarkable."

Evaluation of Ulcerative Colitis in Colectomy Specimens

Surgical treatment with total proctocolectomy and ileal pouch–anal anastomosis (IPAA) is the procedure of choice for UC that is medically refractory or has neoplastic complications.[19] IPAA is contradicted in patients with Crohn disease because of high rates of severe complications and poor pouch outcomes. Most cases are straightforward, and the diagnosis of UC is readily confirmed in colectomy specimens.

FIGURE 26-6. Mucin granuloma. Cluster of histiocytes associated with damaged crypts; this can usually be confirmed by additional sections. **A.** Proximity of histiocytes near a crypt. **B.** Association of histiocytes with damaged crypts on deeper levels. The histiocytes contain pale, foamy cytoplasm.

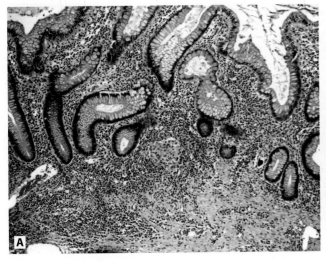
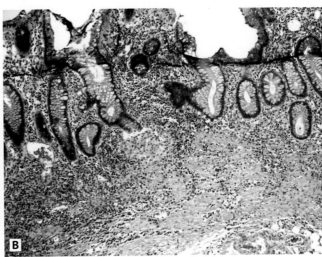

PART SIX

In approximately 5% of IBD cases, a definite diagnosis of UC or Crohn disease cannot be established due to reasons such as insufficient clinical, endoscopic, or radiographic information; prominent overlapping features between these two disorders; or unfamiliarity with or unwillingness to accept atypical features of UC as described previously. Under these circumstances, the term *indeterminate colitis* (IC) had been used as a provisional diagnosis at the time of signing out. In majority of cases, a definite diagnosis may be reached subsequently with increased development of pathologic change[20] or when additional clinical, endoscopic, or radiographic data become available. In occasional resected specimens, atypical features, including discontinuous involvement and rectal sparing, may be seen. Discontinuous involvement may be related to mucosal healing in cases after treatment with either topical or oral agents. Although rectal sparing may be seen in biopsies, histologic rectal sparing is rare when the proctocolectomy specimens are available for more extensive examination.

Diagnosis of fulminant UC on colectomy specimen may be challenging as there may be discontinuous involvement; rectal sparing; deep ulcers, including fissuring; and the presence of transmural inflammation near the deeply ulcerated area.

Indeterminate Colitis in Colectomy Specimens

In 1978, Price introduced the term *indeterminate colitis* to describe cases in which a definitive diagnosis of UC or Crohn disease is not possible in resected specimens.[21] Most of these cases presented as acute fulminant disease in which specific features of either Crohn disease or UC were not fully manifest due to rapid progressive and extensive mucosal necrosis and steroid therapy. The diagnosis of IC should not be applied in biopsies. Instead, for biopsies with equivocal features of UC and Crohn disease, the term *IBD, unclassified* can be used.[22]

Fulminant Colitis

Fulminant colitis is an acute-onset severe inflammation of the colon with associated systemic toxicity.[23] Pathologically, the disease is characterized by marked dilation of the colon, with extensive mucosal necrosis (ulceration). Most cases (89%) are found to have an underlying IBD. Others are due to ischemia or infection. Final elucidation of the underlying etiology depends on postcolectomy clinical course. Features such as skip lesions, rectal sparing, linear ulcers, and terminal ileum involvement were reported in cases that were eventually diagnosed as UC. It had been suggested that in the setting of fulminant colitis, the presence of linear ulcers and deep fissures is not associated with a higher rate of severe pouch complications. However, this may be due to the lower diagnostic threshold for "deep fissures," particularly those occurring in the background of extensive ulceration. Bona fide fissuring ulcers that are typical for Crohn disease usually arise in conjunction with normal background mucosa and are indeed associated with higher rates of complications after IPAA.[24] As discussed previously, when seemingly linear ulcers or fissuring ulcers (Figure 26-7A) and focal transmural inflammation are identified in an extensively ulcerated area (Figure 26-7B), the diagnosis may not need to be changed to Crohn disease or IC if all other evidence supports the diagnosis of UC. Furthermore, for IC, the incidences of pouch complication or failure do not differ from that of UC.[25,26] Except for cases with definitive evidence of Crohn disease in preoperative assessment or in postcolectomy follow-up, patients with IC should not be denied an IPAA procedure.[24]

FIGURE 26-7. Histologic features of fulminant colitis. Fissuring ulceration (**A**) and focal transmural inflammation near a deeply ulcerated area (**B**) are common findings.

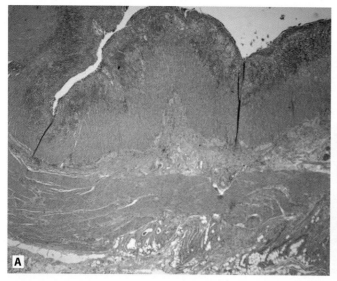
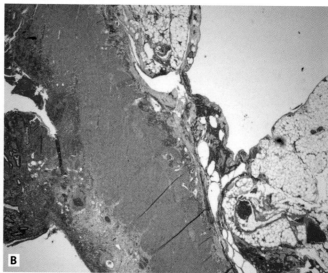

■ DIFFERENTIAL DIAGNOSIS

Crohn Disease

Crohn disease remains the most difficult and critical differential diagnosis for UC. The most appropriate specimens for the distinction are biopsies obtained prior to medical treatment or of colectomy, based on the characteristic gross and microscopic features and disease distribution. Discrete epithelioid granulomas, when not associated with ruptured crypts or foreign material, favor the diagnosis of Crohn disease (see Chapter 4). In the colectomy specimen, relative rectal sparing and segmental sparing (up to one section) are allowed for a diagnosis of UC if the colitis is otherwise diffuse and superficial without transmural inflammation and granulomas. A so-called isolated colonic Crohn disease with UC-like features[27] was introduced recently. This refers to Crohn disease limited to the colonic mucosa without mural involvement such as deep fissuring ulcers, transmural lymphoid aggregates, sinus tracts, or fistulas. However, the involvement is segmental with unequivocal skip lesions, granulomas, or perianal disease clinically. Interestingly, 2 such cases had IPAA procedures and neither developed complications that required resection of the pouch.[27]

Infectious Colitis

Infectious colitis of bacterial or viral etiology sometimes mimics UC clinically. However, infectious colitis usually exhibits a histologic pattern of acute colitis without architectural distortion on biopsies (Figure 26-8). Occasionally, infectious colitis may produce a histologic pattern of chronic active colitis. Correlation with clinical history, patient immunity status, and other laboratory studies will be helpful in the differential diagnosis. Some infections may be superimposed on a background of UC, such as cytomegalovirus (CMV) infection. Therefore, cases of UC with exacerbation should be examined for a superimposed infection, such as with CMV, *Campylobacter*, or *Clostridium difficile*, to name a few. CMV infection can occur particularly in steroid-refractory[28] or steroid-naïve UC[29] or at the onset of UC[30] (Figure 26-9).

FIGURE 26-9. Cytomegaloviral infection superimposed on ulcerative colitis. **A.** Typical features of chronic active colitis. **B.** Cytomegaloviral inclusion on H&E stain. **C.** Cytomegalovirus-infected cells identified by immunohistochemistry.

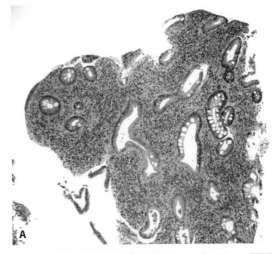

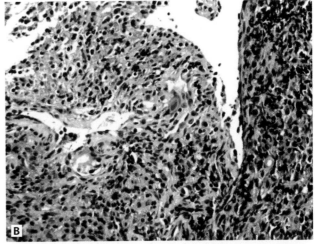

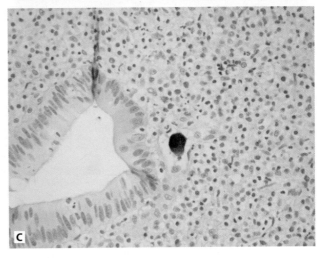

FIGURE 26-8. Acute colitis without architectural distortion and lymphoplasmacytosis is indicative of infectious colitis in many cases.

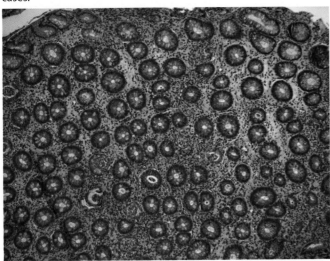

Cord Colitis Syndrome

Recently, a culture-negative, antibiotic-responsive colitis was described in patients receiving cord-blood stem cell transplantation, which may show a pattern of chronic active colitis.[31] In these cases, basal plasmacytosis and architectural distortion are usually not significant. In addition, clinical correlation and a universal excellent response to antibiotic treatment will help in reaching the correct diagnosis.

Drug-Induced Colitis

The GI tract remains a main anatomic site for toxicity by drugs or medications. Although some drug-induced mucosal injury exhibits a toxic-ischemic pattern (see Chapter 1), others demonstrate a histologic pattern of chronic active colitis. For example, nonsteroidal anti-inflammatory drugs (NSAIDs) had been reported to induce five different types of colitis: pseudomembranous colitis, eosinophilic colitis, collagenous colitis, de novo colitis, and reactivation of UC.[32,33]

The key for correct diagnosis is to obtain a detailed medication history with relation to the onset of symptoms and response to cessation of the medication. In transplant patients, the use of mycophenolate is associated with toxicity in the colon, which may manifest as pancolitis and with some UC-like features in about 40% of cases[34,35] (Figure 26-10). Distinction of mycophenolate-induced colitis from UC may be difficult; helpful features include the presence of crypt apoptosis, more prominent involvement of the right colon, and relevant clinical history.

Ischemic Colitis

Although a toxic-ischemic pattern of injury is the most common result of ischemia, chronic or recurrent ischemia sometimes causes significant crypt distortion (Figure 26-11A), Paneth cell metaplasia in the left colon (Figure 26-11B), with superimposed active inflammation. However, there is often hyalinization or fibrosis of the

FIGURE 26-10. Mycophenolate-associated colonic injury may mimic ulcerative colitis by causing significant architectural abnormalities (**A**) and cryptitis (**B**). However, the presence of abundant cryptal apoptotic bodies (**C**) and prominent eosinophilic inflammation in the lamina propria (**D**) would be in favor of mycophenolate-associated colonic injury in the right clinical setting.

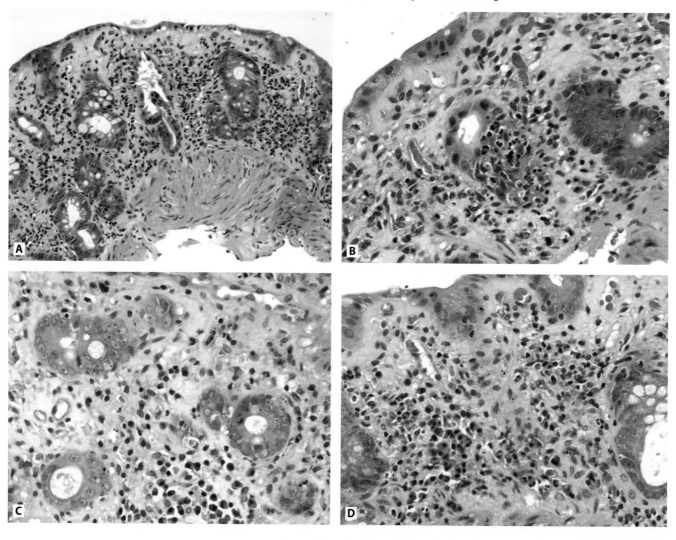

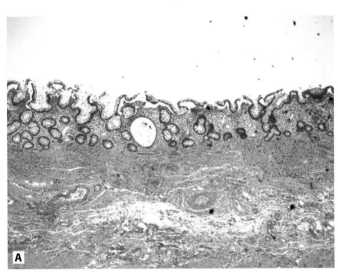
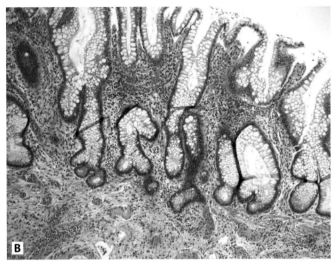

FIGURE 26-11. Chronic ischemic colitis may mimic ulcerative colitis by causing significant architectural abnormalities (**A**) and Paneth cell metaplasia (**B**). The chronic inflammation is usually less prominent than that in ulcerative colitis.

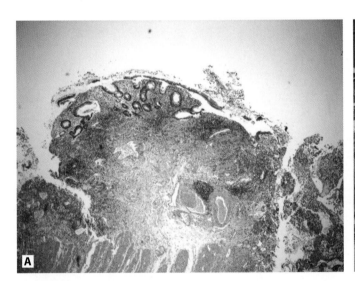
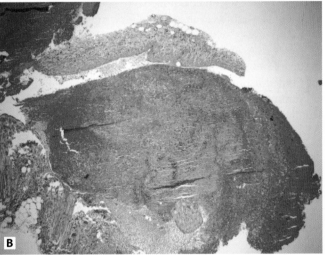

FIGURE 26-12. Severe ulcerative colitis with concurrent mesenteric vein thrombosis. **A.** Severe chronic active colitis with extensive ulceration. **B.** Mesenteric vein thrombus.

lamina propria, and inflammation is rather mild or subtle. On the other hand, UC can induce a hypercoagulative state in genetically predisposed patients, who may develop arterial and venous thrombosis, leading to severe steroid-refractory colitis[36] (Figure 26-12).

■ COMPLICATIONS RELATED TO ILEAL POUCH–ANAL ANASTOMOSIS

Curative treatment of UC is total proctocolectomy with ileostomy and subsequent creation of an IPAA. This procedure is also used in patients with familial adenomatous polyposis and IC.[19] In a large cohort, 33.5% of patients with IPAA experienced early complications and 29.1%, late complications.[19] These complications included acute pouchitis, chronic pouchitis, and more severely, Crohn disease of pouch[37] and neoplasia.[38] Dysplasia and adenocarcinoma arising from the ileal pouch and peripouch region are discussed in Chapter 27 on IBD-associated neoplasia.

Pouchitis

After reestablishment of normal fecal flow through the ileal pouch and anus, some patients develop increased stool frequency, rectal bleeding, and fecal urgency. There are characteristic endoscopic features associated with pouchitis.[37] Microscopically, biopsies from the pouch may show neutrophilic infiltration, cryptitis, crypt abscess, and superficial ulceration. Diagnosis of pouchitis requires clinical, endoscopic, and histological correlation. A pouchitis disease activity index (PDAI) that quantitates clinical findings and endoscopic and histologic features of acute inflammation is commonly used by clinicians.[39] Minimal or mild neutrophilic infiltration by itself is not diagnostic of pouchitis if the patient is clinically asymptomatic and there are no endoscopic abnormalities or before the ileostomy closure.

Classification of pouchitis is necessary before initiating therapy and is primarily based on clinical duration (a cutoff of 4 weeks in duration) and response to antibiotic treatment (antibiotic responsive, antibiotic dependent, and antibiotic resistant). Acute pouchitis usually resolves in 4 weeks after antibiotic treatment. Chronic pouchitis includes chronic relapsing pouchitis (≥3 episodes in a year), chronic antibiotic-dependent pouchitis, and chronic antibiotic-refractory pouchitis. Not uncommonly, acute or chronic pouchitis may have identifiable causes, such as infections, NSAID use, concurrent autoimmune disorder, or pouch ischemia.[37,40,41] Histologic evaluation of biopsies may help diagnose some of these conditions. For example, infectious pouchitis can be diagnosed when cytomegaloviral inclusions or fungal elements are identified.[42,43]

When assessing an ileal pouch biopsy, we apply the same approach as used for evaluating colonic mucosa and report the findings as "within normal range," "active enteritis" (Figure 26-13), or "chronic active enteritis" (Figure 26-14). The degree of neutrophil-mediated epithelial injury is further graded using the scale listed in Table 26-2. In addition, we comment on the presence or absence of pyloric gland metaplasia as it is associated with chronic pouchitis and Crohn disease,[44] in addition to the presence or absence of granuloma and dysplasia (see Chapter 27).

Prepouch Ileitis

Prepouch ileitis is an equivalent of backwash ileitis in patients with an IPAA. It is defined as contiguous inflammation extending proximally from the pouch inlet[45] and

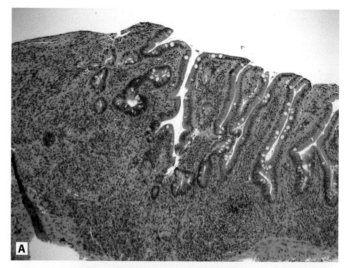
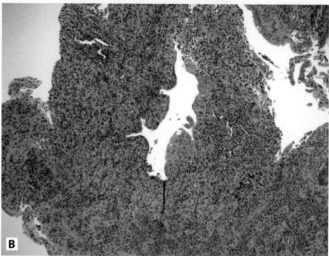
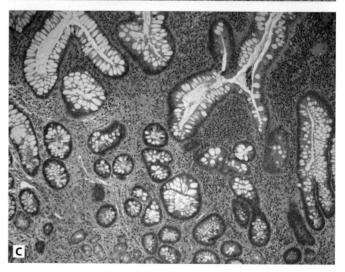

FIGURE 26-14. Pouch biopsy from a patient with clinical impression of chronic pouchitis. **A.** Chronic and active inflammation. **B.** Surface ulceration. **C.** Architectural distortion and pyloric gland metaplasia.

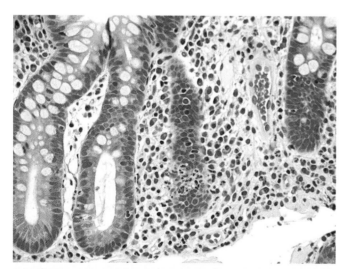

FIGURE 26-13. Pouch biopsy from a patient with clinical and endoscopic evidence of acute pouchitis. Neutrophilic inflammation involving the surface epithelium, crypts, and lamina propria and mild loss of mucin are present.

occurs in about 6% of patients with UC/IC.[46] Most patients have concurrent pouchitis.[45,46] Histological features of pre-pouch ileitis are similar to those of backwash ileitis, which may include partial villous blunting, lymphoplasmacytic inflammation, neutrophilic inflammation (cryptitis and crypt abscess), erosion, or superficial ulceration. Significant architectural distortion and pyloric gland metaplasia are not present. A study with short-term follow-up suggested that it was neither associated with Crohn disease nor predictive of pouch failure.[46]

Cuffitis

Cuffitis is residual UC involving the rectal cuff. It is common in patients with IPAA for UC, especially in those with stapled anastomosis without mucosectomy. Patients with isolated cuffitis may present with symptoms similar to those of pouchitis. Often, they may complain of small-quantity bloody bowel movements.[37] Histology of cuffitis is identical to that of UC.

Crohn Disease of the Pouch

Crohn disease of the pouch occurs with reported cumulative frequencies from 2.7% to 13%.[37] There are three forms of pouch Crohn disease. The first form occurs after an IPAA that is intentionally performed in a selected group of patients with known Crohn diagnosis. The second form arises in unrecognized Crohn disease, in which the colectomy was misinterpreted as UC (ie, features of Crohn disease were present in the colectomy specimen but were not recognized at the time of signing out). The third form is from patients who had bona fide UC but developed de novo Crohn disease of the pouch (reexamination of the colectomy specimen does not reveal features of Crohn disease).[37]

Several risk factors, including a family history of Crohn disease, smoking, and antimicrobial antibodies, were described for the development of de novo pouch Crohn disease.[47-49] However, predicting the development of de novo Crohn disease has been difficult and features studied were mostly unreliable. For example, rigorous histopathological assessment of the colectomy specimens from patients with unclassified IBD failed to find a specific pattern associated with increased risk of developing Crohn disease.[50]

Crohn disease of the pouch can be classified into inflammatory, fibrostenotic, and fistulizing phenotypes.[51] The diagnosis of pouch Crohn disease can be strongly supported if reexamination of the original proctocolectomy specimen showed typical features of Crohn disease or Crohn disease occurred in parts of the GI tract distant from the pouch.[52] Most important, clinical or histologic features such as deep or fissuring ulcers, fistulas, and strictures in the absence of postoperative leak, abscess, and sepsis (Figure 26-15) all support the diagnosis of Crohn disease if other etiologies such as NSAIDs or ischemia can be ruled out. While granulomas are not uncommon in chronic pouchitis without Crohn disease, microscopic identification in pouch biopsies of active enteritis with granulomas (Figure 26-16) or excised pouch

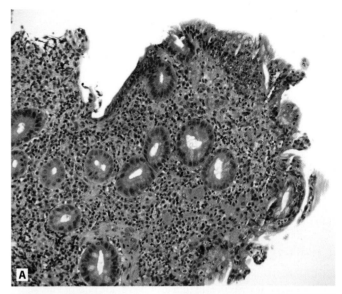

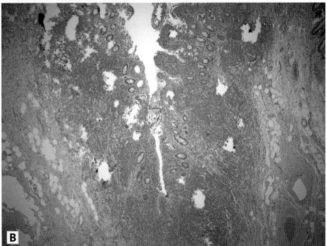

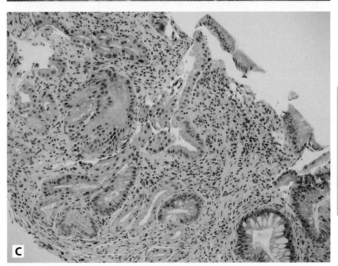

FIGURE 26-15. Crohn disease in an excised failed pouch. **A.** Chronic active inflammation. **B.** Transmural inflammation with fissuring ulcer. **C.** Extensive pyloric gland metaplasia.

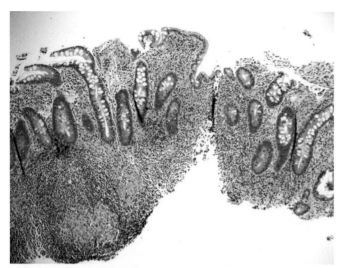

FIGURE 26-16. Pouch biopsy with noncaseating granuloma with patchy chronic active enteritis (not included in the photo). This combination should raise a strong suspicion for pouch Crohn disease if other etiologies of granulomatous inflammation are ruled out.

is highly suggestive for Crohn disease if other etiologies for granulomas, such as extravasated mucin/crypt rupture, foreign material, and infections, can be excluded. Transmural inflammation, pyloric gland metaplasia, and suppurative granulomatous inflammation in the ileal pouch are neither sensitive nor specific for Crohn disease.[44,53,54]

■ REFERENCES

1. Satsangi J, Silverberg MS, Vermeire S, et al. The classification of inflammatory bowel disease: controversies, consensus, and implication. *Gut.* 2006;55:749–753.
2. Gupta RB, Harpaz N, Itzkowitz S, et al. Histologic inflammation is a risk factor for progression to colorectal neoplasia in ulcerative colitis: a cohort study. *Gastroenterology.* 2007;133:1099–1105.
3. Rajwal SR, Puntis JW, McClean P, et al. Endoscopic rectal sparing in children with untreated ulcrative colitis. *J Pediatr Gastroenterol Nutr.* 2004;38:66–69.
4. Markowitz J, Kahn E, Grancher K, et al. Atypical rectosigmoid histology in children with newly diagnosed ulcerative colitis. *Am J Gastroenterol.* 1993;88:2034–2037.
5. Washington K, Greenson JK, Montgomery E, et al. Histopathology of ulcerative colitis in initial rectal biopsy in children. *Am J Surg Pathol.* 2002;26:1441–1449.
6. Glickman JN, Bousvaros A, Farraye FA, et al. Pediatric patients with untreated ulcerative colitis may present initially with unusual morphologic findings. *Am J Surg Pathol.* 2004;28:190–197.
7. D'Haens G, Geboes K, Peeters M, et al. Patchy cecal inflammation associated with distal ulcerative colitis: a prospective endoscopic study. *Am J Gastroenterol,* 1997;92:1275–1279.
8. Ladeforged K, Munck LK, Jorgensen F, et al. Skip inflammation of the appendiceal orifice: a prospective endoscopic study. *Scand J Gastroenterol.* 2005;40:1192–1196.
9. Matsumoto T, Nakamura S, Shimizu M, et al. Significance of appendiceal involvement in patients with ulcerative colitis. *Gastrointest Endosc.* 2002;55:180–185.
10. Mutinga ML, Odze RD, Wang HH, et al. The clinical significance of right-sided colonic inflammation in patients with left-sided chronic ulcerative colitis. *Inflamm Bowel Dis.* 2004;10:215–219.
11. Yang SK, Jung HY, Kang GH, et al. Appendiceal orifice inflammation as a skip lesion in ulcerative colitis: an analysis in relation to medical therapy and disease extent. *Gastrointest Endosc.* 1999;49:743–747.
12. Haskell H, Andrews CW Jr, Reddy SI, et al. Pathologic features and clinical significance of "backwash" ileitis in ulcerative colitis. *Am J Surg Pathol.* 2005;29:1472–1481.
13. Arrossi AV, Kariv Y, Bronner MP, et al. Backwash ileitis does not affect pouch outcome in patients with ulcerative colitis with restorative proctocolectomy. *Clin Gastroenterol Hepatol.* 2011;9:981–988.
14. Mahadeva U, Martin JP, Patel NK, et al. Granulomatous ulcerative colitis: a re-appraisal of the mucosal granuloma in the distinction of Crohn's disease from ulcerative colitis. *Histopathology.* 2002;41:50–55.
15. Scheppach W, Sommer H, Kirchner T, et al. Effect of butyrate enemas on the colonic mucosa in distal ulcerative colitis. *Gastroenterology.* 1992;103:51–56.
16. Bernstein CN, Shanahan F, Anton PA, et al. Patchiness of mucosal inflammation in treated ulcerative colitis: a prospective study. *Gastrointest Endosc.* 1995;42:232–237.
17. Kim B, Barnett JL, Kleer CG, et al. Endoscopic and histological patchiness in treated ulcerative colitis. *Am J Gastroenterol.* 1999;94:3258–3262.
18. Kleer CG, Appelman HD. Ulcerative colitis: patterns of involvement in colorectal biopsies and changes with time. *Am J Surg Pathol.* 1998;22:983–989.
19. Fazio VW, Kiran RP, Remzi FH, et al. Ileal pouch anal anastomosis: analysis of outcome and quality of life in 3707 patients. *Ann Surg.* 2013;257(4):679–685.
20. Meucci G, Bortoli A, Riccioli FA, et al. Frequency and clinical evolution of indeterminate colitis: a retrospective multi-centre study in northern Italy. *Eur J Gastroenterol Hepatol.* 1999;11:909–913.
21. Price AB. Overlap in the spectrum of non-specific inflammatory bowel disease—"colitis indeterminate." *J Clin Pathol.* 1978;31(6):567–577.
22. Martland GT, Shepherd NA. Indeterminate colitis: definition, diagnosis, implications and a plea for nosological sanity. *Histopathology.* 2007;50(1):83–96.
23. Price AB, Morson BC. Inflammatory bowel disease. The surgical pathology of Crohn's disease and ulcerative colitis. *Hum Pathol.* 1975;6:7–29.
24. Gramlich T, Delaney CP, Lynch AC, et al. Pathological subgroups may predict complications but not late failure after ileal pouch-anal anastomosis for indeterminate colitis. *Colorectal Dis.* 2003;5:315–319.
25. Wells AD, McMillan I, Price AB, et al. Natural history of indeterminate colitis. *Br J Surg.* 1991;78:179–181.
26. Tulchinsky H, Hawley PR, Nicholls J. Long-term failure after restorative proctocolectomy for ulcerative colitis. *Ann Surg.* 2003;238:229–234.
27. Soucy G, Wang HH, Farraye FA, et al. Clinical and pathological analysis of colonic Crohn's disease, including a subgroup with ulcerative colitis-like features. *Mod Pathol.* 2012;25:295–307.
28. Domènech E, Vega R, Ojanguren I, et al. Cytomegaloviral infection in ulcerative colitis: a prospective, comparative study on prevalence and diagnostic strategy. *Inflamm Bowel Dis.* 2008;14:1373–1379.
29. Inoue K, Wakabayashi N, Fukumoto K, et al. Toxic megacolon associated with cytomegalovirus infection in a patient with steroid-naïve ulcerative colitis. *Intern Med.* 2012;51:2739–2743.
30. Chiba M, Abe T, Tsuda S, et al. Cytomegaloviral infection associated with onset of ulcerative colitis. *BMC Res Notes.* 2013;6:40.
31. Herrera AF, Soriano G, Bellizzi AM, et al. Cord colitis syndrome in cord-blood stem-cell transplantation. *N Engl J Med.* 2011;365:815–824.
32. Davies NM. Toxicity of nonsteroidal anti-inflammatory drugs in the large intestine. *Dis Rectum.* 1995;38:1311–1321.
33. Kaufmann HJ, Taubin HL. Nonsteroidal anti-inflammatory drugs activate quiescent inflammatory bowel disease. *Ann Intern Med.* 1987;107:513–516.
34. Lee S, de Boer WB, Subramaniam K, et al. Pointers and pitfalls of mycophenolate-associated colitis. *J Clin Pathol.* 2013;66:8–11.

35. Liapis G, Boletis J, Skalioti C, et al. Histological spectrum of mycophenolate mofeti-related colitis: association with apoptosis. *Histopathology*. 2013;63:649–658.

36. Di Fabio F, Obrand D, Satin R, et al. Successful treatment of extensive splanchnic arterial and portal vein thrombosis associated with ulcerative colitis. *Colorect Dis*. 2008;11:653–655.

37. Shen B. Diagnosis and management of postoperative ileal pouch disorders. *Clin Colon Rec Surg*. 2010;23(4):259–268.

38. Jiang W, Shadrach B, Carver P, et al. Histomorphologic and molecular features of pouch and peripouch adenocarcinoma: a comparison with ulcerative colitis-associated adenocarcinoma. *Am J Surg Pathol*. 2012;36(9):1385–1394.

39. Sandborn WJ, Tremaine WJ, Batts KP, Pemberton JH, Phillips SF. Pouchitis after ileal pouch-anastomosis: a Pouchitis Disease Activity Index. *Mayo Clin Proc*. 1994;68(5):409–415.

40. Shen BO, Jiang ZD, Fazio VW, et al. *Clostridium difficile* infection in patients with ileal pouch-anal anastomosis. *Clin Gastroenterol Hepatol*. 2008;6(7):782–788.

41. Kühbacher T, Ott SJ, Helwig U, et al. Bacterial and fungal microbiota in relation to probiotic therapy (VSL#3) in pouchitis. *Gut*. 2006;55(6):833–841.

42. Moonka D, Furth EE, MacDermott RP, Lichtenstein GR. Pouchitis associated with primary cytomegaloviral infection. *Am J Gastroenterol*. 1998;93(2):264–266.

43. Lan N, Patil DT, Shen B. Histoplasma capsulatum infection in refractory Crohn's disease of the pouch on anti-TNF biological therapy. *Am J Gastroenterol*. 2013;108(2):281–283.

44. Agarwal S, Stucchi AF, Dendrinos K, et al. Is pyloric gland metaplasia in ileal pouch biopsies a marker for Crohn's disease? *Dig Dis Sci*. 2013;58:2918–2925.

45. McLaughlin AD, Clark SK, Bell AJ, et al. An open study of antibiotics for the treatment of pre-pouch ileitis following restorative proctocolectomy with ileal pouch-anal anastomosis. *Alimen Pharmacol Ther*. 2008;29(1):69–74.

46. McLaughlin AD, Clark SK, Bell AJ, et al. Incidence and short-term implications of prepouch ileitis following restorative proctocolectomy with ileal pouch-anal anastomosis for ulcerative colitis. *Dis Rectum*. 2009;52(5):879–883.

47. Melmed GY, Fleshner PR, Bardakcioglu O, et al. Family history and serology predict Crohn's disease after ileal pouch-anal anastomosis for ulcerative colitis. *Dis Rectum*. 2008;51(1):100–108.

48. Shen B, Remzi FH, Hammel JP, et al. Family history of Crohn's disease is associated with an increased risk for Crohn's disease of ileal pouch-anal anastomosis. *Inflamm Bowel Dis*. 2009;15(2):163–170.

49. Tyler AD, Milgrom R, Xu W, et al. Antimicrobial antibodies are associated with a Crohn's disease-like phenotype after ileal pouch-anal anastomosis. *Clin Gastroenterol Hepatol*. 2012;10(5):507–512.

50. Nasseri Y, Melmed G, Wang HL, Targan S, Fleshner P. Rigorous histopathological assessment of the colectomy specimen in patients with inflammatory bowel disease unclassified does not predict outcome after ileal pouch-anal anastomosis. *Am J Gastroenterol*. 2010;105(1):155–161.

51. Shen B, Remzi FH, Lavery LC, Lashner BA, Fazio VW. A proposed classification of ieal pouch disorders and associated complications after restorative proctocolectomy. *Clin Gastroenterol Hepatol*. 2008;6(2):145–158.

52. Goldstein NS, Sanford WW, Bodzin JH. Crohn's-like complications in patients with ulcerative colitis after total proctocolectomy and ileal pouch-anal anastomosis. *Am J Surg Pathol*. 1997;21(11):1343–1353.

53. Liu ZX, Deroche T, Remzi FH, et al. Transmural inflammation is not pathognomonic for Crohn's disease of the pouch. *Surg Endosc*. 2011;25(11):3509–3517.

54. So K, Shepherd NA, Mandalia T, Ahmad T. Suppurative granulamatous inflammation in the ileo-anal pouch. *J Crohn's Colitis*. 2013;7(5), e186–e188.

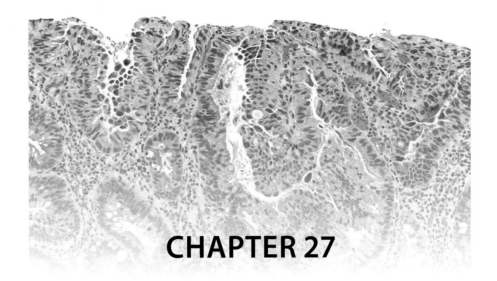

CHAPTER 27

Surveillance Biopsies of Inflammatory Bowel Disease for Dysplasia

Xiuli Liu and Shu-Yuan Xiao

INTRODUCTION

Colorectal cancer (CRC) is a leading cause of mortality in patients with inflammatory bowel disease (IBD) and is responsible for 8% of all deaths in patients with ulcerative colitis.[1] In the last three decades, efforts for cancer prevention in these patients have been directed toward regular colonoscopic surveillance with biopsy to identify dysplasia, which is the most reliable marker of imminent cancer risk (prevalent cancer). Pathological interpretation of these surveillance biopsies is essential to guide clinical management. Patients with small-bowel Crohn disease have a high risk of developing small-bowel adenocarcinomas.[2] However, the value and practicality of endoscopic surveillance of the small bowel remain in question due to difficulty in accessing segments of small bowel in routine procedures.[3] Thus, this chapter only discusses surveillance biopsies from patients with ulcerative colitis (UC) and Crohn colitis.

RISK FOR COLORECTAL CARCINOMA IN IBD

The overall prevalence of CRC in patients with UC is estimated to be 3.7%.[4] The median age at cancer diagnosis is 54.5 years for UC and 43 years for Crohn disease.[5] Extent and duration of disease are the two most important risk factors.[1,4,6] An early onset of UC and Crohn disease (under the age of 25 years)[7] and primary sclerosing cholangitis further increase the risk. The cumulative probabilities of CRC are reported to be 2%, 8%, and 18% at 10 years, 20 years, and 30 years of disease duration,[4] respectively. Understandably, due to the focal or segmental disease and reduced surface area involved by colitis, the overall rate of developing cancers in Crohn patients is much lower; however, the risk of CRC in patients with Crohn disease is similar to that for UC of comparable duration and extent.[7,8]

ADENOCARCINOMA ARISING IN IBD

The CRCs in UC and Crohn colitis tend to be poorly delineated from adjacent inflamed mucosa and may mimic a stricture, fistula, ulcer, or inflammatory polyps. Multifocality (≥2 synchronous tumors) is common, seen in up to 20% of the UC-associated CRCs.[5,6,9] Multifocality is less frequent in CRCs associated with Crohn disease.[9]

Most CRCs in IBD are histologically identical to sporadic (conventional) adenocarcinomas. However, recent studies showed higher rates of mucinous differentiation (Figure 27-1A), tumor heterogeneity, and signet-ring cell component (Figure 27-1B) in IBD-associated CRCs.[5,9] The so-called dirty necrosis is less frequent (Figures 27-1A, 27-1C). Furthermore, well-differentiated adenocarcinomas (low-grade tubuloglandular adenocarcinomas) account for about 10% of IBD-associated CRCs[10] (Figure 27-2), making the biopsy

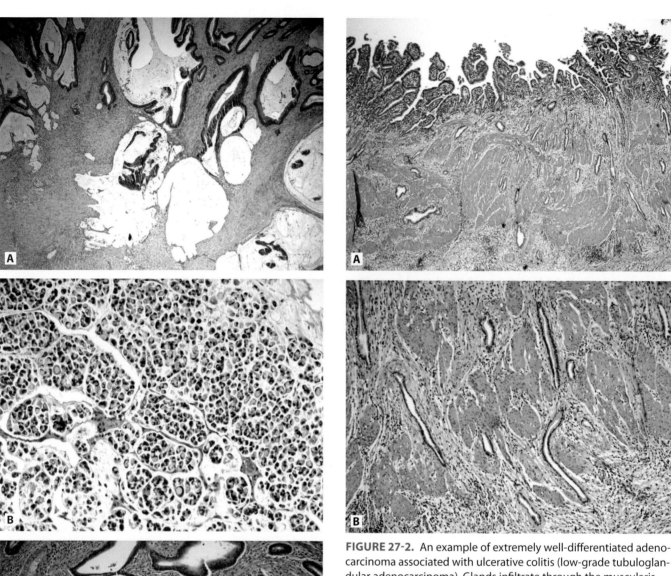

FIGURE 27-1. Colorectal adenocarcinoma associated with ulcerative colitis more often has mucinous differentiation (**A**), has a signet-ring cell component (**B**), and lacks dirty necrosis and is well differentiated (**C**).

FIGURE 27-2. An example of extremely well-differentiated adenocarcinoma associated with ulcerative colitis (low-grade tubuloglandular adenocarcinoma). Glands infiltrate through the muscularis propria (**A**). High power view shows bland cytology of the malignant glands (**B**).

diagnosis challenging in some cases. CRCs in IBD develop in areas of macroscopic disease in 85% of Crohn colitis and 100% of UC. The CRCs in Crohn colitis are evenly distributed in the right and rectosigmoid colon. In contrast, CRCs in UC are predominantly in the rectosigmoid area.[5] In addition, CRCs in Crohn colitis may also be associated with a fistula or arise in a bypassed or excluded segment of bowel.[11]

The CRCs complicating UC and Crohn colitis have comparable 5-year survival rates.[5] In these tumors, high clinical stage and positive margin predict worse survival for sporadic cases, but Crohn-like inflammatory reaction is associated with longer survival.[12]

DYSPLASIA IN IBD

Diagnosis of dysplasia in rectal biopsy was first proposed in 1967 as an aid to cancer control in UC.[13] In this early hallmark article, the authors described two main types of precancerous lesions in UC: the polypoid type and precancerous change in a flat mucosa (flat dysplasia). The prevalence of dysplasia was found to be associated with the duration of disease and reaches 20% for pancolitis with a disease duration of more than 10 years.[13] Dysplasia in UC more commonly occurs in a flat rather than a polypoid mucosa, making it difficult to detect macroscopically. Dysplasia in Crohn colitis is flat in 44% of cases and polypoid in 56% of cases.[14] This is the rationale for establishing surveillance programs, including periodic colonoscopic examination with protocol biopsy (4 biopsies every 10 cm) to detect dysplasia in IBD in addition to sampling endoscopically evident lesions such as a stricture, polyp, or mass.

Dysplasia is defined histologically as unequivocal neoplastic changes of the colonic epithelium that remains limited above the basement membrane.[15] It is synonymous with the term *intraepithelial neoplasia* set forth by the World Health Organization (WHO).[16] Dysplasia is not only a marker of synchronous adenocarcinoma (*prevalent carcinoma*) but also a precursor of carcinoma (*incident carcinoma*). In the landmark 1983 article by Riddell et al,[15] a diagnostic system was proposed to include negative, indefinite, and positive for dysplasia. The last is further classified as low-grade dysplasia (LGD) and high-grade dysplasia (HGD).

Diagnosis of dysplasia is based on a constellation of microscopic features. These features include (1) architectural alteration exceeding that resulting from repair in chronic colitis and (2) cytologic (cellular and nuclear) abnormalities after excluding the possibility of reactive changes due to inflammation.

Negative for Dysplasia

Normal colonic crypts are straight tubular, regularly distributed, and perpendicular to the muscularis mucosae (Figure 27-3A). Mucosa in quiescent colitis shows architectural abnormalities as described previously (Figure 27-3B), often with an increase in mononuclear inflammatory cells in the lamina propria (Figures 27-3C, 27-3D).

In active colitis, injured and regenerating epithelium may show loss of mucin, a feature also seen in dysplasia. However, the presence of neutrophilic infiltration, surface and crypt epithelial damage, gradient maturation toward the surface, lack of nuclear enlargement, and pleomorphism should help to exclude dysplasia (Figures 27-3E, 27-3F). In the resolving phase, there may be no evident inflammation or epithelial injury, yet the epithelial cells may continue to show lack of mucin and variable degrees of nuclear enlargement, hyperchromasia, and nuclear stratification. The mitotic activity may be brisk. It is important to recognize the pattern of regenerative changes in this setting (Figures 27-3G, 27-3H).

Indefinite for Dysplasia

The term *indefinite for dysplasia* (IND) refers to epithelial atypia that are very focal or not severe enough for a firm diagnosis of LGD or focal changes highly suspicious for dysplasia but with evident active inflammation or ulcer. Some other scenarios in which this diagnosis may be appropriate include odd growth pattern, unusually florid inflammation and regeneration, lack of surface epithelium due to erosion/ulceration, or mechanic sloughing off. Sometimes, deeper sections may help resolve the uncertainty, as may the use of several immunohistochemical markers (discussed in the section on HGD). However, for most biopsies that fall into this diagnostic dilemma, it is recommended that the patient undergo treatment of the active disease, followed by repeat examination at a shorter interval.

In some practices, IND is further divided into IND probably negative (Figure 27-4A–27-4D), IND unknown

FIGURE 27-3. Negative for dysplasia includes normal state (**A**, H&E stain, ×100); quiescent colitis (**B**, H&E stain, ×100); chronic inactive colitis (**C**, H&E stain, ×100; **D**, H&E stain, ×200); chronic active colitis (**E**, H&E stain, ×100; **F**, H&E stain, ×200); and resolving phase of ulcerative colitis (**G**, H&E stain, ×100; **H**, H&E stain, ×200). In all scenarios, there is neither atypism nor atypism beyond that expected for reactive changes.

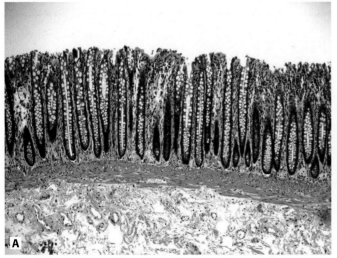

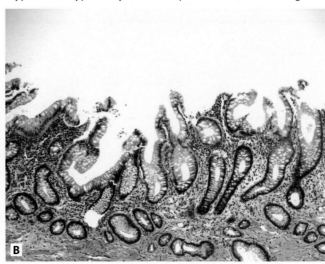

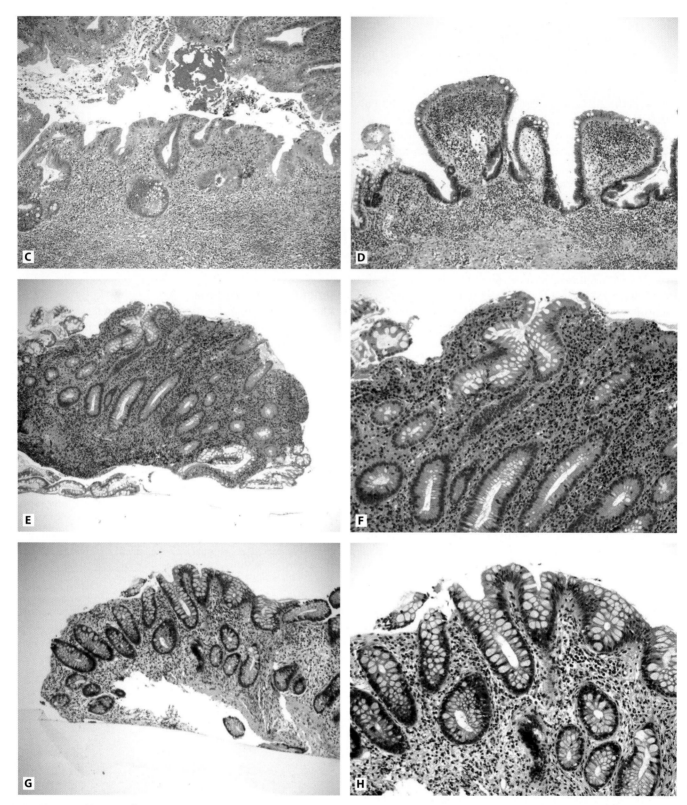

FIGURE 27-3. (*Continued*)

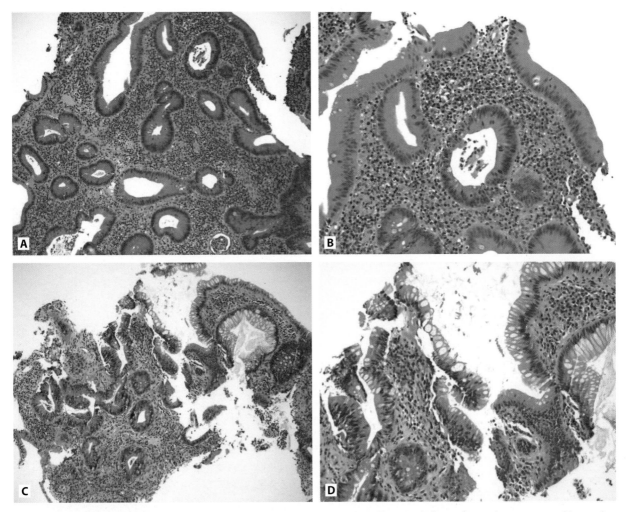

FIGURE 27-4. Epithelial changes indefinite for dysplasia, probably negative. **A, B.** There is slight nuclear enlargement and hyperchromasia in the presence of significant inflammation and nearby ulceration. Most likely, these represent reactive/regenerative changes. **A.** H&E stain, ×100. **B.** H&E stain, ×200. **C, D.** There are nuclear enlargement and hyperchromasia in some crypts; however, surface maturation is present. This biopsy is from a severely inflamed and ulcerated region and most likely represents regenerative changes. **C.** H&E stain, ×100. **D.** H&E stain, ×200.

(Figures 27-5A–27-5D), and IND probably positive (Figures 27-6A–27-6F). It is believed that these subdivisions can be useful in patient management if they are conveyed clearly to the clinician. On the other hand, if diagnostic criteria are followed strictly to keep the pool of IND reasonably small, further division of IND is not encouraged because it only adds to the uncertainty and anxiety.

Low-Grade Dysplasia

Often, LGD is characterized by stratified or pseudostratified hyperchromatic nuclei occupying the basal half of the epithelial layer (Figure 27-7A, 27-7B). The involved crypts show lack of maturation toward the surface (Figures 27-7A–27-7H). However, in some cases, unequivocal dysplasia is seen only in the crypts but not the surface. Therefore, the "surface involvement" rule should not be applied to exclude the diagnosis

of LGD in these cases. In some cases, LGD is accompanied by villiform change, dystrophic goblet cells (Figures 27-7C, 27-7D), endocrine cell hyperplasia, and Paneth cell metaplasia, features easily identified at low-power magnification. Occasionally, changes resembling traditional serrated adenomas may be seen, with cells containing strong eosinophilic cytoplasm (Figures 27-7G, 27-7H). Rarely, the dysplastic cells are uniform and resemble pyloric gland epithelium (Figure 27-7F).

High-Grade Dysplasia

High-grade dysplasia is characterized by cells with hyperchromatic nuclei with significant loss of polarity (Figures 27-8A–27-8D). Other features include marked nuclear membrane irregularity, abnormal mitosis, or architectural complexity of the crypt with cribriform change

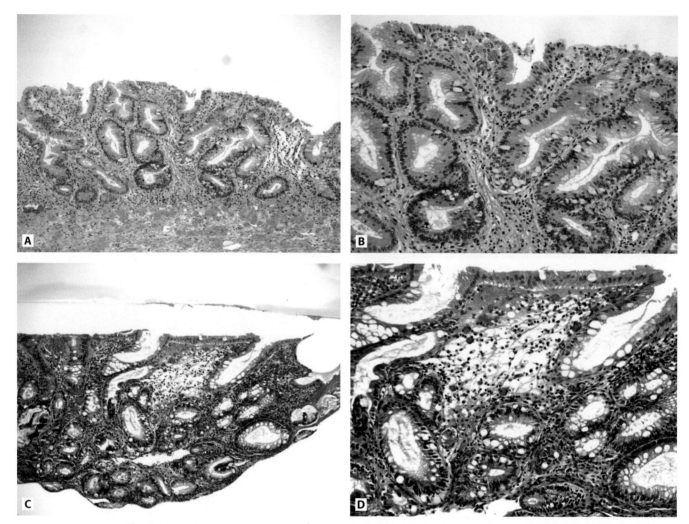

FIGURE 27-5. Epithelial changes indefinite for dysplasia, unknown. **A, B.** This case demonstrates slight hyperchromasia and nuclear enlargement in the epithelium (**A**, H&E stain, ×100; **B**, H&E stain, ×200). There is some degree of surface maturation. In addition, the stroma is slightly fibrotic. **C, D.** Similar features are seen in this case (**C**, H&E stain, ×100; **D**, H&E stain, ×200).

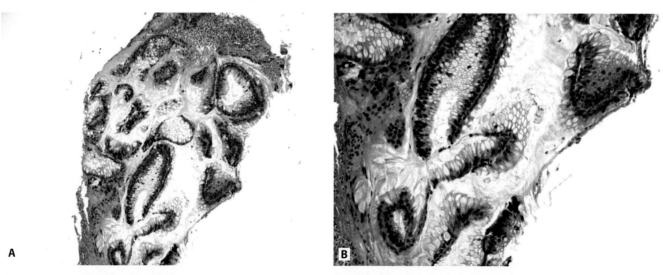

FIGURE 27-6. Epithelial changes indefinite for dysplasia, probably positive. **A, B.** Enlarged nuclei with hyperchromasias and stratification in the detached epithelium (**A**, H&E stain, ×100; **B**, H&E stain, ×200). **C, D.** Mild nuclear enlargement and hyperchromasia (**C**, H&E stain, ×40; **D**, H&E stain, ×100). **E, F.** Glands containing enlarged and hyperchromatic nuclei located at the edge of the tissue fragment (**E**, H&E stain, ×100; **F**, H&E, ×200). There are no surface maturation and an abrupt transition from nonneoplastic epithelium (**F**).

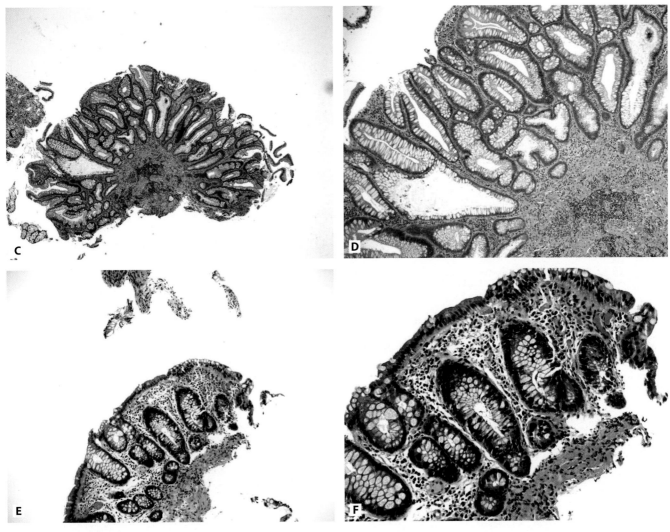

FIGURE 27-6. (*Continued*)

or focal clear cell changes (Figures 27-8E–27-8H). Loss of nuclear polarity, pleomorphism, and marked architectural complexity differentiate HGD from LGD. Rarely, marked inflammation may be present in HGD and may significantly affect the interpretation. Utilization of an immunohistochemical stain, such as p53, may be helpful. A strong and diffuse nuclear staining of p53 in those highly pleomorphic cells provides support for a diagnosis of HGD. However, negative results do not confirm a "nonneoplastic" nature. Because a diagnosis of flat HGD almost always leads to colectomy, concurrence with this diagnosis should be obtained from an expert gastrointestinal pathologist or a second pathologist.

The reproducibility studies for diagnosing and grading dysplasia in IBD showed low interobserver agreement for IND and LGD and good agreement for negative for dysplasia or HGD.[15,17] In these studies, instead of using long-term clinical outcome as end points, a consensus diagnosis was considered the correct diagnosis for data analysis. Therefore, in practice, when surgical treatment is considered as a result of a diagnosis of flat LGD, at least 2 expert gastrointestinal

pathologists should examine the biopsy and reach a consensus diagnosis. Concurrence should also be obtained for a diagnosis of flat HGD because such a diagnosis almost always leads to colectomy. If a consensus cannot be reached, a diagnosis of IND should be given in the hope that the definitive diagnosis can be reached in subsequent biopsies after treatment of active inflammation or better sampling.

As mentioned, immunostains may be considered for diagnostically challenging cases as well, in addition to performing additional levels of sectioning. It has been observed that intense nuclear p53 staining and aberrant CK7 expression occur in dysplastic epithelium[18,19] (Figures 27-9A–27-9I). In cases worrisome for HGD in the presence of marked inflammation or in cases worrisome for LGD in the absence of inflammation, strong and diffuse expression of these markers provides support for the diagnosis (Figures 27-10A, 27-10B). However, it needs to be pointed out that the sensitivities of these markers for dysplasia are low.[19] Biopsies with negative staining should not be automatically "ruled" as negative for dysplasia. Most important, there have been

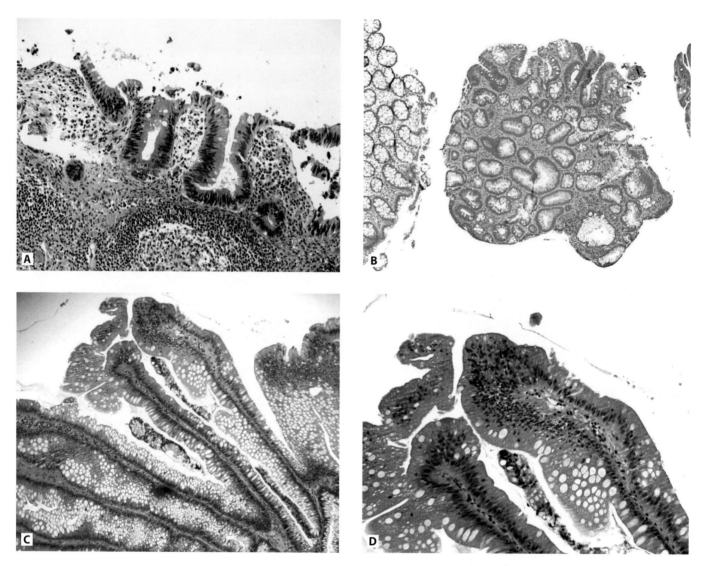

FIGURE 27-7. Epithelium positive for low-grade dysplasia. **A.** Flat low-grade dysplasia. The epithelial cells contain stratified hyperchromatic nuclei without surface maturation (H&E stain, ×100). **B.** Polypoid fragment of low-grade dysplasia. The overall features are similar to that of sporadic adenomas (H&E stain, ×40). **C, D.** A case of low-grade dysplasia with villous configuration and dystrophic goblet cells (**C**, H&E stain, ×100; **D**, H&E stain, ×200). **E.** Flat low-grade dysplasia with villous configuration (H&E stain, ×100). There is no significant pleomorphism or loss of polarity of the nuclei. **F.** Flat low-grade dysplasia with pyloric gland features (H&E stain, ×100). There is uniform, monotonous proliferation of cuboidal cells without surface maturation. **G, H.** Polypoid traditional serrated adenoma (TSA)–like low-grade dysplasia. Some epithelial cells are eosinophilic and resemble that of sporadic traditional serrated adenomas (**G**, H&E stain, ×40; **H**, H&E stain, ×200).

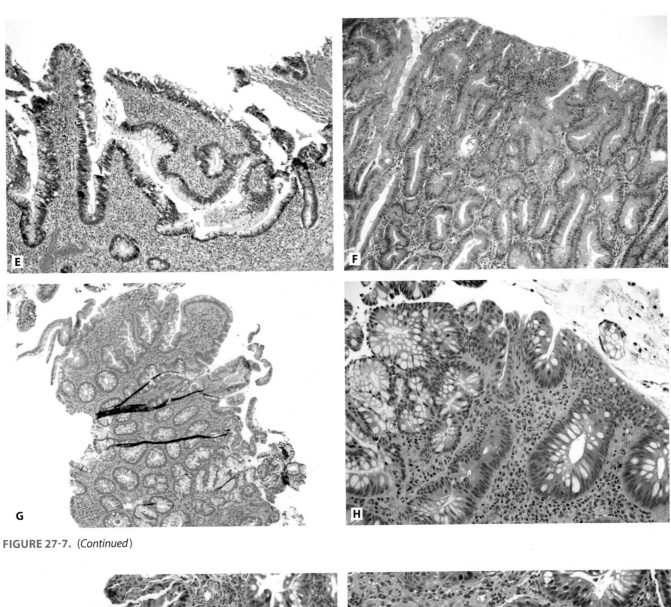

FIGURE 27-7. (*Continued*)

FIGURE 27-8. High-grade dysplasia. **A, B.** Glands with enlarged and hyperchromatic nuclei, extending to the surface (**A**, H&E stain, ×100; **B**, H&E stain, ×400). Pleomorphism is present. **C.** High-grade dysplasia with round cells containing enlarged nuclei. Some of the nuclei are hyperchromatic, but some have open chromatin (H&E stain, ×400). **D.** High-grade dysplasia with marked nuclear pleomorphism (H&E stain, ×400). This degree of pleomorphism is sufficient for a diagnosis of high-grade dysplasia despite the presence of acute inflammation. **E, F.** High-grade dysplasia with serrated features (**E**, H&E stain, ×100; **F**, H&E stain, ×200). In addition, there is architectural complexity (**F**). **G, H.** High-grade dysplasia with architectural complexity and focal clear cell changes (**G**, H&E stain, ×100; **H**, H&E stain, ×400).

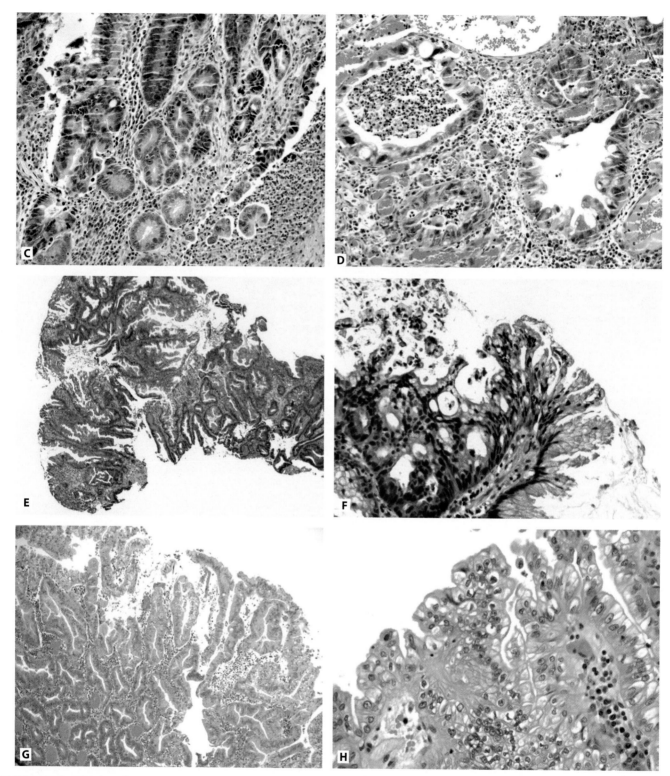

FIGURE 27-8. (*Continued*)

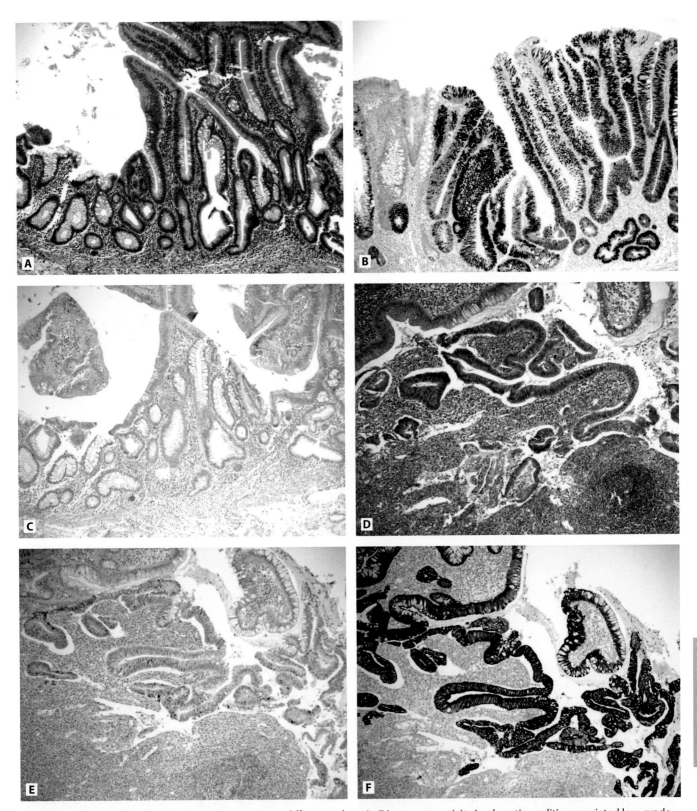

FIGURE 27-9. Strong p53 nuclear immunoreactivity or diffuse cytokeratin 7 immunoreactivity in ulcerative colitis–associated low-grade dysplasia. **A–C.** A case of low-grade dysplasia with strong nuclear p53 staining but negative CK7 immunoreactivity (**A**, H&E stain, ×100; **B**, immunostain for p53, ×100; **C**, immunostain for CK7, ×100). **D–F.** A case of low-grade dysplasia with negative p53 nuclear staining but strong and diffuse immunoreactivity for CK7 (**D**, H&E stain, ×100; **E**, immunostain for p53, ×100; **F**, immunostain for CK7, ×100). **G–I**. A case of low-grade dysplasia with positive p53 nuclear staining and immunoreactivity for CK7 (**G**, H&E stain, ×100; **H**, immunoperoxidase stain for p53, ×100; **I**, immunoperoxidase stain for CK7, ×100).

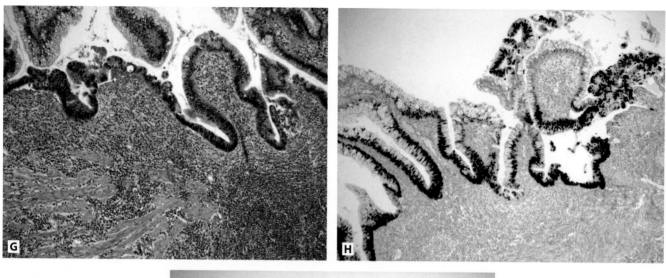

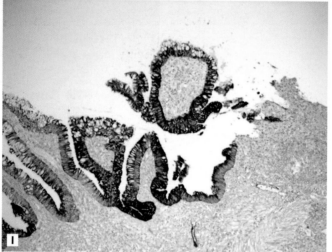

FIGURE 27-9. (*Continued*)

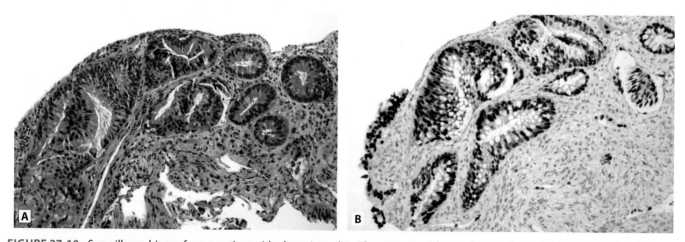

FIGURE 27-10. Surveillance biopsy from a patient with ulcerative colitis. There is a small focus of atypical glands with enlarged and hyper-chromatic nuclei (**A**). Surface maturation cannot be evaluated due to tangential sectioning. Strong and diffuse nuclear p53 staining (**B**) supports the diagnosis of low-grade dysplasia in this case.

no rigorously tested or uniformly accepted algorithms in interpretation of these immunostains despite several excellent studies that were institutionally based.[19,20] Therefore, its use should be considered, with discretion of the individual pathologist, purely as an ancillary test. It cannot be overemphasized that assessment for dysplasia should primarily rely on high-quality H&E stained sections, and no single immunohistochemical or molecular markers can replace the good practice of careful and objective H&E examination.

Dysplasia Identified in Endoscopically Apparent Lesions

Dysplasia identified in a polyp or mass has been traditionally termed as a *dysplasia-associated lesion or mass* (DALM).[21] More recent findings indicated that the so-called DALM may be further divided into 3 categories based on endoscopic appearance and location of the lesion: (1) sporadic adenoma if the polyp looks like a usual adenoma both endoscopically and histologically and is located outside the areas of histologically proven colitis; (2) IBD-associated adenoma-like polypoid dysplasia if the lesion looks like an adenoma but is located in the areas of colitis; and (3) IBD-associated nonadenomatous dysplasia (true DALM) if the elevated lesion is irregular and broadly based or forms a mass in the areas of colitis. This classification is necessary for further management as sporadic adenomas can be removed by polypectomy followed by routine surveillance colonoscopy, and those with IBD-associated adenoma-like dysplasia can undergo polypectomy with regular or increased frequency of surveillance.[22,23] The rationale for this type of practice is that (1) these lesions likely behave as adenomas occurring in patients without IBD, and (2) the location of polypectomy can be tracked and easily recognized in follow-up examinations, so colectomy is considered unnecessary without other indications for surgery.

However, for IBD-associated nonadenomatous dysplasia (DALM lesion, LGD or HGD), flat LGD, flat HGD, colectomy is preferred due to a higher risk for both prevalent and incident carcinoma and because flat lesions are difficult to locate in subsequent follow-up. It should be kept in mind that, in reality, it is often challenging on histological grounds alone to distinguish adenoma-like polypoid dysplasia from nonadenoma-like DALM. Clinical correlation with the extent of colitis, the location of the polypoid lesion, and the endoscopic appearance of the polypoid lesion are essential in this process. In addition, biopsy of the mucosa surrounding the polyp and attention to the epithelial lining of the stalk of the polyp are important for the judgment.

Serrated Crypts in Flat Mucosa or Other Atypical Endoscopic Lesions

Typical hyperplastic polyps occur outside the areas of colitis in patients with IBD and should be diagnosed as such when recognized. When the superficial portion of the crypts exhibits a serrated pattern similar to that of a hyperplastic polyp in mucosa involved by colitis, it should be recorded

as "serrated change" if it is prominent, with the understanding that its significance is still under study, and anecdotal evidence suggests there may be increased risk for cancer. However, focal serrated change in the absence of cytological atypia (Figure 27-11A) may not be associated with increased risk of incident neoplasia (our unpublished observation). However, if there is mild concurrent cytologic atypia, this change is best interpreted as IND (Figure 27-11B). A typical sessile serrated polyp (SSP) outside the areas of colitis in

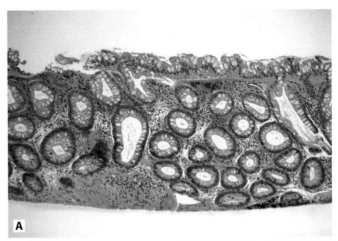

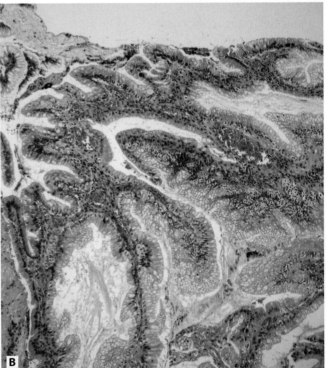

FIGURE 27-11. Focal serrated features resembling early hyperplastic polyp is noted in this surveillance colonic biopsy from a patient with ulcerative colitis. This alone, in the absence of cytological atypia, should not be interpreted as indefinite for dysplasia (**A**). However, when there is accompanying mild cytological atypia, this change should be interpreted as epithelial changes indefinite for dysplasia (**B**).

PART SIX

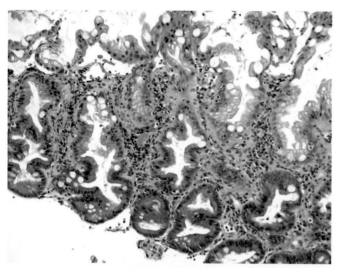

FIGURE 27-12. Sessile serrated polyp occurring in the region of colitis. This is indistinguishable from a sporadic sessile serrated polyp.

patients with IBD should be diagnosed as such when recognized. However, when an SSP occurs in the region of colitis (Figure 27-12), it should be completely removed by polypectomy and the patient continued on surveillance as there are only a few clinical follow-up studies on this entity.[24]

Invasive Adenocarcinoma

Occasionally, a more severe lesion, such as invasive adenocarcinoma (Figure 27-13A), may be diagnosed on the screening and surveillance biopsies. These lesions can be flat without endoscopically evident lesions or present as a mass. The diagnosis relies on the presence of infiltrative or haphazardly arranged malignant glands, infiltrating single malignant

cells, and desmoplasia. Often, dysplasia and chronic colitis may be found in adjacent tissue (Figure 27-13B). The presence of dysplasia and chronic colitis adjacent to the invasive adenocarcinoma supports a diagnosis of colitis-associated CRC.

■ SURVEILLANCE BIOPSIES AND CLINICAL MANAGEMENT

Clinical management of patients with UC in a surveillance program depends on several factors. It is recommended that both HGD and DALM carry higher risk (about 40% for HGD and 30% for DALMs) for prevalent CRC or short-term progression to CRC (about 25%); therefore, immediate colectomy is warranted.[25,26] The natural history of LGD is more controversial. In some studies, LGD was associated with a 20% risk of prevalent CRC in patients who underwent immediate colectomy or colectomy within 6 months and a 14.5% to 19.4% risk of progressing to CRC in patients if followed.[26,27] However, in some institutions, the progression rate of LGD may be much lower (7.8%).[28] There are no clinical features to predict progression among these patients.[27] Our recent study showed that, for UC with mucosal changes IND, there was a significant risk for prevalent HGD (27%) and a significant progression rate to dysplasia (3.2 cases/100 person-years) or advanced neoplasia (1.5 cases/100 person-years).[29]

The current approach to surveillance in UC is to perform a colonoscopy after 8–10 years of left-sided or extensive colitis and repeat colonoscopy every 1–3 years. The current guidelines for management are listed in Table 27-1.[15,23,29,30] For patients with chronic extensive Crohn colitis, similar colonoscopic surveillance has been used and reportedly detected prevalent neoplasia in 8% of patients and incident neoplasia in an additional 14% of patients.[31]

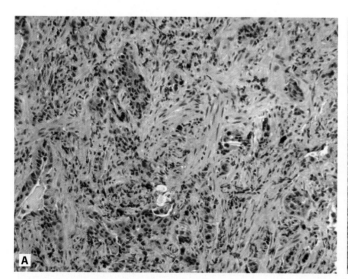

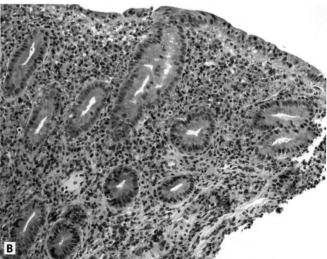

FIGURE 27-13. Invasive adenocarcinoma in surveillance colonic biopsy from a patient with ulcerative colitis. Angulated malignant glands infiltrating desmoplastic stroma (**A**). A small focus of dysplasia is noted in adjacent mucosa (**B**).

TABLE 27-1. Clinical management in patients with ulcerative colitis and extensive chronic Crohn colitis in surveillance program.

Histology in colonic biopsy	Endoscopic finding	Need for confirmation by an experienced gastrointestinal pathologist	Recommended management
Negative for dysplasia	N/A	No	Continue regular surveillance
Indefinite for dysplasia, probably negative	Absence of lesion	No	Continue regular surveillance
Indefinite for dysplasia, unknown	Presence of lesion	No	Repeat biopsy at short intervals within days or months[a]
	Absence of lesion	No	Repeat biopsy at short intervals within months[a]
Indefinite for dysplasia, probably positive	Presence of lesion	May be helpful	Repeat biopsy at short intervals within days or months[a]
	Absence of lesion	May be helpful	Repeat biopsy at short intervals within months[a]
LGD	Polyp that can be completely removed endoscopically	No	Polypectomy followed by regular surveillance
	Sessile/mass lesion that cannot be completely removed endoscopically	Yes	Colectomy
	Absence of lesion (flat)	Yes	Surveillance at short interval if unifocal flat LGD[a,b]; colectomy if multifocal flat LGD[b] or if flat LGD spreads to other regions or progresses in patients initially choose continued surveillance
HGD	Polyp that can be completely removed endoscopically	No	Polypectomy
	Either sessile/mass lesion that cannot be completely removed endoscopically or absence of lesion (flat)	Yes	Colectomy

Abbreviations: HGD, high-grade dysplasia; LGD, low-grade dysplasia; N/A, not applicable.

[a]Intervals may be days or months depending on clinical impression and endoscopic findings, but should not be longer than 1 year.[15,29] If interpretational difficulties are due to active inflammation, it is useful to repeat biopsy after the disease activity has subsided.[15]

[b]Unifocal flat LGD is defined as only 1 specimen showing flat LGD. Multifocal flat LGD is defined as 2 or more specimen jars contained biopsy samples with flat LGD.[27]

◼ NEOPLASIA IN THE POUCH AND PERIPOUCH REGION

Approximately 30% of the patients with UC would ultimately require colectomy for medically refractory UC or UC-associated neoplasia. Restorative ileal pouch–anal anastomosis (IPAA) after proctocolectomy has become the surgical treatment of choice for these patients.[32] Neoplasia can occur in the pouch or the peripouch region[33] but occurrence is relatively low, with reported incidence rates of 1.6% and 1.8% in two studies.[34,35] Risk factors of developing pouch neoplasia include prior colorectal neoplasia.[34,35] Pouch and peripouch adenocarcinoma (Figure 27-14) is histomorphologically similar to UC-associated adenocarcinoma.[33] Mortality associated with pouch cancer appears to be high.[33]

Endoscopic surveillance with biopsy has been conventional for patients with UC with IPAA, especially patients with prior colorectal neoplasia, but the performance is suboptimal as dysplasia is only noted in biopsy in 33% of patients with pouch and peripouch adenocarcinoma.[33]

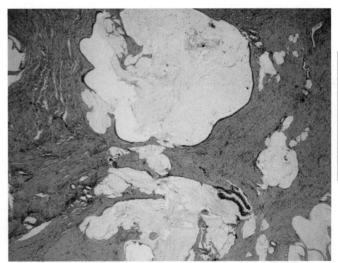

FIGURE 27-14. Pouch biopsy with invasive adenocarcinoma. Dysplastic gland with associated extracellular mucin invading muscularis propria, consistent with a well-differentiated mucinous adenocarcinoma.

PART SIX

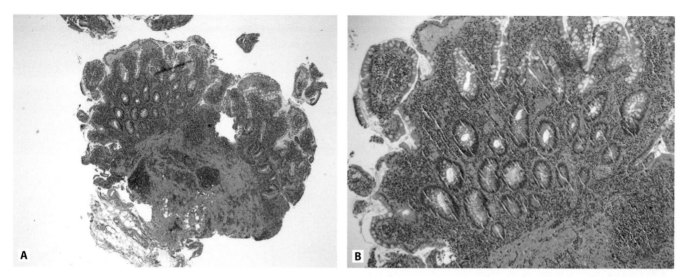

FIGURE 27-15. Pouch biopsy negative for dysplasia. **A, B.** This pouch biopsy shows chronic active inflammation but no evidence of dysplasia.

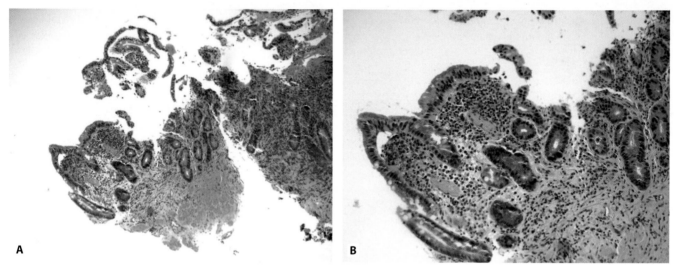

FIGURE 27-16. Pouch biopsy with indefinite for dysplasia. **A, B.** There are a few glands with hyperchromatic and slightly enlarged nuclei, which are more than would be expected for the degree of inflammation.

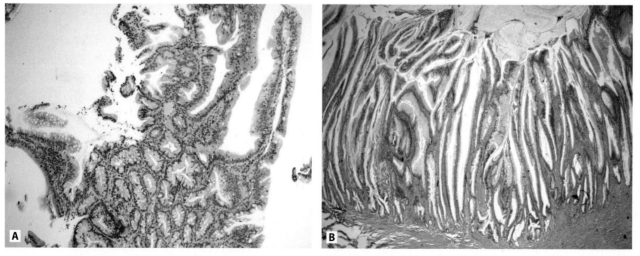

FIGURE 27-17. Pouch biopsy with low-grade dysplasia. **A.** This pouch biopsy shows proliferation of uniform cells with mildly enlarged and hyperchromatic nuclei without surface maturation. **B.** This pouch biopsy shows features identical to villous adenoma.

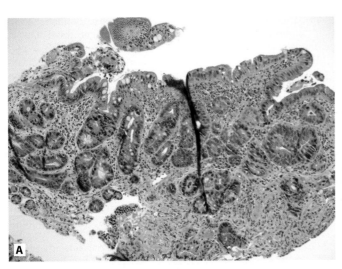
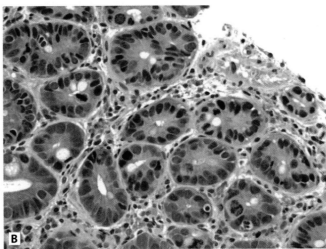

FIGURE 27-18. Pouch biopsy with high-grade dysplasia. **A, B.** This biopsy shows proliferation of glands lined by epithelium with marked hyperchromatic and enlarged nuclei.

This may be related to postoperative anatomic complexity in this region. Regardless, the diagnosing and grading of prepouch ileal, pouch, and rectal cuff/anal transitional zone biopsy are similar to those used in patients with UC. Specifically, this is a diagnostic system that includes negative, indefinite, and positive for dysplasia; the last is further classified as LGD and HGD and should be used for the interpretation of biopsies from these regions in patients with IBD with IPAA. Examples of pouch biopsies with epithelia changes negative for dysplasia, IND, positive for LGD, and positive for HGD are shown in Figures 27-15 to 27-18.

▇ REFERENCES

1. Jess T, Loftus EV Jr, Harmsen WS, et al. Survival and cause specific mortality in patients with inflammatory bowel disease: a long term outcome study in Olmsted County, Minnesota, 1940–2004. *Gut.* 2006;55:1248–1254.
2. Whitcomb E, Liu X, Xiao SY. Crohn's-associated small bowel adenocarcinomas exhibit gastric differentiation. *Hum Pathol.* 2014;45(2):359–367.
3. Simpson S, Traube J, Riddell RH. The histologic appearance of dysplasia (precarcinomatous change) in Crohn's disease of the small and large intestine. *Gastroenterology.* 1981;81:492–501.
4. Eaden JA, Abrams KR, Mayberry JF. The risk of colorectal cancer in ulcerative colitis: a meta-analysis. *Gut.* 2001;48:526–535.
5. Choi PM, Zelig MP. Similarity of colorectal cancer in Crohn's disease and ulcerative colitis: implications for carcinogenesis and prevention. *Gut.* 1994;35:950–954
6. Harpaz N, Polydorides AD. Colorectal dysplasia in chronic inflammatory bowel disease: pathology, clinical implications, and pathogenesis. *Arch Pathol Lab Med.* 2010;13:876–895.
7. Gillen CD, Walmsley RS, Prior P, et al. Ulcerative colitis and Crohn's disease: a comparison of the colorectal cancer risk in extensive colitis. *Gut.* 1994;35:1590–1592.
8. Bernstein CN, Blanchard JF, Kliewer E, et al. Cancer risk in patients with inflammatory bowel disease: a population-based study. *Cancer.* 2001;91:854–862.
9. Liu X, Goldblum JR, Zhao Z, et al. Distinct clinicohistologic features of inflammatory bowel disease-associated colorectal adenocarcinoma. *Am J Surg Pathol.* 2012;36:1228–1233.
10. Levi GS, Harpaz N. Intestinal low-grade tubuloglandular adenocarcinoma in inflammatory bowel disease. *Am J Surg Pathol.* 2006;30(8):1022–1029.
11. Traube J, Simpson S, Riddell RH, Levin B, Kirsner JB. Crohn's disease and adenocarcinoma of the bowel. *Dig Dis Sci.* 1980;25(12):939–944.
12. Lewis B, Lin J, Wu X, et al. Crohn's disease-like reaction predicts favorable prognosis in colitis-associated colorectal cancer. *Inflamm Bowel Dis.* 2013;19:2190–2198.
13. Morson BC, Pang LSC. Rectal biopsy as an aid to cancer control in ulcerative colitis. *Gut.* 1967;8:423–434.
14. Friedman S, Rubin PH, Bodian C, et al. Screening and surveillance colonoscopy in chronic Crohn's colitis: results of a surveillance program spanning 25 years. *Clin Gastroenterol Hepatol.* 2008;6:993–998
15. Riddell RH, Goldman H, Ransohoff DF, et al. Dysplasia in inflammatory bowel disease: standardized classification with provisional clinical application. *Hum Pathol.* 1983;14:931–968.
16. Hamilton SR, Aaltonen LA, eds. *World Health Organization Classification of Tumours.* Vol. 2. *Pathology and Genetics of Tumours of the Digestive System.* Lyon, France: IARC Press; 2000.
17. Eaden J, Abrams K, McKay H, et al. Inter-observer variation between general and specialist gastrointestinal pathologists when grading dysplasia in ulcerative colitis. *J Pathol.* 2001;194:152–157.
18. Walsh SV, Loda M, Torres CM, et al. P53 and beta catenin expression in chronic ulcerative colitis—associated polypoid dysplasia and sporadic adenomas: an immunohistochemical study. *Am J Surg Pathol.* 1999;23(8):963–969.
19. Xie H, Xiao S-Y, Pai R, et al. Diagnostic utility of TP53 and cytokeratin immunohistochemistry in idiopathic inflammatory bowel disease-associated neoplasia. *Mod Pathol.* 2014;27(2):303–313.
20. Marx A, Wandrey T, Simon P, et al. Combined alpha-methylacyl coenzyme A racemase/p53 analysis to identify dysplasia in inflammatory bowel disease. *Hum Pathol.* 2009;40(2):166–173.
21. Blackstone MO, Riddell RH, Rogers BHG, et al. Dysplasia-associated lesion or mass (DALM) detected by colonoscopy in long-standing ulcerative colitis: an indication for colectomy. *Gastroenterology.* 1981;8:366–374.
22. Rubin PH, Friedman S, Harpaz N, et al. Colonoscopic polypectomy in chronic colitis: conservative management after endoscopic resection of dysplastic polyps. *Gastroenterology.* 1999;117(6):1295–1300.

PART SIX

23. Farraye FA, Odze RD, Eaden J, et al. AGA technical review on the diagnosis and management of colorectal neoplasia in inflammatory bowel disease. *Gastroenterology*. 2010;138:746–774.

24. Ko HM, Harpaz N, Polydorides AD. Classification and significance of serrated colorectal polyps in inflammatory bowel disease. *Mod Pathol*. 2013;26(Suppl 2):160A.

25. Bernstein CN, Shanahan F, Weinstein WM. Are we telling patients the truth about surveilance colonoscopy in ulcerative colitis? *Lancet*. 1994;107:934–944.

26. Rutter MD, Saunders BP, Wilkinson KH, et al. Thirty-year analysis of a colonoscopic surveillance program for neoplasia in ulcerative colitis. *Gastroenterology*. 2006;130:1030–1038.

27. Ullman T, Croog V, Harpaz N, et al. Progression of flat low-grade dysplasia to advanced neoplasia in patients with ulcerative colitis. *Gastroenterology*. 2003;125:1311–1319.

28. Pekow JR, Hetzel JT, Rothe JA, et al. Outcome after surveillance of low-grade and indefinite for dysplasia in patients with ulcerative colitis. *Inflamm Bowel Dis*. 2010;16(8):1352–1356.

29. Lai KK, Wang Y, Xie H, et al. Clinical otucome after the diagnosis of indefinite for dysplasia in patients with idiopathic inflammatory bowel disease. *Mod Pathol*. 2013;26(Suppl 2):163A.

30. Farraye FA, Odze RD, Eaden J, et al. AGA medical position statement on the diagnosis and management of colorectal neoplasia in inflammatory bowel disease. *Gastroenterology*. 2010;138:738–745.

31. Friedman S, Rubin PH, Bodian C, et al. Screening and surveillance colonoscopy in chronic Crohn's colitis: results of a surveillance program spanning 25 years. *Clin Gastroenterol Hepatol*. 2008;6:993–998.

32. Fazio VW, Kiran RP, Remzi FH, et al. Ileal pouch anal anastomosis: analysis of outcome and quality of life in 3707 patients. *Ann Surg*. 2013;257(4):679–685.

33. Jiang W, Shadrach B, Carver P, et al. Histomorphologic and molecular features of pouch and peripouch adenocarcinoma: a comparison with ulcerative colitis-associated adenocarcinoma. *Am J Surg Pathol*. 2012;36(9):1385–1394.

34. Kariv R, Remzi FH, Lian L, et al. Preoperative colorectal neoplasia increases risk for pouch neoplasia in patients with restorative proctocolectomy. *Gastroenterology*. 2010;139:806–812.

35. Derikx LAAP, Kievit W, Drenth JP, et al. Prior colorectal neoplasia is associated with increased risk of ileoanal pouch neoplasia in patients with inflammatory bowel disease. *Gastroenterology*. 2014;146:119–128.

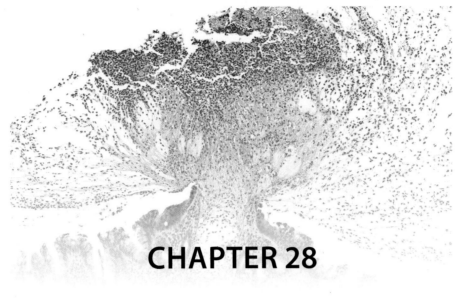

CHAPTER 28

Infectious and Other Colitis

Nhu Thuy Can and Shu-Yuan Xiao

INTRODUCTION

In general, the term *colitis* refers to colonic mucosal injury with infiltration by inflammatory cells. Inflammatory bowel disease (IBD; discussed in other chapters) and colitis of infectious etiology fit this description. However, several other types of mucosal injury exist that are not remarkable for inflammatory infiltration, such as pure radiation-induced damage or ischemic injury, unless there is neutrophilic infiltration secondary to surface erosions. Nevertheless, the term *colitis* has been used for these diseases as well. Both ischemic and radiation colitis are discussed in Chapter 1. Several drug-induced colitides are discussed in Chapter 2 due to their frequent occurrence in transplant settings. However, for the purpose of comparison, some of these are further described in this chapter as well.

INFECTIOUS COLITIS

Some authors use the terms *acute self-limited colitis* and *infectious colitis* interchangeably. However, several forms of fungal or parasitic colitis are neither acute nor self-limited. Infectious colitis includes both acute self-limited colitis (mostly bacterial) and more severe or prolonged colitis. In our practice, the term acute self-limited colitis is applied to some of the bacterial colitis that are transient and not associated with significant mucosal architectural abnormalities. They are usually accompanied by bloody diarrhea that resolves approximately 1–2 weeks after onset without recurrence on follow-up examinations.[1,2] By this definition, acute

self-limited colitis does not manifest histologically as chronic crypt injury and thus is usually not confused with IBD. On the other hand, infectious colitides that are chronic or have a prolonged clinical course may display histological findings that overlap with IBD, leading to potential misdiagnosis. In addition, patients with IBD are at increased risk for infectious colitis due to immunosuppressive therapy, further complicating the diagnosis.[1,2] Thus, an infectious etiology should always be considered in patients with IBD who are refractory to therapy or during acute exacerbations.[3]

Viral Colitis

Viral infections of the colon are overwhelmingly more common in immunocompromised individuals but can affect immunocompetent patients as well.[4,5] Up to 30% of acute exacerbations of IBD may be related to viral infection.[6]

Cytomegalovirus (CMV) colitis is the most common form of viral colitis in the immunocompromised setting and typically presents with diarrhea, abdominal pain, and ulceration with bleeding or perforation.[5,7,8] One study found that up to 25% of patients with CMV colitis had normal-appearing mucosa on endoscopy.[5] CMV colitis may mimic an acute episode of IBD, and it is also a known complication of immunosuppressive therapy.[9–11] Histologically, the colonic mucosa demonstrates a mixed inflammatory infiltrate, with activity and granulation tissue in more severe cases (ulceration). Crypt apoptosis may be evident in some cases (Figure 28-1A). CMV-induced cytopathic changes are characterized by intranuclear inclusions surrounded by a

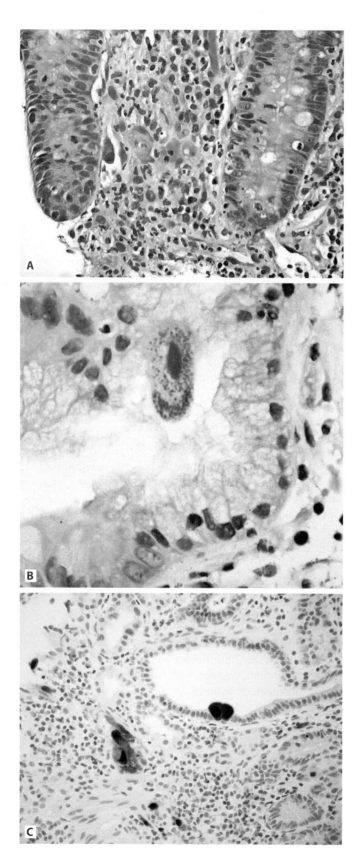

FIGURE 28-1. Cytomegalovirus (CMV) colitis. **A.** Acute CMV colitis with inflammatory cellular infiltration, crypt apoptosis, and multiple inclusion bodies. **B.** An infected epithelial cell with nuclear and cytoplasmic inclusions (purple cytoplasmic granules). **C.** Immunostain for CMV.

clear halo and granular intracytoplasmic inclusion bodies (Figure 28-1B). The cytopathic changes can be seen in both endothelial cells and epithelial cells. A CMV immunostain (Figure 28-1C) may be useful in identifying the organisms to either confirm the infection when inclusion bodies are rare and hard to find or in cases that are highly suspicious for CMV infection clinically but show no evidence of the infection on hematoxylin and eosin (H&E) sections. In colitis of longer duration, there may be marked crypt loss accompanied by fibrosis (Figure 28-2). Chronic changes sometimes can be difficult to distinguish from IBD. To make the situation more complex, it is not uncommon to see superimposed CMV infection in the background of IBD (Figure 28-3).

Adenovirus colitis is another common form of infectious colitis in immunosuppressed patients, particularly those with AIDS.[8,12,13] Adenovirus is also a major cause of acute diarrhea in children, accounting for 3.2% to 12.5% of cases.[14] However, it is not commonly associated with acute exacerbations in patients with IBD.[15,16] The virus typically infects the epithelium, producing amphophilic-to-eosinophilic intranuclear inclusions that are irregular and crescent or sickle shape (Figure 28-4B). Sometimes, mild epithelial degenerative change may mimic adenoviral inclusions. Immunostain for adenovirus can help to confirm the diagnosis (Figure 28-4D). Coinfection with CMV is a common occurrence, with studies reporting up to 75% of adenovirus cases exhibiting coinfection with CMV.[12,13] In addition, coinfection with other agents, such as histoplasmosis, is not uncommon (Figure 28-4).

Herpes simplex virus (HSV) typically causes acute proctitis in immunosuppressed patients. Friable colonic mucosa as well as necrotic ulcers may be evident on colonoscopy. Histologically, there is a marked mixed inflammatory cellular infiltrate with lymphocytes and plasma cells. Epithelial

FIGURE 28-2. Chronic colitis due to cytomegalovirus infection in a patient who had a hematopoietic stem cell transplant. Severe loss of crypts is seen as well as fibrosis in the lamina propria and submucosa. It is not possible to completely exclude the possibility that the crypt loss is due to another etiology, such as chronic GVHD (no evidence of ongoing GVHD identified in this case).

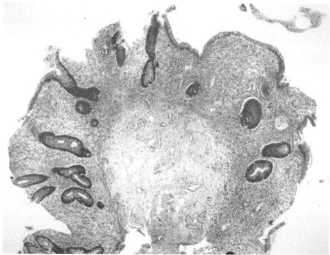

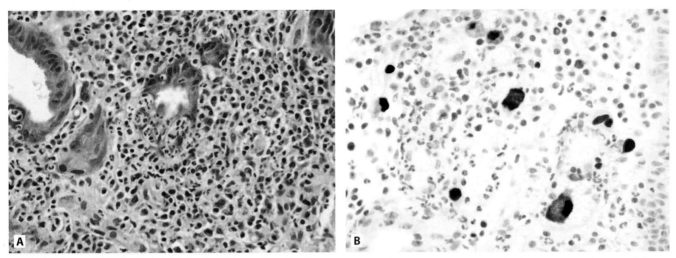

FIGURE 28-3. Cytomegalovirus (CMV) infection in a background of ulcerative colitis. **A.** The background exhibits crypt architectural distortion and crypt loss with mixed inflammatory infiltration and cryptitis; however, several epithelial cells and stroma cells contain CMV inclusions. **B.** Immunostain for CMV.

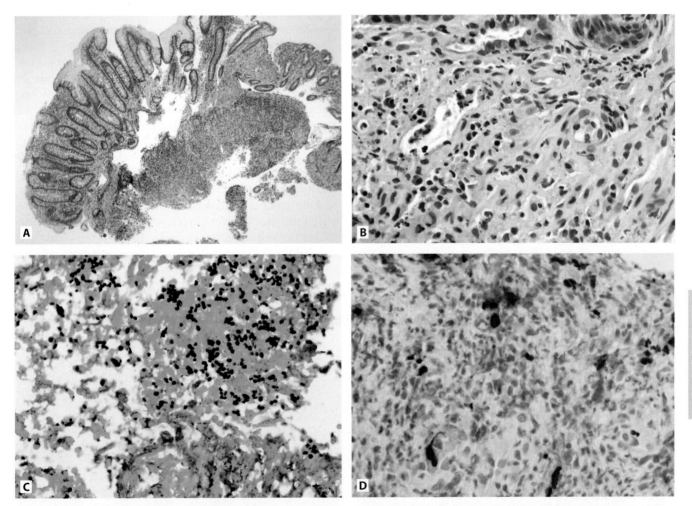

FIGURE 28-4. Colitis due to adenovirus and histoplasmosis coinfection. **A.** The mucosa exhibits hyperplastic changes in reaction to the inflammatory infiltration in the lamina propria. The submucosa contains a large epithelioid granuloma. **B.** Several epithelial cells and stromal cells contain dark, smudged nuclei, suggestive of adenoviral cytopathic changes. **C.** Gomori methamine silver (GMS) stain highlights numerous intracellular fungal yeast. **D.** Immunostain for adenovirus.

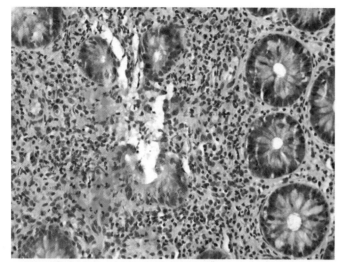

FIGURE 28-5. Acute self-limited colitis. There are no changes of chronicity, such as crypt branching or loss. There is a ruptured crypt due to cryptitis.

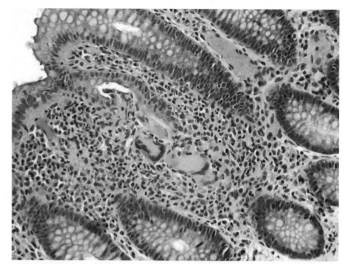

FIGURE 28-7. Multinucleated giant cells associated with a ruptured crypt in a case of acute infectious colitis.

cells contain eosinophilic intranuclear inclusions with multinucleation and margination of chromatin, which imparts a ground-glass appearance. Immunohistochemistry for HSV is useful if dense inflammation obscures the viral inclusions.

Bacterial Colitis

Most bacterial colitides manifest as an acute self-limited colitis. Infection may occur through ingestion of contaminated raw or undercooked food. The common clinically significant organisms include *Campylobacter, Shigella, Salmonella, Yersinia,* and *Escheria coli* O157:H7, although in most cases the precise organism cannot be identified. Mild acute self-limited colitis manifests histologically as a patchy neutrophilic infiltrate in the lamina propria and surface epithelium (Figure 28-5). The lamina propria also contains a mixed inflammatory cellular infiltration, sometimes with lymphoid follicles (Figure 28-6A). More severe cases have cryptitis,

crypt abscesses, or even ulceration, such as in *Salmonella* colitis (Figure 28-6).[1] Rarely, mucin granulomas can be seen associated with a ruptured crypt in acute infectious colitis (Figure 28-7). Unlike IBD, the normal crypt architecture is preserved in acute self-limited infectious colitis.

Histologic findings of more severe forms of acute colitis can sometimes help to identify the causative agents. For instance, infection by *E. coli* O157:H7 leads to a histologic pattern similar to that seen in early ischemic colitis, with superficial mucosal necrosis and fibrin thrombi in the capillaries of the lamina propria, which are components of the microangiopathic hemolytic anemia induced by the secreted Shiga toxins[17–20] (Figure 28-8).

Clostridium difficile colitis is associated with antibiotic use and is a major cause of diarrhea in hospitalized or institutionalized patients. The characteristic findings in *C. difficile* colitis are marked superficial mucosal necrosis (erosions), with overlying mushroom- or volcano-shape pseudomembranes

FIGURE 28-6. *Salmonella* colitis. **A.** Large lymphoid follicles with an adjacent ulcer. **B.** Crypt dilation and crypt abscesses may also be present.

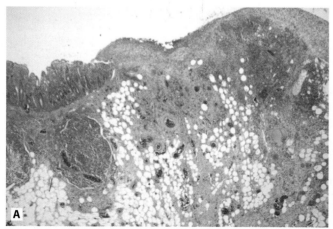

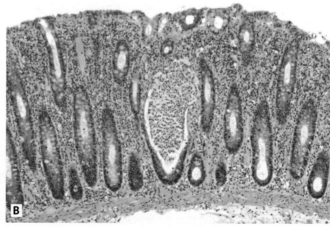

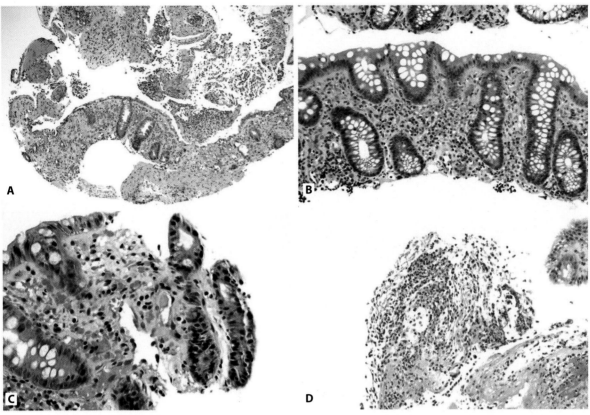

FIGURE 28-8. Enterohemorrhagic *Escherichia coli* O157:H7 colitis. **A.** The colonic mucosa exhibits crypt withering and dropout, superficial erosion, and marked lamina propria fibrosis. **B.** There is a paucity of inflammatory cellular infiltration. **C.** Microthrombi. **D.** Focal fibrinopurulent exudate (pseudomembrane).

consisting of mucin, neutrophils, and necroinflammatory debris (Figure 28-9). It should be emphasized that not all pseudomembranous colitis is caused by *C. difficile*, and some *C. difficile* colitis may not be accompanied by typical pseudomembranes, depending on the stage of disease. Some cases of *C. difficile* colitis without pseudomembranes can have nonspecific findings of acute self-limited colitis. In more severe cases, the mucosal necrosis may involve the full thickness of mucosa (Figure 28-10A), with focal features mimicking acute ischemic colitis (Figure 28-10B).

Mycobacterial infections are commonly seen in immunosuppressed individuals, including patients with IBD on immunosuppressive therapy. *Mycobacterium tuberculosis* predominantly involves the ileocecal region and manifests with mucosal ulcerations and caseating granulomas (see Chapter 20), while *M. avium-intracellulare* is characterized by aggregates of macrophages with abundant foamy cytoplasm in the lamina propria. AFB (acid-fast bacteria) stains will confirm the diagnosis in both diseases (Figure 28-11).

Fungal Colitis
Clinically significant fungal infections of the colon are predominantly seen in immunosuppressed patients but can be seen rarely in immunocompetent patients. The most common causes of fungal colitides are *Histoplasma*, *Aspergillus*,

Candida, and *Cryptococcus*.[8,21] In general, a high index of suspicion is required to make the diagnosis of fungal colitis as the findings may overlap with bacterial colitis.[8,21] Granulomas are considered characteristic of histoplasmosis (Figure 28-4) and cryptococcal infection. *Aspergillus* and *Candida* can both cause extensive angioinvasion with transmural infarction of the bowel wall.[21] In suspected specimens, special stains (periodic acid–Schiff [PAS] and Gomori methamine silver [GMS]) will help in diagnosing most cases.

Parasitic Colitis
Entamoeba histolytica is a protozoan parasite that causes colitis and amoebic liver abscesses. This infection is more common in developing countries and is especially prevalent in patients who are immunocompromised and have AIDS. About 90% of those infected with *E. histolytica* are asymptomatic.[22–24] Infants, elderly patients, and pregnant women are susceptible to fulminant disease. Infection with this organism can rarely form a mass mimicking a malignant neoplasm with gastrointestinal bleeding and obstruction.[22] The endoscopic appearance includes single or multiple irregular, flask-shaped ulcerated lesions with exudates, more commonly seen in the cecum, sigmoid, and rectum (Figure 28-12). Microscopic identification of typical amebic trophozoites is the key to tissue diagnosis (Figure 28-13). The colitis is characterized by

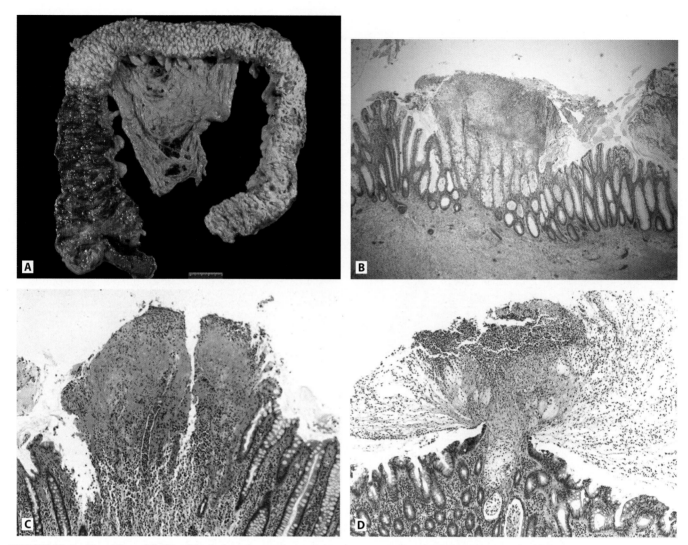

FIGURE 28-9. *Clostridium difficile* colitis. **A.** Pseudomembranous exudates extending from the rectum to the distal ascending colon, with focal polypoid configuration. The proximal colon exhibits hemorrhagic changes of mucosal necrosis. **B.** Multifocal superficial mucosal necrosis with characteristic necroinflammatory exudates forming "caps." **C.** A denser fibrinopurulent exudate is attached to the underlying inflamed and necrotic crypts. **D.** Volcano-type eruption of necroinflammatory exudate from a single damaged crypt.

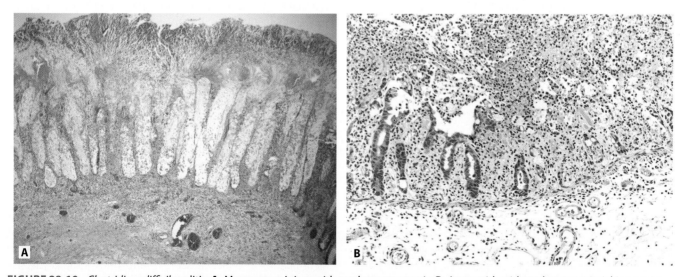

FIGURE 28-10. *Clostridium difficile* colitis. **A.** More severe injury with total crypt necrosis. **B.** Areas with withered crypts mimicking acute ischemic colitis.

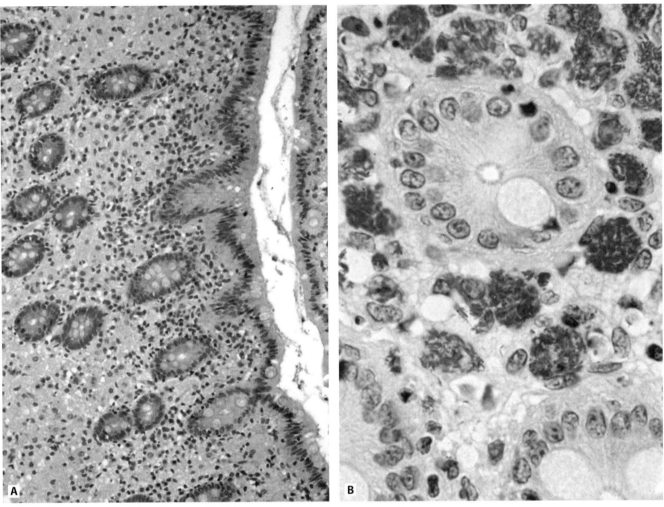

FIGURE 28-11. *Mycobacterium avium-intracellulare* colitis. **A.** The lamina propria is expanded by large foamy macrophages. **B.** Acid-fast stain highlights numerous intracellular bacilli organisms.

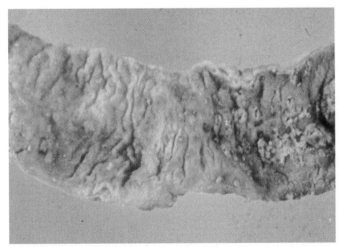

FIGURE 28-12. Macroscopic appearance of *Entamoeba histolytica* colitis showing many discrete small ulcers with exudates.

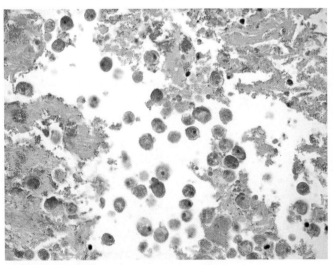

FIGURE 28-13. *Entamoeba histolytica* trophozoites.

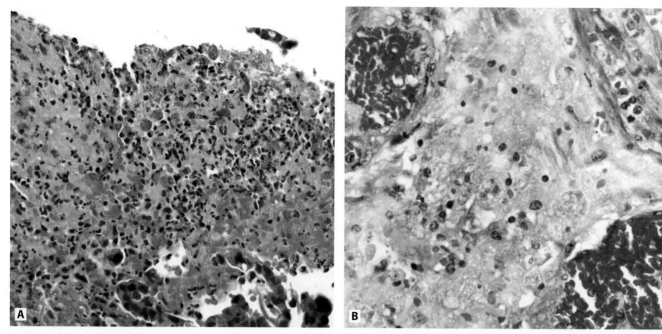

FIGURE 28-14. *Entamoeba histolytica.* **A.** Trophozoites in necrotic tissue. **B.** Trichrome stain can highlight the organisms.

a diffuse mixed inflammatory infiltrate, with lymphocytes, plasma cells, eosinophils, and neutrophils; amoebic trophozoites can be seen in necrotic tissue or debris (Figure 28-14). The trophozoites contain a single nucleus with intracytoplasmic erythrocytes that are positive by PAS stain or trichrome stain (Figure 28-14B). However, trophozoites may be absent in biopsies in up to two-thirds of cases; multiple biopsies may be necessary to establish the diagnosis.

Colonic schistosomiasis is most often caused by *Schistosoma japonicum* and *S. mansoni* and usually involves the sigmoid colon and rectum.[25,26] Mature adult schistosome worms do not elicit an inflammatory reaction, but schistosome ova will cause a granulomatous reaction, with inflammation consisting of eosinophils or neutrophils. Calcification of the schistosome ova as well as mucosal atrophy and fibrosis can be seen in chronic cases (Figure 28-15).

FIGURE 28-15. *Schistosoma* ova in lamina propria of colon.

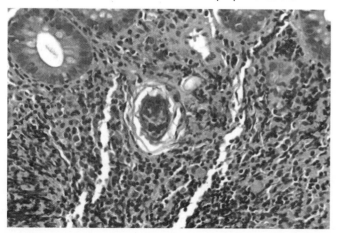

Strongyloides colitis is a severe form of disseminated infection by *Strongyloides stercoralis* and has a high mortality rate. Colonic infection with this parasite may mimic IBD, but it usually lacks significant crypt architectural distortion.[27–29] Hyperinfection with *Strongyloides* can be seen in patients with malnutrition, malignancy, diabetes, and immunodeficiency.[30] Colonoscopy reveals friable, ulcerated mucosa with yellow-white nodular lesions; larvae can sometimes be grossly identified.[27,29] Granulomas surrounding larvae with thick cuticles are seen in the mucosa, muscularis propria, or serosa (see Chapter 20). Eosinophilic microabscesses may be present.

Sexually Transmitted Disease–Associated Proctitis

There has been a recent rise in proctocolitis or proctitis related to sexually transmitted infections as a result of anorectal intercourse and oroanal sex.[31–33] It is thought to be an underrecognized disease due to lack of awareness as well as clinical and histologic overlap with manifestations of IBD. Up to 85% of patients who have gonorrheal or chlamydial proctitis have reported having a complete absence of symptoms.[31] The most common causative infection is gonorrhea, accounting for 30% of cases, followed by chlamydia (19%), herpes (16%), and syphilis (2%). An infectious source cannot be identified in the remaining 45% of cases.[33] It may be difficult to distinguish these forms of sexually transmitted proctitis from IBD due to endoscopic and histologic overlap; a high level of suspicion is required to make the diagnosis. Infectious proctitis should be considered as part of the differential diagnosis in patients initially diagnosed with IBD who are not responding to standard therapy.[33] Histologically, there is no specific pattern of injury. Cryptitis, crypt abscesses, and granulomas may be seen in lymphogranuloma venereum colitis (*Chlamydia trachomatis*) (Figure 28-16).

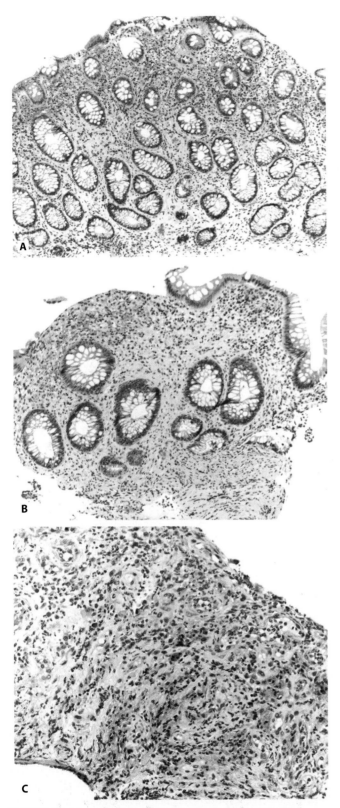

FIGURE 28-16. Lymphogranuloma venereum proctitis. The changes are rather nonspecific, with a mixed inflammatory cellular infiltration, including numerous eosinophils and patchy crypt damage (**A**). There is slight crypt architectural irregularity and lamina propria fibrosis (**B**). Focal mucosal ulceration may be evident, accompanied by a denser inflammatory infiltrate, including plasma cells and neutrophils (**C**).

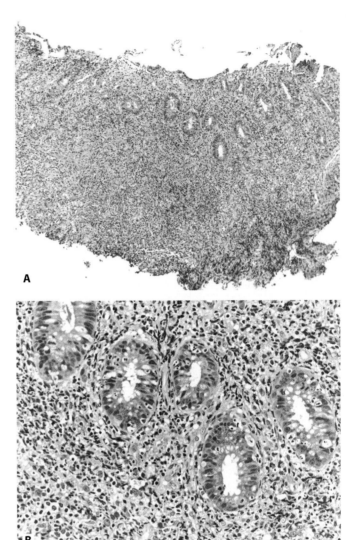

FIGURE 28-17. Syphilis proctitis. **A.** Dense mononuclear cellular infiltrate of the lamina propria displacing crypts. **B.** Cryptitis and crypt apoptosis are both evident. In addition, the lamina propria infiltration comprises many larger histiocytes and scattered small rod-like organisms.

In cases associated with syphilis, abundant plasma cells can be seen (Figure 28-17), with immunostains readily demonstrating the organism (Figure 28-18).

DRUG-RELATED COLITIS

A wide spectrum exists of medications that may cause injury to the large intestine. The heterogeneous histologic features of drug-induced colitis may overlap with other colitides, including microscopic colitis, infectious and necrotizing enterocolitis, pseudomembranous colitis, and ischemic colitis.[34] For example, nonsteroidal anti-inflammatory drugs (NSAIDs) are some of the most commonly used medications and commonly cause ulcers in the right colon.[34] Histologically, NSAIDs-related colitis manifests as a patchy active

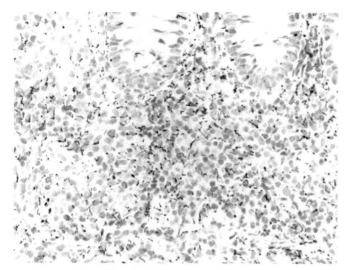

FIGURE 28-18. Immunostain for *Treponema pallidum*.

colitis with increased intraepithelial lymphocytes, prominent eosinophils, and crypt apoptosis.

Many cases of drug-induced colitis exhibit the toxic-ischemic pattern as described in Chapter 1, characterized by epithelial necrosis that is most prominent at the surface and spares the crypt bases, imparting a withered appearance, which is accompanied by hyalinization or fibrosis of the lamina propria (Figure 28-19). Examples of drugs with this pattern of injury include digitalis and diuretics, as well as narcotics. Estrogens may cause mesenteric vein thrombosis, and ergotamine and cocaine can cause vasoconstriction, leading to the pattern of toxic-ischemic injury. Pancreatic enzyme replacement containing methacrylic acid, used in the treatment of children with cystic fibrosis, has been reported to cause fibrosis that results in strictures, mainly in the right colon.[34]

FIGURE 28-19. Narcotic-induced ischemic colitis. There is severe surface epithelial attenuation, diffuse and dense lamina propria fibrosis, and multifocal erosions with necroinflammatory exudates.

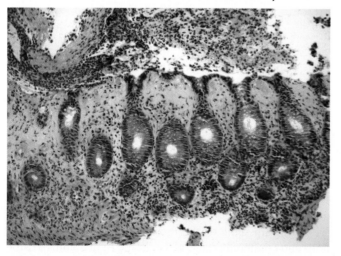

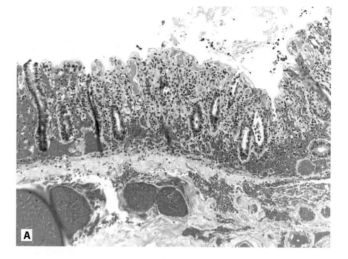

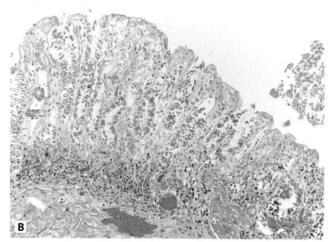

FIGURE 28-20. Neutropenic colitis (typhlitis). Right colectomy from a patient with neutropenic fever and septic shock, with computed tomographic scan demonstrating acute circumferential thickening of cecum. The patient was status post chemotherapy for acute leukemia that had transformed from myelodysplastic syndrome. **A.** Extensive mucosal hemorrhage with superficial necrosis and intracapillary thrombosis. Note the increased intraepithelial lymphocytes in residual crypts and the total lack of neutrophils in lamina propria. **B.** Full-thickness mucosal necrosis with intramucosal capillary thrombosis.

Chemotherapy-Related Colitis

Chemotherapy may cause significant neutropenia, leading to neutropenic enterocolitis (typhlitis) involving the ileum and cecum, sometimes requiring colectomy (Figure 28-20). Histologically, there is florid bacterial or fungal colonization, hemorrhage, and necrosis with an absence of active inflammation.[34] There may be increased intraepithelial lymphocytosis (Figure 28-20A) and extensive intramucosal thrombosis (Figure 28-20B). Typhlitis has been associated with cytosine arabinoside, cisplatin, vincristine, adriamycin, 5-fluorouracil, and mercaptopurine.[34] Treatment with cyclosporin may lead to atypical changes in the colonic epithelium, concerning for dysplasia, but the cells will have nuclear maturation with increasing cytoplasm toward the surface.[34]

Mycophenolate Mofetil–Related Colitis

Mycophenolate mofetil (MMF) is a commonly used immunosuppressant in solid-organ transplantation and autoimmune disorders. This drug is known to cause gastrointestinal toxicity, with diarrhea as the most commonly reported side effect.[35-38] There is a spectrum of histologic findings that may mimic graft-vs-host disease (GVHD), ischemia, or IBD. IBD-like changes are related to prolonged crypt injury, leading to focal or extensive crypt loss, crypt branching, and crypt shortening. Superimposed active inflammation with neutrophilic infiltration (cryptitis and focal crypt abscesses) may also occur as a secondary response to mucosal injury, mimicking active IBD. However, marked crypt apoptosis with withering and sparse lamina propria infiltration are features that favor MMF colitis (see Chapter 2). Intraepithelial lymphocytes and increased eosinophils are also commonly associated with MMF colitis.[35,38,39] In addition, MMF-associated colitis has been reported to be more severe in the right colon than in other portions of the large bowel.[36,39] Concurrent CMV colitis and other coinfections are not uncommon due to immunosuppression.[36] The main challenge is the distinction between MMF colitis and GVHD in the setting of bone marrow transplantation (see Chapter 2).

Anti-CTLA-4 Enterocolitis

Ipilimumab is a humanized monoclonal antibody that targets the CTLA-4 (anticytotoxic T-lymphocyte–associated antigen 4) antigen expressed mostly on CD4+ regulatory T cells. By suppressing the function of the target cells, it promotes the activity of cytotoxic T cells to enhance antitumor activity in vaccine treatment of melanoma and other malignancies.[40] However, the increased T-cell immunity also leads to immune-mediated injury to gastrointestinal mucosa, causing severe refractory diarrhea in some cases.[41-43] The mechanism and pathologic changes of anti-CTLA-4 enterocolitis are similar to that of autoimmune enterocolitis (see Chapter 3). Histologically, there is prominent infiltration of the lamina propria by lymphocytes, plasma cells, and varying numbers of other inflammatory cells.[41] An increase in intraepithelial lymphocytes may also be noted. Most cases exhibit increased epithelial apoptosis in the crypts. Due to reduced mucosal immunity, there may be a secondary neutrophilic reaction in the form of cryptitis or crypt abscesses (Figure 28-21).

■ DIVERSION COLITIS

Diversion colitis may develop in any portion of colon that has been excluded from the fecal stream as a result of surgical diversion, such as a Hartmann pouch, for management of malignancy, IBD, trauma, or diverticular disease.[44-46] Diversion colitis can occur within months to years after the surgery, and it typically resolves within 3–6 months of reestablishment of the fecal stream.

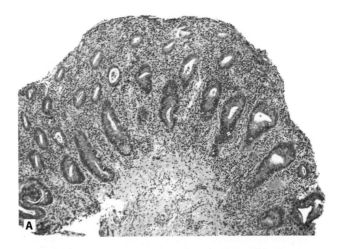

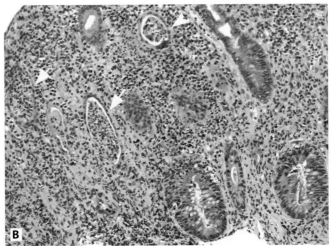

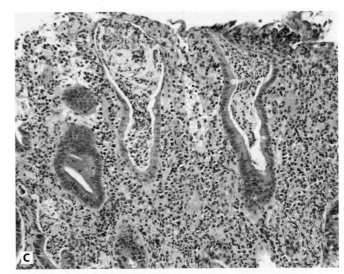

FIGURE 28-21. Ipilimumab colitis. **A.** There is a lymphoplasmacytic dominant infiltrate in the lamina propria and an increase in intraepithelial lymphocytes. Crypt apoptosis is also evident. **B.** Several features are evident: withered crypts with crypt abscesses (arrows) cryptitis, and prominent apoptosis. **C.** Higher power view showing withered crypts containing apoptotic debris and neutrophils.

PART SIX

Depending on the endoscopic diagnostic criteria, between 50% and 100% of patients may develop diversion colitis, but most are asymptomatic. The involved segment appears granular and nodular when viewed endoscopically; some cases demonstrate erosions or aphthous ulcers. Histologically, nearly all cases manifest with prominent lymphoid follicular hyperplasia in the diverted segment, corresponding to the endoscopic nodularity as well as a background of lymphoplasmacytic infiltration in the lamina propria. This suggests that lymphoid hyperplasia is a uniform change of diversion that does not necessarily represent colitis. However, in some patients, particularly symptomatic ones, there is also neutrophilic infiltration—with cryptitis, crypt abscesses, and erosions—changes that evidently correspond to bona fide diversion colitis. Mild crypt architectural distortion may also be present.

In patients who have undergone total colectomy for ulcerative colitis, the temporarily diverted rectum is uniformly involved by the underlying disease. When the distal rectum is further resected at the time of ileal pouch–anal anastomosis, it exhibits prominent lymphoid hyperplasia, severe crypt architectural distortion, and other features of active colitis. It is impossible to determine if these last features are due to the underlying UC or diversion colitis. In this situation, it is preferable to render the diagnosis of ulcerative colitis with superimposed diversion changes (Figure 28-22).

In patients who had an ileostomy or colostomy for indications other than IBD, such as diverticular disease and tumors, inflammation in the diverted segment is best attributed to diversion colitis.

MICROSCOPIC COLITIS

Lymphocytic colitis and collagenous colitis are the two main forms of microscopic colitis. Both diseases exhibit fairly characteristic microscopic features that are familiar to most practicing pathologists. Clinically, most patients present with watery diarrhea, usually with negative endoscopic findings. Many excellent texts, including recent reviews, provide adequate and updated descriptions of microscopic colitis.[47–49] Therefore, it was decided not to include a detailed discussion in this chapter. However, it is worth noting that, in many cases, lymphocytic colitis or collagenous colitis merely represents a diagnostic "pattern," and that the underlying disease may be a drug-induced colitis, such as seen with NSAIDs, olmesartan, and the like.

SYSTEMIC CONDITIONS INVOLVING THE GASTROINTESTINAL TRACT

Many systemic diseases involve the GI tract, including the large intestine, such as Behçet disease, Henoch-Schonlein purpura, chronic granulomatous disease, Hermansky-Pudlack syndrome, Langerhans cell histiocytosis, idiopathic hypereosinophilic syndrome, common variable immune deficiency (CVID) syndrome, and systemic mastocytosis (SM). The last two conditions are discussed next. Behçet disease shares many features with Crohn disease and is discussed as part of the differential diagnosis in Chapter 4.

Common Variable Immune Deficiency Syndrome

When encountered in colonic biopsies, knowing the patient's clinical history and having a high index of suspicion will aid in making the correct diagnosis. The common histologic changes for CVID include prominent lymphoid aggregates, crypt apoptosis, and, most importantly, lack or have a paucity of plasma cells (Figure 28-23). The last feature can be easily missed if the pathologist is not aware of this entity.[50] Due to a lack or paucity of plasma cells with associated reduction in mucosal immunity, the GI tract mucosa may have a variety

FIGURE 28-22. Diversion colitis in background of ulcerative colitis. **A.** Prominent lymphoid follicles mostly in the mucosa of the diverted segment of colon. **B.** Prominent lymphoid infiltrate in the background of ulcerative colitis of a remnant rectum before completion proctocolectomy. In this setting, it is not possible to determine the role of diversion vs the underlying ulcerative colitis, thus the term *diversion change* is more appropriate than *diversion colitis*.

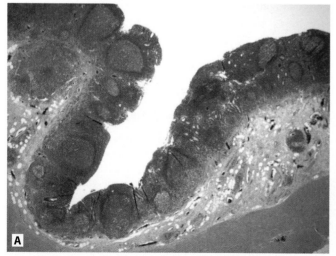
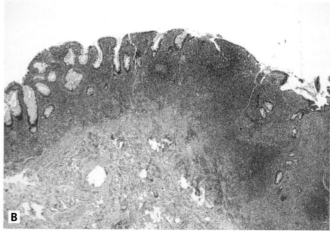

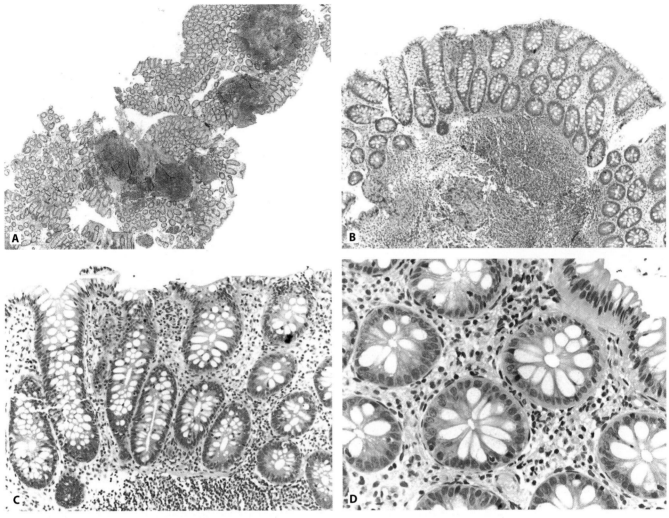

FIGURE 28-23. Common variable immune deficiency syndrome (CVID), colon biopsy. **A.** Several fragments contain prominent lymphoid follicles. **B.** Essentially normal mucosa, with prominent submucosal lymphoid follicle. **C.** The lamina propria appears "empty." However, there is an increase in intraepithelial lymphocytes. **D.** Higher-power view demonstrates a lack of plasma cells.

of changes, including increased inflammation, superimposed CMV or cryptosporidium infection,[50] or active enterocolitis.

Mast Cell–Related Colitis

Colonic involvement is a well-known component of cutaneous mastocytosis (CM, or urticaria pigmentosa) and SM. The latter is characterized by neoplastic mast cells accumulating in the bone marrow and other sites. There is also evidence to suggest that an isolated increase in mast cell infiltration of small-bowel and colonic mucosa may be associated with intractable chronic diarrhea.[51-53] In biopsies from patients with SM, the colonic mucosa is characterized by mixed inflammatory cellular infiltration, often with prominent eosinophils (Figure 28-24A). On careful scrutiny, another cell population becomes evident, resembling either plasma cells or macrophages but containing much darker nuclei (Figure 28-24B). Correlation with clinical

history and performing immunostains for mast cell markers (see next discussion) help in reaching the correct diagnosis of colonic involvement by SM.

Using an immunostain for mast cell tryptase (MCT) and comparing patients with idiopathic diarrhea with control groups, Jakate suggested that more than 20 mast cells per high-power field (using an average of ten 40× objective fields) is specifically related to clinically intractable diarrhea in patients without SM and has suggested the term *mastocytic enterocolitis* for this condition.[53] This finding was further supported by more recent studies[54] (Figure 28-25).

Immunostains for MCT, CD25, and CD117 have been used to help identify mast cells in the colonic mucosa and to diagnose mast cell–related colitis. For example, an increased CD25+ mast cell population seems to correlate well with SM,[55] as opposed to other mast cell conditions.

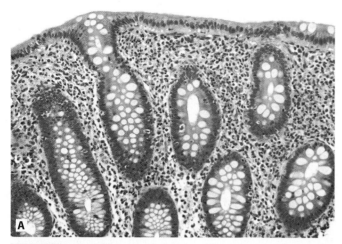

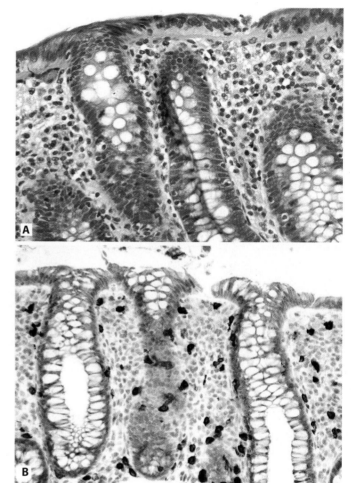

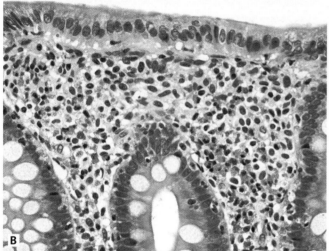

FIGURE 28-24. Colitis in systemic mastocytosis. **A.** The crypt architecture is normal. However, there is a dense inflammatory cellular infiltration, with prominent eosinophils. There is also a focal increase in intraepithelial lymphocytes. **B.** Higher magnification showing that most of the mononuclear cells are mast cells, with dark nuclei and a perinuclear halo (fried egg appearance). There are no cytoplasmic granules.

FIGURE 28-25. Mastocytic enterocolitis. **A.** This biopsy was from a patient with chronic diarrhea. The colonic biopsy shows no active colitis, but there is a dense inflammatory infiltration in lamina propria with lymphocytes, plasma cells, eosinophils, and suspected mast cells. Similar to the previous example, there is a mild increase in intraepithelial lymphocytes. **B.** An immunostain for CD117 highlights greater than 25 mast cells per high-power field.

■ REFERENCES

1. Cerilli LA, Greenson JK. The differential diagnosis of colitis in endoscopic biopsy specimens: a review article. *Arch Pathol Lab Med.* 2012;136:854–864.
2. Kumar NB, Nostrant TT, Appelman HD. The histopathologic spectrum of acute self-limited colitis (acute infectious-type colitis). *Am J Surg Pathol.* 1982;6:523–529.
3. Schunter MO, Walles T, Fritz P, et al. Herpes simplex virus colitis complicating ulcerative colitis: a case report and brief review on superinfections. *J Crohns Colitis.* 2007;1:41–46.
4. Blair SD, Forbes A, Parkins RA. CMV colitis in an immunocompetent adult. *J R Soc Med.* 1992;85:238–239.
5. Dieterich DT, Rahmin M. Cytomegalovirus colitis in AIDS: presentation in 44 patients and a review of the literature. *J Acquir Immune Defic Syndr.* 1991;4(Suppl 1):S29–S35.
6. el-Serag HB, Zwas FR, Cirillo NW, Eisen RN. Fulminant herpes colitis in a patient with Crohn's disease. *J Clin Gastroenterol.* 1996;22:220–223.
7. Lin WR, Su MY, Hsu CM, et al. Clinical and endoscopic features for alimentary tract cytomegalovirus disease: report of 20 cases with gastrointestinal cytomegalovirus disease. *Chang Gung Med J.* 2005;28:476–484.
8. Dixon MR. Viral and fungal infectious colitides. *Clin Colon Rectal Surg.* 2007;20:28–32.
9. Iida T, Ikeya K, Watanabe F, et al. Looking for endoscopic features of cytomegalovirus colitis: a study of 187 patients with active ulcerative colitis, positive and negative for cytomegalovirus. *Inflamm Bowel Dis.* 2013;19:1156–1163.
10. Shepherd NA. Pathological mimics of chronic inflammatory bowel disease. *J Clin Pathol.* 1991;44:726–733.
11. Dixon LR, Crawford JM. Early histologic changes in fibrosing cholestatic hepatitis C. *Liver Transplant.* 2007;13:219–226.
12. Yan Z, Nguyen S, Poles M, Melamed J, Scholes JV. Adenovirus colitis in human immunodeficiency virus infection: an underdiagnosed entity. *Am J Surg Pathol.* 1998;22:1101–1106.
13. Thomas PD, Pollok RC, Gazzard BG. Enteric viral infections as a cause of diarrhoea in the acquired immunodeficiency syndrome. *HIV Med.* 1999;1:19–24.

14. Liu L, Qian Y, Zhang Y, Deng J, Jia L, Dong H. Adenoviruses associated with acute diarrhea in children in Beijing, China. *PloS One*. 2014;9:e88791.

15. Kangro HO, Chong SK, Hardiman A, Heath RB, Walker-Smith JA. A prospective study of viral and mycoplasma infections in chronic inflammatory bowel disease. *Gastroenterology*. 1990;98:549–553.

16. Masclee GM, Penders J, Pierik M, Wolffs P, Jonkers D. Enteropathogenic viruses: triggers for exacerbation in IBD? A prospective cohort study using real-time quantitative polymerase chain reaction. *Inflamm Bowel Dis*. 2013;19:124–131.

17. Cleary TG. *Escherichia coli* that cause hemolytic uremic syndrome. *Infect Dis Clin North Am*. 1992;6:163–176.

18. Tarr PI. *Escherichia coli* O157:H7: clinical, diagnostic, and epidemiological aspects of human infection. *Clin Infect Dis*. 1995;20:1–8; quiz 9–10.

19. Cleary TG. The role of Shiga-toxin-producing *Escherichia coli* in hemorrhagic colitis and hemolytic uremic syndrome. *Semin Pediatr Infect Dis*. 2004;15:260–265.

20. Melnyk AM, Solez K, Kjellstrand CM. Adult hemolytic-uremic syndrome. A review of 37 cases. *Arch Intern Med* 1995;155:2077–2084.

21. Prescott RJ, Harris M, Banerjee SS. Fungal infections of the small and large intestine. *J Clin Pathol*. 1992;45:806–811.

22. Lin CC, Kao KY. Ameboma: a colon carcinoma-like lesion in a colonoscopy finding. *Case Rep Gastroenterol*. 2013;7:438–441.

23. Kawazoe A, Nagata N. Fulminant amebic colitis with an atypical clinical presentation successfully treated by metronidazole. *Clin Gastroenterol Hepatol*. 2012;10:e91.

24. Haque R, Kabir M, Noor Z, et al. Diagnosis of amebic liver abscess and amebic colitis by detection of *Entamoeba histolytica* DNA in blood, urine, and saliva by a real-time PCR assay. *J Clin Microbiol*. 2010;48:2798–2801.

25. Cao J, Liu WJ, Xu XY, Zou XP. Endoscopic findings and clinicopathologic characteristics of colonic schistosomiasis: a report of 46 cases. *World J Gastroenterol*. 2010;16:723–727.

26. Liu W, Zeng HZ, Wang QM, et al. Schistosomiasis combined with colorectal carcinoma diagnosed based on endoscopic findings and clinicopathological characteristics: a report on 32 cases. *Asian Pac J Cancer Prev*. 2013;14:4839–4842.

27. Qu Z, Kundu UR, Abadeer RA, Wanger A. Strongyloides colitis is a lethal mimic of ulcerative colitis: the key morphologic differential diagnosis. *Hum Pathol*. 2009;40:572–577.

28. Báez-Vallecillo L, Stewart BD, Kott MM, Bhattacharjee M. Strongyloides hyperinfection as a mimic of inflammatory bowel disease. *Am J Gastroenterol*. 2013;108:622–623.

29. Sridhara S, Simon N, Raghuraman U, Crowson N, Aggarwal V. *Strongyloides stercoralis* pancolitis in an immunocompetent patient. *Gastrointest Endosc*. 2008;68:196–199.

30. Gutierrez Y, Bhatia P, Garbadawala ST, Dobson JR, Wallace TM, Carey TE. *Strongyloides stercoralis* eosinophilic granulomatous enterocolitis. *Am J Surg Pathol*. 1996;20:603–612.

31. Hamlyn E, Taylor C. Sexually transmitted proctitis. *Postgrad Med J*. 2006;82:733–736.

32. Rompalo AM. Diagnosis and treatment of sexually acquired proctitis and proctocolitis: an update. *Clin Infect Dis*. 1999;28(Suppl 1):S84–S90.

33. Hoentjen F, Rubin DT. Infectious proctitis: when to suspect it is not inflammatory bowel disease. *Dig Dis Sci*. 2012;57:269–273.

34. Parfitt JR, Driman DK. Pathological effects of drugs on the gastrointestinal tract: a review. *Hum Pathol*. 2007;38:527–536.

35. Papadimitriou JC, Cangro CB, Lustberg A, et al. Histologic features of mycophenolate mofetil-related colitis: a graft-versus-host disease-like pattern. *Int J Surg Pathol*. 2003;11:295–302.

36. Lee S, de Boer WB, Subramaniam K, Kumarasinghe MP. Pointers and pitfalls of mycophenolate-associated colitis. *J Clin Pathol*. 2013;66:8–11.

37. Selbst MK, Ahrens WA, Robert ME, Friedman A, Proctor DD, Jain D. Spectrum of histologic changes in colonic biopsies in patients treated with mycophenolate mofetil. *Mod Pathol*. 2009;22:737–743.

38. Star KV, Ho VT, Wang HH, Odze RD. Histologic features in colon biopsies can discriminate mycophenolate from GVHD-induced colitis. *Am J Surg Pathol*. 2013;37:1319–1328.

39. Liapis G, Boletis J, Skalioti C, et al. Histological spectrum of mycophenolate mofetil-related colitis: association with apoptosis. *Histopathology*. 2013;63:649–658.

40. Berman D, Parker SM, Siegel J, et al. Blockade of cytotoxic T-lymphocyte antigen-4 by ipilimumab results in dysregulation of gastrointestinal immunity in patients with advanced melanoma. *Cancer Immun*. 2010;10:11.

41. Beck KE, Blansfield JA, Tran KQ, et al. Enterocolitis in patients with cancer after antibody blockade of cytotoxic T-lymphocyte-associated antigen 4. *J Clin Oncol*. 2006;24:2283–2289.

42. Lord JD, Hackman RC, Moklebust A, et al. Refractory colitis following anti-CTLA4 antibody therapy: analysis of mucosal FOXP3+ T cells. *Dig Dis Sci*. 2010;55:1396–1405.

43. Pessi MA, Zilembo N, Haspinger ER, et al. Targeted therapy-induced diarrhea: a review of the literature. *Crit Rev Oncol Hematol*. 2014;90:165–179.

44. Murray FE, O'Brien MJ, Birkett DH, Kennedy SM, LaMont JT. Diversion colitis. Pathologic findings in a resected sigmoid colon and rectum. *Gastroenterology*. 1987;93:1404–1408.

45. Haque S, West AB. Diversion colitis—20 years a-growing. *J Clin Gastroenterol*. 1992;15:281–283.

46. Violi V, Cobianchi F, Adami M, Torri T, Ferraro G, Roncoroni L. Human defunctionalized colon: a histopathological and pharmacological study of muscularis propria in resection specimens. *Dig Dis Sci*. 1998;43:616–623.

47. Mahajan D, Goldblum JR, Xiao SY, Shen B, Liu X. Lymphocytic colitis and collagenous colitis: a review of clinicopathologic features and immunologic abnormalities. *Adv Anat Pathol*. 2012;19:28–38.

48. Langner C, Aust D, Ensari A, et al. Histology of microscopic colitis—review with practical approach for pathologists. *Histopathology*. 2015;66(5):613–626.

49. Verhaegh BP, Jonkers DM, Driessen A, et al. Incidence of microscopic colitis in the Netherlands. A nationwide population-based study from 2000 to 2012. *Dig Liver Dis*. 2015;47:30–36.

50. Daniels JA, Lederman HM, Maitra A, Montgomery EA. Gastrointestinal tract pathology in patients with common variable immunodeficiency (CVID): a clinicopathologic study and review. *Am J Surg Pathol*. 2007;31:1800–1812.

51. Thonhofer R, Siegel C, Trummer M, Langner C. Mastocytic enterocolitis as a rare cause of chronic diarrhea in a patient with rheumatoid arthritis. *Wien Klin Wochenschr*. 2011;123:297–298.

52. Ogilvie-McDaniel C, Blaiss M, Osborn FD, Carpenter J. Mastocytic enterocolitis: a newly described mast cell entity. *Ann Allergy Asthma Immunol*. 2008;101:645–646.

53. Jakate S, Demeo M, John R, Tobin M, Keshavarzian A. Mastocytic enterocolitis: increased mucosal mast cells in chronic intractable diarrhea. *Arch Pathol Lab Med*. 2006;130:362–367.

54. Akhavein MA, Patel NR, Muniyappa PK, Glover SC. Allergic mastocytic gastroenteritis and colitis: an unexplained etiology in chronic abdominal pain and gastrointestinal dysmotility. *Gastroenterol Res Pract*. 2012;2012:950582.

55. Hahn HP, Hornick JL. Immunoreactivity for CD25 in gastrointestinal mucosal mast cells is specific for systemic mastocytosis. *Am J Surg Pathol*. 2007;31:1669–1676.

PART SIX

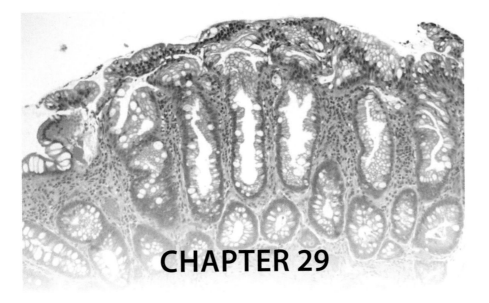

CHAPTER 29

Colon Polyps

Xiuli Liu and Shu-Yuan Xiao

■ INTRODUCTION

Colorectal polyps can be grouped based on the tissue component mainly involved (epithelial or stromal) and can be either neoplastic or nonneoplastic. For practical consideration, in this chapter colon polyps are reviewed individually without a strict classification hierarchy: hyperplastic polyps; adenomas; sessile serrated polyps (SSPs); hamartomatous polyps; inflammatory polyps; extrinsic polyps (metastatic tumor, foreign body, sarcoidosis); and mesenchymal lesions that present as a mucosal polyp.

■ HYPERPLASTIC POLYPS

Hyperplastic polyps are small and innocuous lesions. While recent data suggest that hyperplastic polyps harbor various genetic and cell-cycle regulatory defects, most hyperplastic polyps are of no clinical consequence.[1] However, large hyperplastic polyps in the right colon may give rise to sporadic colonic adenocarcinomas that exhibit the phenotype with high levels of microsatellite instability (MSI-H).

Pathologic Features

Histologically, hyperplastic polyps are characterized by a saw-tooth (or serrated) luminal surface contour (Figure 29-1A) of the crypts, with no dysplasia in the epithelium. The base of the crypts is normal. On cross sections, hyperplastic polyps demonstrate a "starfish" appearance (Figure 29-1B).

Two major differential diagnoses for hyperplastic polyps are adenomas when there are marked regenerative changes in the deep portion of the polyp and SSPs (see further discussion in this chapter) when there is architectural distortion toward the basal portion of the polyp due to prolapse (Figure 29-2). Finding evidence of orderly maturation helps distinguish a hyperplastic polyp from adenoma, and the presence of prolapse changes helps distinguish it from an SSP. Another lesion that has morphologic overlap with the hyperplastic polyp is the traditional serrated adenoma (TSA). The TSA is characterized by enlarged, cigar-shape nuclei without surface maturation (see discussion in a following section).

Clinical Consideration

Small (<10-mm) hyperplastic polyps located in the rectum or sigmoid colon are considered innocuous lesions that are not associated with increased risk for colorectal adenocarcinoma (CRC), and subsequent colonoscopies can be performed at intervals of 10 years.[1] However, hyperplastic polyps in the setting of hyperplastic polyposis may pose increased risk for developing CRC and require increased surveillance.

■ ADENOMAS

Most patients with an adenoma are asymptomatic, but large adenomas may cause bleeding and lead to anemia. The prevalence of adenomas increases with age. An individual's likelihood of developing adenomas is strongly influenced by family history.

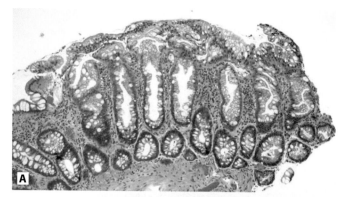

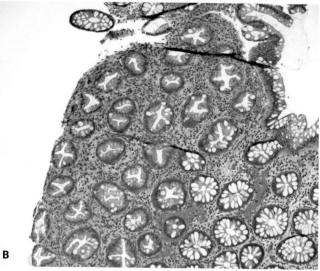

FIGURE 29-1. Hyperplastic polyp. The hyperplastic polyp is characterized by a sawtooth (or serrated) luminal surface contour of the crypts, without dysplasia. The base of the crypts is normal without architectural abnormalities (**A**). On cross sections, the hyperplastic polyp demonstrates a "starfish" appearance (**B**).

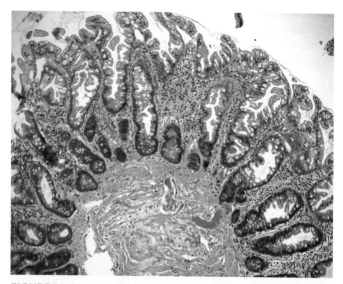

FIGURE 29-2. Hyperplastic polyp (HP) with prolapse changes. There is mild architectural distortion at the base of the crypts. However, the presence of fibromuscular proliferation in the lamina propria supports a diagnosis of HP with prolapse changes.

Pathologic Features

Adenomas are defined as dysplastic clonal proliferations of the epithelium. Based on gross appearance, adenomas can be classified as flat, sessile, and pedunculated (with a stalk). Rare variants manifest as filiform and multilobulated polyps.

Microscopically, adenomas are classified as tubular, tubulovillous, and villous (Figure 29-3). When each of the tubular and villous elements exceeds 25% of the entire polyp, the designation of tubulovillous is warranted. The villous component is considered "advanced" histology associated with a relative risk of 1.26 to 1.40 for subsequent development of advanced adenoma or carcinoma.[2,3] Therefore, in the current guidelines, the presence of a villous component requires follow-up surveillance in 3 years.[1]

By definition, all adenomas have at least low-grade dysplasia; some have high-grade dysplasia (carcinoma in situ). We do not encourage using the term *carcinoma in situ* for fear of overinterpretation by the clinician. Low-grade dysplasia is characterized by parallel arrangement of proliferating glands (Figure 29-4) without back-to-back, cribriform, or complex budding. The proliferating glands are lined by epithelium containing pseudostratified or partially stratified pencil-shape nuclei (Figure 29-4). High-grade dysplasia is characterized by either marked architectural complexity (Figure 29-5A) or marked cytologic atypia (Figure 29-5B), including severe pleomorphism; loss of polarity and abnormal mitoses; and back-to-back, cribriform, or complex glands (Figure 29-5A). In addition, "open" or "vesicular" nuclei are features of high-grade dysplasia.

The interobserver agreement has been suboptimal among expert gastrointestinal (GI) pathologists from major academic medical centers regarding grading of dysplasia. In addition, there have been insufficient data regarding clinical significance of high-grade dysplasia or carcinoma in situ once the polyp has been completely removed by polypectomy. More importantly, as there are variable levels of understanding among surgeons regarding the meaning of high-grade dysplasia, such a diagnosis has occasionally led to overtreatment (colectomy). Therefore, in our own practice and some other institutions, a diagnosis of adenoma is made with only size and villous component mentioned when applicable, without providing a grade.

Colonic adenoma may show differentiation toward other cell types (a metaplastic phenomenon), such as Paneth cell metaplasia[4] and squamous metaplasia (Figures 29-6A, 29-6B). In rare situations, there may be endocrine cell metaplasia, which may detach from the adenoma and "drop" into the lamina propria as individual cells or small nests, mimicking invasive "poorly" differentiated adenocarcinoma[5–7] (Figure 29-6C). Patients with an adenoma and microcarcinoids have a benign clinical course.[6]

Occasionally, an adenoma may be found to contain invasion into the lamina propria by dysplastic epithelium in the form of single-cell or a small cluster of dysplastic epithelium, which is considered as progression to intramucosal

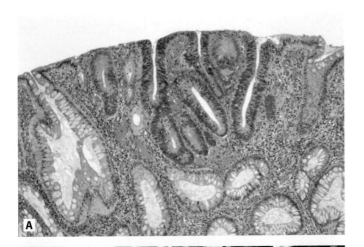

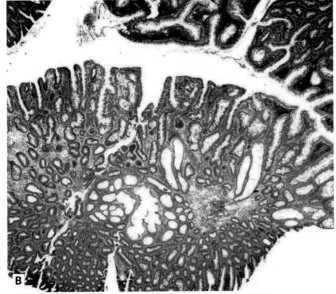

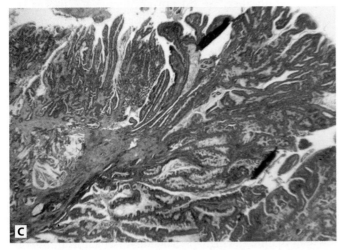

FIGURE 29-3. Colonic adenoma. **A.** Tubular adenoma. **B.** Tubulovillous adenoma. **C.** Villous adenoma.

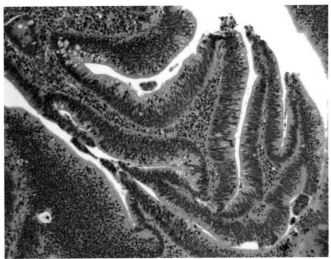

FIGURE 29-4. Colonic adenoma with low-grade dysplasia. Low-grade dysplasia is characterized by hyperchromatic, pencil-shape, stratified nuclei.

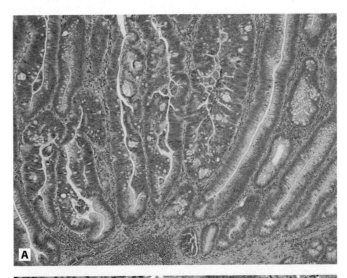

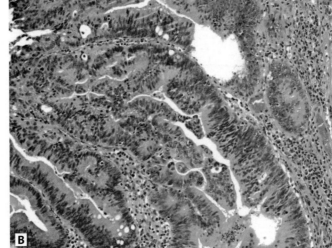

FIGURE 29-5. Colonic adenoma with high-grade dysplasia. High-grade dysplasia is characterized by severe cytologic abnormalities (**A**) and glandular complexity (**B**).

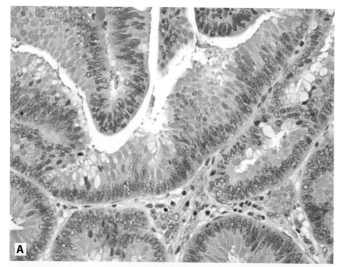

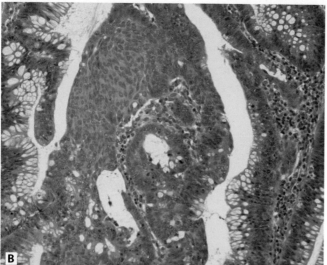

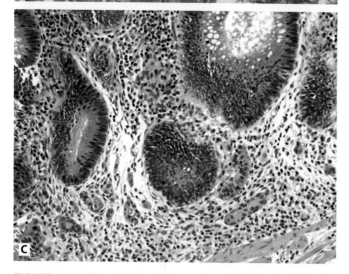

FIGURE 29-6. Colonic adenoma may show differentiation toward other cell types (metaplasia), including Paneth cell metaplasia (**A**), squamous metaplasia (**B**), and neuroendocrine metaplasia (**C**).

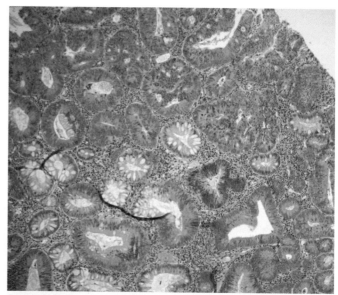

FIGURE 29-7. Adenoma with intramucosal invasion. The glands with high-grade dysplasia exhibit irregular contour with focal "pointed" growth. However, a desmoplastic reaction is lacking.

adenocarcinoma (Figure 29-7). In a polypectomy specimen with adequate margin, a distinction from high-grade dysplasia may not be critical, as many studies have shown a lack of metastatic potential for these lesions. However, in a small biopsy from a mass that shows invasion into the lamina propria or muscularis mucosae, the diagnosis of intramucosal adenocarcinoma or "at least intramucosal adenocarcinoma" may be used by some pathologists. In such cases, a comment should be given and direct communication with the clinician may be necessary.[8] However, due to the lack of proven clinical significance, we do not encourage the use of the terms *carcinoma in situ* or *intramucosal carcinoma* in colonic specimens.

Adenomas may have ulceration and inflammation. Some pedunculated adenomas may contain dilated and ruptured crypts with mucin extraversion in the lamina propria. Some of these may have misplacement in the submucosa mimicking invasion (see following discussion).

Clinical Consideration

Colonoscopic surveillance interval is based on assessment of risk for future advanced adenomas and carcinoma. Table 29-1 lists current guidelines for colonoscopy surveillance after screening and polypectomy.[1] It recognizes 2 major risk groups: low-risk adenomas, defined as 1–2 tubular adenomas less than 10 mm; and high-risk adenomas, which are those with a villous component, high-grade dysplasia, a size of 10 mm or more, or 3 or more adenomas.

Malignant Polyps

A malignant polyp is a pedunculated adenoma with an invasive component into the submucosa of the "head" or

TABLE 29-1. Recommended postpolypectomy colonoscopic surveillance intervals in individuals with baseline average risk and adenoma.[a]

Risk factor	Surveillance interval (years)
1–2 small (<10-mm) tubular adenoma	5–10
3–10 tubular adenomas	3
>10 adenomas	<3
1 or more tubular adenomas ≥ 10 mm	3
1 or more villous adenomas	3
Adenoma with high-grade dysplasia	3

[a]Adapted with permission from Lieberman DA, Rex DK, Winawer SJ, et al. Guidelines for colonoscopy surveillance after screening and polypectomy: a consensus update by the US Multi-Society Task Force on Colorectal Cancer. *Gastroenterology.* 2012;143(3):844–857.[1]

stalk (Figure 29-8). The presence of submucosal invasion in a flat or sessile polyp is considered a polypoid invasive adenocarcinoma. These last lesions are associated with higher risk of lymph node metastasis, positive endoscopic resection margin, and a worse outcome compared to pedunculated ones[9–12]; therefore, they require additional surgery after polypectomy.

For a pedunculated malignant polyp, further management depends on the histologic features of the invasive component and the margin status. The decision to proceed with additional surgery also relies on clinical factors such as the level of tumor if in the rectum, and age and general health status of patients. Important histologic features include (1) completeness of polypectomy; (2) grade of differentiation; and (3) presence of angiolymphatic invasion.[9,13] A positive resection margin is defined as the presence of tumor cells within 1 mm of the free edge of the submucosa containing diathermic changes.[14] For grading, poor differentiation (grade 3) is determined by the least-differentiated area of carcinoma. Lymphatic/vascular invasion is defined as the presence of cancer cells in the lymphatic or venous microvessels. An evolving body of evidence supports the stratification of malignant polyps into low risk and high risk based on these parameters.[12–14] The presence of one of these features (ie, positive resection margin, poor differentiation, and lymphatic/vascular invasion) qualifies the polyp as high risk[14] (Figures 29-9A to 29-9C), and the patient should be evaluated for colectomy, particularly when there is lymphovascular invasion.

A diagnostic pitfall in interpretation of malignant polyps is placement of dysplastic glands in the submucosa in a pedunculated polyp as a result of mucosa injury with epithelial herniation (Figure 29-10). Several histologic features are helpful in differentiating this from true invasion (Table 29-2).

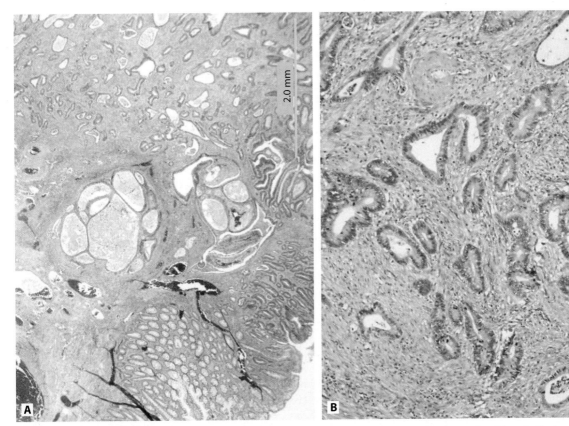

FIGURE 29-8. Malignant polyp (adenocarcinoma arising from an adenoma). **A.** Adenomatous change is evident in the lower right corner; the remaining surface is replaced by invasive adenocarcinoma. **B.** Submucosal invasion with marked stromal desmoplastic change. This polyp had a clear stalk resection margin (not shown).

PART SIX

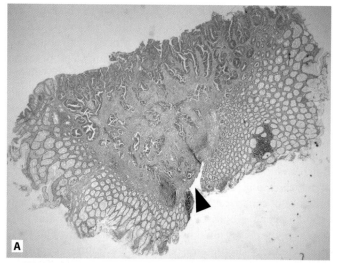

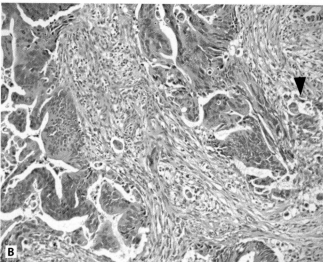

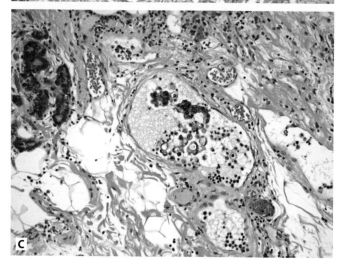

FIGURE 29-9. Malignant polyps with "high-risk" features. **A.** Positive resection margin (arrowhead). **B.** Poor differentiation (arrowhead). **C.** Lymphatic invasion.

TRADITIONAL SERRATED ADENOMAS

The term *serrated adenoma* was initially used to describe a then-new type of polyp characterized by architectural serration and cytological dysplasia.[15] Subsequently, another polyp characterized by marked serration extending to the base of the crypts and without cytologic dysplasia was described and termed *sessile serrated adenoma* (SSP; see the next section). To avoid confusion, polyps originally called serrated adenomas are now termed *traditional serrated adenomas*.

The TSAs are rare, making up less than 1% of all colon polyps. They are usually pedunculated but can be sessile.[16,17] Histologically, a TSA is characterized by an overall protuberant configuration and a complex villous growth pattern.[16,17] The villi of TSAs are lined with a distinct cell type: tall columnar cells with a narrow pencillate nucleus and eosinophilic cytoplasm (Figure 29-11A). In some TSAs, the narrow pencillate nuclei may exhibit pseudostratification, and there may be micropapillary formation by the surface epithelium[16] (Figure 29-11B). Another reported feature for TSAs is the so-called ectopic crypts, which lack anchoring to the underlying muscularis mucosae[18] (Figure 29-11C). However, the evaluation of this feature depends on optimal orientation of the specimen, is not always observed, and thus is not required for diagnosis.

BRAF or *KRAS* mutation can be found in up to 75% to 89% of TSAs.[17,19] However, they do not show methylation of MLH1 and are not associated with CpG island methylator phenotype (CIMP-H) MSI carcinomas.

Regarding clinical management, the 2012 American Gastroenterological Association (AGA) guidelines recommended a surveillance interval of 3 years for patients with TSA detected on screening colonoscopy and polypectomy[1] (Table 29-3).

SESSILE SERRATED POLYPS

Sessile serrated polyps are associated with sporadic MSI-H colorectal carcinomas. They are said to occur more frequently in older women, in the right colon. SSPs have been increasingly diagnosed and accepted as an important precursor lesion for colonic adenocarcinoma involving the serrated pathway of carcinogenesis.[20,21]

Architectural changes that characterize SSPs include prominent dilation, serration, and branching at the base of the crypts and asymmetric proliferative zone (Figure 29-12A). Nuclear atypia is minimal or subtle and mainly manifests as vesicular nuclei with prominent nucleoli and mitotic activity involving the upper third of crypts[22] (Figure 29-12B). Most SSPs have more than two contiguous crypts demonstrating these features[22] (Figure 29-12A). Occasionally, small SSPs can be identified involving diverticula (Figures 29-12C, 29-12D).

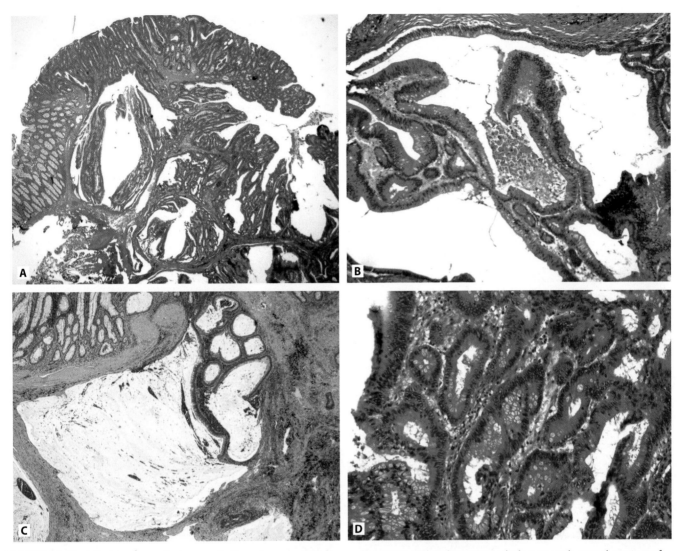

FIGURE 29-10. Misplacement of adenoma in the submucosa. Features supporting such a diagnosis include a smooth, round contour of the lesion (**A**), the presence of lamina propria around the crypts in the deep portion of the lesion (**B**), the presence of hemosiderin (**C**), and a cytologic similarity between the deep portion and the surface portion of the lesion (**D**).

TABLE 29-2. Histologic features helpful for distinguishing adenomatous epithelial misplacement vs submucosal invasion (adenocarcinoma).

Features	Adenomatous epithelial misplacement	Invasive adenocarcinoma
Pedunculation	Usually	May be absent
Architecture at low-power view	Lobular, round, or smooth contour	Irregular shape; haphazard distribution
Hemosiderin	Yes	No
Lamina propria around crypts	Yes	No
Mucin pools	Round, smooth, lined by dysplastic epithelia at periphery	Irregular, floating cells may be present
Small nests or single cells	No	Maybe
Desmoplasia	No	Yes

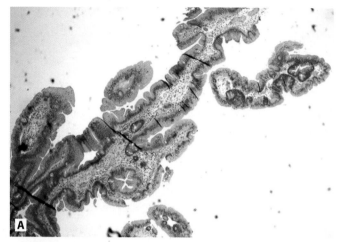

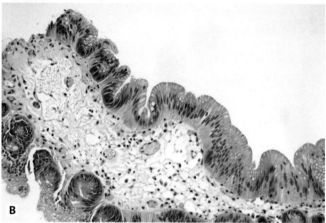

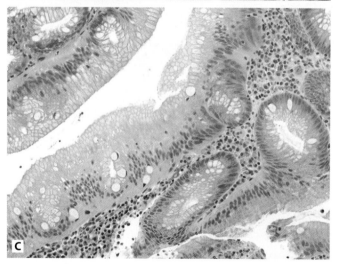

FIGURE 29-11. Traditional serrated adenoma. Villous architecture and serration of the adenoma are evident (**A**) and there is micropapillary formation (**B**). The adenoma has pencil-shape nuclei and demonstrates "ectopic" crypts (**C**).

When the SSP was first described, cytological dysplasia was not a feature. However, it has been recognized that some SSPs may exhibit dysplasia (Figure 29-13). These likely include the polyps that had been previously referred to as "mixed hyperplastic polyp and adenoma." We use the term

TABLE 29-3. Recommended postpolypectomy colonoscopic surveillance intervals in individuals with baseline average risk and serrated polyp.[a]

Risk factor	Surveillance interval (years)	Comment
Rectosigmoid hyperplastic polyps < 10 mm	10	
SSP < 10 mm without dysplasia	5	
SSP ≥ 10 mm or with dysplasia	3	
Traditional serrated adenoma	3	
Serrated polyposis	1	WHO definition

Abbreviations: SSP, sessile serrated polyp; WHO, World Health Organization.

[a]Data from Lieberman DA, Rex DK, Winawer SJ, et al. Guidelines for colonoscopy surveillance after screening and polypectomy: a consensus update by the US Multi-Society Task Force on Colorectal Cancer. *Gastroenterology.* 2012;143(3):844–857.[1]

sessile serrated polyp with conventional adenomatous change for these lesions.

The natural history of SSPs is unknown. Early longitudinal outcome studies had shown an increased risk for subsequent right-sided colorectal carcinoma. Patients with SSPs are also significantly more likely to develop subsequent SSPs.[23] Currently, as these polyps are considered premalignant, the patients are recommended to undergo regular surveillance as listed in Table 29-3.

◼ SERRATED POLYPOSIS

Serrated polyposis was previously termed hyperplastic polyposis. The diagnostic criteria include (1) at least 5 serrated or hyperplastic polyps proximal to the sigmoid colon, with 2 or more greater than 10 mm in size; (2) any number of serrated polyps proximal to the sigmoid colon in an individual who has a first-degree relative with serrated polyposis; or (3) more than 20 serrated polyps of any size, but distributed throughout the colon.[22]

◼ JUVENILE POLYPS

Juvenile polyps occur either sporadically or in the setting of juvenile polyposis syndrome (JPS), and mostly occur in children. However, polyps morphologically indistinguishable from those of JPS can occur in adults and are often referred to as *retention* or *inflammatory polyps.*

Juvenile polyposis syndrome is the most common GI hamartomatous polyposis syndrome. It was first described by McColl et al.[23] The diagnostic criteria are as follows: (1) more than 3 juvenile polyps in the colon or rectum; (2) juvenile polyps throughout the GI tract; or (3) any number of juvenile polyps with a family history of juvenile polyposis. JPS is associated with germline mutations

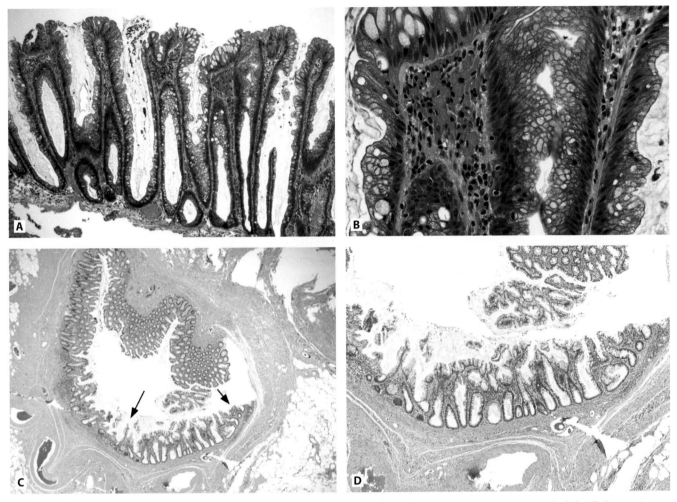

FIGURE 29-12. Sessile serrated polyp (SSP). There is serration and crypt dilation at the base of the crypts. The epithelial cells have microvesicular mucin and nondysplastic nuclei (**A**). Mitotic figures may be seen in the upper third of the crypt (**B**). **C.** A small focus of an SSP (between the two arrows) in a colon diverticulum. **D.** Higher magnification of an SSP in a colon diverticulum.

in *DPC4/SMAD4* or *BMPR1A* genes.[24] Congenital birth defects are reported in about 20% of patients with JPS.[25]

Pathologic Features

Isolated juvenile polyps are most common in the rectosigmoid but can occur anywhere in the GI tract. The polyps have a smooth and round surface and are unilobate. The cut surface is multicystic. Histologically, the polyps are characterized by numerous cystically dilated or tortuous crypts (Figures 29-14A, 29-14B). The surface frequently shows erosion, often associated with regenerative and reactive changes of the adjacent epithelium (Figure 29-14C). The lamina propria is edematous and expanded by inflammatory cells. Occasionally, a juvenile polyp can be filiform (Figure 29-15), and larger juvenile polyps may be multilobulated, giving rise to the appearance of several polyps attached to a single stalk. Dysplasia can be seen up to 31% of the syndromic polyps but almost never occurs in an isolated juvenile polyp[26] (Figure 29-16).

Clinical Consideration

Patients with sporadic juvenile polyps are not predisposed to the development of new juvenile polyps or increased risk of cancer. However, patients with JPS have increased risk for GI malignancy.[25] Surveillance by upper and lower endoscopy is thus recommended by age 15 and should be repeated annually.[24,27] If diffuse polyposis cannot be controlled by endoscopic polypectomy or if there is a family history of GI carcinoma or dysplasia, prophylactic colectomy or gastrectomy should be considered.[27]

■ PEUTZ-JEGHERS POLYPS

Peutz-Jeghers syndrome (PJS) is an autosomal dominant syndrome characterized by mucocutaneous pigmentation and hamartomatous polyps of the small intestine, colon, and stomach. Mutation of the *LKB1/STK1* gene on chromosome 19p13.3 can be found in about 60% of familial and 50% of sporadic cases.[28] Patients with PJS have an increased

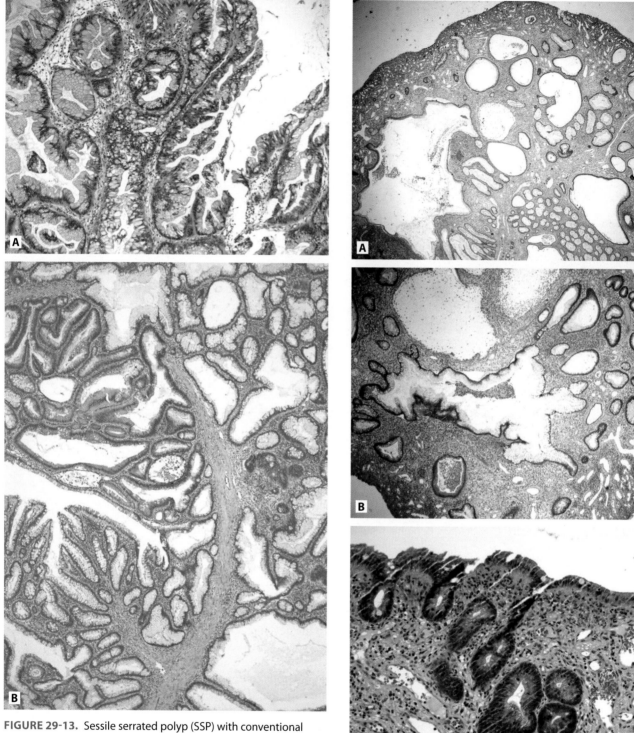

FIGURE 29-13. Sessile serrated polyp (SSP) with conventional adenomatous change. **A.** This polyp contains architecturally complex glands with nuclear enlargement and hyperchromasia. **B.** Typical low-grade adenomatous epithelium within the background of architectural SSP crypt dilation.

FIGURE 29-14. Juvenile polyp. This polyp has many cystically dilated or tortuous crypts and an eroded surface (**A**). The lamina propria is slightly edematous and expanded by inflammatory cells (**B**). Regenerative and reactive changes of the epithelium are commonly seen adjacent to erosion (**C**).

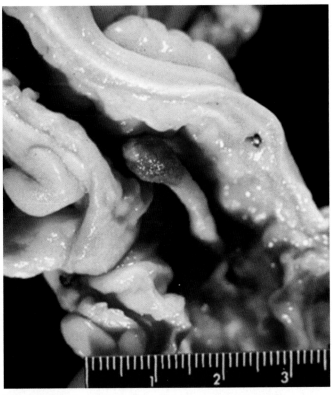

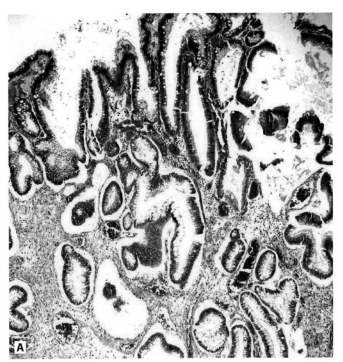

FIGURE 29-15. A filiform juvenile polyp with a long stalk.

risk for both intestinal and extraintestinal malignancies. Most patients are diagnosed in the second or third decades of life.[29]

Pathologic Features

Hamartomatous polyps of PJS may occur throughout the GI tract but are more common in the small bowel, followed by the colon and stomach.[29,30] Well-developed polyps in the intestine tend to be pedunculated and may be mulberry-like. Histologically, PJS polyps are characterized by arborizing smooth muscle bundles derived from the underlying muscularis mucosae; the lamina propria is otherwise normal or mildly inflamed (Figure 29-17). In colonic PJS polyps, the epithelium may show overgrowth or hyperplasia (Figure 29-17). Some PJS polyps may progress through a hamartoma/dysplasia (adenoma)/carcinoma sequence.[30]

Clinical Consideration

The polyps of PJS may cause intussusception of the small bowel, leading to abnormal pain, obstruction, and GI bleeding. Prolapse of a pedunculated PJS polyp through the rectum may also occur.[31] As mentioned, PJS is associated with increased risk of both GI and extraintestinal neoplasms,[31–33] including cancers of the stomach, small bowel, colon, cervix, and pancreas.[32,33] A retrospective study from the Mayo Clinic showed that 18 of 34 (57%) patients with PJS developed non-cutaneous cancers at a mean age of 39 years. The cumulative

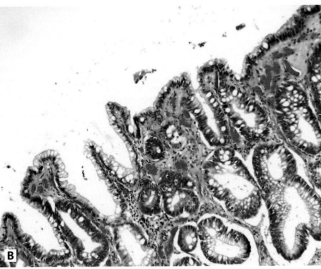

FIGURE 29-16. Juvenile polyp with low-grade dysplasia. **A.** Epithelia at the surface showing enlarged and hyperchromatic nuclei. **B.** Higher magnification view of dysplasia. The presence of dysplasia in a juvenile polyp is strongly suggestive of juvenile polyposis syndrome.

risk of malignancy is 93% in patients 15 to 64 years of age, including breast, pancreatic, gastric, ovarian, and small-intestinal cancer.[34] Therefore, surveillance for patients with PJS is warranted for removal of polyps and for early cancer detection.[35] Colonoscopy and upper endoscopy are recommended every 1 to 2 years beginning in adolescence. In addition, breast examination, mammography, and pancreatic ultrasound are advocated.[35]

PART SIX

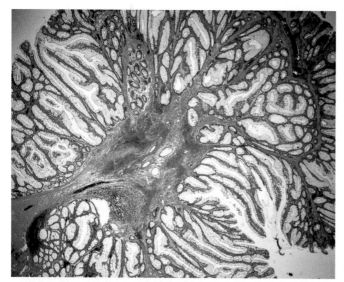

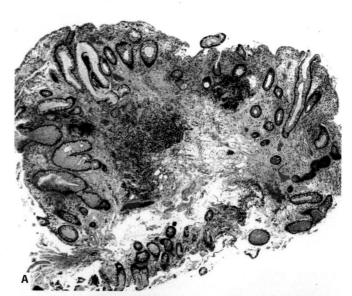

FIGURE 29-17. The Peutz-Jeghers polyp is characterized by arborizing smooth muscle bundles derived from the underlying muscularis mucosae, with glandular overgrowth; the lamina propria is otherwise normal.

COWDEN POLYPS

Cowden syndrome is an autosomal dominant hamartoma/ neoplastic syndrome that bears the family name of the original patient described in 1963 by Lloyd and Dennis[36] and is associated with germline mutations in the *PTEN* gene.[37] Currently, Cowden syndrome and other related conditions (such as Bannayan-Riley-Ruvalcaba syndrome) are collectively referred to as *PTEN* hamartoma tumor syndrome (PHTS).

Hamartomas in Cowden syndrome affect all three germ cell layers but most commonly arise from ectodermal and endodermal elements. Almost all patients have mucocutaneous lesions, including trichilemmomas, acral keratoses, and oral papillomas.[37,38] Breast lesions, including fibroadenomas, fibrocystic changes, and adenocarcinomas, affect most female patients; 25%–50% of them also develop breast cancer.[38]

Pathologic Features

Gastrointestinal lesions in Cowden syndrome include esophageal mucosal glycogen acanthosis and polyps in the stomach, small bowel, and colon. These include hyperplastic, hamartomatous, and inflammatory/retention polyps[39,40] (Figure 29-18A). Other lesions that can occur in the colon include lipoma, fibrolipoma, fibroma, ganglioneuroma (Figure 29-18B), and adenomas.

Clinical Consideration

There are no definitive data regarding increased risk of GI malignancies. Some patients may develop colon cancer at a younger age[41]; thus, endoscopic surveillance is recommended.[37] Surveillance for other types of cancer, including of the breast and thyroid, is also recommended.

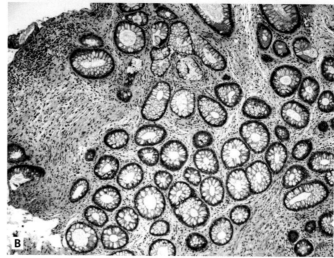

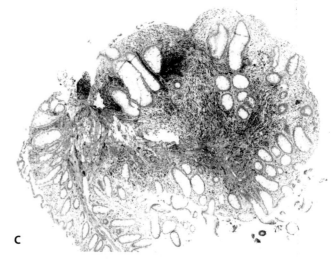

FIGURE 29-18. Colonic polyps in Cowden disease include a hamartomatous polyp (**A**) and a ganglioneuroma (**B**, H&E stain; **C**, immunostain for S-100 protein).

CRONKHITE-CANADA SYNDROME POLYPS

Cronkhite-Canada syndrome (CCS) is a rare, nonhereditary polyposis syndrome of unknown etiology, first described in 1955 by Cronkhite and Canada.[42] Patients are usually in middle age and present with diarrhea, weight loss, nausea and vomiting, anorexia, and GI bleeding. Diarrhea may be profound, leading to severe electrolyte imbalance. Other associated disorders include alopecia, dystrophy of nails, and skin hyperpigmentation.[42]

Pathologic Features

Polyps in CCS occur throughout the GI tract. Histologically, the polyps are hyperplastic and may resemble juvenile polyps in the colon, with cystically dilated and tortuous glands filled with inspissated mucin. The distinguishing feature of CCS polyps is abnormality in the intervening nonpolypoid mucosa, including edema, and cystically dilated glands, which are not seen in other types of polyp.

Clinical Consideration

Cronkhite-Canada syndrome is not easy to recognize clinically without a high degree of suspicion because of the nonspecific presentation, but it is associated with a high mortality rate, approaching 50%.[44] Treatment includes nutritional support, antibiotics, corticosteroids, or surgical resection of the involved segments, such as gastrectomy. The malignant potential of colonic CCS is unknown due to the rarity of cases. Some studies reported a 14.5% progression to GI carcinomas.[43]

INFLAMMATORY POLYPS

There are no strict clinical and pathologic criteria for inflammatory polyps except for those occurring in the background of inflammatory bowel diseases (IBDs). These polyps show no distinct features in the surface or crypt epithelium except for minimal or focal crypt branching or elongation and mild lamina propria inflammation. Some inflammatory polyps represent a small mucosal prolapse or redundant mucosa adjacent to a diverticulum (Figure 29-19). Polyps microscopically resemble juvenile polyps in adults and are also referred to as inflammatory polyps, as discussed previously. Other variants include inflammatory myoglandular polyps.

Inflammatory bowel disease, particularly ulcerative colitis, predisposes the development of multiple inflammatory polyps, some resulting from inflammatory pseudopolyps (see next section) after healing of the ulcerated mucosa. These are also referred to as *postinflammatory polyps* endoscopically. As part of the underlying IBD, inflammatory polyps in this setting exhibit marked crypt architectural distortion, often with surface villiform transformation, in contrast to the subtle changes in other inflammatory polyps (eg, prolapse). Recognizing this distinction, inflammatory polyps in a non-IBD setting are sometimes referred to as *inflammatory-type polyps*.

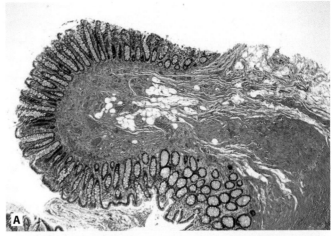

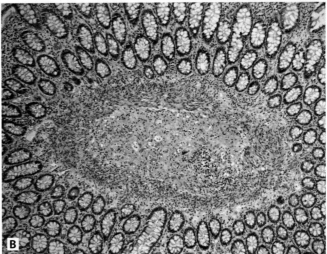

FIGURE 29-19. Some inflammatory polyps only show subtle abnormalities. This polyp shows normal colonic epithelium overlying a fibrovascular core without significant inflammation (**A**). On cross section, the fibrovascular core shows increased fibrosis with interspersed ganglion cells and disorganized smooth muscle bundles (**B**).

INFLAMMATORY PSEUDOPOLYPS

Inflammatory pseudopolyps are polypoid projections of inflamed and regenerating mucosa above the level of the surrounding ulcerated mucosa. By definition, these develop in IBD.[44,45] The pathogenesis is related to severe ulceration of the mucosa, followed by regenerative hyperplasia and inflammation of the intervening residual mucosa. Inflammatory pseudopolyps may also occur in the background of ischemic colitis, infectious colitis, and neonatal necrotizing enterocolitis.[46]

Pathology Features

Inflammatory pseudopolyps may be sessile, pedunculated, or filiform. They can be solitary or multiple and may be localized or diffusely distributed.[45] Microscopically, the lesions are composed of inflamed lamina propria with distorted crypts, which are often dilated, branched, and hyperplastic; cryptitis and crypt abscess may be present (Figure 29-20).

PART SIX

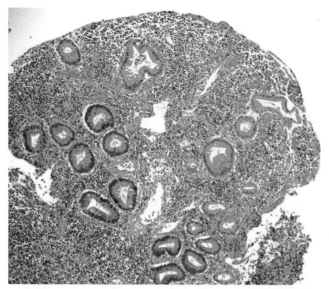

FIGURE 29-20. Inflammatory pseudopolyp. This polyp consists of inflamed and regenerating mucosa above the level of the surrounding ulcerated mucosa. The lamina propria is markedly inflamed, and the epithelium shows regenerative changes.

The diagnosis of inflammatory pseudopolyps is straightforward in a proper clinical setting. As they are often associated with marked regenerative changes or atypia, distinction from true dysplasia may become an issue. This is discussed in detail in Chapter 27. Another diagnostic pitfall is the presence of bizarre-shaped, large, or multinucleated stromal cells, which mimic sarcoma.[47] These cells may be spindled or epithelioid and often aggregate toward the surface of a polyp in areas of ulceration with granulation tissue.[47]

Clinical Consideration

Inflammatory pseudopolyps tend to persist even after the surrounding mucosa has healed; therefore, they are frequently found in quiescent ulcerative colitis. There polyps are not associated with increased risk for neoplastic transformation.[45]

■ MESENCHYMAL POLYPS

Stromal tissue is the main component of mesenchymal polyps. These may include inflammatory fibroid polyps; benign or malignant tumors of adipose tissue, smooth muscle, vascular tissue, or neural tissue; and gastrointestinal stromal tumors (GISTs). Only lesions that present endoscopically as mucosa polyps are discussed here.

Ganglioneuroma

A ganglioneuroma arises in the GI tract in three clinical settings: (1) solitary polypoid intramucosal ganglioneuroma; (2) ganglioneuroma polyposis; (3) diffuse (transmural) ganglioneuromas. The intramucosal ganglioneuroma is most commonly found in the colon and rectum[48] as a sessile or pedunculated polyp and consists of nerve fibers, Schwann cells, and ganglion cells.

Pathologic Features

The polyp is characterized by disorganized crypt architecture with cystic glands, expanded lamina propria, and clusters of spindle cells with mature ganglion cells (Figures 29-21A, 29-21B). Ganglion cells are not a component of normal lamina propria. Their presence in mucosa thus warrants further attention, including additional sectioning, so that a ganglioneuroma is not missed. On the other hand, ganglion cells may migrate into the lamina propria in response to mucosal injury, such as in Crohn disease, but these foci of "ectopic" ganglion cells lack proliferation of spindle cells.[49] Similar lesions in which ganglion cells are not found are termed *intramucosal neuromas.*

Clinical Consideration

Solitary intramucosal ganglioneuromas have no systemic disease association; thus, long-term follow-up is not required. However, ganglioneuromatous polyposis may be associated

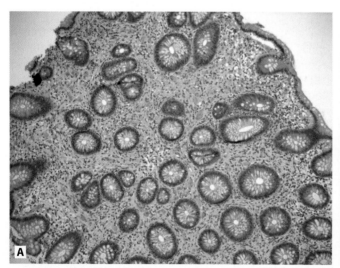

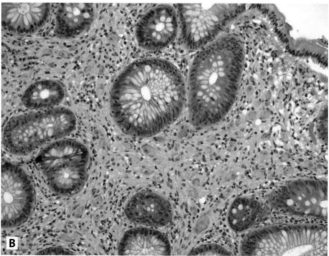

FIGURE 29-21. Ganglioneuroma. This polyp is characterized by disorganized crypt architecture, expanded lamina propria, and unremarkable surface epithelium (**A**). Clusters of spindle cells with mature ganglion cells are evident with a higher-magnification view (**B**).

with multiple cutaneous lipomas and skin tags, Cowden disease, juvenile polyposis, adenoma or carcinoma, or von Recklinghausen neurofibromatosis.[48,50] Diffuse ganglioneuromas occur in patients with multiple endocrine neoplasia (MEN) 2b, von Recklinghausen neurofibromatosis, multiple intestinal neurofibroma, or neurogenic sarcoma. Of these, the association between diffuse ganglioneuromas with MEN 2b is most strong.[51] Ganglioneuromatous polyposis is characterized by the presence of many (dozens) to innumerable polyps in the colon.[48] Patients are often symptomatic, with pain, bleeding, and irritable bowel syndrome.[48] Patients with diffuse ganglioneuromatosis are universally symptomatic, with abnormal pain, rectal bleeding, or megacolon.[48]

Benign Nerve Sheath Tumors (Neurofibroma, Perineurioma, Schwann Cell Hamartoma)

Benign nerve sheath tumors are occasionally encountered as GI polyps. These include neurofibroma or neuroma, Schwann cell hamartoma, perineurioma, and hybrid schwannoma/perineurioma. Distinction among these lesions depends on immunohistochemical study. Neurofibromas occur either sporadically or as part of neurofibromatosis type 1 (NF-1) or von Recklinghausen disease. Isolated GI tract neurofibromas outside the setting of NF-1 are rare.

Neuromas

Some investigators consider neuromas as nonneoplastic overgrowth of nerve fibers and Schwann cells. They may arise in the submucosa and extend into the lamina propria, forming polypoid lesions. Histologically, the tumor consists of proliferating bundles of spindle cells with wavy dark nuclei, strands of collagen, varying amounts of myxoid matrix, and scattered neurites. Schwann cells and fibroblasts may be present. Immunohistochemically, the tumor is marked by positive staining for CD68 (Schwann cells turned phagocytes), S-100, neurofilament, and CD34.

Schwann Cell Hamartomas

Schwann cell hamartomas refer to proliferation of nerve sheath cells in the lamina propria that lack ganglion cells. There are no associations with NF1, MEN 2B, or Cowden syndromes.[52] The polyps are sessile and small (1–6 mm in size). Histologically, the proliferation consists of uniform bland spindle cells with elongated, tapering nuclei and abundant dense eosinophilic cytoplasm (Figure 29-22). There may

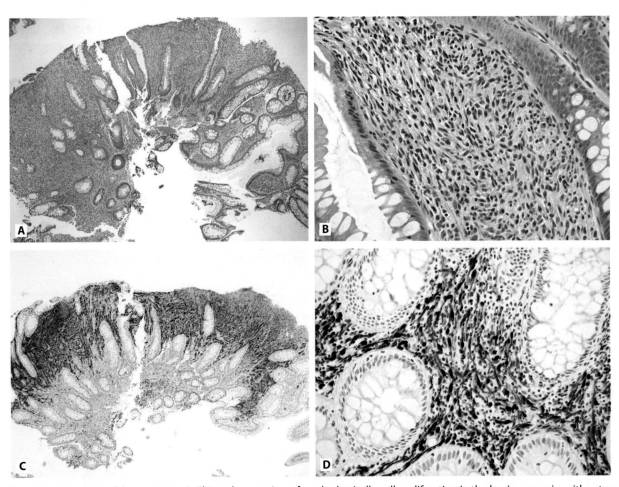

FIGURE 29-22. Schwann cell hamartoma. **A.** This polyp consists of marked spindle cell proliferation in the lamina propria, without complete displacement of the crypts. **B.** High-power view revealing cells with schwannian morphology, with scattered inflammatory cells, such as mast cells and eosinophils. **C.** Immunostain for S-100 highlights the entire spindle cell component. **D.** High-power view showing strong nuclear staining and less-intensive staining of the cellular processes.

be entrapped adjacent glands. Immunostaining for S-100 is strongly positive. A rare axon may be present (positive for neurofilament stain). But, staining for epithelial membrane antigen (EMA) is negative.

Perineuriomas

A perineurioma is composed of a proliferation of bland spindle cells of perineurium origin (Figure 29-23), which stain positive for EMA but negative for S-100 immunohistochemically. Intramucosal perineuriomas have no other clinical consequences. Some lesions may be accompanied by hyperplastic/serrated epithelial changes, are termed *perineurial-like stromal proliferations in serrated polyps*,[53] and are positive for *BRAF* V600E mutation.[53]

Hybrid Schwannomas/Perineuriomas

The hybrid schwannoma/perineurioma may rarely occur in the colon.[54] Histologically, this lesion is composed of spindle cells with plump, tapering nuclei and palely eosinophilic cytoplasm, arranged in a storiform, whorled, or lamellar architecture. Antoni A and B zonation and hyaline vessels, typical features of schwannomas, are absent. Immunohistochemical stain shows mixed components of S-100–positive Schwann cells and EMA-positive perineurial cells. There is no association with neurofibromatosis.

Features of the benign neurogenic polyps are summarized in Table 29-4.

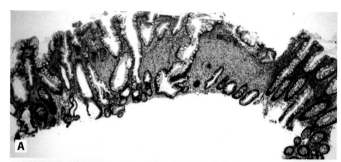
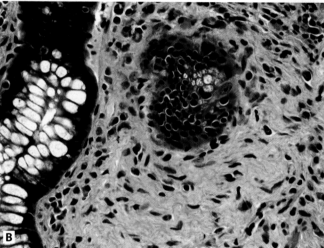

FIGURE 29-23. Perineurioma. This polyp shows proliferation of bland spindle cells separating hyperplastic/serrated crypts (**A**). The spindle cells are closely associated with crypts (**B**).

TABLE 29-4. Benign colorectal intramucosal neurogenic and fibroblastic nodules.

Type	Median age (range)	M/F	Mean size, mm (range)	Histology	Immunophenotype	Syndromic association
Neurofibroma (neuroma)	Variable	N/A	Variable	Spindle cells, variable cellularity	Focal S-100+ Scattered NF+ axons Scattered CD68+ Scattered CD34+	Some associated with NF-1
Schwann cell hamartoma	60 (46–88)	10/16	2.5 (1–6)	Proliferation of uniformly bland spindle cells with elongated, tapering nuclei and abundant, eosinophilic cytoplasm, entrapping adjacent crypts	Strong S-100+ EMA− Neurofilament−	None
Perineurioma	56.5 (44–87)	11/9	5.1 (3–15)	Bland spindle cells with delicate cytoplasmic processes; focal whorled growth pattern, forming concentric rings around crypts, which may be serrated	EMA+ S-100−	None
Perineurial-like stromal proliferation in serrated polyp	69 (54–78)	7/6	12.5 (4–25)	Similar to perineurioma	Same as above	None
Hybrid schwannoma/ perineurioma	48	M	50	Spindle cells with plump, tapering nuclei and pale eosinophilic cytoplasm, arranged in a storiform, whorled, or lamellar architecture	60%–70% cells positive for S100 and 30%–40% cells positive for EMA (mutually exclusive)	None
Fibroblastic polyp	58.5 (37–84)	6/8	5.1 (2–15)	Bland spindle cells	Vimentin+ Focally and weakly positive for CD34 and SMA Negative for S-100 and EMA	None

Abbreviations: EMA, epithelial membrane antigen; F, female; M, male; NF, neurofilament; NF-1, neurofibromatosis type 1; SMA, smooth muscle actin.

TABLE 29-5. Diagnostic features for serrated polyps.

Features	HP	SSP	TSA
Serration or dilation			
Upper crypt	+++	+++	+++
Lower crypt	−	+++	++
Architectural abnormalities			
Horizontal crypts	Rare	Common	Often
Crypt branching	Rare	Common	Often
Ectopic crypts	Rare	Rare	Common
Mitosis			
Upper crypts	−	+	++
Lower crypts	++	++	++
Goblet cells			
Upper crypt	+++	+++	+++
Lower crypt	+	+	+
Gastric-type epithelium	±	±	±
Nuclear features			
Hyperchromasia	−	+	+++
Elongation	−	+	+++
Pseudostratification	−	+	+++
Vesicular nucleus	±	+	+
Prominent nucleolus	+	++	++
Cytoplasmic eosinophilia	±	+	+++

Abbreviations: HP, hyperplastic polyp; SSP, sessile serrated polyp; TSA, traditional serrated adenoma.

SUMMARY AND PRACTICAL CONSIDERATIONS

Specimen Handling

All polyps removed endoscopically are submitted for histology, as endoscopic appearance is unreliable for classification. Polyps with a stalk or larger than 1 cm in size should be trisected after the stalk or deep margin is inked; adenomas larger than 1 cm are associated with higher risk of harboring an invasive component ("malignant polyp"). Optimal orientation should be attempted for proper evaluation of the deep portion of a "sessile" polyp, which is essential for differentiation between hyperplastic polyps and SSPs.

Differential Diagnosis of Polyps with Serration (Serrated Polyps)

The diagnostic agreement among pathologists regarding serrated polyps (note: no "sessile" here) has improved in recent years, with better understanding and morphological definition, although these were originally poor.[55,56] The diagnostic criteria for serrated polyps are listed in Table 29-5. The pathologist should compare the size of the polyp on the slide with the gross description to make sure the sections represent the entire lesion; otherwise, additional deeper levels should be prepared and examined before the diagnosis of hyperplastic polyp is given.

REFERENCES

1. Lieberman DA, Rex DK, Winawer SJ, Giardiello FM, Johnson DA, Levin TR. Guidelines for colonoscopy surveillance after screening and polypectomy: a consensus update by the US multi-society task force on colorectal cancer. *Gastroenterology*. 2012;143:844–857.
2. Saini SD, Kim HM, Schoenfeld P. Incidence of advanced adenomas at surveillance colonoscopy in patients with a personal history of colon adenomas: a meta-analysis and systemic review. *Gastrointest Endosc*. 2006;64:614–626.
3. Martinez ME, Baron JA, Lieberman DA, et al. A pooled analysis of advanced colorectal neoplasia diagnoses following colonoscopic polypectomy. *Gastroenterology*. 2009;136:832–841.
4. Pai RK, Rybicki LA, Goldblum JR, et al. Paneth cells in colonic adenomas: association with male sex and adenoma burden. *Am J Surg Pathol*. 2013;37:98–103.
5. Pulitzer M, Xu R, Suriawinata AA, et al. Microcarcinoids in large intestinal adenomas. *Am J Surg Pathol*. 2006;30:1531–1536.
6. Lin J, Goldblum JR, Bennett AE, et al. Composite intestinal adenoma-microcarcinoid. *Am J Surg Pathol*. 2012;36:292–295.
7. Salaria SN, Abu Alfa AK, Alsaigh NY, et al. Composite intestinal adenoma-microcarcinoid clues to diagnosing an under-recognised mimic of invasive adenocarcinoma. *J Clin Pathol*. 2013;66:302–306.
8. Macdonald AW, Tayyab M, Arsalani-Zadeh R, et al. Intramucosal carcinoma on biopsy reliably predicts invasive colorectal cancer. *Ann Surg Oncol*. 2009;16:3267–3270.
9. Muller S, Chesner IM, Egan MJ, et al. Significance of venous and lymphatic invasion in malignant polyps of the colon and rectum. *Gut*. 1989;30:1385–1391.
10. Park YJ, Kim WH, Paeng SS, et al. Histological analysis of early colorectal cancer. *World J Surg*. 2000;24:1029–1035.
11. Boenicke L, Fein M, Sailer M, et al. The concurrence of histologically positive resection margins and sessile morphology is an important risk factor for lymph node metastasis after complete endoscopic removal of malignant colorectal polyps. *Int J Colorectal Dis*. 2010;25:433–438.
12. Hassan C, Zullo A, Risio M, et al. Histologic risk factors and clinical outcome in colorectal malignant polyp: a pooled-data analysis. *Dis Colon Rectum*. 2005;48:1588–1596.
13. Morson BC, Whiteway JE, Jones EA, et al. Histopathology and prognosis of malignant colorectal polyps treated by endoscopic polypectomy. *Gut*. 1984;25:437–444.
14. Di Gregorio C, Bonetti LR, de Gaetani C, et al. Clinical outcome of low- and high-risk malignant colorectal polyps: results of a population-based study and meta-analysis of the available literature. *Intern Emerg Med*. 2014;9(2):151–160.
15. Longacre TA, Fenoglio-Preiser CM. Mixed hyperplastic adenomatous polyps/serrated adenomas. A distinct form of colorectal neoplasia. *Am J Surg Pathol*. 1990;14:524–537.
16. Torlakovic E, Skovlund E, Snover DC, Torlakovic G, Nesland JM. Morphologic reappraisal of serrated colorectal polyps. *Am J Surg Pathol*. 2003;27:65–81.

PART SIX

17. Kim M-J, Lee E-J, Suh J-P, et al. Traditional serrated adenoma of the colorectum: clinicopathologic implications and endoscopic findings of the precursor lesions. *Am J Clin Pathol.* 2013;140:898–911.

18. East JE, Saunders BP, Jass JR. Sporadic and syndromic hyperplastic polyps and serrated adenomas of the colon: classification, molecular genetics, natural history, and clinical management. *Gastroenterol Clin North Am.* 2008;37:25–46.

19. Fu B, Yachida S, Morgan R, et al. Clinicopathologic and genetic characterization of traditional serrated adenomas of the colon. *Am J Clin Pathol.* 2012;138:356–366.

20. Oh K, Redston M, Odze RD. Support for hMLH1 and MGMT silencing as a mechanism of tumorigenesis in the hyperplastic-adenoma-carcinoma (serrated) carcinogenic pathway in the colon. *Hum Pathol.* 2005;36:101–111.

21. Goldstein NS. Small colonic microsatellite unstable adenocarcinomas and high-grade epithelial dysplasias in sessile serrated adenoma polypectomy specimens: a study of eight cases. *Am J Clin Pathol.* 2006;125:132–145.

22. Snover DC, Ahnen DJ, Burt RW, et al. Serrated polyps of the colon and rectum and serrated polyposis. In: Bosman FT, Carneiro F, Hruban RH, Theise ND, eds. *WHO Classification of Tumors of the Digestive System.* 4th ed. Lyon, France: International Agency for Research on Cancer; 2010:160–165.

23. McColl I, Busxey HJ, Veale AM, Morson BC. Juvenile polyposis coli. *Proc R Soc Med.* 1964;57: 896–897.

24. Merg A, Howe JR. Genetic conditions associated with intestinal juvenile polyps. *Am J Med Genet C Semin Med Genet.* 2004;129C:44–55.

25. Latchford AR, Neale K, Phillips RKS, Clark SK. Juvenile polyposis syndrome: a study of genotype, phenotype, and long-term outcome. *Dis Colon Rectum.* 2012;55:1038–1043.

26. Wu T-T, Rezai B, Rashid A, et al. Genetic alterations and epithelial dysplasia in juvenile polyposis syndrome and sporadic juvenile polyps. *Am J Pathol.* 1997;150:939–947.

27. Wirtzfeld DA, Perelli NJ, Rodriguez-Bigas MA. Hamartomatous polyposis syndrome: molecular genetics, neoplastic risk, and surveillance recommendations. *Ann Surg Oncol.* 2001;8:319–327.

28. Ylikorkala A, Avizienyte E, Tomlinson IPM, et al. Mutations and impaired function of LKB1 in familial and non-familial Peutz-Jeghers syndrome and a sporadic testicular cancer. *Hum Mol Genet.* 1999;8:45–51.

29. Jeghers H, McKusick VA, Katz KH. Generalized intestinal polyposis and melanin spots of the oral mucosa, lips, and digits—a syndrome of diagnostic significance. *N Engl J Med.* 1949;241:993–1005.

30. Entius MM, Westerman AM, Giardiello FM, et al. Peutz-Jeghers polyps, dysplasia, and K-ras codon 12 mutations. *Gut.* 1997;41:320–322.

31. Westerman AM, Entius MM, de Baar E, et al. Peutz-Jeghers syndrome: 78-year follow-up of the original family. *Lancet.* 1999;353:1211–1215.

32. Resta N, Pierannunzio D, Lenato GM, et al. Cancer risk associated with STK1/LKB1 germline mutations in Peutz-Jeghers syndrome patients: results of an Italian multicenter study. *Dig Liver Dis.* 2013;45:606–611.

33. van Lier MGF, Wagner A, Mathus-Vliegen EMH, et al. High cancer risk in Peutz-Jeghers syndrome: a systemic review and surveillance recommendations. *Am J Gastroenterol.* 2010;105:1258–1264.

34. Giardiello FM, Brensinger JD, Tersmette AC, et al. Very high risk of cancer in familial Peutz-Jeghers syndrome. *Gastroenterology.* 2000;119:1447–1453.

35. Giardiello FM, Trimbath JD. Peutz-Jeghers syndrome and management recommendations. *Clin Gastroenterol Hepatol.* 2006;4:408–415.

36. Lloyd KM II, Dennis M. Cowden's disease. A possible new symptom complex with multiple system involvement. *Ann Intern Med.* 1963;58:136–142.

37. Hobert JA, Eng C. PTEN hamartoma tumor syndrome: an overview. *Genet Med.* 2009;11:687–694.

38. Bubien V, Bonnet F, Brouste V, et al. High cumulative risks of cancer in patients with PTEN hamartoma tumour syndrome. *J Med Genet.* 2013;50:255–263.

39. Levi Z, Baris HN, Kedar I, et al. Upper and lower gastrointestinal findings in PTEN mutation-positive Cowden syndrome patients participating in an active surveillance program. *Clin Transl Gastroenterol.* 2011;2:e5

40. Stanich PP, Owens VL, Sweetser S, et al. Colonic polyposis and neoplasia in Cowden syndrome. *Mayo Clin Proc.* 2011;86:489–492.

41. Heald B, Mester J, Rybicki L, et al. Frequent gastrointestinal polyps and colorectal adenocarcinomas in a prospective series of PTEN mutation carriers. *Gastroenterology.* 2010;139:1927–1933.

42. Cronkhite LW, Canada WJ. Generalized gastrointestinal polyposis. an unusual syndrome of polyposis, pigmentation, alopecia and onychotrophia. *N Engl J Med.* 1955;252:1011–1015.

43. Daniel ES, Ludwig SL, Lewin KJ, et al. The Cronkhite-Canada syndrome. An analysis of clinical and pathologic features and therapy in 55 patients. *Medicine (Baltimore).* 1982;61:293–309.

44. Lumb G. Pathology of ulcerative colitis. *Gastroenterology.* 1961;40: 290–297.

45. Teague RH, Read AE. Polyposis in ulcerative colitis. *Gut.* 1975;16: 792–795.

46. Kim H-S, Lee KY, Kim YW. Filiform polyposis associated with sigmoid diverticulitis in a patient without inflammatory bowel disease. *J Crohns Colitis.* 2010;4(6):671–673.

47. Jessurun J, Paplanus SH, Nagle RB, et al. Pseudosarcomatous changes in inflammatory pseudopolyps of the colon. *Arch Pathol Lab Med.* 1986;110:833–836.

48. Shekitka KM, Sobin LH. Ganglioneuromas of the gastrointestinal tract. Relation to von Recklinghausen disease and other multiple tumor syndromes. *Am J Surg Pathol.* 1994;18:250–257.

49. Tunru-Dinh V, Wu ML. Intramucosal ganglion cells in normal adult colorectal mucosa. *Int J Surg Pathol.* 2007;15:31–37.

50. Chan OTM, Haghighi P. Hamatomaous polyps of the colon: ganglioneuromatous, stromal, and lipomatous. *Arch Pathol Lab Med.* 2006;130:1561–1566.

51. Carney JA, Go VLW, Sizemore GW, Hayles AB. Alimentary-tract ganglioneuromatosis. A major component of the syndrome of multiple endocrine neoplasia, type 2b. *N Engl J Med.* 1976;295(23):1287–1291.

52. Gibson JA, Hornick JL. Mucosal Schwann cell "hamartoma": clinicopathologic study of 26 neural colorectal polyps distinct from neurofibromas and mucosal neuromas. *Am J Surg Pathol.* 2009;33:781–787.

53. Pai RK, Mojtahed A, Rouse RV, et al. Histologic and molecular analyses of colonic perineurial-like proliferations in serrated polyps: perineurial-like stromal proliferations are seen in sessile serrated polyps. *Am J Surg Pathol.* 2011;35:1373–1380.

54. Hornick JL, Bundock EA, Fletcher CD. Hybrid schwannoma/perineurioma: clinicopathologic analysis of 42 distinctive benign nerve sheath tumors. *Am J Surg Pathol.* 2009;33:1554–1561.

55. Farris AB, Misdraji J, Srivastava A, et al. Sessile serrated adenoma: challenging discrimination from other serrated colonic polyps. *Am J Surg Pathol.* 2008;32(1):30–35.

56. Gonzalo DH, Lai KK, Shadrach B, et al. Gene expression profiling of serrated polyps identifies annexin A10 as a marker of a sessile serrated adenoma/polyp. *J Pathol.* 2013;230(4):420–429.

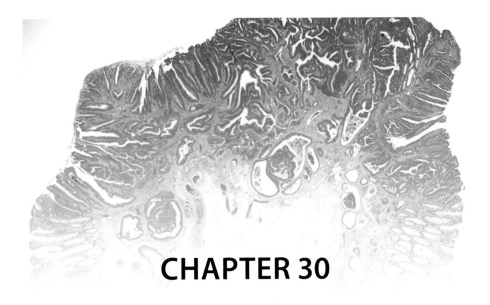

CHAPTER 30

Colorectal Carcinomas

■ INTRODUCTION

As one of the most common malignancies, colonic carcinomas are frequently encountered in daily diagnostic practice. For most specimens, either biopsy or resection, the diagnosis is straightforward. Information regarding diagnosis, histologic grading and subtyping, and tumor staging are readily available in other sources and well understood by practicing pathologists. Therefore, a detailed systematic review in this chapter is unnecessary. Instead, a few practical issues that frequently arise in routine sign-out are discussed, as outlined in Table 30-1.

■ ADENOCARCINOMA ARISING IN AN ADENOMATOUS POLYP (MALIGNANT POLYP)

Malignant polyps are described in Chapter 29, but are discussed here with different emphasis. Once in a while in a polypectomy specimen, a focus of dysplastic gland is located in the submucosa of the polyp head or stalk. Two questions have to be resolved in this situation. First, is this dysplastic focus a result of gland herniation into the submucosa, tangential sectioning, or does it represent true invasion? The lesion is designated as a malignant polyp if the submucosal glands are determined to represent invasion (Figure 30-1). Second, what are the important parameters that need to be

communicated to the clinician if it is determined to be a malignant polyp? For both questions, it is critical that optimal specimen orientation is achieved, with the specimen submitted entirely for histology.

Distinction between True Submucosal Invasion and Herniation or Tangential Sectioning

The distinction between true submucosal invasion and herniation or tangential sectioning may be one of the most challenging diagnostic tasks. There are no optimal or uniformly accepted ancillary tests to address this question, but a set of microscopic features should be used in combination to reach a conclusion. First, a well-fixed, well-oriented specimen is most essential for proper assessment (Figure 30-1). When there is difficulty, additional levels of sections should be prepared (Figure 30-2). If the orientation of the specimen is determined to be improper, the paraffin block can be melted and the specimen reembedded for better orientation. Deeper sectioning, with or without reembedding, usually helps resolve the question of tangential sectioning artifact (Figure 30-3).

Herniated dysplastic glands in submucosa usually retain the smooth contour of noncancerous glands and are associated with typical lamina propria surrounding the glands (Figure 30-3). These foci are often accompanied by hemosiderin-laden macrophages. In contrast, true invasive

TABLE 30-1. Issues to be discussed for colon cancers.

Adenocarcinoma arising in adenoma

Polypectomy and endoscopic mucosal resection specimens

Histologic tumor types

    Mucinous

    Medullary

    Adenocarcinomas with neuroendocrine features

    Adenosquamous carcinoma

    Squamous carcinoma

    Distinction from *metastatic* carcinoma

Issues related to tumor grading and staging

    Histologic grading: degree of differentiation

    T4a vs radial margin: different segments

    Regional lymph nodes

    Vascular invasion (R0/R1/R2)

    Intramucosal lymphatics: do they exist?

Issues related to microsatellite instability (MSI) features

    Mainly associated with Lynch syndrome

    Sporadic tumors with high levels of MSI more common in the elderly and have serrated features; thus, the revised Bethesda criteria will not include these features

glands lack lamina propria and are often associated with desmoplasia. The last is characterized by fibrosis with increased cellularity, sometimes with a myxoid appearance due to freshly produced collagenous protein (Figure 30-4). In addition, invasive glands often exhibit an irregular or angulated growth pattern, forming "pointing" or "abortive" glands, with single-cell infiltration, as illustrated in Figure 30-5. As mentioned,

FIGURE 30-1. Adenocarcinoma arising in an adenoma (polyp). Well-oriented intact polyp (low power). In addition, the resection margin (outside the field of image) is clear of invasive carcinoma or dysplasia.

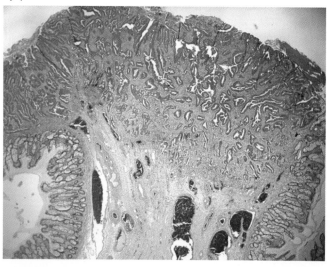

abundant hemosiderin-laden macrophages usually accompany herniated glands. However, finding these cells in the vicinity of glands or cells in the submucosa does not necessarily exclude invasion, as this can be seen in some cases (Figure 30-5D).

Resection Margin

It is usually not required to comment on the margin status of adenomas. If the polypectomy specimen is found to harbor invasive carcinoma, resection with negative margin must be achieved. In daily practice, the possibility of an occult invasive carcinoma is presumed to exist in all routine polypectomy and endoscopic mucosal resection (EMR; for larger lesions) specimens. Therefore, not only should a specimen be submitted in its entirety, but also an attempt should be made to identify and ink a resection margin grossly, whenever possible. This of course does not apply to fragmented specimens. Trying to "force" out an assessment of the margin status in fragmented specimens likely leads to misinformation. For tumors without lymphovascular invasion (LVI), a negative margin status may spare the patient a colectomy. This is defined by the front of invasive carcinoma being 1 mm or more from the cauterized (inked) margin (Figure 30-1), and the tumor is considered completely excised (Figure 30-1). Otherwise, the margin is considered positive (Figure 30-6). For specimens with suboptimal orientation or processing, with a margin status that cannot be assessed with certainty, but without LVI, a repeat colonoscopy may be performed for additional resection of the polypectomy site with an EMR. It is understood and accepted that most of these reassessments yield a negative result. This is not considered unnecessary treatment but has value in ensuring completeness of treatment. Surgical resection may be considered for lesions with a positive margin or if deeper invasion is identified in repeat colonoscopic evaluation of the polypectomy site.

Lymphovascular Invasion

Once the diagnosis of malignant polyp is made, the presence or absence of lymphatic invasion should also be assessed. This is particularly important for tumors of the lower rectum (distal one-third). For tumors of other regions of the colon, including the lower anterior resection of the proximal rectum, a decision for colectomy is relatively easier for the patient to make, since an anastomosis can be performed without a colostomy. However, for lower-rectum adenocarcinoma, the curative treatment requires an abdominoperineal resection (APR), which will result in a permanent colostomy, with a much less-desirable quality of life. It is not an easy choice unless the indications for the procedure are compelling.

For a polypoid lesion, because complete resection can be achieved with EMR or endoscopic submucosal dissection (ESD) with negative margins, the most important factor that leads to colectomy is the presence of LVI (Figure 30-7A). For proper evaluation of this parameter, the specimen needs to be well fixed and properly processed, which will minimize peritumoral tissue retraction artifact that can be mistaken

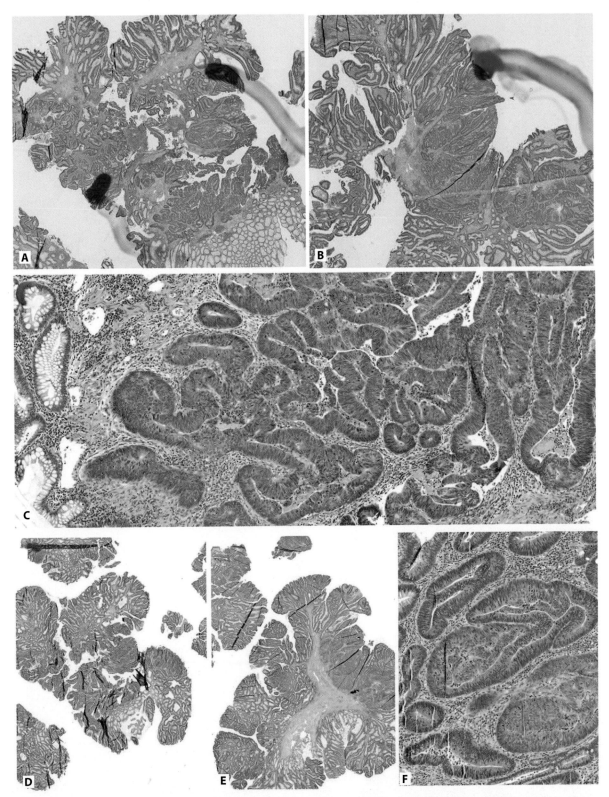

FIGURE 30-2. A polyp suspicious for submucosal invasion. **A–C.** Original section: central portion in (**A**) and (**B**) appeared as placement of dysplastic glands in submucosa. Higher magnification showed some irregular configuration of the glands (**C**). **D–F.** Additional deeper sections showed lack of submucosal invasion. Higher-power view showed glands similar to that in (**C**), both surrounded by loose connective tissue of normal lamina propria. The suspicion in the initial section was due to tangential sectioning.

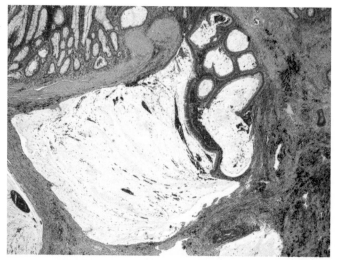

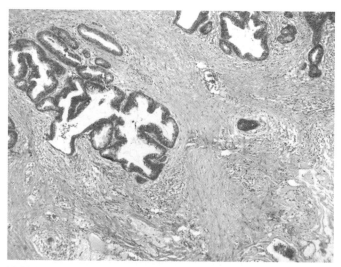

FIGURE 30-3. Herniation. Dysplastic glands along with extracellular mucin of a villous adenoma were displaced to the submucosa, along with prominent hemosiderin-laden macrophages. There is no desmoplasia.

FIGURE 30-4. Invasive glands surrounded by desmoplasia with myxoid appearance.

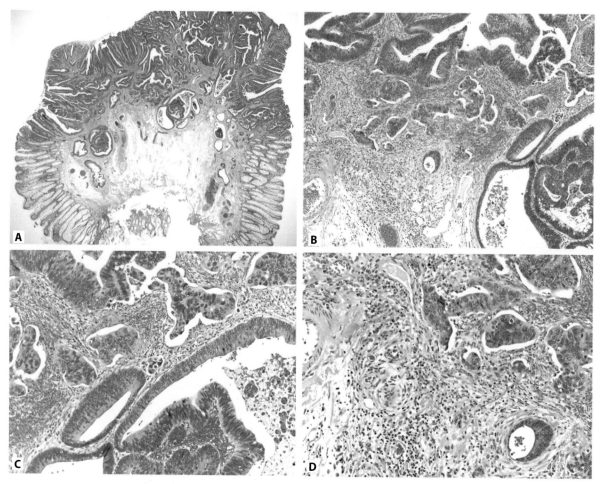

FIGURE 30-5. Invasive adenocarcinoma arising from a tubular adenoma. **A.** Complete polypectomy, with the inked, cauterized margin clear of carcinoma and flanked by nondysplastic mucosa. **B.** Small, irregular, and angulated glands or cell clusters with infiltrative growth pattern. **C.** Higher-power view of invasive component, with cellular desmoplasia and focal retraction artifact. **D.** Occasionally, invasion may also be associated with hemosiderin in nearby stroma.

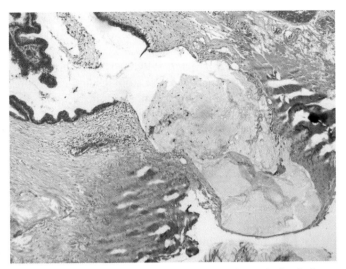

FIGURE 30-6. Positive resection (polypectomy) margin. Pool of mucin with associated epithelium extending to the cauterized edge.

FIGURE 30-7. Lymphovascular invasion (LVI) in a polypoid carcinoma. **A.** True invasion should have readily recognizable endothelial cells. **B.** Tissue retraction mimicking LVI.

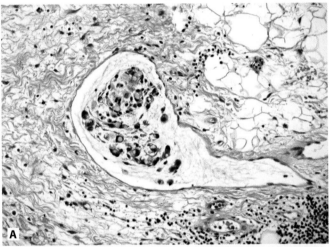

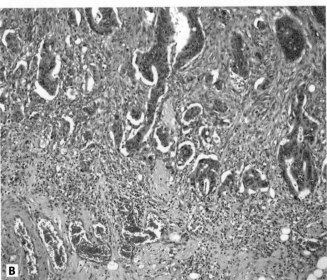

for LVI (Figure 30-7B). When a focus is suspicious for LVI, multiple levels of sections may be helpful.

Degree of Differentiation

Another relatively independent parameter used for treatment decision-making is the grade or differentiation of the carcinoma. If the tumor is graded as poorly differentiated (G3) or worse, the malignant lesion is considered to have a high risk for progression after polypectomy. Most malignant polyps contain well- or moderately differentiated carcinoma. Rare cases may have a poorly differentiated component despite the small size of the tumor. There is a question of reproducibility associated with grading of tumors (see the next section). Therefore, it is advisable that for cases with a small focus suspicious for poor differentiation, discussion with a colleague and an attempt to reach a consensus should take place.

■ COLORECTAL CARCINOMA: HISTOLOGIC TYPES

There are several systems for typing or classification of colorectal carcinomas. A true taxonomic system should rely on a single set of uniform criteria for each level of classification in a hierarchical manner. For example, based on an assumed origin of cell type or lineage of differentiation, these tumors are classified as adenocarcinoma, squamous carcinoma, adenosquamous carcinoma, mixed adenoendocrine carcinomas (MAECs), and so on. Adenocarcinomas are further divided based on pattern of growth, whether glandular, diffuse, mucinous, and so on. Some of these growth patterns are also used for grading (see below). Table 30-2 provides a list of histologic types (histotypes), which provide the basis for the following discussions. Some of the official or comprehensive classifications are readily available in the World

TABLE 30-2. Colorectal carcinoma histologic tumor types.
Adenocarcinoma
Usual type (NOS)
Well, moderate, or poorly differentiated
Mucinous
Well or poorly differentiated
Medullary
Signet ring
Squamous and adenosquamous carcinoma
Carcinomas with neuroendocrine component
Poorly differentiated neuroendocrine carcinoma (small-cell carcinoma)
Adenocarcinoma with focal neuroendocrine features
Focal synaptophysin positive, but chromogranin negative
Mixed adenoneuroendocrine carcinoma (MANEC)

Abbreviation: NOS, not otherwise specified.

PART SIX

Health Organization (WHO) classification and other excellent publications.

Adenocarcinoma not otherwise specified (NOS) consists mainly of a glandular component, with simple or complex glands, various solid areas, or other components, depending on the level of differentiation. When these other components/features become predominant (consisting of 50% or more of the tumor), the tumor should be labeled accordingly as specific histotype, such as mucinous, signet ring, and so on, recognizing that these unique types carry pathologic and clinical significance. For example, the medullary type may be predictive of microsatellite instability (MSI) status (see below). Rarely, the same tumor may exhibit multidirectional differentiation, including glandular, endocrine, squamous, or mesenchymal differentiations.[1]

Mucinous carcinoma is characterized by abundant mucin production (>50%) (Figure 30-8), which expands or dissects the structure where it resides or invades. The tumor mucin contains individual or clusters of tumor cells with mild-to-marked cytologic atypia, which corresponds to poor differentiation (Figure 30-8B). Some mucinous tumors may be lined by low-grade goblet cell strips, which should represent a well-differentiated tumor.

Signet-ring cell carcinoma (SRCC) is less common in the colorectum as compared to the stomach and constitutes less than 1% of all colorectal adenocarcinomas. Signet-ring cells should constitute more than 50% of the tumor.[2] These tumors usually have scirrhous infiltration, with strong desmoplasia, or predominantly are a lymphangiosis type without significant stromal desmoplasia (Figure 30-9).[2,3] However, it is not uncommon to see signet-ring cells in a tumor that is otherwise classified as a high-grade mucinous carcinoma (Figure 30-10). SRCCs demonstrate much shorter survival, with about one-third presenting with metastasis (more commonly lymphatics and peritoneal).[4,5]

FIGURE 30-8. Mucinous carcinoma. **A.** A large mucinous adenocarcinoma of the distal rectum. **B.** Mucinous carcinoma with high-grade tumor epithelium.

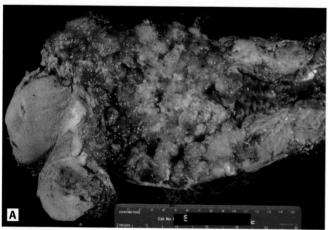

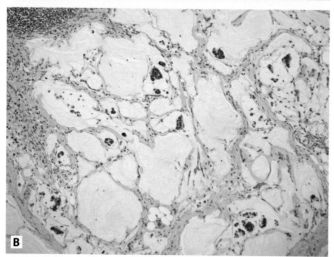

FIGURE 30-9. Signet-ring cell carcinoma of colon. **A.** Solid pattern of signet-ring cell infiltration among benign residual crypts. **B.** Signet-ring carcinoma arising from a villous adenoma in the cecum. Tumor cells are infiltrating dense fibrous tissue with a minor mucinous component.

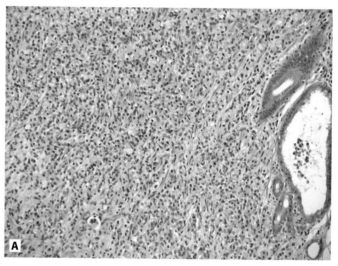

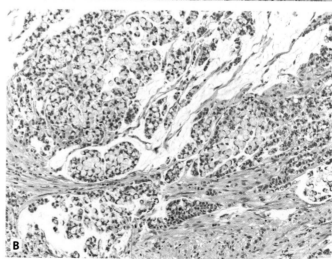

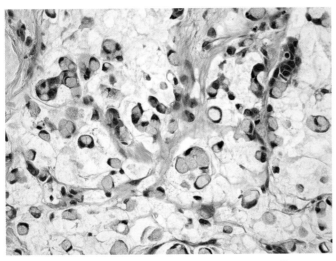

FIGURE 30-10. Mucinous carcinoma with signet-ring cells.

Despite similar morphology to gastric SRCCs, most cases of colorectal SRCC have a CK7-/CK20+ immunohistochemistry (IHC) pattern.[6]

Medullary carcinoma is characterized by nests or sheets of tumor cells with a minimal glandular component. The tumor cells have large nuclei with open chromatin and prominent nucleoli. The cells often form a syncytial pattern and are infiltrated by intratumoral reactive lymphocytes (Figure 30-11). Immunohistochemically, the tumor cells are negative for the endocrine markers synaptophysin and chromogranin.[7] In contrast to medullary carcinoma of the esophagus or stomach,

colonic medullary carcinoma is rarely related to the presence of Epstein-Barr virus (EBV).[8] However, it has a high predictive association with MSI status.[9] Those with medullary carcinomas seem to have better survival when compared to individuals with other solid, poorly differentiated CRCs.[7,10] Immunohistochemically, medullary carcinomas express calretinin in 73% of cases.[11] Loss of MLH1 and CDX2 was found in nearly 80% of cases.[11]

Squamous cell carcinoma (SCC) and *adenosquamous carcinoma* of the colon are extremely rare. Some cases may represent metastasis or direct extension (when in the rectum) from the anal canal. Occasional cases may appear as SCC but are found to be adenosquamous as they express IHC markers for adenocarcinoma instead of squamous markers (Figure 30-12). Adenosquamous carcinoma represents 0.01%–0.18% of the usual adenocarcinoma.[12-16] By definition, both the adeno- and squamous components should be malignant (Figure 30-13). In contrast, there are adenocarcinomas that contain focal benign squamous metaplasia, which should not be given the diagnosis of adenosquamous carcinoma. Due to their rarity, the clinicopathologic behavior of these tumors is unknown. Some cases may secrete parathyroid hormone with associated hypercalcemia.[17-19] In limited studies, adenosquamous carcinomas had a higher rate of metastasis at presentation[13,15,20] and thus a worse prognosis in terms of survival as compared to adenocarcinoma.[14,16] Whether there is an association between colorectal squamous, adenosquamous, adenocarcinoma, and human papilloma virus (HPV) infection is under debate, as some studies using in situ hybridization or IHC resulted in negative findings.[15,21]

FIGURE 30-11. Medullary carcinoma. This was a right colon mass in a 32-year-old male patient. **A.** There is a well-differentiated glandular component, intermixed with solid sheets of tumor cells forming syncytial pattern. There is tumor necrosis. The cells have indistinct cell borders, but with large vesicular nuclei and prominent nucleoli. **B.** There is mild intratumoral lymphocytic infiltration. Immunohistochemically, the tumor exhibits loss of MSH2 and MSH6 (not shown).

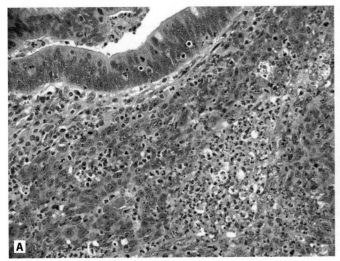

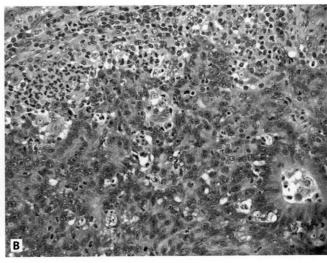

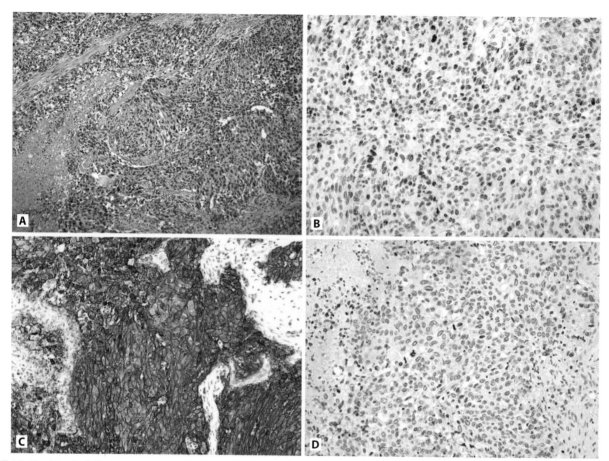

FIGURE 30-12. Poorly differentiated adenocarcinoma mimicking a squamous cell carcinoma. This right colon carcinoma has no gland formation and exhibits a squamous cell morphology (**A**). Immunohistochemically, the intestinal lineage is demonstrated by diffuse expression of CDX2 (**B**). However, the tumor is strongly positive for MOC31 (**C**) and completely negative for p63 (**D**). The tumor lacked staining for CK20 and CK7.

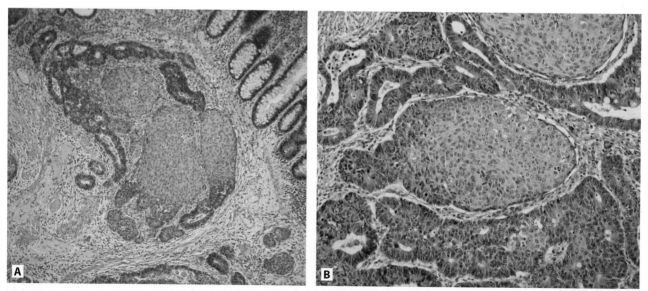

FIGURE 30-13. Adenosquamous carcinoma. **A.** Tumor with overlying colonic mucosa. **B.** Transition between the two components is evident.

CARCINOMAS WITH A NEUROENDOCRINE COMPONENT

Adenocarcinoma with focal neuroendocrine differentiation. Some poorly differentiated adenocarcinomas may exhibit focal positive staining for neuroendocrine markers, such as synaptophysin, which should not prompt a change of diagnosis to neuroendocrine carcinoma (NEC) or MAEC.

Mixed adenoendocrine carcinoma. The best example of MAEC is the appendiceal goblet cell carcinoid, with or without various components of gland-forming conventional adenocarcinoma, mucinous carcinoma, or SRCCs. Ample evidence supports the concept that, despite the name, goblet cell carcinoid is a "bridging entity" between neuroendocrine tumor and conventional adenocarcinoma. It behaves like adenocarcinoma, and should be staged as such in the TNM staging protocol.[22] For other types of MAEC, there are two readily identifiable morphologic components; both are malignant.[1] Molecular profiling in limited cases demonstrated common mutations in both adeno- and neuroendocrine components.[23]

Poorly differentiated neuroendocrine carcinoma. Excluding morphologically typical well-differentiated neuroendocrine tumors (carcinoid tumors), true NECs constitute less than 1% of all colorectal carcinomas, with over 60% presenting with metastasis.[24] The important morphologic aspects of this type of tumor include markedly increased nucleus-to-cytoplasm (N/C) ratio (Figure 30-14) and positivity for the endocrine marker synaptophysin. It must be pointed out that only a subset of these tumors is positive for the neuroendocrine markers chromogranin or synaptophysin, and diagnosis has to rely on hematoxylin and eosin (H&E) morphology and electron microscopy in negative cases.[25] These tumors are high grade and poorly differentiated (Figure 30-14) and behave as the usual poorly-differentiated adenocarcinoma, with

high mortality.[24–27] One of the diagnostic pitfalls is positive immunostaining for CD117 in a subset of colorectal NECs, potentially leading to erroneous diagnosis of GIST.[28]

ISSUES RELATED TO STAGING PARAMETERS

The complete list and descriptions of the TNM staging parameters can be found in the *AJCC Cancer Staging Manual* (7th edition).[22] Only selected parameters are discussed in this section, as questions often arise in daily practice.

Level of Differentiation and Tumor Grade

Tumor differentiation or grade is provided routinely in the pathology report and seems a straightforward task. Clinicians often place much emphasis on this information, to an extent that treatment decisions are sometimes made based on it. However, for many tumors, grading is subjective and not straightforward. A colonic adenocarcinoma can be graded as well, moderately, or poorly differentiated or undifferentiated, corresponding to G1, G2, G3, and G4, respectively. Pure gland formation clearly makes it well differentiated (G1). A tumor with little gland formation and mostly consisting of a solid component or widely infiltrated discohesive cells is evidently poorly differentiated (G3). However, most of the rest are hard to classify and may be placed into any of the 3 categories: well, moderately, or poorly differentiated. It is recommended (WHO classification) that a percentage cutoff is used for grading: G1 (>95% gland formation), G2 (50%–95% gland formation), and G3 (<50% gland formation). However, it is also recommended (WHO classification) that in tumors with heterologous morphology (which probably include most large tumors), the grading should be based on the least-differentiated component. Even when a single grading system was used, the interobserver agreement was poor. Discrepancies like this may account for the lack of meaningful association between tumor grade and clinical

FIGURE 30-14. Neuroendocrine carcinoma (NEC). **A.** The rectal tumor consists of solid sheets and nests of monotonous cells with large nucleus-to-cytoplasm ratio. **B.** Small-cell carcinoma of the rectum. Tumor cells exhibit large nuclei with stippling chromatin, frequent mitotic figures, and necrosis.

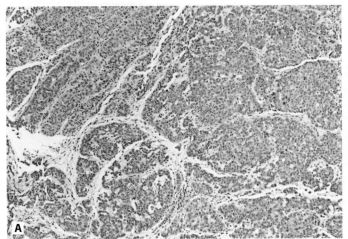
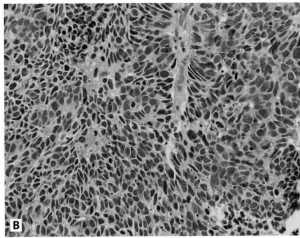

TABLE 30-3. Grading of colorectal carcinoma.

Low grade

    Well (G1) or moderately differentiated (G2)

    Gland formation ≥ 50% of the tumor

High grade

    Poorly or undifferentiated

    Gland formation < 50% of the tumor

    Signet-ring cell carcinoma

    Poorly differentiated neuroendocrine carcinoma (including small-cell carcinoma)

    Sarcomatoid carcinoma

    Squamous or adenosquamous

Grade not assigned[a]

    Medullary carcinoma

    Mucinous carcinoma

[a]World Health Organization classification recommends those medullary carcinomas or mucinous carcinomas with a high-level microsatellite instability status be considered low grade.

outcome in many studies. For these reasons, currently the College of American Pathologists (CAP) cancer protocol and WHO classification further recommend the simplified two-tier system of low and high grade, with low grade referring to 50% or more gland formation and high grade less than 50% gland formation (Table 30-3). However, for tumors with around 50% glandular component, the separation between low and high grade is still problematic.

Some of the special histotypes described are high grade by default: SRCC, small-cell carcinoma, and undifferentiated carcinoma (Table 30-3). Medullary carcinoma, despite being histologically poorly differentiated, is said to be associated with better prognosis and had been placed with the low-grade tumors. However, the notion of "better prognosis" was only relative to most "poorly differentiated" adenocarcinomas. Both morphologically and clinically, this should still be considered as a high-grade tumor. For mucinous tumors, there are examples for which the epithelium exhibits low-grade cytology and should be considered as low grade (or if MSI-H), despite the fact that most mucinous carcinomas show poorly

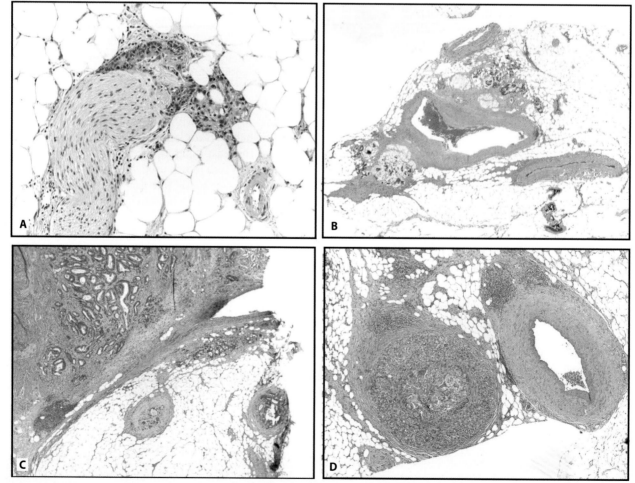

FIGURE 30-15. Tumor deposits. **A.** Extramural tumor spread along a nerve bundle. **B.** Perivascular spreading. **C.** Venous invasion. **D.** Large-vessel invasion, with tumor replacing the vascular wall as well as the lumen, mimicking lymph node metastasis.

differentiated or high-grade cytologic features. Therefore, grading of these tumors should be based on the individual case.

If grading is based on the representative or predominant component, it should be avoided on biopsies because the tumor focus in the biopsy may be too limited to be representative.

Tumor Deposits

Another important feature for TNM tumor parameters is the number of tumor deposits. These are defined as foci or nodules of tumor cells in the pericolic fat, away from the leading edge of the main tumor. They may represent a lymph node completely replaced by tumor, tumor spread along the blood vessels either intravascularly or perivascularly, or perineural spread (Figure 30-15).

Vascular Invasion

Venous invasion. This refers to tumor in venous vessels located in extramural adipose tissue, with V1 denoting microscopic invasion (Figures 30-15C, 30-15D) and V2 macroscopic invasion.

Lymphovascular invasion. Biologically, almost all invasive carcinomas have tumor cells invading into the lymphovascular system, therefore posing a risk for metastasis. However, as a prognostic factor that is measurable reproducibly and has clinical relevance, only frank LVI should be reported. That is, after careful microscopic examination of good-quality H&E-stained sections, the focus is deemed unequivocal for LVI (Figure 30-16). Therefore, immunostain for endothelial markers, such as D2-40, should not be used for this purpose. If the focus cannot be confidently recognized as true LVI on H&E staining, it should not be considered as such. Otherwise, the

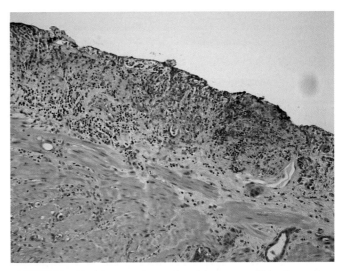

FIGURE 30-17. Adenocarcinoma involving serosa (T4a change).

threshold is too low in specificity to yield a meaningful assessment.

To reemphasize, from a biological point of view, all invasive carcinomas are considered to contain LVI that is not visible in routine microscopic examination. From an extreme scenario, these biological or "occult" LVIs are not what diagnostic pathologists should worry about because outcome studies were performed based on "overt" LVIs. Adding ancillary techniques to increase the sensitivity of detecting LVIs will provide misleading information.

T4 Status vs Circumferential (Radial) Margin: Different Segment

Despite the seemingly straightforward descriptions regarding what constitutes serosal involvement (pT4) (Figure 30-17) or circumferential margin (Figure 30-18), accurate assessment may sometimes be difficult. Definitive distinction very much relies on good "grossing" technique. The circumferential or radial margin may be one of the most challenging parameters to evaluate.

FIGURE 30-16. Lymphatic invasion. A submucosal lymphatic containing tumor cell clusters with matching contour is seen next to an arterial vessel.

FIGURE 30-18. Positive circumferential margin of rectal adenocarcinoma.

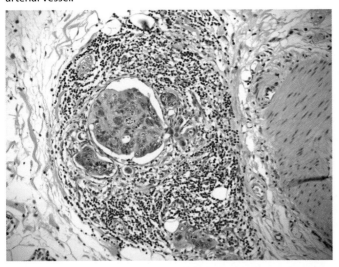

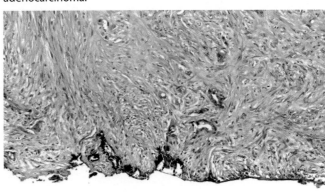

PART SIX

TABLE 30-4. T4 status vs circumferential margin.

Segment	Peritoneal lining	T4a	Circumferential margin
Cecum	Complete	Maybe	No
Ascending	Partial	Maybe	Posterior
Transverse	Complete	Maybe	No
Descending	Partial	Maybe	Posterior
Sigmoid	Complete	Maybe	No
Upper rectum	Partial	Maybe	Lateral and posterior
Lower rectum	No	No	All around

Due to the difference in peritoneal (serosal) covering in different segments of the colon (Table 30-4), correct identification of tumor location is the first important step. The segment involved by tumor should be carefully inspected on fresh specimen to identify peritoneum (serosa) covering. Areas not covered by peritoneum or epiploica fat are where the bowel was separated from retroperitoneal tissue and represent the circumferential (radial) margin. In an ideal situation, direct involvement by the surgeon may greatly facilitate the correct identification. Other than the radial margin, tumor extending to the surface of the bowel is interpreted as an invasion of the serosa and thus is staged as pT4a (Figures 30-17 and 30-19). Mesothelial cover is often disrupted or lost during processing; therefore, identifying the mesothelium itself in the sections is not required. Clear identification regarding what the tissue section represents is necessary, which often relies on an accurate gross description (Figure 30-19).

In a segment completely invested by peritoneum (appendix, cecum, transverse colon, eg), there is a mesenteric margin, which should be clearly identified and assessed.

Parameters such as intactness of the mesorectum, completeness of resection (R0, complete resection; R1, residual tumor [positive margin] microscopically; R2, positive margin macroscopically), and lymph node status are not further discussed in this chapter.

■ REFERENCES

1. Ouban A, Nawab RA, Coppola D. Diagnostic and pathogenetic implications of colorectal carcinomas with multidirectional differentiation: a report of 4 cases. *Clin Colorectal Cancer.* 2002;1(4):243–248. PMID: 12450423.
2. Messerini L, Palomba A, Zampi G. Primary signet-ring cell carcinoma of the colon and rectum. *Dis Colon Rectum.* 1995;38(11):1189–1192. PMID: 7587762.
3. Shirouzu K, Isomoto H, Morodomi T, Ogata Y, Akagi Y, Kakegawa T. Primary linitis plastica carcinoma of the colon and rectum. *Cancer.* 1994;74(7):1863–1868. PMID: 8082091.
4. Nissan A, Guillem JG, Paty PB, Wong WD, Cohen AM. Signet-ring cell carcinoma of the colon and rectum: a matched control study. *Dis Colon Rectum.* 1999;42(9):1176–1180. PMID: 10496558.
5. Thota R, Fang X, Subbiah S. Clinicopathological features and survival outcomes of primary signet ring cell and mucinous adenocarcinoma of colon: retrospective analysis of VACCR database. *J Gastrointest Oncol.* 2014;5(1):18–24. PMID: 24490039. PMCID: 3904029.
6. Goldstein NS, Long A, Kuan SF, Hart J. Colon signet ring cell adenocarcinoma: immunohistochemical characterization and comparison with gastric and typical colon adenocarcinomas. *Appl Immunohistochem Mol Norphol.* 2000;8(3):183–188. PMID: 10981869.
7. Jessurun J, Romero-Guadarrama M, Manivel JC. Medullary adenocarcinoma of the colon: clinicopathologic study of 11 cases. *Hum Pathol.* 1999;30(7):843–848. PMID: 10414504.
8. Delaney D, Chetty R. Lymphoepithelioma-like carcinoma of the colon. *Int J Clin Exp Pathol.* 2012;5(1):105–109. PMID: 22295155. PMCID: 3267494
9. Alexander J, Watanabe T, Wu TT, Rashid A, Li S, Hamilton SR. Histopathological identification of colon cancer with microsatellite instability. *Am J Pathol.* 2001;158(2):527–535. PMID: 11159189. PMCID: 1850324.

FIGURE 30-19. T4a status of a tumor in the upper rectum. **A.** The upper anterior aspect of the specimen is covered by peritoneum and epiploica fat (inked), with tumor in the subserosal zone (arrowhead). **B.** Microscopically, the tumor cells extend to the surface. This could be mistakenly interpreted as positive circumferential margin due to lack of mesothelial lining in the section if it were not clearly labeled during gross examination.

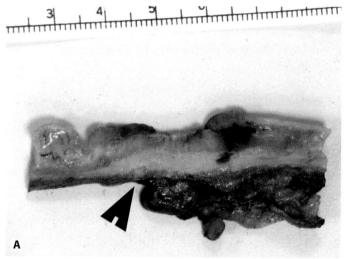

A

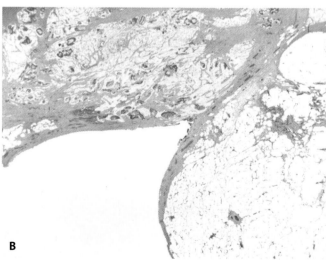

B

10. Wick MR, Vitsky JL, Ritter JH, Swanson PE, Mills SE. Sporadic medullary carcinoma of the colon: a clinicopathologic comparison with nonhereditary poorly differentiated enteric-type adenocarcinoma and neuroendocrine colorectal carcinoma. *Am J Clin Pathol.* 2005;123(1):56–65. PMID: 15762280.

11. Winn B, Tavares R, Fanion J, et al. Differentiating the undifferentiated: immunohistochemical profile of medullary carcinoma of the colon with an emphasis on intestinal differentiation. *Hum Pathol.* 2009;40(3):398–404. PMID: 18992917. PMCID: 2657293.

12. Crissman JD. Adenosquamous and squamous cell carcinoma of the colon. *Am J Surg Pathol.* 1978;2(1):47–54. PMID: 637188.

13. Petrelli NJ, Valle AA, Weber TK, Rodriguez-Bigas M. Adenosquamous carcinoma of the colon and rectum. *Dis Colon Rectum.* 1996;39(11):1265–1268. PMID: 8918436.

14. Cagir B, Nagy MW, Topham A, Rakinic J, Fry RD. Adenosquamous carcinoma of the colon, rectum, and anus: epidemiology, distribution, and survival characteristics. *Dis Colon Rectum.* 1999;42(2):258–263. PMID:10211505.

15. Frizelle FA, Hobday KS, Batts KP, Nelson H. Adenosquamous and squamous carcinoma of the colon and upper rectum: a clinical and histopathologic study. *Dis Colon Rectum.* 2001;44(3):341–346. PMID: 11289278.

16. Masoomi H, Ziogas A, Lin BS, et al. Population-based evaluation of adenosquamous carcinoma of the colon and rectum. *Dis Colon Rectum.* 2012;55(5):509–514. PMID: 22513428. PMCID: 3330249.

17. Chevinsky AH, Berelowitz M, Hoover HC Jr. Adenosquamous carcinoma of the colon presenting with hypercalcemia. *Cancer.* 1987;60(5):1111–1116. PMID: 3300949.

18. Berkelhammer CH, Baker AL, Block GE, Bostwick DG, Michelassi F. Humoral hypercalcemia complicating adenosquamous carcinoma of the proximal colon. *Dig Dis Sci.* 1989;34(1):142–147. PMID: 2910674.

19. Moll UM, Ilardi CF, Zuna R, Phillips ME. A biologically active parathyroid hormone-like substance secreted by an adenosquamous carcinoma of the transverse colon. *Hum Pathol.* 1987;18(12):1287–1290. PMID: 3679201.

20. Juturi JV, Francis B, Koontz PW, Wilkes JD. Squamous-cell carcinoma of the colon responsive to combination chemotherapy: report of two cases and review of the literature. *Dis Colon Rectum.* 1999;42(1):102–109. PMID: 10211528.

21. Audeau A, Han HW, Johnston MJ, Whitehead MW, Frizelle FA. Does human papilloma virus have a role in squamous cell carcinoma of the colon and upper rectum? *Eur J Surg Oncol.* 2002;28(6):657–660. PMID: 12359204.

22. Edge SB BD, Compton CC, et al, eds. *AJCC Cancer Staging Manual.* 7th ed. New York, NY: Springer; 2010.

23. Vanacker L, Smeets D, Hoorens A, et al. Mixed adenoneuroendocrine carcinoma of the colon: molecular pathogenesis and treatment. *Anticancer Res.* 2014;34(10):5517–5521. PMID: 25275049.

24. Bernick PE, Klimstra DS, Shia J, et al. Neuroendocrine carcinomas of the colon and rectum. *Dis Colon Rectum.* 2004;47(2):163–169. PMID:15043285.

25. Gaffey MJ, Mills SE, Lack EE. Neuroendocrine carcinoma of the colon and rectum. A clinicopathologic, ultrastructural, and immunohistochemical study of 24 cases. *Am J Surg Pathol.* 1990;14(11):1010–1023. PMID: 2173427.

26. Wick MR, Weatherby RP, Weiland LH. Small cell neuroendocrine carcinoma of the colon and rectum: clinical, histologic, and ultrastructural study and immunohistochemical comparison with cloacogenic carcinoma. *Hum Pathol.* 1987;18(1):9–21. PMID: 2434408.

27. Saclarides TJ, Szeluga D, Staren ED. Neuroendocrine cancers of the colon and rectum. Results of a ten-year experience. *Dis Colon Rectum.* 1994;37(7):635–642. PMID: 8026228.

28. Akintola-Ogunremi O, Pfeifer JD, Tan BR, et al. Analysis of protein expression and gene mutation of c-kit in colorectal neuroendocrine carcinomas. *Am J Surg Pathol.* 2003;27(12):1551–1558. PMID: 14657715.

PART SIX

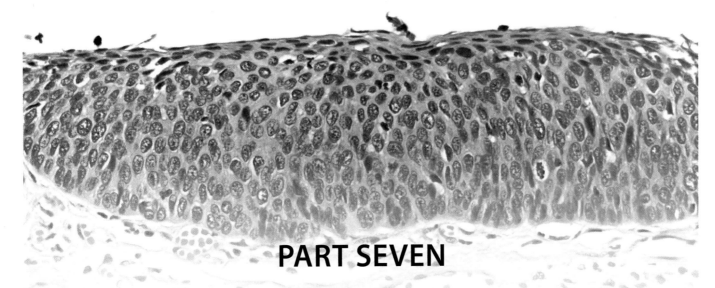

PART SEVEN

ANUS

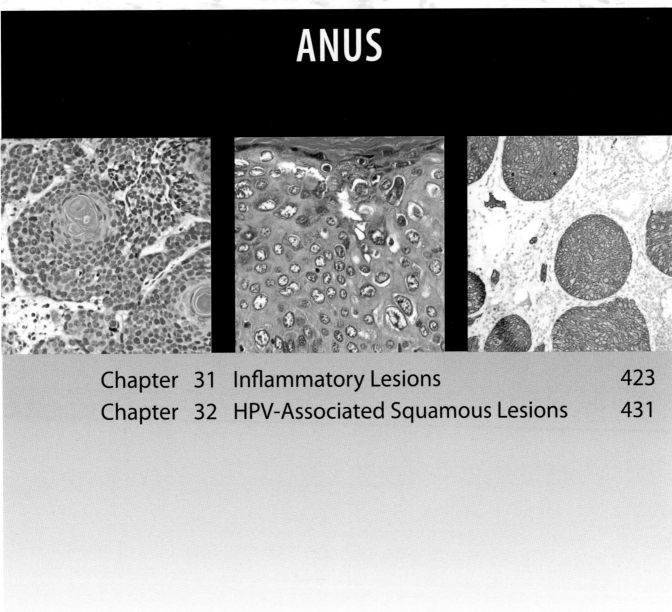

421

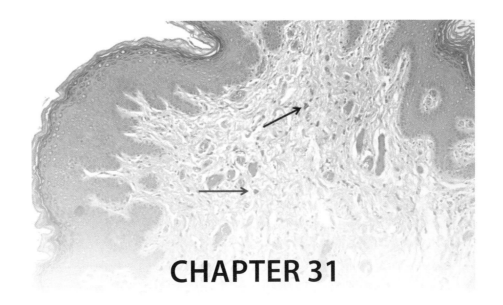

CHAPTER 31

Inflammatory Lesions

Shriram Jakate

INTRODUCTION

Anal inflammatory lesions are varied and reflect the distinct anatomical and physiological diversity of this relatively restricted part of the lowermost gastrointestinal tract. Anatomically, the anal region is a short sequential tract starting at the distal rectal mucosa and progressing caudally to cloacogenic anal transition zone mucosa and nonkeratinizing squamous anal canal mucosa (beginning at the dentate line) and extending through the anal orifice (or verge) into keratinizing, hair-bearing anal and perianal skin. Within the walls of the anal region are the internal and external sphincter muscles, anal mucinous as well as specialized perianal apocrine glands with their ducts and submucosal cushions with rich vasculature. Some inflammatory lesions are peculiar to these precise anatomical locations, such as inflammatory cloacogenic polyps occurring at the anal transition zone, hydradenitis suppurativa originating in the perianal apocrine glands, and hemorrhoids arising from the anal submucosal vascular cushions. In addition to these anatomical correlates, physiological factors play an equally crucial role in anal inflammatory lesions. Fecal matter passing through the anus may be hard or forceful and potentially traumatic, resulting in an anal fissure. Fecal incontinence creates a perpetual source of sepsis (and hindrance for healing) for perianal abscess, fistulas, and pilonidal disease. In addition, anal sexual activity may result in anal and perianal sexually transmitted diseases. In Crohn disease, anal involvement may be a marker for a specific phenotype and create significant medical and surgical therapeutic challenges.

HEMORRHOIDS

Hemorrhoids are the most common anal disease, affecting 4.4% of the US population.[1] Hemorrhoids may be defined as symptomatic vascular distention and abnormal downward displacement of the anal vascular and mucosal cushions. Physiologically, there are 3 primary anal cushions (right anterior, right posterior, and left lateral) that, along with the anal sphincter muscles, help to prevent incontinence. Age-related degenerative changes in the supportive connective tissue of the anal cushions may be just as crucial as vascular hyperplasia and distention in the development of hemorrhoids.[2,3] Risk factors for hemorrhoids include aging, constipation with prolonged straining, pregnancy, and chronic diarrhea. It is important to distinguish hemorrhoids as a distinctly separate entity from the anorectal varices that may occur in portal hypertension. The variceal vascular distention due to portal hypertension generally occurs in the lower rectum and upper anal canal above the dentate line. Vascular compressibility similar to esophageal varices may be observed, and there generally is no prolapse. Hemorrhoids, on the other hand, are unrelated to portal hypertension, often prolapse below the dentate line, and show no vascular compressibility.[4]

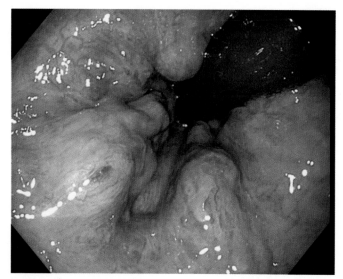

FIGURE 31-1. Internal hemorrhoids visualized endoscopically (retroflexion) showing distended subepithelial vessels and maintaining the lobulations of anal cushions.

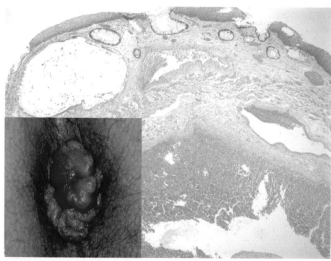

FIGURE 31-2. Microscopic low-magnification view of hemorrhoids showing markedly dilated, focally thick-wall vessels and a covering of anorectal junction mucosa (internal hemorrhoid). Inset shows grade IV prolapse, also maintaining the lobulations of anal cushions.

Hemorrhoids are classified as internal or external depending on whether they originate above or below the dentate line. Internal hemorrhoids are further subclassified as grades I through IV depending on the degree and reducibility of their prolapse (grade I, nonprolapsing; grade II, prolapsing but spontaneously reducing; grade III, prolapsing, requiring manual reduction; grade IV, prolapsing, nonreducible). Grade IV internal hemorrhoids may also present with thrombosis and incarceration. Extensive hemorrhoidal disease may involve both internal and external hemorrhoids. Most hemorrhoids retain the lobulations of the anal cushions: right anterior, right posterior, and left lateral (Figure 31-1). While bleeding with bowel movements is the principal symptom of hemorrhoids, spontaneous bleeding, pain, discomfort, and itching may occur depending on complications, such as inflammation, ulceration, thrombosis, strangulation, and infarction.

Hemorrhoidectomy specimens for pathological examination are only received when hemorrhoids are treated by surgical excision (typically grades III or IV of internal hemorrhoids, or internal or external hemorrhoids complicated by thrombosis). Lower grades of internal hemorrhoids are generally treated conservatively with bowel management and nonresective office procedures such as rubber-band ligation, infrared coagulation, or sclerotherapy.[5] On gross examination, the covering surface (tan-color rectal, smooth and glistening white nonkeratinizing anal squamous or anal skin) and any ulceration need to be described.

Sampling for microscopy should include sufficient representation of the covering mucosal surface and any thrombosis or necrosis visible on the cut surface. Microscopically, typical hemorrhoids show dilated, variably proliferated, and congested submucosal anal cushion vessels with variable intervening hemorrhage, inflammation, and fibrosis

(Figure 31-2). Thrombosis, ulceration, and infarction may or may not be present. Detailed documentation of all pathological findings provides correlation with the clinical grade, presentation, and complications of hemorrhoids.

It is critically important not to overlook incidental clinically unanticipated lesions in the overlying squamous or transitional zone mucosa, such as dysplasia or carcinoma in situ. Occasionally, hemorrhoidectomy is performed with the clinical misdiagnosis of hemorrhoids. The lesion may instead turn out to be melanoma or carcinoid or basal cell carcinoma. Their dark, firm appearance may be mistaken for thrombosed hemorrhoids.

ANAL FISSURE

An anal fissure is a linear tear in the squamous epithelial lining of the anal canal starting proximally at or just below the dentate line and extending distally to the anal verge skin (anoderm). An anal fissure typically causes severe pain during defecation. The most common location of an anal fissure is along the midline (posterior midline in about 90% of cases and anterior midline in about 10% of cases).[6,7] Anterior midline fissures are more likely to occur in females and younger patients. The pathogenesis of an anal fissure is multifactorial, including anal trauma from hardened fecal material in constipation, hypertonia of the internal anal sphincter muscle, and hypoperfusion of the anal canal. Constipation and hard stools account for over 90% of cases, while hypertonia of the internal anal sphincter muscle is the cause in most others.

Most fissures heal with simple methods of bowel management, including high-fiber diet, fiber supplements, fluids, stool softeners, and warm baths. Management options for patients with hypertonicity are targeted toward reducing anal tone (ie, glyceryl trinitrate ointment, calcium channel

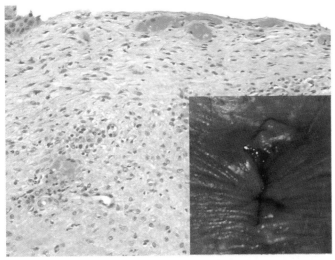

FIGURE 31-3. High-magnification microphotograph of chronic anal fissure showing nonspecific changes of fibrosis and inflammatory granulation tissue. Inset shows midline chronic anal fissure with prominent sentinel anal tag at the outer apex.

blocker cream, botulinum toxin, sphincterotomy, and rarely, fissurectomy). When an anal fissure is atypical, such as off the midline, painless, irregular, or multiple, perianal Crohn disease (PCD) should be a consideration (particularly when associated with an abscess or fistula).

Anal fissures are classified as acute (lasting 4–6 weeks or less) or chronic (>6 weeks). Chronic anal fissures often have the additional findings of a nodule at each end: hypertrophied anal papilla arising from the dentate line at the internal apex and a sentinel skin tag below the lower end at the anal verge (Figure 31-3 inset).[8] Although most chronic anal fissures are due to persistence or recurrence of an acute anal fissure, occasionally they may be associated with HIV infection, Crohn disease, syphilis, tuberculosis, or underlying malignancy.

Tissue specimens for pathological examination are not procured for acute anal fissures because the clinical picture is characteristic, and most heal without surgery. Chronic anal fissures may be biopsied or excised to histologically assess for infections, Crohn disease, or malignancy. Apart from ulceration, inflammatory granulation tissue, and fibrosis (Figure 31-3), the microscopic changes will vary depending on the etiology.

ANAL ABSCESS AND FISTULA

Anal abscess and fistula are best regarded as two phases of the same inflammatory process. Most anal abscesses begin as an infection and suppurative inflammation of the anal glands deep in the anal canal wall. With progression, the purulent process tracks along the paths of least resistance, either along the duct and draining internally within the anal canal (at the dentate line) or along the various perianal tissue planes to exit externally through the perianal skin. Such progression of

an abscess to a fistula occurs in at least one-third of all cases.[9] Thus, an abscess may be considered an early phase and a fistula as a late phase of the same disorder. Anal abscesses may develop in various locations within the perianal and perirectal tissues, depending on the location of the involved anal gland and the direction that the infection dissects out.

Abscesses are anatomically classified as superficial or perianal, submucosal if they progress up along the rectal wall plain, intersphincteric between the internal and external sphincter muscle layers, ischiorectal when outside the sphincters but below the levator muscles, and high or supralevator when above the pelvic floor muscles.[10] Only one draining site may be present, which is more accurately described as a sinus. However, often two draining sites develop, one internally, usually at the dentate line at the site of the original duct opening, and the other externally through the skin, creating a classical "fistula-in-ano." Complex and high fistulas are harder to treat surgically because the tracts traverse the sphincter complex. The higher the tract, the more risk of incontinence there is with a surgical fistulotomy. Other current approaches to a fistula include a two-stage fistulotomy using a seton as a drain between stages, advancement flap repair, collagen plug repair, or the LIFT (ligation of the internal fistula tract) procedure.

The most common cause of anal abscess is believed to be infection of anal glands due to overgrowth of bacteria when the draining anal ducts become obstructed—the cryptoglandular theory. Histologically, an anal abscess shows generic abscess-related suppurative inflammation of the gland and cavity wall. Fistula tracts show linear strips of acute and chronic inflammation with granulation tissue. Residual duct structures with epithelial proliferative changes in the duct lining epithelium and squamous metaplasia may also be seen. Supralevator abscesses may also result from pelvic sepsis sources, such as pelvic inflammatory disease, appendicitis, or diverticulitis. A subset of patients with Crohn disease will develop perianal problems, including complex anal abscesses and fistulas, ulcers, and swollen skin tags. This is discussed under PCD.

Suppurative inflammation of specialized perianal apocrine glands leads to the specific condition of hidradenitis suppurativa.[11] Hidradenitis suppurativa, a chronic recurring and occasionally debilitating disorder, may affect axillary, inguinal, labial, perineal, and perianal apocrine glands. Multiple subcutaneous perianal abscesses occur with arborizing sinus tracts, malodorous discharge, and prominent scarring (Figure 31-4). The perineal process spares the anal canal because it is devoid of apocrine glands. The pathogenesis of hidradenitis involves keratinous occlusion of apocrine gland ducts and resultant inflammation of glands. This typically occurs only after puberty, and as such, hormonal secondary sexual development likely has a role. The underlying cause is unknown. Another specific perianal abscess-forming condition is pilonidal disease; hair follicles in the natal cleft become infected and produce characteristic midline pits.[12] Exfoliated hair shafts may enter these pits, inciting foreign

PART SEVEN

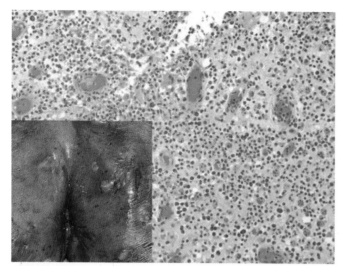

FIGURE 31-4. Numerous acute and chronic inflammatory cells are seen in this high-magnification microphotograph of a hidradenitis suppurativa abscess, representing destroyed anal apocrine glands. Inset shows prominent scarring and multiple discharging sinuses.

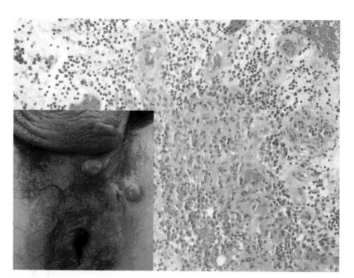

FIGURE 31-6. Microphotograph of perianal Crohn disease in high magnification showing patchy chronic inflammation and lymphohistiocytic clusters. Inset shows multiple manifestations, including large anal skin tags, irregular scarring representing a healed atypical fissure, and multiple fistulous openings, including one in the scrotum.

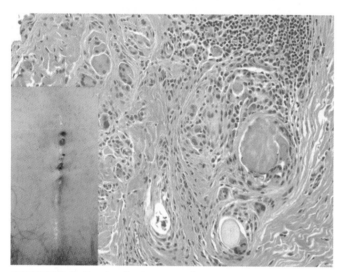

FIGURE 31-5. Foreign-body giant-cell reaction to hair shaft material is seen in pilonidal disease (high-magnification microphotograph). Inset shows characteristic midline pits in the natal cleft where exfoliated hair shafts are trapped, causing recurrent inflammation.

body reaction and infection. Hirsute young adult men are most prone to this disorder, although young women are also at risk. Associated conditions include obesity and sedentary occupations. Histologically, pilonidal disease shows abscesses with hair debris and sinus tracts lined by granulation tissue (Figure 31-5).

■ PERIANAL CROHN DISEASE

Perianal disease in the setting of inflammatory bowel disease (IBD) is strongly linked to Crohn disease and likely represents a Crohn phenotype prone to fistulization.[13,14]

Occasional occurrence of perianal disease in ulcerative colitis is incidental and in the form of conventional anal fissure or abscess. The association of complex perianal disease and Crohn disease is so specific that in patients whose colitis cannot be definitely determined to be ulcerative colitis or Crohn disease ("indeterminate IBD colitis"), the presence of perianal disease is equivalent to a definitive diagnosis of Crohn disease.[15] The spectrum of PCD includes multiple manifestations, including swollen, bluish anal tags, anal ulcers, and deep fissures, abscesses, fistulas, and anal strictures or stenosis (Figure 31-6 inset).[16] Apart from the multiplicity of manifestations, many lesions tend to be atypical or complex compared to isolated lesions in patients without Crohn disease. Anal fissures in patients with Crohn disease are often atypical (off midline, painless, irregular, multiple, and deep). Anal abscesses are deep, and fistulas arising from these are often complex. Fistulas may have multiple tracts and may develop into rectovaginal or rectovesical fistulas. In the literature, the reported frequency of PCD in Crohn disease varies greatly (13%–62%) due to lack of standardized data and definitions. However, it is estimated that overall 25% of patients with Crohn disease display some perianal disease, and about 15% of patients with Crohn disease have severe manifestations, including abscesses and fistulas.[16] Clinical features may include anal pain, swelling, masses, large skin tags, itching, bleeding, purulent discharge, and incontinence. Yet, in some patients, despite severe perianal disease, symptoms may be absent. PCD is associated with younger age at diagnosis and ileal or rectal involvement. There may be a genetic link with NCF4 (neutrophil cytosolic factor 4).[17] In the majority of cases, bowel involvement precedes PCD; however, about 5% of patients with an ultimate diagnosis of Crohn disease present with an anal manifestation first.[18] Histological changes in tissue from PCD are nonspecific and similar to individual disorders such as fissure, abscess, tag, fistula, and stricture.

The diagnosis of PCD is best made by correlating the clinically atypical and complex perianal findings with Crohn disease elsewhere in the gastrointestinal tract. Occasionally, persuasive features of Crohn disease, such as a patchy peri-lymphoid inflammatory pattern, lymphohistiocytic clusters (Figure 31-6), and granulomas, may be present in perianal tissues. In patients with seemingly isolated PCD, it is crucial to determine if there is intestinal involvement (which may be clinically cryptic). Other diagnoses, such as Behçet disease or hidradenitis suppurativa, may be considered if there is no intestinal Crohn disease. Clinically, PCD presents additional challenges to the management of Crohn disease, which may include early use of immune-suppressive medical or modulating therapy and surgical management. There is also a long-term risk of perianal dysplasia and carcinoma.

ANAL NONNEOPLASTIC POLYPS

Polypoid inflammatory and reactive anal projections are assigned specific names depending on their precise level of origin within the anal region and their covering epithelium. At the highest level above the dentate line, mucosal prolapse with a covering of anal transition zone or anorectal junction mucosa is an *inflammatory cloacogenic polyp*. A little lower, at the dentate line and often atop an anal fissure, a reactive projection is an *anal papilla* lined by nonkeratinizing squamous epithelium. Lowest, outside the anal verge and covered with keratinizing squamous epithelium or skin, is the *anal skin tag* or fibroepithelial polyp. The anal tag is identical to any other skin tag elsewhere on the body. When the same anal skin tag develops at the caudal end of an anal fissure, it is given the name *sentinel tag*. The pathogenesis of each of these polyps is similar: reactive inflammatory proliferation of epithelial and subepithelial mesenchymal structures in response to injury, irritation, or infection. Small anal inflammatory polyps are usually asymptomatic and common in the population. However, when these polyps enlarge, prolapse, or erode, they may become symptomatic, causing bleeding, pruritus, foreign body sensation, a feeling of a mass within the anus, discharge, and a sense of incomplete evacuation. While the pathogenesis is similar, these polyps have distinct clinical and morphological differences.

An inflammatory cloacogenic polyp is within the spectrum of *mucosal prolapse syndrome*, analogous to solitary rectal ulcer syndrome.[19] Endoscopically, it is at the anorectal junction and best detected through deliberate anorectal examination by retroflexion (Figure 31-7). It may be clinically mistaken for adenomatous polyp or prolapsed hemorrhoid. Histologically, it shows hyperplastic and nondysplastic anorectal junction or anal transition zone mucosa at the surface and common features of mucosal prolapse, such as thin vertical strands of smooth muscle between elongated crypts, vascular ectasia, and thickened muscularis mucosa (Figure 31-8). Often, there is an increase in mixed

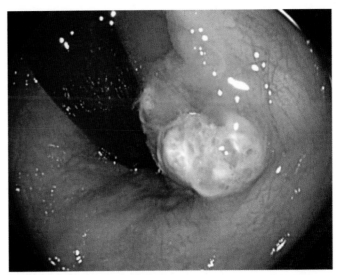

FIGURE 31-7. Endoscopically detected polyp at the anorectal junction (on retroflexion), which histologically showed an inflammatory cloacogenic polyp.

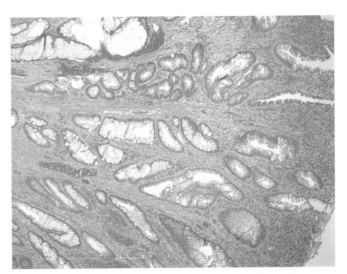

FIGURE 31-8. Medium-level magnification microphotograph of inflammatory cloacogenic polyp showing surface erosion (right edge) with granulation tissue and mixed inflammatory cells. Features of prolapse include thin muscle bands between elongated crypts and dilated vessels.

inflammatory cells in the lamina propria (hence the term *inflammatory*). An anal papilla is a small projection located within the anal canal at the dentate line. It has a covering of nonkeratinizing and nondysplastic anal squamous mucosa with variable hyperplasia (Figure 31-9). The underlying stroma may show variable fibrosis, vascularity, and inflammation. Occasionally, the papilla may enlarge and even prolapse and protrude out through the anus (Figure 31-9 inset). Clinically, it may be mistaken for a prolapsed hemorrhoid or neoplastic polyp. An anal fibroepithelial polyp or anal verge skin tag shows all the usual features of a typical skin tag, such as growth of subepithelial loose edematous fibroconnective

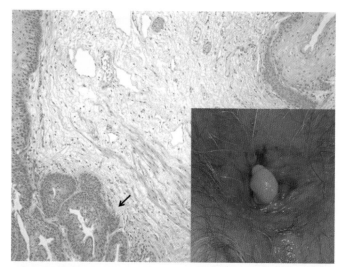

FIGURE 31-9. Low-magnification microphotograph of anal papilla showing a covering of nonkeratinizing squamous epithelium of the anal canal, including focal anal transition zone mucosa (arrow). Inset shows prolapsed anal papilla visible through the anal verge.

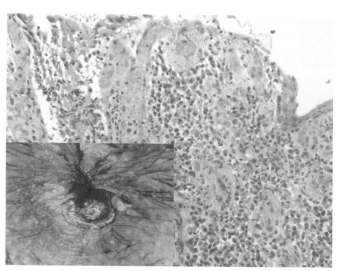

FIGURE 31-11. Histologically nonspecific findings in syphilis that include granulation tissue and abundant plasma cells (high magnification). Inset shows circular ulcer or chancre of primary syphilis.

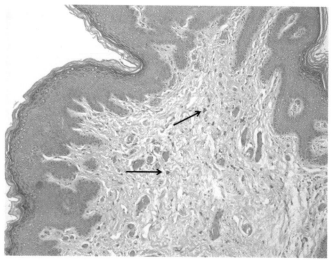

FIGURE 31-10. Microphotograph of low magnification of anal skin tag or fibroepithelial polyp with a covering of keratinized squamous epithelium and scattered subepithelial multinucleated stromal cells (arrows).

tissue, scattered stellate or multinucleated atypical stromal cells (but without mitotic activity), and a covering of keratinized nondysplastic squamous epithelium (Figure 31-10).

ANAL INFECTIOUS DISEASES

The vast majority of anal infectious diseases are sexually transmitted. The most common among these is caused by human papilloma virus (HPV; condyloma acuminatum). This is discussed separately. A few selected common infections are discussed here.

The anus can be a site of inoculation of the *Treponema pallidum* spirochete, causing the classical chancre of primary syphilis within 3–6 weeks after inoculation. This is a dark papule rapidly converting into a circular shallow ulcer (Figure 31-11) with indurated base and edges. This is soon followed by bilateral inguinal lymphadenopathy and disappearance of the chancre. Only 30%–40% of cases are diagnosed clinically at this primary stage of syphilis because a serological response is not yet established.[20] Therefore, the diagnosis is dependent on clinicopathological awareness and identification of the pathogen. The spirochetes may be found in the secretion fluid over the chancre. Immediate dark-field microscopy and detection of characteristic movement by an experienced microbiologist will identify the pathogen.[20] The histological features of the chancre are nonspecific, with ulceration, necrotic exudate, and dense inflammatory granulation tissue rich in plasma cells (Figure 31-11). Organisms are not visualized on routine hematoxylin and eosin (H&E) stain, and unless clinicopathologically suspected, the diagnosis of syphilis is usually not entertained. Silver stains (such as Warthin-Starry and Steiner) may highlight the organisms, but heavy staining of tissues in the background may hinder detection. Immunohistochemical staining for *T. pallidum* successfully demonstrates the organisms in the majority of cases.[21]

Anal ulceration may also be caused by genital herpes or herpes simplex virus (HSV) infection (more often HSV-2 than HSV-1), which presents as a cluster of painful vesicles that break and coalesce into a superficial ulcer (Figure 31-12 inset). Initial infection is associated with systemic symptoms, such as fever and lymphadenopathy. The virus, which is transported to the sensory nerve roots, may be repeatedly reactivated in patients with decreased immunity. The virus may be identified in culture studies of the blister fluid

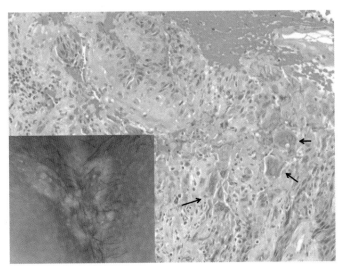

FIGURE 31-12. Inset shows characteristic cluster of merging ruptured vesicles in perianal herpes simplex virus infection. Microscopically, multinucleated squamous cells with pale, molded nuclei and peripherally pushed chromatin are characteristic (arrows).

and by serological testing. However, histological features are characteristic in making the diagnosis. The edges of the ulcer show typical HSV intranuclear viral inclusions. These consist of large squamous cells with multiple, often pale, molded nuclei that have native chromatin pushed peripherally (Figure 31-12). Immunostains for HSV are confirmatory.

■ REFERENCES

1. Johanson JF, Sonnenberg A. The prevalence of hemorrhoids and chronic constipation. An epidemiologic study. *Gastroenterology.* 1990;98(2):380–386.
2. Lohsiriwat V. Hemorrhoids: from basic pathophysiology to clinical management. *World J Gastroenterol.* 2012;18(17):2009–2017.
3. Lohsiriwat V. Approach to hemorrhoids. *Curr Gastroenterol Rep.* 2013;15(7):332-013-0332-6.
4. Maslekar S, Toh EW, Adair R, Bate JP, Botterill I. Systematic review of anorectal varices. *Colorectal Dis.* 2013;15(12):e702–e710.
5. Sanchez C, Chinn BT. Hemorrhoids. *Clin Colon Rectal Surg.* 2011;24(1):5–13.
6. Zaghiyan KN, Fleshner P. Anal fissure. *Clin Colon Rectal Surg.* 2011;24(1):22–30.
7. Herzig DO, Lu KC. Anal fissure. *Surg Clin North Am.* 2010;90(1): 33–44, Table of Contents.
8. Madoff RD, Fleshman JW. AGA technical review on the diagnosis and care of patients with anal fissure. *Gastroenterology.* 2003;124(1):235–245.
9. Rizzo JA, Naig AL, Johnson EK. Anorectal abscess and fistula-in-ano: evidence-based management. *Surg Clin North Am.* 2010;90(1):45–68, Table of Contents.
10. Abcarian H. Anorectal infection: abscess-fistula. *Clin Colon Rectal Surg.* 2011;24(1):14–21.
11. Mitchell KM, Beck DE. Hidradenitis suppurativa. *Surg Clin North Am.* 2002;82(6):1187–1197.
12. Velasco AL, Dunlap WW. Pilonidal disease and hidradenitis. *Surg Clin North Am.* 2009;89(3):689–701.
13. Tarrant KM, Barclay ML, Frampton CM, Gearry RB. Perianal disease predicts changes in Crohn's disease phenotype-results of a population-based study of inflammatory bowel disease phenotype. *Am J Gastroenterol.* 2008;103(12):3082–3093.
14. Sachar DB, Bodian CA, Goldstein ES, et al. Is perianal Crohn's disease associated with intestinal fistulization? *Am J Gastroenterol.* 2005;100(7):1547–1549.
15. North American Society for Pediatric Gastroenterology, Hepatology, and Nutrition, Colitis Foundation of America, Bousvaros A, et al. Differentiating ulcerative colitis from Crohn disease in children and young adults: report of a working group of the North American Society for Pediatric Gastroenterology, Hepatology, and Nutrition and the Crohn's and Colitis Foundation of America. *J Pediatr Gastroenterol Nutr.* 2007;44(5):653–674.
16. de Zoeten EF, Pasternak BA, Mattei P, Kramer RE, Kader HA. Diagnosis and treatment of perianal Crohn disease: NASPGHAN clinical report and consensus statement. *J Pediatr Gastroenterol Nutr.* 2013;57(3):401–412.
17. Eglinton TW, Roberts R, Pearson J, et al. Clinical and genetic risk factors for perianal Crohn's disease in a population-based cohort. *Am J Gastroenterol.* 2012;107(4):589–596.
18. Lewis RT, Maron DJ. Anorectal Crohn's disease. *Surg Clin North Am.* 2010;90(1):83–97, Table of Contents.
19. Abid S, Khawaja A, Bhimani SA, Ahmad Z, Hamid S, Jafri W. The clinical, endoscopic and histological spectrum of the solitary rectal ulcer syndrome: a single-center experience of 116 cases. *BMC Gastroenterol.* 2012;12:72230X-12-72.
20. Lautenschlager S. Diagnosis of syphilis: clinical and laboratory problems. *J Dtsch Dermatol Ges.* 2006;4(12):1058–1075.
21. Martin-Ezquerra G, Fernandez-Casado A, Barco D, et al. *Treponema pallidum* distribution patterns in mucocutaneous lesions of primary and secondary syphilis: an immunohistochemical and ultrastructural study. *Hum Pathol.* 2009;40(5):624–630.

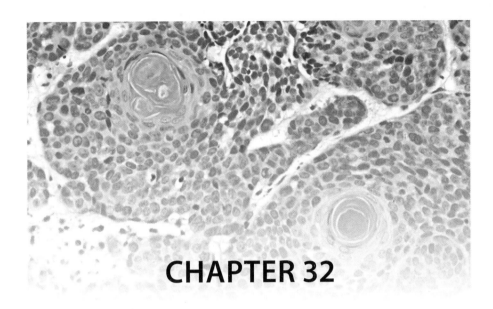

CHAPTER 32

HPV-Associated Squamous Lesions

Jingmei Lin

■ INTRODUCTION

Squamous cell carcinoma (SCC) comprises more than 70% of anal malignancies.[1,2] Epidemiologic studies have established an association between SCC and its precursor lesions with human papilloma virus (HPV) infection, especially genotypes 16, 18, 31, and 33.[3–13] In this chapter, the discussion is focused on HPV-associated squamous lesions.[14,15] Until recently, the nomenclature for anal squamous lesions had been rather confusing, demanding standardized diagnostic criteria and terminology for pathological reporting. Therefore, the recently proposed terminology, including condyloma, anal intraepithelial neoplasia (AIN), and SCC are explained, along with the histological criteria and prognostic and therapeutic implications.

■ CONDYLOMA ACUMINATUM

Condyloma acuminatum, also known as anal wart, is a common HPV-associated benign squamous lesion.

Pathologic Features

Condyloma acuminatum presents as single or multiple polypoid, cauliflower-shape, pedunculated excrescences in the anal canal. Histologically, it is composed of acanthotic papillomatous squamous epithelia with variable degrees of hyperkeratosis and parakeratosis (Figure 32-1A). Koilocytic atypia, the key feature, is characterized by perinuclear clearing, irregular nuclear membrane, binucleation, and nuclear

atypia—similar to that of cervical intraepithelial neoplasia (Figure 32-1B). However, the absence of koilocytic change is not rare due to subsidence of HPV infection, which should not cast doubt in diagnosing condyloma.[16] Orderly progression of epithelial maturation is often preserved, with rare mitotic figures. However, dysplasia, and even microscopic foci of invasive carcinoma, can be seen in condylomata.[17,18] Therefore, careful gross and histologic examinations are critical.

Prognosis

Studies have shown that condylomata without dysplasia or with mild (low-grade) dysplasia are associated with low-risk HPV (subtypes 6 and 11). For this reason, anal condylomata are generally considered low-risk lesions with an "innocent" clinical course.[19] However, condylomata with high-grade dysplasia are associated with high-risk HPV (subtypes 16 and 18) and are likely to be associated with high-grade AIN or invasive SCC.[11,19] The variable risk associated with HPV subtypes raises the question of whether HPV should be subtyped in an anal condyloma. So far, a cost-effective approach to balance HPV subtyping and accurate prognostic prediction has not been reached.

■ ANAL INTRAEPITHELIAL NEOPLASIA

Multiple nomenclatures were previously used to describe these lesions, including squamous cell dysplasia, SCC in situ, bowenoid papulosis, and Bowen disease of the anus.

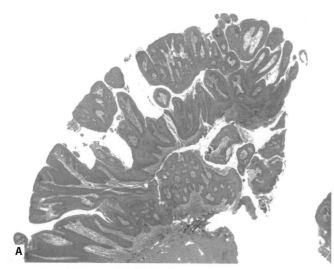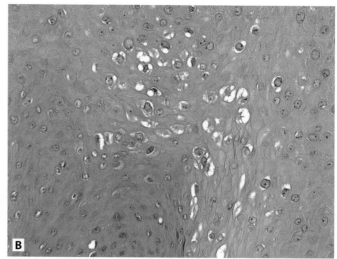

FIGURE 32-1. Anal condyloma acuminatum. **A.** Low-power view showing a papillomatous squamous proliferation with cauliflower-shape pedunculated excrescence. **B.** High-power view showing koilocytes characterized by perinuclear clearing, enlarged nuclei, and irregular nuclear membrane.

These led to much confusion for clinical management and for understanding research data. To simplify the terminology, the World Health Organization (WHO) facilitated the use of AIN, which is used in this chapter.[20]

Clinical Background

Anal intraepithelial neoplasia can occur either in the context of a condyloma acuminatum or as a flat lesion. Incidentally, AIN may be found in hemorrhoid specimens.[7,17,18] Multifocality is common.[21] AIN is usually located in the anal canal but can also be encountered in the perianal skin. HPV is commonly detected in these lesions.[22]

Individuals infected with HIV are at particularly high risk for AIN.[23,24] Other risk factors for AIN include increasing age, receptive anal intercourse, heavy smoking, history of sexually transmitted diseases, immunosuppression, fistulas in patients with Crohn disease, and the presence of lower genital tract squamous neoplasia in females.[3, 21, 25–28]

Histopathology

Histologically, AIN is analogous to that of cervical intraepithelial neoplasia (Figures 32-2A–32-2C). It is characterized by nuclear pleomorphism, enlargement, hyperchromasia, increased nuclear-to-cytoplasmic (N/C) ratio, and mitosis. Koilocytes are usually present. Depending on the severity of dysplasia, AIN is divided into three morphologic grades: AIN 1 (mild dysplasia), AIN 2 (moderate dysplasia), and AIN 3 (severe dysplasia). However, for reporting purposes, a two-tier system is used: *Low grade* is equivalent to mild dysplasia (AIN 1), and *high grade* includes moderate-to-severe dysplasia (AIN 2 and AIN 3). This two-tier system is based on the morphological features similarly graded in cervical intraepithelial neoplasia.

The AIN grade distinction is based on the proportion of the epithelial thickness occupied by dysplastic cells.

In AIN 1, dysplasia involves the lower one-third of the epithelium (Figure 32-2A). In AIN 2, the dysplasia comprises up to two-thirds of the epithelial thickness (Figure 32-2B). Dysplastic cells involve the upper one-third of the epithelium in AIN 3 (Figure 32-2C). In questionable specimens, due to either thermal artifact or unsatisfied orientation, ancillary stains for p16 (Figure 32-3) (see also Chapter 7) or Ki-67 may be of help.[29–33] More important, when it is difficult to distinguish between AIN 3 and a mimic lesion, such as immature squamous metaplasia, unusual repair, and tangential sectioning, a diffuse and band-like staining pattern for p16 will strengthen the diagnosis of dysplasia.

In daily practice, the distinction between AIN and condyloma acuminatum may not always be straightforward, especially in biopsy specimens that are small. Architecturally, condyloma acuminatum is polypoid or pedunculated; therefore, clinical impression is essential. AIN can occur in either a condyloma or a flat lesion. Dysplasia is a required feature for AIN. As mentioned, a condyloma may lack dysplasia due to the subsidence of viral infection, but an AIN by definition has at least low-grade dysplasia. An algorithm is listed in Table 32-1 as a reference for the distinction. Clinically, high-grade dysplasia on top of condyloma is not rare and should be reported either as condyloma with high-grade dysplasia or as condyloma with high-grade AIN.

Treatment

The classification to low- and high-grade AIN has therapeutic implications. In general, low-grade lesions (AIN 1 or mild dysplasia) are managed by topical agents, such as imiquimod, an immunomodulatory drug.[34–36] Other modalities include fulguration or clinical monitoring. High-grade lesions (AIN 2 and 3, moderate and severe dysplasia, respectively) require excision. Surgical excision, infrared coagulation, and photodynamic therapy have been effective in both HIV-positive

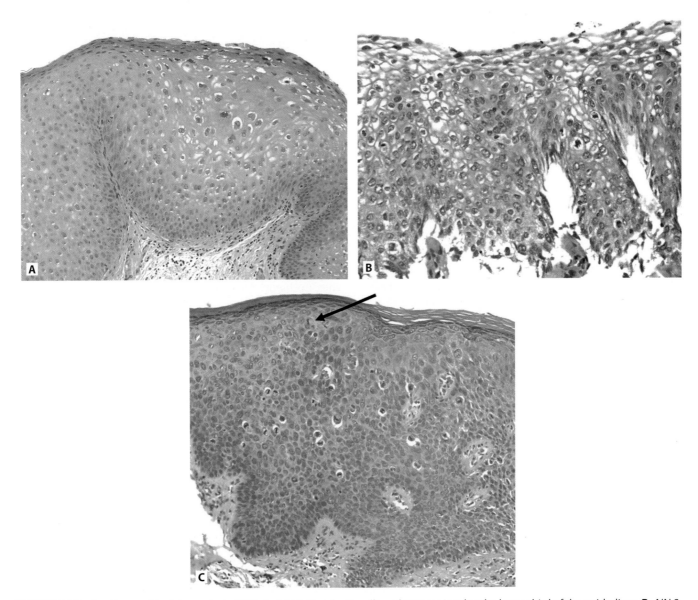

FIGURE 32-2. Anal intraepithelial neoplasia (AIN). **A.** AIN 1. Dysplastic cells and mitoses involve the lower third of the epithelium. **B.** AIN 2. **C.** AIN 3. Distinction between them is based on the proportion of the epithelial thickness occupied by dysplasia (see text). Note the mitoses (indicated by arrow) involving the full thickness of the squamous mucosa with complete loss of squamous maturation in AIN 3.

and HIV-negative patients; however, variable resistance and recurrence exist.[37–42]

Studies have shown that treatment of AIN is difficult particularly in HIV-positive patients, for whom recurrence rates are high.[37,43] It seems that HIV-negative patients respond much better to treatment than HIV-positive patients.[37] AIN 1 is likely to regress spontaneously, but high-grade AIN tends to recur or resist.[43] Currently, different centers offer variable treatment options for AIN. The choice of treatment may depend on preference and experience due to the lack of standardized therapy.[44–46] However, a unanimous consensus is to prevent progression to SCC, especially in the high-risk population, such as the HIV-positive patients with high-grade AIN.

ANAL SQUAMOUS CELL CARCINOMA

In this chapter, all squamous tumors of the anal canal are designated as SCC. Many other terms have been used previously, including cloacogenic carcinoma, verrucous carcinoma (giant condyloma of Buschke-Löwenstein), transitional carcinoma, large-cell keratinizing carcinoma, large-cell nonkeratinizing carcinoma, and basaloid carcinoma. Studies had shown a poor consensus or reproducibility in recognizing the many subtypes of SCC, even among experienced pathologists.[44] In addition, tissue sampling adds to the subjectivity in diagnosis. Last, prevalent HPV infection in all anal squamous tumors and the lack of evidence between prognosis and the histological subtypes support a single

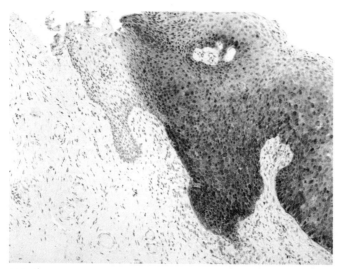

FIGURE 32-3. p16 expression in high-grade AIN. Strong band-like expression of p16 highlights the dysplastic component in high-grade AIN. Note the abrupt transition between the dysplastic and nondysplastic epithelia.

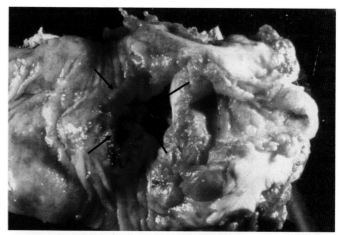

FIGURE 32-4. Gross image of anal squamous cell carcinoma. The tumor is ulcerated, with hemorrhage and necrosis involving the anus. The border is irregular and thickened. (Used with permission of Dr. Henry D. Appelman from the University of Michigan Department of Pathology.)

terminology.[23,47,48] Based on these, the WHO recommends simplifying the generic term SCC to include all squamous tumors of the anal canal.[20]

Clinical Background

Anal SCC is uncommon in the general population, with age-standardized annual incidence rates of 1–2 per 100,000.[1,2] However, the incidence rate increases by 1%–3% per year in the United States and Europe.[1,49] Most anal SCC occurs in patients in the sixth or seventh decade, with a male-to-female ratio of 0.81.[50–52]

Recent studies have identified risk factors for anal SCC to include HPV infection, immunodeficiency due to HIV infection, immunosuppression, receptive anal intercourse, and tobacco smoking.[2,53] Epidemiologic studies have indicated an association between SCC and HPV infection (especially genotypes 16, 18, 31, and 33), with genotype 16 the most prevalent.[7–11, 54–56] High-risk HPV types can be detected in 80%–90% of all anal SCCs, ranking it second only to cervical SCC in its association with HPV.[57]

Clinically, anal SCC may cause anal pruritus, discomfort in the sitting position, sensation of a pelvic mass, change in bowel movement, incontinence, bleeding, and pain. However, these symptoms are not specific. Examination reveals a lump, mass, or ulcer.

Pathologic Features

Anal SCC may invade deeply into the rectal wall or extend into perianal tissue. Gross examination reveals an ulcer or indurated mass with irregularly thickened borders (Figure 32-4).

Histologically, anal SCC may exhibit two dominant growth patterns. The first pattern is conventional SCC with a variable degree of keratinization (Figure 32-5A). Similar to SCC of other sites, such as the uterine cervix, the degree of differentiation designates the grade of tumor. The second pattern is a basaloid variant, characterized by nests of small, crowded, poorly differentiated tumor cells, mimicking those of cutaneous basal cell carcinoma (Figures 32-5B, 32-5C). There is peripheral palisading with abundant intraepithelial lymphocytosis. Microcyst formation may also be prominent, with frequent central necrosis or microabscess formation.

Most basaloid SCCs also contain variable components of squamous differentiation, such as keratinizing pearls in nests of small basaloid tumor cells (Figure 32-5D), a useful feature to distinguish it from direct extension of basal cell carcinoma originating in perianal skin. In addition, tumor cells in the latter are usually small and relatively uniform, lack microcyst formation, and are mitotically less active. In practice,

TABLE 32-1. Clinicopathological features to distinguish condyloma acuminatum and anal intraepithelial neoplasia (AIN).

	Condyloma	AIN
Gross feature	Polypoid, cauliflower-shape, or pedunculated excrescences	Occur in condyloma or flat lesion/plaque
Dysplasia	Present or absent	Always present
Acanthotic papillomatous	Present	Present or absent
Hyperkeratosis and parakeratosis	Often present	Present or absent
Koilocytic atypia	Present or absent	Often present
Mitosis	May or may not be present	Often present, involving partial or full thickness of epithelium depending on the degree of dysplasia

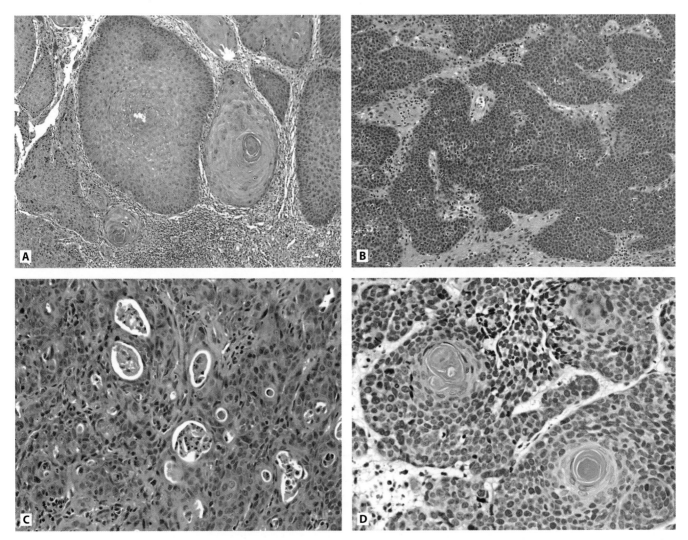

FIGURE 32-5. Anal squamous cell carcinoma. **A.** Well-differentiated squamous cell carcinoma with keratinizing pearl formation. **B.** Basaloid growth pattern with peripheral palisading and intraepithelial lymphocytosis. **C.** Microcyst formation and central microabscesses in basaloid variants of squamous cell carcinoma. **D.** Squamous keratinization in basaloid variants of squamous cell carcinoma.

immunohistochemical markers may be required to confirm the epithelial differentiation of poorly differentiated SCC, as well as exclude other less-common tumor types, such as melanocytic, hematologic and lymphoid, or neuroendocrine malignancy.

Diagnosis of anal SCC is rendered based on tumor invasion in the stroma, usually without difficulties. However, the diagnosis may be challenging under certain conditions, such as in evaluating the edge of excision during intraoperative consultation (frozen sectioning). Complete epithelial denudation, fragmentation (Figure 32-6A), poor orientation (Figure 32-6B), and severe cauterization (Figure 32-6C) could hamper a distinction between dysplasia and invasion. In lesions highly suspicious for invasion, deeper sectioning, communication with clinicians for close follow-up, or rebiopsy is recommended.

Prognosis and Treatment

The most important prognostic factor related to the outcome of anal SCC is stage, which includes depth of invasion, status of regional lymph nodes, and presence or absence of distant metastases.[58] Morphological subtypes lacked specificity in prognosis. According to the seventh edition of the *AJCC Cancer Staging Manual*, T1 tumors are 2 cm or less in greatest dimension, T2 tumors are greater than 2 cm but less than 5 cm, T3 tumors are greater than 5 cm, and a T4 tumor is of any size that invades an adjacent organ.[58]

Abdominoperineal resection (APR) was once the main treatment of anal SCC. Currently, this tumor is treated mainly with radiation and chemotherapy.[59,60] Therefore, an accurate tumor stage is defined by imaging modalities given the variable histological regression of tumor in resection specimens after adjuvant therapy.[58]

PART SEVEN

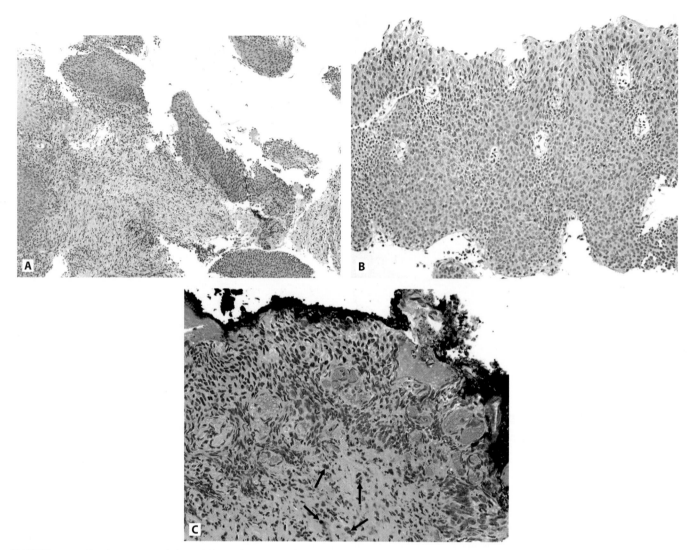

FIGURE 32-6. Conditions may defer a definite diagnosis of anal squamous cell carcinoma in biopsy specimens. The diagnosis of invasion may be challenging when the specimen is fragmented (**A**) or poorly oriented (**B**). Severe cauterization also prevents reliable distinction of individual atypical cells in stroma (**C**, arrows). An immunostain for cytokeratin may help to rule out invasion.

Prophylactic HPV vaccination is now licensed and recommended worldwide.[61] The US Centers for Diseases Control and Prevention (CDC) currently recommends HPV vaccination for all HIV-infected adults up to age 26 years.[62] HPV vaccination appears to hold great promise for anal cancer prevention, but its efficacy in reducing morbidity takes time to measure.

OTHER NONSQUAMOUS ANAL CANAL CARCINOMAS

Nonsquamous anal carcinomas include adenocarcinoma, neuroendocrine carcinoma (including small-cell carcinoma), and undifferentiated carcinoma in the anal canal. Association with HPV infection has been reported in rare cases of anal adenocarcinoma or anal neuroendocrine carcinoma.[63,64]

However, given the high prevalence of HPV, a true association needs further studies.

REFERENCES

1. Joseph DA, Miller JW, Wu X, et al. Understanding the burden of human papillomavirus-associated anal cancers in the US. *Cancer.* 2008;113(10 Suppl):2892–2900. PMID: 18980293. PMCID: 2729501.
2. Grulich AE, Poynten IM, Machalek DA, Jin F, Templeton DJ, Hillman RJ. The epidemiology of anal cancer. *Sex Health.* 2012;9(6):504–508. PMID: 22958581.
3. Noffsinger A, Witte D, Fenoglio-Preiser CM. The relationship of human papillomaviruses to anorectal neoplasia. *Cancer.* 1992; 70(5 Suppl):1276–1287. PMID: 1324782. English.
4. Palefsky JM. Human papillomavirus-associated anogenital neoplasia and other solid tumors in human immunodeficiency virus-infected individuals. *Curr Opin Oncol.* 1991;3(5):881–885. PMID: 1661170.

5. Palefsky JM, Holly EA, Gonzales J, Berline J, Ahn DK, Greenspan JS. Detection of human papillomavirus DNA in anal intraepithelial neoplasia and anal cancer. *Cancer Res.* 1991;51(3):1014–1019. PMID: 1846314.

6. Wu X, Watson M, Wilson R, Saraiya M, Cleveland JL, Markowitz L. Human papillomavirus-associated cancers—United States, 2004–2008. *MMWR Morb Mortal Wkly Rep.* 2012;2012(61):258–261.

7. Foust RL, Dean PJ, Stoler MH, Moinuddin SM. Intraepithelial neoplasia of the anal canal in hemorrhoidal tissue: a study of 19 cases. *Hum Pathol.* 1991;22(6):528–534. PMID: 1650751.

8. Taxy JB, Gupta PK, Gupta JW, Shah KV. Anal cancer. Microscopic condyloma and tissue demonstration of human papillomavirus capsid antigen and viral DNA. *Arch Pathol Lab Med.* 1989;113(10):1127–1131. PMID: 2552954.

9. Gal AA, Saul SH, Stoler MH. In situ hybridization analysis of human papillomavirus in anal squamous cell carcinoma. *Mod Pathol.* 1989;2(5):439–443. PMID: 2554279.

10. Zaki SR, Judd R, Coffield LM, Greer P, Rolston F, Evatt BL. Human papillomavirus infection and anal carcinoma. Retrospective analysis by in situ hybridization and the polymerase chain reaction. *Am J Pathol.* 1992;140(6):1345–1355. PMID: 1318640. PMCID: 1886536.

11. Puy-Montbrun T, Denis J, Ganansia R, Mathoniere F, Lemarchand N, Arnous-Dubois N. Anorectal lesions in human immunodeficiency virus-infected patients. *Int J Colorectal Dis.* 1992;7(1):26–30. PMID: 1588221.

12. Wong AK, Chan RC, Aggarwal N, Singh MK, Nichols WS, Bose S. Human papillomavirus genotypes in anal intraepithelial neoplasia and anal carcinoma as detected in tissue biopsies. *Mod Pathol.* 2010;23(1):144–150. PMID: 19838162.

13. Scholefield JH, Kerr IB, Shepherd NA, Miller KJ, Bloomfield R, Northover JM. Human papillomavirus type 16 DNA in anal cancers from six different countries. *Gut.* 1991;32(6):674–676. PMID: 1648029. PMCID: 1378887.

14. Jin F, Stein AN, Conway EL, et al. Trends in anal cancer in Australia, 1982–2005. *Vaccine.* 2011;29(12):2322–2327. PMID: 21255682.

15. Daling JR, Madeleine MM, Johnson LG, et al. Human papillomavirus, smoking, and sexual practices in the etiology of anal cancer. *Cancer.* 2004;101(2):270–280. PMID: 15241823.

16. Rock B, Shah KV, Farmer ER. A morphologic, pathologic, and virologic study of anogenital warts in men. *Arch Dermatol.* 1992;128(4):495–500. PMID: 1316102.

17. Grodsky L. Unsuspected anal cancer discovered after minor anorectal surgery. *Dis Colon Rectum.* 1967;10(6):471–478. PMID: 6066372.

18. Fenger C. Anal canal tumors and their precursors. *Pathol Annu.* 1988;23(Pt 1):45–66. PMID: 2838795.

19. Caruso ML, Valentini AM. Different human papillomavirus genotypes in ano-genital lesions. *Anticancer Res.* 1999;19(4B):3049–3053. PMID: 10652591.

20. Bosman FT, Carneiro F, Hruban RH, Theise ND. *WHO Classification of Tumours of the Digestive System.* 4th ed. *Tumours of the Anal Canal.* Lyons, France: International Agency for Research on Cancer; 2010;9:184–193.

21. Scholefield JH, Hickson WG, Smith JH, Rogers K, Sharp F. Anal intraepithelial neoplasia: part of a multifocal disease process. *Lancet.* 1992;340(8830):1271–1273. PMID: 1359331.

22. Surawicz CM, Kirby P, Critchlow C, Sayer J, Dunphy C, Kiviat N. Anal dysplasia in homosexual men: role of anoscopy and biopsy. *Gastroenterology.* 1993;105(3):658–666. PMID: 8359638.

23. Fenger C. Anal neoplasia and its precursors: facts and controversies. *Semin Diagn Pathol.* 1991;8(3):190–201. PMID: 1656504.

24. Kiviat NB, Critchlow CW, Holmes KK, et al. Association of anal dysplasia and human papillomavirus with immunosuppression and HIV infection among homosexual men. *AIDS.* 1993;7(1):43–49. PMID: 8382927.

25. Buchman AL, Ament ME, Doty J. Development of squamous cell carcinoma in chronic perineal sinus and wounds in Crohn's disease. *Am J Gastroenterol.* 1991;86(12):1829–1832. PMID: 1962632.

26. Frisch M, Glimelius B, van den Brule AJ, et al. Sexually transmitted infection as a cause of anal cancer. *N Engl J Med.* 1997;337(19):1350–1358. PMID: 9358129.

27. Daling JR, Weiss NS, Hislop TG, et al. Sexual practices, sexually transmitted diseases, and the incidence of anal cancer. *N Engl J Med.* 1987;317(16):973–977. PMID: 2821396.

28. Palefsky JM, Gonzales J, Greenblatt RM, Ahn DK, Hollander H. Anal intraepithelial neoplasia and anal papillomavirus infection among homosexual males with group IV HIV disease. *J Am Med Assoc.* 1990;263(21):2911–2916. PMID: 2160023.

29. Cotter MB, Kelly ME, O'Connell PR, et al. Anal intraepithelial neoplasia: a single centre 19 year review. *Colorectal Dis.* 2014;16(10):777–782. PMID: 24888873.

30. Walts AE, Lechago J, Bose S. P16 and Ki67 immunostaining is a useful adjunct in the assessment of biopsies for HPV-associated anal intraepithelial neoplasia. *Am J Surg Pathol.* 2006;30(7):795–801. PMID: 16819320.

31. Lu DW, El-Mofty SK, Wang HL. Expression of p16, Rb, and p53 proteins in squamous cell carcinomas of the anorectal region harboring human papillomavirus DNA. *Mod Pathol.* 2003;16(7):692–699. PMID: 12861066.

32. Samama B, Lipsker D, Boehm N. p16 expression in relation to human papillomavirus in anogenital lesions. *Hum Pathol.* 2006;37(5):513–519. PMID: 16647947.

33. Longacre TA, Kong CS, Welton ML. Diagnostic problems in anal pathology. *Adv Anat Pathol.* 2008;15(5):263–278. PMID: 18724100.

34. Kaspari M, Gutzmer R, Kaspari T, Kapp A, Brodersen JP. Application of imiquimod by suppositories (anal tampons) efficiently prevents recurrences after ablation of anal canal condyloma. *Br J Dermatol.* 2002;147(4):757–759. PMID: 12366425.

35. Wieland U, Brockmeyer NH, Weissenborn SJ, et al. Imiquimod treatment of anal intraepithelial neoplasia in HIV-positive men. *Arch Dermatol.* 2006;142(11):1438–1444. PMID: 17116834.

36. Kreuter A, Potthoff A, Brockmeyer NH, et al. Imiquimod leads to a decrease of human papillomavirus DNA and to a sustained clearance of anal intraepithelial neoplasia in HIV-infected men. *J Invest Dermatol.* 2008;128(8):2078–2083. PMID: 18273049.

37. Chang GJ, Berry JM, Jay N, Palefsky JM, Welton ML. Surgical treatment of high-grade anal squamous intraepithelial lesions: a prospective study. *Dis Colon Rectum.* 2002;45(4):453–458. PMID: 12006924.

38. Pineda CE, Berry JM, Jay N, Palefsky JM, Welton ML. High resolution anoscopy in the planned staged treatment of anal squamous intraepithelial lesions in HIV-negative patients. *J Gastrointest Surg.* 2007;11(11):1410–1415; discussion 1415–1416. PMID: 17710507.

39. Goldstone SE, Kawalek AZ, Huyett JW. Infrared coagulator: a useful tool for treating anal squamous intraepithelial lesions. *Dis Colon Rectum.* 2005;48(5):1042–1054. PMID: 15868241.

40. Goldstone SE, Hundert JS, Huyett JW. Infrared coagulator ablation of high-grade anal squamous intraepithelial lesions in HIV-negative males who have sex with males. *Dis Colon Rectum.* 2007;50(5):565–575. PMID: 17380365.

41. Stier EA, Goldstone SE, Berry JM, et al. Infrared coagulator treatment of high-grade anal dysplasia in HIV-infected individuals: an AIDS malignancy consortium pilot study. *J Acquir Immune Defic Syndr.* 2008;47(1):56–61. PMID: 18156992.

42. Webber J, Fromm D. Photodynamic therapy for carcinoma in situ of the anus. *Arch Surg.* 2004;139(3):259–261. PMID: 15006881.

43. Fox PA, Nathan M, Francis N, et al. A double-blind, randomized controlled trial of the use of imiquimod cream for the treatment of anal canal high-grade anal intraepithelial neoplasia in HIV-positive MSM on HAART, with long-term follow-up data including the use of open-label imiquimod. *AIDS.* 2010;24(15):2331–2335. PMID: 20729710.

44. Orchard M, Roman A, Parvaiz AC. Anal intraepithelial neoplasia—is treatment better than observation? *Int J Surg.* 2013;11(6):438–441. PMID: 23643642.

PART SEVEN

45. Fox PA. Treatment options for anal intraepithelial neoplasia and evidence for their effectiveness. *Sex Health.* 2012;9(6):587–592. PMID: 22951292.

46. Macaya A, Munoz-Santos C, Balaguer A, Barbera MJ. Interventions for anal canal intraepithelial neoplasia. *Cochrane Database Syst Rev.* 2012;12:CD009244. PMID: 23235673.

47. Schraut WH, Wang CH, Dawson PJ, Block GE. Depth of invasion, location, and size of cancer of the anus dictate operative treatment. *Cancer.* 1983;51(7):1291–1296. PMID: 6825051.

48. Fenger C, Frisch M, Jass JJ, Williams GT, Hilden J. Anal cancer subtype reproducibility study. *Virchows Arch.* 2000;436(3):229–233. PMID: 10782881.

49. Jemal A, Siegel R, Ward E, et al. Cancer statistics, 2008. *CA Cancer J Clin.* 2008;58(2):71–96. PMID: 18287387.

50. Frisch M, Melbye M, Moller H. Trends in incidence of anal cancer in Denmark. *Br Med J (Clin Res Ed).* 1993;306(6875):419–422. PMID: 8461721. PMCID: 1676495.

51. Cook MB, Dawsey SM, Freedman ND, et al. Sex disparities in cancer incidence by period and age. *Cancer Epidemiol Biomarkers Prev.* 2009;18(4):1174–1182. PMID: 19293308. PMCID: 2793271.

52. Melbye M, Rabkin C, Frisch M, Biggar RJ. Changing patterns of anal cancer incidence in the United States, 1940–1989. *Am J Epidemiol.* 1994;139(8):772–780. PMID: 8178790.

53. Uronis HE, Bendell JC. Anal cancer: an overview. *Oncologist.* 2007;12(5):524–534. PMID: 17522240.

54. Tachezy R, Smahelova J, Salakova M, Arbyn M, Rob L, Skapa P, et al. Human papillomavirus genotype distribution in Czech women and men with diseases etiologically linked to HPV. *PLoS One.* 2011;6(7):e21913. PMID: 21765924. PMCID: 3135602.

55. Abramowitz L, Jacquard AC, Jaroud F, et al. Human papillomavirus genotype distribution in anal cancer in France: the EDiTH V study. *Int J Cancer.* 2011;129(2):433–439. PMID: 20839262.

56. Hoots BE, Palefsky JM, Pimenta JM, Smith JS. Human papillomavirus type distribution in anal cancer and anal intraepithelial lesions. *Int J Cancer.* 2009;124(10):2375–2383. PMID: 19189402.

57. De Vuyst H, Clifford GM, Nascimento MC, Madeleine MM, Franceschi S. Prevalence and type distribution of human papillomavirus in carcinoma and intraepithelial neoplasia of the vulva, vagina and anus: a meta-analysis. *Int J Cancer.* 2009;124(7):1626–1636. PMID: 19115209.

58. Edge SB, Byrd Dr, Compton CC, Fritz AG, Greene FL, Trotti A. *AJCC Cancer Staging Manual.* 7th ed. New York, NY: Springer-Verlag; 2010:165–173.

59. Bartelink H, Roelofsen F, Eschwege F, et al. Concomitant radiotherapy and chemotherapy is superior to radiotherapy alone in the treatment of locally advanced anal cancer: results of a phase III randomized trial of the European Organization for Research and Treatment of Cancer Radiotherapy and Gastrointestinal Cooperative Groups. *J Clin Oncol.* 1997;15(5):2040–2049. PMID: 9164216.

60. Bosset JF, Pavy JJ, Roelofsen F, Bartelink H. Combined radiotherapy and chemotherapy for anal cancer. EORTC Radiotherapy and Gastrointestinal Cooperative Groups. *Lancet.* 1997;349(9046):205–206. PMID: 9111560.

61. Frazer IH, Leggatt GR, Mattarollo SR. Prevention and treatment of papillomavirus-related cancers through immunization. *Annu Rev Immunol.* 2011;29:111–138. PMID: 21166538.

62. Centers for Disease Control and Prevention. Recommended adult immunization schedule—United States. *MMWR Morbid Mortal Wkly Rep.* 2012;2012(61):1–7.

63. Koulos J, Symmans F, Chumas J, Nuovo G. Human papillomavirus detection in adenocarcinoma of the anus. *Mod Pathol.* 1991;4(1):58–61. PMID: 1850518.

64. Ohtomo R, Sekine S, Taniguchi H, Tsuda H, Moriya Y, Kushima R. Anal canal neuroendocrine carcinoma associated with squamous intraepithelial neoplasia: a human papillomavirus 18-related lesion. *Pathol Int.* 2012;62(5):356–359. PMID: 22524667.

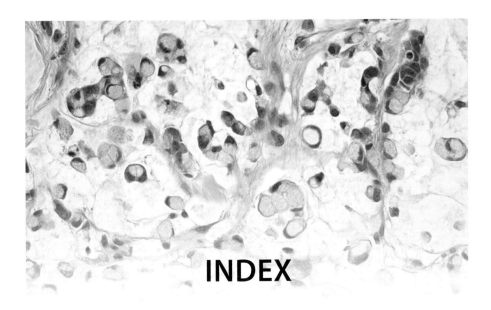

INDEX

Page numbers followed by "*f*" denote figures and "*t*" denote tables